Nutrition of the
Chicken

Fourth Edition

Steven Leson PhD
Professor of Animal Nutrition

John D Summers PhD
Professor Emeritus
Department of Animal and Poultry Science
University of Guelph
Guelph, Ontario, Canada N1G 2W1

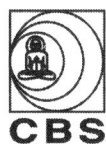

CBS

CBS Publishers & Distributors Pvt Ltd

New Delhi • Bengaluru • Chennai • Kochi • Kolkata • Mumbai
Bhopal • Bhubaneswar • Hyderabad • Jharkhand • Nagpur
• Patna • Pune•Uttarakhand • Dhaka (Bangladesh)

Nutrition of the
Chicken

CBS Reprint: 2019
Fourth Edition: 2001
First Indian Reprint: 2002

ISBN-13   978-81-85860-91-6
ISBN-10   81-85860-91-2

Published by Satish Kumar Jain and produced by Varun Jain for

CBS Publishers & Distributors Pvt Ltd
204 FIE, Patparganj Industrial Area, Delhi 110 092
E-mail: delhi@cbspd.com, cbspubs@airtelmail.in
Ph: 4934 4934   Fax: 4934 4935   Website: www.cbspd.com
e-mail: publishing@cbspd.com;
publicity@cbspd.com

Branches

- **Bengaluru:** Seema House 2975, 17th Cross, K.R. Road, Banasankari 2nd Stage, Bengaluru 560 070, Karnataka
  Ph: +91-80-26771678/79   Fax: +91-80-26771680   e-mail: bangalore@cbspd.com
- **Chennai:** 7, Subbaraya Street, Shenoy Nagar, Chennai 600 030, Tamil Nadu
  Ph: +91-44-26260666, 26208620   Fax: +91-44-42032115   e-mail: chennai@cbspd.com
- **Kochi:** 42/1325, 1326, Power House Road, Opp KSEB Power House, Ernakulam 682 018, Kochi, Kerala
  Ph: +91-484-4059061-65   Fax: +91-484-4059065   e-mail: kochi@cbspd.com
- **Kolkata:** No. 6/B, Ground Floor, Rameswar Shaw Road, Kolkata-700014 (West Bengal), India
  Ph: +91-33-2289-1126, 2289-1127, 2289-1128   e-mail: kolkata@cbspd.com
- **Mumbai:** 83-C, Dr E Moses Road, Worli, Mumbai-400018, Maharashtra
  Ph: +91-22-24902340/41   Fax: +91-22-24902342   e-mail: mumbai@cbspd.com

Representatives

• Bhopal	0-8319310552	• Bhubaneswar	0-9911037372	• Hyderabad	0-9885175004
• Jharkhand	0-9811541605	• Nagpur	0-9421945513	• Patna	0-9334159340
• Pune	0-9623451994	• Uttarakhand	0-9716462459		
• Dhaka (Bangladesh)	01912-003485				

Printed at India Binding House, Noida, UP (India)

Preface

Nutrition of the Chicken was first published in 1969 authored by Scott, Nesheim and Young at Cornell University. The book was unique in that it pioneered the compilation of current information on nutritional sciences as applied to poultry production. A second edition was printed in 1976 and the third edition was released in 1982. Since this time, the original authors have either retired or moved to areas outside of poultry nutrition. The idea for a revision of the book followed a lunch meeting with Dr. Dave Austic, also from Cornell, during the Latin American Poultry Congress in Lima, Peru. Enquiring about Dr Scott, Dave indicated that there were no plans for anyone to produce a 4th edition of the book and that Dr Scott was pursuing other writing endeavors including a book on Nutrition of the dog.

On returning to Guelph, we contacted Dr Scott, and were delighted with his enthusiastic support of our suggestion of revising this classic book. Over the last 2 years, we have worked on this new 4th edition, attempting to maintain the quality and intent so wonderfully achieved by Drs Scott, Nesheim and Young in their previous editions. Hopefully the readers of this 4th edition will be as inspired and educated as we have become in its preparation. It has been necessary for us to delve into somewhat infamiliar topics of poultry nutrition, and this quickly becomes a rewarding personal experience. We have attempted to include as much recent relevant information on poultry nutrition as possible, while at the same time retaining a balance with the many classical aspects so expertly researched and described in the original editions. Certainly many topics are new and we have reluctantly decided to dealt some of the older information of lesser historical importance. The reader is presented with a range of referenced material that spans the last 100 years. Our intended audience for this book is undergraduate and graduate students of poultry nutrition, together with professionals in the poultry and feed industries.

We are once again indebted to Wendy Bauer for her contrition in the layout of the chapters and to Laurie Parr for invaluable assistance in scanning and design of many of the new figures. Our thanks to Linda Caston and Diane Spratt for their conscientious and meticulous proofing of may manuscript editions.

The final chapter 10 was the inspiration of Dr. Gonzalo Diaz, Departmento de Ciencias Fisiolagiras, Universidad Nacional de Columbia. Gonzalo has co-authored one of our previous books and when he heard of our re-write of this book, he suggested a section on natural toxicants in feed. Virtually all the material in Chapter 10 was prepared and researched by Dr Diaz.

Lastly, out thanks to all the researchers listed in the various reference sections. Their research interests and ideas form the basis of this book

Steven Leeson and John Summers
Guelph, April, 2001

Contents

Digestion and Nutrient Availability

1.1 INTRODUCTION

Diets are composed of complex organic and inorganic molecules that must be reduced in size so as to enable absorption. Carbohydrates, proteins and fat provide the overwhelming substrates for digestion, although mineral complexes and some forms of vitamins may also require molecular cleavage prior to uptake in the jejunum. Most enzyme secretion occurs in the proventriculus or duodenum, and then absorption of digested nutrients occurs primarily in the jejunum. The bird does not have any teeth, and so there is no feed particle size reduction prior to swallowing as occurs in most mammals. In wild gallinaceous birds, the gizzard is responsible for particle size reduction, although in domesticated poultry, the gizzard is often rudimentary and provides little grinding action. In essence, the milling of feed during manufacture replaces the need for meaningful gizzard activity. Likewise, the crop serves little function in most birds today, unless there are severe limitations on feed availability as occurs with young broiler breeders.

There are some age-related issues in digestion, and particularly the inability of young birds to adequately digest saturated fats. A schematic picture of the avian digestive system and associated organs is shown in Fig 1.1 while general enzyme activity as occurs throughout the gastro-intestinal tract is summarized in Table 1.1

TABLE 1.1 Digestive enzyme activity				
Location	pH	Enzyme (or secretion)	Substrate	Product
Mouth	7.0 to 7.5	Saliva	Lubricates and softens feed	
		Amylase (ptyalin)	Starch	Dextrin
			Dextrin	Glucose
Crop	4.5	Mucus	Lubricates and softens feed	
Gizzard and proventriculus	2.5	HCl	Lowers digesta pH, initiates protein cleavage	
		Pepsin	Protein	Polypeptides
		Lipase	Triglyceride	Fatty acids, monoglycerides
Duodenum	6.0 to 6.8	Amylase (amylopsin)	Starch Dextrin	Maltose Glucose
		Trypsin, chymotrypsin and Elastases	Proteins, peptides	Peptides, amino acids
		Carboxypeptidases Collagenase	Peptides Collagen	Amino acids Peptides
		Bile	Emulsification of fats	
		Lipase	Fat	Fatty acids, monoglycerides, diglycarides
		Cholesterol esterase	Cholesterol Esters	Fatty acids, Cholesterol
Jejunum	5.8 to 6.8	Maltase and Isomaltase	Maltose Isomaltose	Glucose Glucose
		Sucrase	Sucrose	Glucose, Fructose
		Lactase	Lactase	Glucose, Galactose
		Peptidases	Peptides	Dipeptides, Amino acids
		Polynucleotidase	Nucleic acids	Mononucleotides
Ceca	5.7 to 5.9	Microbial activity	Cellulose, polysaccharides, starches, sugars	Volatile fatty acids, vitamin K, B-vitamins

Development of the digestive tract of young birds has been extensively reviewed by Jin *et al.*, (1998). There seems to be a general consensus of an increase in production and/or activity of enzymes during the first 14d of development, although it is unclear if enzyme production in the hatchling chick in any way limits growth. One confusing area in the literature is the non-standard methods of describing enzyme

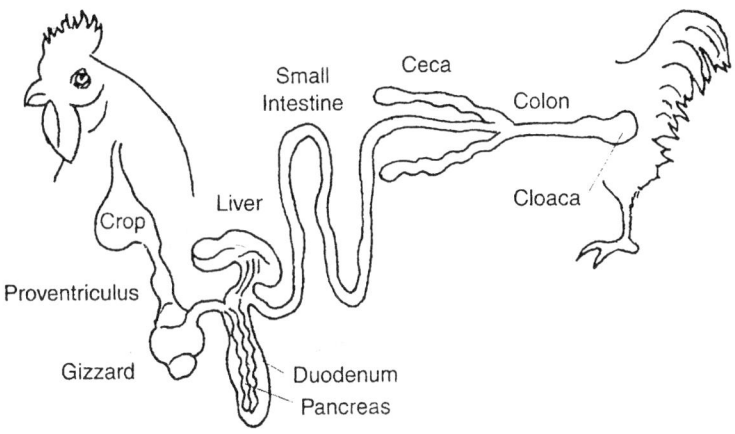

Figure 1.1 Schematic of avian digestive system.

activity, which make comparisons very difficult. Certainly endocrine organs such as the pancreas do increase in size faster than does general body weight, and so this factor must also be taken into account when reviewing enzyme activity data. Another confounding factor is diet, where increased supply of a particular substrate seems to induce increased production of target enzymes. At this time, it is concluded that endogenous enzyme production is not a rate-limiting step to growth. Croom *et al.*, (1999) in fact, suggests that it may be the process of absorption, rather than digestion, which potentially limits growth in birds such as the broiler chicken.

1.2 CARBOHYDRATES

Normal digestion processes

The major storage carbohydrate in grains is starch, and this usually exists as insoluble granules that resist digestion. However, these starch granules can be easily disrupted by physical action and wetting, as can occur in the crop, and this activity greatly speeds up subsequent digestion. Birds produce up to 15-20 ml of saliva each day and this contains small quantities of amylase enzyme, which initiates starch digestion. If feed is held in the crop for any length of time, then starch digestion can commence, although it is unclear as to how much of this digestion is due to amylase vs. the action of microbes such as lactobacilli.

Most carbohydrate digestion occurs in the jejunum. Alpha-amylase is secreted by the pancreas into the duodenum and during this process the 1,4α-linkages on both sides of the 1,6 attachment sites are hydrolysed, yielding maltose and some oligosaccharides such as isomaltose. Maltose is subsequently further cleaved by maltase (α-glucosidase) and together with isomaltase, produced by the intestinal mucosa, yields glucose, which is readily absorbed. The jejunal brush border membrane also produces other disaccharidases that cleave the more complex sugars into their component monosaccharides ready for absorption. Sucrase hydrolyses any sucrose present yielding glucose and fructose while any milk derived carbohydrates are hydrolysed by lactase to yield glucose and galactose.

There is considerable variance in reports concerning amylase concentration in the jejunum, although in part, this may be due to different assay methods being used. For example Nitsan *et al.*, (1991), suggest an amylase concentration of just 0.3 units/g intestinal contents in day-old chicks, while Ritz *et al.*, (1995) indicate 40 units/g. While enzyme activity does increase with bird age, there is variability in reported values. The above two research groups suggest a 3x and 6x increase in amylase activity up to 20d of age. Working with turkey poults, Sell and co-workers at Iowa State University suggest a 100% increase in amylase activity through to 32d of age, while for sucrase and isomaltase the increased activity is even greater at 300%. The greatest activity of most amylase and other carbohydrate digesting enzymes is in the jejunum, followed by the ileum and the duodenum.

Once digested, the monosaccharides will be absorbed by an energy dependent active system. The Na^+ dependent transport system is functional in late stage embryo's although activity and efficiency of the system increases during the first 20-30d of the chick's life. Sodium ion concentration within the intestinal contents is critical for monosaccharide absorption and low concentrations can reduce sugar absorption. Some hexoses and pentoses are absorbed by passive diffusion, although their overall contribution to energy metabolism of the bird is quite small. Unabsorbed sugars provide a readily fermentable substrate for microbes in the large intestine and ceca, potentially leading to proliferation of pathogenic strains and/or diarrhea.

Digestibility values

Most carbohydrates are readily digested, although cellulose and lignin are indigestible. About 60-70% of starch in cereals is in the form of mono- or disaccharides by the time digesta reaches the proximal ileum, while up to 95% is digested by the time digesta reaches the terminal ileum. Unlike the situation in most mammals, the milk sugar lactose is poorly digested because of limited production of lactase enzyme. Virtually all the glucose that is hydrolyzed from complex carbohydrates is absorbed, starting in the duodenum with most occurring in the jejunum. The digestibility of starch and some sugars is shown in Table 1.2.

TABLE 1.2 Gross energy digestible energy metabolizable energy of starch and sugars (kcal/kg)			
	ENERGY		
	Gross	Digestible	Metabolizable
Starch	3750	3550	3350
Glucose	3430	3400	3330
Maltose	3600	3390	3250
Fructose	3000	2875	2750
Sucrose	3950	3875	3750

Factors affecting digestion

The major factor influencing carbohydrate digestion, is the content of complex polysaccharides such as cellulose and lignin. There is usually very little lignin in ingredients fed to birds, and so cellulose becomes the major limitation to digestibility. Although up to 10% of ingested cellulose may disappear in the digestive tract, most of this loss relates to microbial activity in the large intestine and ceca, where products of digestion are of limited use to the bird. Other polysaccharides of more interest to poultry nutritionists, are hemicelluloses, pentosans, β-glucan and the oligosaccharides such as stachyose and raffinose found more commonly in the oilseed meals. Most recently these carbohydrates have been referred to as non-starch polysaccharides (NSP's) which in many instances equate to the older terminology of "crude fibre".

Hemicelluose refers to plant components that are insoluble in water but readily hydrolysed by dilute acids. Of particular significance are the xylans, the most abundant being the arabinoxylans in wheat. Although birds do not possess a xylanase enzyme, there is some hydrolysis due to the action of HCl in the gizzard and proventriculus. Another complex polysaccharide that is poorly digested is β-glucan, found in most cereals, but being particularly abundant in barley and rye. There is usually a negative correlation between carbohydrate digestibility and the content of pentosans and β-glucans. Unfortunately these undigested polysaccharides have the adverse side effect of binding large quantities of water from the digesta, leading to a more viscous medium. This increased digesta viscosity reduces physical mixing in the digesta and transport of products to the brush border. Consequently there is less chance for contact of substrates with enzymes, while any digested products may not reach the microvilli of the intestine. These complex carbohydrates can therefore lead to reduce digestibility of all nutrient classes in the digesta, and not just the carbohydrate component. This action of pentosans and β-glucans is responsible for the 'sticky' excreta commonly seen when feeding high levels of barley and some varieties of wheat and especially rye. Fortunately there are now exogenous xylanase and β-glucanase enzymes that can be added to the feed, that virtually eliminate problems of digesta viscosity, and so lead to improved nutrient digestibility (see Chapter 6).

Although high levels of barley and wheat are only used in certain regions of the world, soybean meal is more common to most poultry diets and here again there are some complex carbohydrates that are poorly digested. Alpha-galactosaccharides, commonly called oligosaccharides can represent up to 12% of the carbohydrates in soybean meal. The most common components are stachyose, raffinose and cellebiose. Although extracted by ethanol, these oligosaccharides are not removed by normal hexane fat extraction of soybeans, and their residue is partly responsible for the relatively low energy digestibility of soybean meal for poultry. Pigs can digest these carbohydrates more efficiently, and this partly explains the higher metabolizable energy value seen for soybean meal in pigs vs. poultry. Due to absence of α-galactosidase activity in the intestinal mucosa, there is interest in adding such exogenous enzymes to the feed, and/or extracting the polysaccharides with ethanol. Alternatively we may see new varieties of soybeans that are low in raffinose, stachyose and sucrose. Apart from improving soybean AME, these new varieties may be less prone to Maillard Reaction loss of lysine. During normal heat treatment of soybeans, there is some destruction of lysine due to irreversible linkage with sucrose and other soluble sugars. Pectins in vegetable proteins also cause a more viscous digesta, the degree of which is affected by their concentration (usually 1-2%), while Langhout and Schutte (1996) indicate that degree of esterification is also important in influencing pectin digestibility.

Ingredient pretreatment and feed processing can both influence digestibility of carbohydrates. The classical situation is seen with raw potato starch, which is very poorly digested by poultry and most other animals. The presence of phosphate groups in potato starch forms a barrier to α- and β-amylase degradation resulting in two or three residues being unhydrolysed on either side of the phosphorylated glucose molecule. Cooking of potato starch results in cleavage of the phosphate bonding, and the starch is then readily digestible. The effects of heat treatment on starch digestibility in more commonly used grains are quite variable. There is some indication of improved energy utilization from coarse grains such as barley and rye, due to steam cooking. Unfortunately the release of any free sugars during these procedures, increases the risk of Maillard Reaction with lysine as previously described for soybeans. Moisture content of grains and vegetable proteins is important during cooking or steam treatment. As with studies of field peas, it has been shown that high temperature moist heat treatment is beneficial, while similar temperatures with no added moisture actually causes loss in digestibility. Tonroy and Perry (1975) reported that dry heat treatment does not cause the starch granule to swell sufficiently enough to cause rupture. The improvement in starch digestibility associated with steam pelleting is therefore partly a result of gelatinization, which improves starch solubility, together with increased surface area for action by the amylase enzymes. The stronger the intermolecular bonding of starch, then the greater the potential improvements in digestibility due to steam pelleting. Thus steam pelleting is known to improve the AMEn of peas by 5-7%, while maize and wheat are little affected. The starch in peas is more intricate with stronger intermolecular bonding of glucose. It is also possible that steam pelleting destroys any residual lectins in peas.

1.3. PROTEINS AND AMINO ACIDS

Normal digestion process

There is no meaningful digestion of protein in the mouth or crop, and consequently the proventriculus is the first site of protein degradation. Immediately upon the ingestion of food, there is a reflex stimulation of the vagus nerves of the gastric mucosa, which initiates the secretion of gastric juice into the proventriculus. Secretions from the proventriculus include hydrochloric acid and the enzyme precursor, pepsinogen, which is converted to the active enzyme pepsin as the pH declines, with digesta movement through the proventriculus and gizzard. Rise in pepsinogen concentration slightly precedes the rise in hydrochloric acid production. Before entrance of feed into the proventriculus and gizzard, the pH of the secretions present in these organs may be as low as 1.5-2, but under the buffering effects of the feed, the pH rises to about 3.5-5. When the partially digested chyme passes into the small intestine, the decrease in free acidity and possibly other mechanisms, cause the liberation of the hormone, gastrin, which stimulates further secretion of hydrochloric acid. The hydrochloric acid of the proventriculus (at pH values below 5) causes an autocatalytic conversion of the pepsinogen to pepsin. This conversion involves the splitting off of a peptide chain and peptide fragments, which prevents pepsinogen from having any effective enzyme activity. Pepsin is known to hydrolyze several different peptide linkages. Its most pronounced effect is between leucine and valine, tyrosine, and leucine, or between the aromatic amino acids such as phenylalanine-phenylalanine or phenylalanine-tyrosine. It has been suggested that pepsin is a single enzyme with two active centers each of which attack a different substrate site maximally at a different pH. However, as many as 5 separate pepsinogens have been detected in crude extract from the chicken proventriculus. The object of proteolysis in the proventriculus and gizzard, is to make available peptide molecules, which are readily susceptible to further hydrolysis by the proteolytic enzymes of the intestine. The low specificity of the pepsin enzyme complex greatly increases the likelihood that at least some of the bonds in most proteins will be hydrolyzed, resulting in denaturation and solubilization of the peptide linkages of most dietary proteins.

Level of dietary protein has an effect upon the emptying rate of the stomach in rats. Low protein diets tend to cause the feed to move rapidly through the stomach while high protein diets produce feedback mechanisms which slow the emptying of the stomach, thereby allowing time for denaturation and solubilization of the raw proteins being consumed. Since the chicken is a "nibbler" rather than a meal eater, one might expect the mechanisms controlling the emptying of the proventriculus and gizzard to differ from those that have been found to occur in rats and other simple-stomach mammals. However, when one considers that the feed consumed by the chicken passes into the crop, it could be that periodic ejection of feed from the crop into the proventriculus, evokes a gastric secretion and stomach emptying mechanism similar to that occurring in mammals such as the rat. Many proteins in the feed are often quite resistant to attack by enzymes and must be denatured so that the three-dimensional form of the protein is broken down into single structures in order to expose each peptide linkage to attack. Hydrochloric acid effectively serves to denature such proteins, although this action is aided by modern high-temperature heat treatment of feed as occurs with expanding, extrusion, thermal cooking and to a lesser extent high-temperature pelleting.

In the gizzard, the ingesta is further mixed with the fluid secreted by the proventriculus. There is also mechanical grinding of the feed facilitated by ingredients such as insoluble grit, that may be added to the diet. Grit provides additional surfaces for grinding as well as acting to stimulate motility in the gizzard. The digestibility of coarse feed particles, such as whole grains, grain with a minimal amount of processing, or pelleted feed, is improved by addition of grit in the diet. However, protein digestibility of ground feed is little affected by the absence of a fully developed gizzard.

Once proteolysis has been initiated by pepsin, a rapid increase occurs in accessibility of peptide bonds to hydrolysis by the proteolytic enzymes of the small intestine. Polypeptides resulting from pepsin digestion in the proventriculus and the gizzard, are broken down further in the intestine by trypsin, chymotrypsin and elastase. The action of these enzymes releases numerous terminal peptide bonds, which are attacked by aminopeptidases, carboxypeptidases and other specific peptidases present in the lumen or mucosa of the small intestine. Each enzyme must play its part in the sequential hydrolysis of the protein. In many cases, the hydrolysate resulting from the action of one enzyme provides the substrate for the next. Thus, inhibition of any of the proteolytic enzymes, particularly of the initial enzymes, pepsin or trypsin, will result in a marked decrease in digestion of the dietary proteins.

The pancreas produces fluids containing zymogens that are converted to their active enzyme forms at the sites of digestion. Trypsinogen is activated to trypsin in the duodenum by enterokinase, an enzyme secreted from the intestinal mucosa. Once started, this process is autocatalytic and the newly formed trypsin initiates activation of other zymogens. Trypsin is therefore central in the development of adequate protein digestion. The consequence of trypsin inhibitors found in certain legumes and cereals is poor digestibility of dietary proteins. Trypsin, chymotrypsin and elastase, catalyse the break down of proteins, peptones and peptides into smaller peptides and amino acids in the duodenum. Trypsin catalyzes breakdown of bonds which involve lysine and/or arginine, whereas bonds involving aromatic amino acid residues are susceptible to chymotrypsin catalysis. Elastases are relatively non-specific with regard to the type of peptide bonds.

The pancreas also secretes exopeptidases containing carboxypeptidases A and B, which catalyze the hydrolysis of the terminal bonds in polypeptide chains. They hydrolyze the carboxyl-terminal ends of the peptides, thereby removing the amino acid residues in sequence. Carboxypeptidase A is inhibited in sequence hydrolysis by the proximity of charged side-chains and by proline, while carboxypeptidase B is also inhibited by proline but requires cationic side-chains for maximal activity. The pancreatic secretion also contains certain collagenases that catalyse the hydrolysis of collagen to small peptides. The jejunal wall secretes the proteolytic enzymes peptidase (erepsin) and polynucleotidase which catalyse the hydrolysis of small peptides into amino acids and dipeptides, and also convert nucleic acids to mononucleotides, respectively, which can then be absorbed.

There seems to be an increase in enzyme activity as the bird gets older. Nitsan et al. (1991) and Nir et al. (1993), suggest trypsin activity in the intestinal contents to increase around 10-fold up to 30 days of age. Trypsin activities of 2-4 units/g intestinal contents were recorded at 1d of age, while values of around 30 units/g were seen at 15-20d. Comparable values for chymotrypsin reported by these same authors were 2-5 units/g at 1d, and 6-14 units/g at 15-20d. Krogdahl and Sell (1989) also reported a 70% increase in trypsin activity of birds from 1-21d of age.

The endopeptidases secreted in the proventriculus, and by the pancreas, are capable of degrading proteins to small peptides containing from 2 to 6 amino acids (oligopeptides) and some free amino acids. The hydrolysis of these small peptides must then occur through the action of numerous peptidases located in the intestinal mucosa, rather than in the lumen. Any hydrolysis that does take place in the lumen occurs by the action of peptidases that are present in desquamated mucosal cells. Some peptide hydrolysis occurs at the surface of microvilli of the intestinal cells.

Evidence exists suggesting that the intestinal mucosal cells of a number of animals contain an external coating synthesized and secreted by these cells. This surface coat is most prominent at the tips of the microvilli, and is shown to contain a number of digestive and other enzymes. The function of the surface coat-plasma membrane complex is not established, although it is the site of initial contact between nutrients in the gut lumen and the absorption cells. The presence of numerous digestive enzymes (disaccharidases, alkaline phosphatase, aminopeptidase) supports the role of the brush border membrane as the digestive-absorptive surface in which the components responsible for both digestion and absorption are aligned.

Peptides are absorbed into the mucosal cell by active transport involving Na^+, with different carrier systems for various amino acid categories. Peptidases located in the cytoplasm of the intestinal mucosal cell complete the hydrolysis of the peptides to free amino acids. Certain amino acids have been shown to be absorbed much more rapidly when given in the form of peptides than when present as free amino acids. Multiple systems appear to exist for amino acid entry into mucosal cells, either as free amino acids or as small peptides. The amino acids enter the blood stream from the mucosal cells as free amino acids since only trace amounts of peptides can be detected in plasma. Peptide uptake is most rapid in the jejunum, whereas amino acid uptake is most rapid in the ileum. The natural isomers of amino acids (L-amino acids) are generally absorbed more rapidly than the D-forms. A common but L-preferring site exists for the transport of both isomers of methionine. Other neutral L-amino acids have a high affinity for this site, whereas the D-isomers, except for D-methionine, have a very low affinity. The overall capacity of the gastrointestinal tract to digest protein is very high since levels of protein up to 60-70% of the diet are apparently digested as well as are lower levels. It seems difficult to exceed the digestive capacity of an animal with a diet composed of readily digested components.

Endogenous protein. A considerable amount of endogenous protein enters the digestive tract. This protein is contained in the saliva, gastric juice, pancreatic juice, desquamated epithelial cells of intestinal mucosa, and mucins that are produced and secreted by cells throughout the gastrointestinal tract. This endogenous protein increases the total amount of protein digestion that takes place in the digestive tract. Even when birds consume a protein-free diet, or one in which free amino acids supply all the nitrogen, considerable amounts of endogenous protein must be digested. This endogenous protein is not to be confused with the endogenous nitrogen losses in urine, since the intestinal endogenous protein is digested and utilized by the animal, while the endogenous nitrogen loss in urine must be replaced each day by additional dietary protein.

Amino acid transport. As previously described, the uptake of most free amino acids occurs by "active" processes which are able to transport amino acids against a concentration gradient. These transport mechanisms require energy and show specificity for the L-forms of the amino acids. D-amino acids generally are absorbed much more slowly than corresponding L-forms. Three separate transport mechanisms have been detected in intestinal mucosa. One system is specific for the monoamino-monocarboxylic or neutral amino acids, another for arginine, lysine and other basic amino acids as well as cystine, and a third transport system for the dicarboxylic or acidic amino acids. Although active transport of glutamic and aspartic acid has not been demonstrated, some specific system for their absorption seems to be present. Within these transport systems, competition for transport among individual amino acids apparently exists. Large excesses of some amino acids may influence the site of absorption of other amino acids that share the same transport system. Because the small intestine has such a large absorptive area, and concentrations of amino acids from the diet change as the feed traverses the intestinal tract, excesses of single amino acids are quickly neutralized by absorption and probably do not influence the total *in vivo* absorption of an amino acid mixture.

Reabsorption of amino acids, in the kidney tubule is also quite efficient, as very low levels of amino acids are normally present in urine. However, competition between amino acids for reabsorption in the kidney can be demonstrated. When high levels of lysine are infused or fed, urinary arginine losses generally increase. Some D-amino acids are not efficiently reabsorbed by the kidney tubule. The kidney, for example, does not reabsorb D-tryptophan, so large amounts of this amino acid are found in the urine of chickens when DL-tryptophan is fed. This appears to be the main reason that the D-form of tryptophan is not used efficiently by chicks as a source of tryptophan.

Portal blood shows a marked rise in free amino acids during digestion. Some amino acids liberated at the intestinal membrane are incorporated into proteins of the mucosal cells, while other amino acids are metabolized within the epithelium of the small intestine. For these reasons, and since they have been mixed with amino acids of endogenous origin during the digestion and absorption process, the amino acids present in the portal vein do not completely reflect the amino acid pattern of the diet.

Digestibility values

Feedstuffs commonly used in poultry diets vary widely in content and digestibility of protein and amino acids. There is also significant variance in values reported for protein digestibility of the same feedstuff. Digestibility of protein in different samples of hydrolysed feather meal for example, was estimated to range from 32-70% (Han and Parsons, 1998). Such variability highlights the effect of thermal processing on protein digestibility, with a similar effect seen with vegetable proteins or cereals that have been heat-treated. There is no indication of major variability in protein or amino acid digestibility across varieties within a given plant species.

Dietary supplementation with synthetic amino acids, or their analogues, is a common practice with commercial poultry diets. Results of many studies show that the digestibility of such additives is much higher than for comparable amino acids fed as intact proteins. Sibbald and Wolynetz (1985), using cockerels compared synthetic lysine (L-lysine HCl) to lysine provided by conventional ingredients and obtained bioavailability of 93% for the synthetic form as opposed to 88% for the natural form of lysine. Even higher digestibility (up to 97%) has been shown for synthetic lysine when fed to broiler chickens. Table 1.3 shows some average values for ileal digestibility of protein, and some important amino acids, in various feed ingredients. In most instances, ileal digestibility values are determined with surgically modified adult roosters, although comparable values are found with young broilers when samples are taken from the ileum of birds fed inert markers. Age (after 7-10d) does not seem to be a large factor in digestibility of amino acids, probably due to the large digestive capacity and absorptive area of the intestine as already eluded to.

TABLE 1.3 Normal crude protein contents and digestibilities of common poultry feedstuffs					
Feedstuff	Crude Protein (%)	Illeal digestibility (%)			
		Crude Protein	Lys	Met	Cys
Vegetable sources (cereals):					
Corn	8	82-86	81	91	85
Wheat	12	78-82	81	87	87
Barley	10	70-82	78	79	81
Sorghum	10	67-72	78	89	83
Vegetable sources (oil seed meals):					
Peanut meal	49	88-91	83	88	78
Soybean meal	46	83-87	91	92	82
Cottonseed meal	43	61-76	67	73	73
Animal sources:					
Blood meal	88	82-92	86	91	76
Fish meal	66	86-90	88	92	73
Meat meal	60	75-80	79	85	58
Feather meal	87	36-77	66	76	59

Factors affecting digestion

A number of dietary ingredients contain anti-nutritional compounds that influence protein and amino acid digestibility. A classic example is the tannins present in sorghum that can bind and precipitate both dietary proteins and digestive enzymes (Butler et al. 1984). With tannins as high as 5% on a dry matter basis, there is reduced digestibility of both protein (Halley et al., 1986) and amino acids (Longstaff and McNab, 1991), although there does seem to be an age effect, with older birds being more immune. Feeding raw soybeans has long been known to cause poor growth rate, the result of inefficient digestibility of proteins (Zhang and Parsons, 1993). Anti-trypsins in soybeans inhibit the enzyme trypsin, which leads to impairment in the utilization of other enzymes that cleave smaller peptide units. While in rats, this adverse effect is mainly related to utilization of methionine, all amino acids seem to be affected in poultry. Fortunately the heat treatment applied during normal solvent extraction of soybeans is adequate to destroy the trypsin inhibitor (Anderson-Hefermann et al., 1993).

Cottonseed also contains a natural toxin known as gossypol, which can affect protein utilization. For this toxin, heat treatment is not always beneficial, as there can be formation of indigestible complexes with free lysine, similar to the Maillard Reaction, described previously for some carbohydrates. Proteins found in animal hide, scales, hair, feather, and bone are not easily digested as they contain high concentrations of keratin and collagen. The major component of feather meal protein, for example, is keratin, which necessitates that it be prehydrolysed to make it digestible by poultry. Moran et al., (1966) reported that heating feather meal results in cleavage of disulfide bonds of cystine, allowing better digestion by proteases with growing chicks. As previously described, variable processing conditions are responsible for the unprecedented range in amino acid digestibility seen for different samples of products such as feather meal. For these types of ingredients, total amino acid analyses can be very misleading as a basis for formulation.

While protein and amino acid digestibilities of many ingredients are improved by judicious heat processing, overheating invariably reduces availability. Heat stability of potential toxins, and availability of amino acids in ingredients and feeds, are both influenced by the balance between processing temperatures and processing time. Fairly innocuous temperatures (70-80°C) maintained for long time periods (hours) can be as deleterious as high temperature (e.g. 150°C) maintained for very short times. For example Parsons et al., (1992) reported that the true digestibility of several amino acids in soybean meal decreased linearly with time when processing at around 120°C, with lysine and histidine being most susceptible. Such a large decrease in lysine digestibility can be largely attributed to the formation of Maillard Reaction products formed during heat treatment (Hurrell, 1990). Many of the Maillard products result from the nonenzymatic Browning reactions between lysine and oligosaccharides such as fructose, stachyose, sucrose and raffinose. Soybean meal contains substantial quantities of these soluble sugars, making it very susceptible to Maillard Reactions during heat treatment (Araba et al., 1994). Chemical treatments, such as ethanol extraction of soybean meal have been reported to remove the oligosaccharides, thereby decreasing the potential for lysine destruction occurring during heat treatment (Hanock et al., 1990).

Measures of amino acid availability are further confounded by production of so-called early Maillard Reaction products known as Amadori rearrangement compounds. Many of the amino acids in Amadori compounds are released during acid hydrolysis and therefore detectable by ion-exchange chromatography, however, they are unavailable to birds for protein synthesis (Carpenter, 1973). These compounds have been isolated in heated soybean meal (Parsons *et al.*, 1992) and have a specific effect on the availability of lysine, cystine and histidine. Cystine digestibility may also be affected by heat treatment through its conversion to lanthionine, a cross-linked sulfur amino acid that is apparently indigestible (Parsons *et al.*, 1992).

Although steam pelleting is widely used in the production of poultry feeds, there are some inconsistencies in performance of birds fed mash vs. pelleted diets (Araba and Dale, 1990). This effect has been attributed to occurrence of Maillard Reaction between free sugars and free lysine under the hot, moist conditions of pelleting (Dale, 1992). The discrepancies in the response of feeding pelleted diets may be due to differences in pelleting conditions and the soluble sugar content of the feedstuffs. A commonly used protein source, like soybean meal, that contains over 6% sucrose and other oligosaccharides, may therefore, be more susceptible to reduced lysine digestibility during pelleting.

1.4 FATS AND FATTY ACIDS

Normal digestion processes

There is no evidence for hydrolysis of fats in the upper alimentary tract of poultry, although by analogy with the human, a limited acid-catalyzed hydrolysis in the proventriculus and gizzard cannot be precluded. In carnivore avian species such as raptors however, there is secretion of lipase from the walls of the stomach, which suggest the beginning of fat digestion. The digestion and absorption of fats in the chicken occurs mainly in the small intestine. While there is significant lipase secretion in the chick from a very early age, activity increases very rapidly during the first three weeks. Duodenal activity of lipase for example, was shown to increase almost 100 fold between 4 and 21 days post-hatch (Noy and Sklan, 1994). Fat digestion is enhanced by emulsification with bile salts, secreted into the lumen of the small intestine, from the gall bladder. Lipases act at an oil-water interface and this explains why emulsification is required for fat digestion. Pancreatic lipase breaks down the emulsified fats into fatty acids, monoglycerides and glycerol while cholesterol esterase, also secreted from the pancreas, hydrolyses cholesterol-fatty acid esters into cholesterol and free fatty acids. Short-chain fatty acids and free glycerol are then absorbed directly into the mucosa of the small intestine and transported to the portal circulation. Other free fatty acids, monoglycerides and cholesterol molecules are emulsified by bile salts, forming micelles, which are essential for normal fat absorption. Water-insoluble compounds such as polar unsaturated fatty acids and monoglycerides, that cannot form micelles alone, readily form stable mixed micelles with conjugated bile salts. Saturated fatty acids such as palmitic and stearic acids on the other hand, which are non-polar and have high melting points, are only slightly soluble in emulsions with bile salts. They are, however, markedly solubilized in the presence of a mixed micelle. In this form, the fatty acids and other lipid-like materials are solubilized in the aqueous phase of the lumen and are transported to the mucosal cell membrane. Consequently, the balance of dietary saturated:unsaturated fatty acids and amount of bile salt secreted are important factors in fat absorption. Figure 1.2 shows the relationship between fat digestion and content of saturated and unsaturated fatty acids.

Fat digestion is optimized when there is at least 80% unsaturated fatty acid content. Fat digestibility is also affected by other factors, most notably bird age and also the content of free fatty acids.

Nitsan *et al.* (1991) reported levels of lipase in contents of jejunal digesta to increase from 4 units/g at 1d of age, up to 8 units/g at 20d. Nir *et al.* (1993) reported comparable values of 0.8 and 2 units/g for 1d and 15d old birds, respectively.

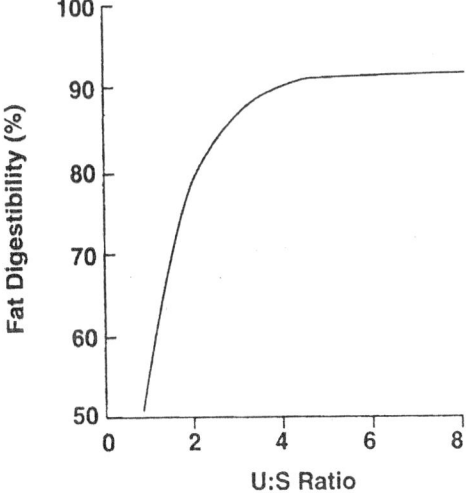

Figure 1.2 Shows the relationship between fat digestion and content of saturated and unsaturated fatty acids. *Adapted from Ketels and DeGroote (1989)*

This age-related change may be influenced by diet fat content, since Krogdahl and Sell (1989) showed a 100% increase in intestinal lipase activity in birds fed a high fat diet, while there was little change over time for birds on a low fat diet. Green and Kellogg (1987) also indicated a relatively high level of bile salts (13.9 mM/L) in intestinal contents of 2d old birds and while this value doubled over a 44d period there was a noticeable decline (8.2 mM/L) at 9d of age.

Pancreatic lipase shows specificity for the fatty acids esterified to glycerol in the 1- and 3-positions. This specificity of lipase leads first to 1,2-diglycerides, then to 2-monoglycerides. The 2-monoglycerides cannot be hydrolyzed as such, but may be broken down only if they are isomerized to 1-monoglycerides. The degree of unsaturation or chain length of the fatty acids involved does not alter the specificity of pancreatic lipase for the primary ester linkages of glycerides. Using isotopically labeled monglycerides, it has been shown that unhydrolyzed monoglycerides are absorbed intact. Fifty to seventy-eight per cent of the dietary triglyceride molecules are hydrolyzed to 2-monoglycerides and absorbed in this form.

The formation of a lipid-bile salt micelle is an important physiochemical prerequisite for fat absorption. Conjugated bile salts possess dissymmetric polar and non-polar regions and so are capable of reducing surface tension of aqueous solutions and behave as detergents. Certain water-insoluble compounds such as monoglycerides and unsaturated fatty acids cannot form micelles alone, but they readily form stable mixed micelles with the conjugated bile salts. These mixed micelles have the ability to solubilize significant amounts of the nonpolar fatty acids and fat-soluble vitamins. Compounds in the micelles are oriented with their polar groups extending out to the micellar surface. In contrast to large oil-water emulsion droplets, micelles form spontaneously and are only 30-100 Å in diameter, forming solutions that are optically clear and very stable. An important feature of the micelle is the ability to take-up relatively large amounts of nonpolar compounds within its liquid nonpolar interior. Thus, palmitic acid and stearic acid, which are water-insoluble, nonpolar fatty acids with high melting points, are only slightly soluble in bile salts in emulsion form but are markedly solubilized in the presence of a mixed micelle. In this form the fatty acids and other lipid-like materials, are solubilized within the aqueous phase of the lumen and are transported to the mucosal cell membrane. The process of fat absorption can be summarized as shown in Fig 1.3.

Dietary lipids, composed primarily of triglycerides, enter the duodenum and become emulsified upon contact with the conjugated bile salts. At the surface of this fairly large emulsion droplet (5000 Å) the activity of pancreatic lipase is greatly accelerated. The fatty acids in the 1- and 3-positions of the triglycerides project into the aqueous phase of the intestinal contents and are readily acted upon by the pancreatic lipase (Fig 1.3). A portion of the released monoglycerides and the

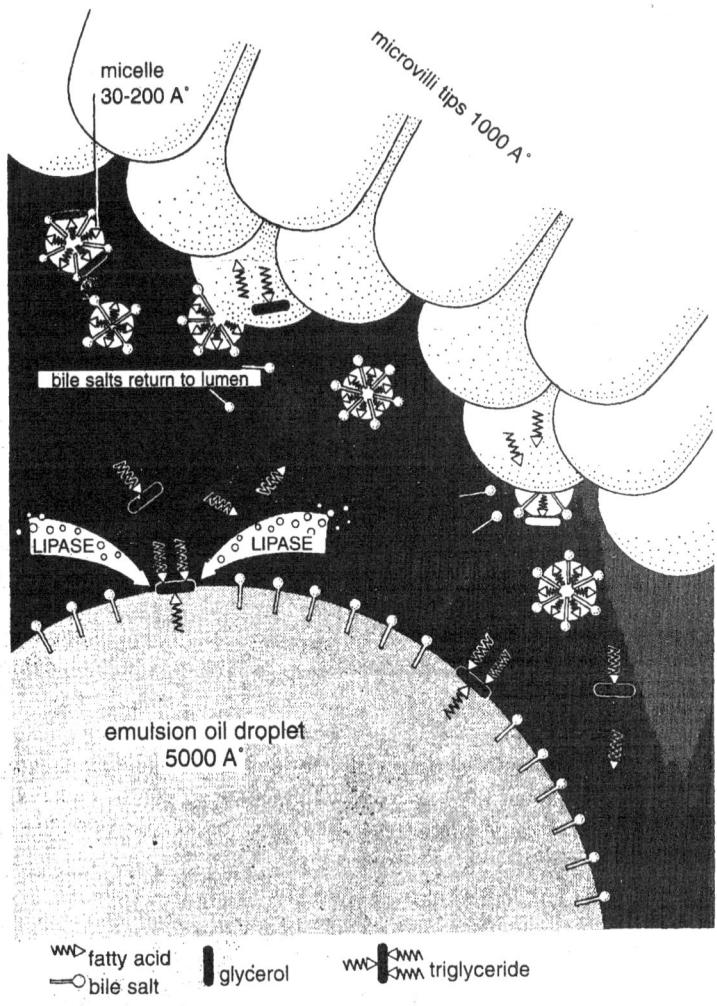

Figure 1.3 Schematic representation of fat digestion and absorption.

unsaturated fatty acids aid in the formation and stabilization of smaller emulsion droplets while most of the monoglycerides and unsaturated fatty acids, together with the conjugated bile salts, spontaneously form mixed micelles. These tiny particles, only 30 to 100 Å in diameter, become highly dispersed in the aqueous medium of the intestinal lumen. They solubilize the nonpolar dietary fatty acids such as palmitic and stearic acids. In this form the fatty acids and the monoglycerides are readily brought into contact with the microvilli. Monoglycerides and fatty acids pass across this membrane into the mucosal cells. Since bile salts are not absorbed in the upper small intestine, they are continuously re-utilized for subsequent micelle formation and are eventually absorbed in the lower jejunum.

At the microvilli surface, the digested lipids face two barriers, namely the unstirred water layer and secondly the lipid membrane itself. The former barrier may be the rate-limiting step to absorption while the second introduces an energy dependent transport system. The bile salts may also cross into the jejunal enterocyte, although this seems to be a two-way transport system and there are substantial quantities of bile acids in the feces, especially for young birds. A fatty acid binding protein has been isolated in jejunal enterocytes and other tissues such as the liver, ovary and retina. There is some speculation that availability of this protein may limit fat absorption in young birds, although liver concentrations seem to be at their highest in very young birds (Sewell *et al.*, 1990).

Once inside the mucosal cells, the monoglycerides and fatty acids are re-esterified, and together with free and esterified cholesterol, lipoproteins and phospholipids, are assembled into chylomicrons. There are two re-esterification pathways in the intestinal mucosal cells. One requires monoglycerides as the initial acceptor, the other being glycerol. The chylomicrons formed within the cells contain a central core of re-esterified triglycerides surrounded by a membrane-like structure composed of protein, cholesterol and phospholipids. It is in this form that the re-esterified triglycerides are transported from the intestinal mucosal cells to the systemic circulation of the body.

Sklan *et al.*, (1996) indicate that up to 15% of fatty acids present in the lumen will be catabolized in the mucosal epithelium. Such action, similar to the metabolism of glucose and some amino acids in this tissue, contributes to the "maintenance" cost of a functional digestive system. Most digested fat will however, be transported to the liver for subsequent catabolism or redirection to storage adipose tissue. Chickens, unlike mammals do not have a specialized lacteal system that transports fat to the liver. For chickens, transport of chylomicrons (sometimes called portomicrons) occurs via the portal venous system. The newly resynthesized hydrophobic triglycerides coalesce into small droplets and are coated with amphiphilic compounds such as phosphatidylcholine, cholesterol and proteins known as apoproteins. These physical chylomicron mixtures are stable enough to be transported in the aqueous portal system environment.

Digestibility values

Fats and fatty acids differ significantly as sources of available energy for the chicken. The magnitude of this difference has been quantitatively demonstrated by determining the percentage absorbability of a variety of intact fats, monoglycerides and fatty acids. These values are shown in Table 1.4.

TABLE 1.4 Digestibility values of various fatty acids, monoglycerides, triglycerides and hydrolyzed triglycerides			
		Digestibility (%)	
		3-4 wks	> 8 wks
Fatty acids:			
Lauric	12:0	65	-
Myristic	14:0	25	29
Palmitic	16:0	2	12
Stearic	18:0	0	4
Oleic	18:1	88	94
Linoleic	18:2	91	95
Monoglycerides:			
Monocaprylic	8:0		100
Monocaprin	10:0		93
Monolaurin	12:0		89
Monomyristin	14:0		67
Monopalmitin	16:0		55
Monostearin	18:0		41
Monoelaidin	18:1 (trans)		93
Monoolein	18:1 (cis)		98
Monolinolein	18:2		96
Triglycerides:			
Soybean oil		96	96
Corn oil		84	95
Lard		92	93
Beef tallow		70	76
Menhaden oil		88	97
Restaurant grease		87	96
Hydrolyzed triglycerides:			
Soybean oil fatty acids		88	93
Corn oil fatty acids		90	92
Lard fatty acids		82	83
Beef tallow fatty acids		82	83
*When monoglycerides were fed the pancreatic ducts were ligated to eliminate pancreatic lipase from the lumen			

Fat digestibility is influenced by the following factors: (1) The chain length of the fatty acids; (2) the number of double bonds in the fatty acid; (3) the presence or absence of ester linkages, or whether the fat is in the form of triglyceride or as a free fatty acid; (4) the specific arrangement of the saturated and unsaturated fatty acids on the glycerol moiety of a triglyceride molecule; (5) age of the chicken; (6) the ratio of unsaturated to saturated fatty acids in the mixture of free fatty acids; (7) the intestinal microflora; (8) the composition of the diet in which the fatty acids are fed; and (9) the amount and type of triglycerides in the dietary fat mixture.

It appears that oleic and linoleic acids, and various monoglycerides, readily form mixed micelles with bile salts and these mixed micelles solubilize the saturated fatty acids. Thus, there is an improvement in absorption of palmitic acid when fed with increasing amounts of oleic acid or monoolein. Also monoolein is more than twice as effective as oleic acid in improving the absorption of palmitic acid. This appears to be due to the fact that monoolein forms a mixed micelle which will solubilize larger amounts of palmitic acid. Thus, in a feeding situation, where the major portion of the fat in a feed happened to be saturated, improvement in absorbability and therefore in energy value, would result from addition to the feed of a small amount of vegetable oil containing a preponderance of unsaturated fatty acids.

Several investigators have reported that a mixture of tallow and a vegetable oil, resulted in a metabolizable energy value greater than the sum of the individual **fats.** This situation is often referred to as fatty acid synergism and is responsible **for the fact** that stearic acids and similar saturates are utilized fairly well in mixed fats. A saturated fatty acid is also absorbed quite readily if it happens to be in the 2- position of the triglyceride, since monoglycerides of saturated fatty acids are better absorbed than are the free saturated fatty acids (Table 1.4.). This phenomenon is responsible for the very high absorbability of the palmitic acid in lard in which this fatty acid is present largely in the 2- position, as compared with the poor absorbability of palmitic and stearic acid in tallow, where these fatty acids are distributed throughout the 1- and 3- positions of the triglyceride.

Factors affecting digestion

Impurities and non-saponifiables. Impurities are most often referred to collectively as M.I.U. (moisture, impurities and unsaponifiables). Most of these compounds will have little nutritional value, and so obviously digestibility values must be adjusted corresponding to total fat content. During oxidation at both high and low temperatures, a vast range of unusual polymers can be produced, and Wiseman (1986) has extensively described their structure and formation and the adverse effect of feeding such polymers in oxidized fats. Wiseman (1986) cites evidence for the dramatic effect of oxidation of a fat, caused by overheating, on available energy, where loss in digestibility can reach up to 30%. A number of naturally occurring fatty acids can also adversely affect overall fat utilization, although their mode of action is most likely via general well-being of the animal rather than through any specific mode of action related to digestion or absorption etc. Two such components are erucic acid present in rapeseed oils and some other Brassica sp., and the cyclopropenoid fatty acids in cottonseed.

Fatty acid composition and bile salts. As previously described, the content of fatty acids within a fat can have a marked effect on digestibility. Generally, the unsaturates are more readily digested than are saturates, although combinations of the two result in some synergism. Lewis (1989) concludes that maximum synergism occurs with fats added at about 3% of the diet and that ME values determined from digestibility studies, rather than conventional ME studies, are "unrealistic". Similarly Ketels and DeGroote (1989) determined the optimum ratio of unsaturates:saturates in terms of overall fat digestibility and ME. Contrary to the conclusion of Lewis (1989), Ketels and DeGroote (1989) show a similar ratio for optimum fat digestibility and fat ME at around 4:1 (unsaturated:saturated).

While unsaturated fatty acid content of a diet, has a marked effect on overall fat digestion, there is often concern over a fat's content of free-fatty acids. Although a large proportion of fatty acids are released in the lumen after hydrolysis, the presence of monoglycerides plays an important part in solubilizing non-polar long-chain saturates. Sklan (1979) also showed that overall absorption of fatty acids was highest in 3-week old chicks fed triglycerides and lowest when pure fatty acids were fed. This may be due to less efficient micelle formation, or less bile production. Sklan (1979) suggests that when products high in FFA content are used, such problems may be corrected by supplying a source of monoglyceride. Wiseman and Salvador (1991) indicate that free fatty acid content of fats influences digestibility depending upon saturation and bird age. In most situations digestibility is reduced when high levels of free fatty acids are fed to young birds (Fig 1.4)

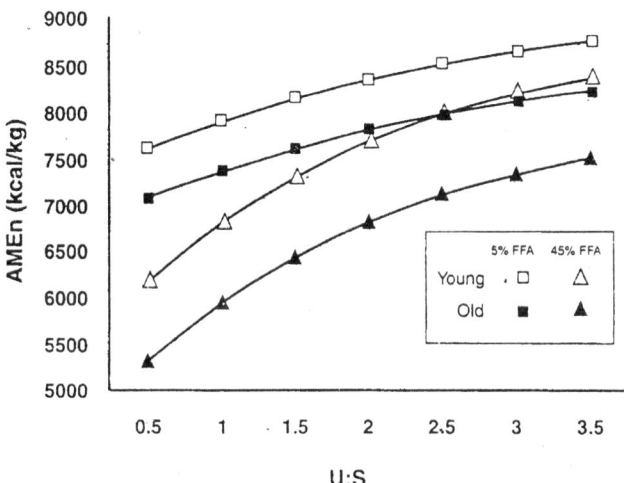

Figure 1.4 Effect of free fatty content and degree of saturation on fat digestion in young and older broilers.
Adapted from Wiseman and Salvador (1991)

Another important factor associated with micelle formation is availability of bile salts. The age-related effect on digestion of fats is partly accounted for by inefficient bile-salt recycling in very young birds. Atteh and Leeson (1985) clearly showed the advantage to be gained by adding cholic acid (bile salt) to the diet of broiler chickens (Table 1.5). With approximately 8% palmitate in the diet or 8% of an oleic/palmitate mixture there was a dramatic increase in bird performance and fat utilization in response to added cholic acid. Unfortunately the use of 0.2% cholic acid in the diet, as used in this study, is not economically viable.

TABLE 1.5 Influence of synthetic bile acid on fat digestion in young broilers		
	Apparent fat retention (%)	
Diet type	Control	+0.2% cholic acid
Control diet (2% fat)	77.0	78.8
+8% palmitic acid	32.3	41.3
+8% oleic/palmitic acid	52.7	68.6
		Adapted from Atteh and Leeson (1985)

Intestinal factors, rate of passage and interaction with other ingredients. Status of the intestinal lumen will obviously have an effect on the digestion and/or absorption of any nutrient. Digesta pH can influence fat digestion, because acidic conditions reduce micellar solubilization. In rats, fat digestibility is reduced when the diet contains lactic acid. This concept warrants further study considering the use of organic acid mold inhibitors and the use of various feed additives to modify gut pH. A fatty acid-albumin complex has been shown to be absorbed less efficiently than are micellar fatty acids and the formation of a complex of these fatty acids with undigested protein maybe partly responsible for the poorer fat digestion seen when animals are fed improperly processed soybean meal.

Birds infected with coccidiosis often exhibit inferior fat digestibility. Steatorrhoea occurring with intestinal coccidiosis may, therefore, result from the loss of reconstituted fat globules following the rupture of parasitized epithelial cells. Fat *per se* and linoleic acid in particular, may also affect the microbial population in the intestine, since a reduction in coliform bacterial population has been seen in layers fed corn oil. Fat digestion also seems to be adversely affected by high levels of indigestible fibre (Cherry and Jones, 1982). Increased levels of cellulose apparently result in reduced fat digestion, possibly through complexing of fibre with bile salts.

Diet fat *per se* can affect rate of passage of digesta, and this can influence overall diet digestibility. Sell and co-workers at Iowa State University have used this argument to account for the so-called "extra-metabolic" effect of fat. These workers suggest that fats and oils, likely delay proventricular emptying and intestinal digesta movement. However, this effect is influenced by diet constituents, the rate of passage being more affected when the diet contains sucrose vs. starch (Mateos and Sell, 1981). Delayed rate of passage suggests that digesta spends more time in contact with digestive enzymes, carriers or co-factors and absorptive sites, etc. Addition of fats to the diet may, therefore, lead to increased digestion of non-fat components of the diet.

Bird age. The fact that young birds cannot digest fats as well as do older birds has been documented for many years, and yet this fact has rarely been incorporated in formulation matrices. Sell *et al.* (1986) demonstrated the ability of young turkeys to metabolize various fat sources, where from 2 to 8 weeks of age the energy contribution of tallow increased by 25%. Katongole and March (1979) likewise show a 20-30% improvement in digestion of tallow for 6 vs. 3 week-old broilers and Leghorns. The effect of age on the ability to digest fats is most pronounced for the saturates (Table 1.6).

TABLE 1.6 Effect of bird age on digestion of fats and fatty acids						
		Digestion (%)				
Fat type	Bird age (d)	Fat	16:0	18:0	18:1	18:2
Corn oil	14	96	90	-	95	95
	56	98	96	-	100	47
Tallow	14	57	51	49	94	-
	56	74	84	83	98	-
				Adapted from (Whitehead and Fisher, 1975)		

The reason why adult birds are better able to digest fats, and particularly saturated fats, is not clear. Young birds recycle bile salts less efficiently, and this may be a factor as described previously. Also there is an indication that fatty acid binding protein is not produced in adequate quantities by young birds. Both Sell *et al.*, (1986) and Katongole and March (1979) cite evidence for up to 5x increase in FABP with chicks from hatch through 8 weeks of age.

Soap formation Once fats have been digested, free-fatty acids have the opportunity of reacting with other nutrients within the digesta. One such possible association is with minerals to form soaps that may or may not be soluble. If insoluble soaps are formed, there is the possibility that both the fatty acid and the mineral will be unavailable to the bird. Atteh and Leeson (1984) indicate substantial soap formation in the digesta of broiler chicks and that this is most pronounced with saturated fatty acids and with high levels of diet minerals. Differences in fat digestibility were mirrored in changes in fecal soap formation. In other studies, Atteh and Leeson (1983) indicated such increased fecal soap production is associated with reduced bone ash and bone calcium content of broilers. Soap production seems to be less of a problem with older birds, and this situation is of importance to laying hens that are fed high levels of calcium. In addition to calcium, other minerals such as magnesium can form soaps with saturated fatty acids. In older birds and some other animals, there is an indication that while soaps develop in the upper digestive tract, they are subsequently solubilized in the lower tract due to changes in pH. Under these conditions both the fatty acid and mineral are available to the bird. Control over digesta pH may, therefore, be an important parameter for control over soap formation.

1.5 VITAMINS

Normal digestion process

D igestion and absorption of fat- and water-soluble vitamins must be considered separately, because their solubility characteristics dictate the general mechanisms by which they are absorbed. The fat soluble vitamins, A, D, E and K, undergo similar digestive processes as do dietary triglycerides, mainly in the small intestine, and these processes have been described previously for fats. The processes briefly include emulsification, which is enhanced by bile salts, action of pancreatic lipase and formation of mixed micelles, which are prerequisites for their absorption into the intestinal cells. Depending upon the dietary forms of the vitamins, digestion of vitamins A and E involves the action of retinyl and tocopherol esterases respectively. These enzymes hydrolyse fatty acid esters of retinol and tocopherol into their free forms, namely retinol and tocopherol and also free fatty acids (Linder, 1985). Retinol, tocopherol and β-carotene become dispersed in mixed micelles similar to products of fat digestion. The mixed micelles comprised of bile salts, monoglycerides and long-chain fatty acids together with vitamins A, D, E and K, and β-carotene facilitate their absorption into the mucosal cells.

Absorption takes place mostly at the proximal site of the small intestine with little uptake for vitamins D and K at the more distal sites. Under normal conditions, where there is adequate bile and monoglycerides, both d- and L-α-tocopherol are shown to be well absorbed, but equal dietary levels produce a lower blood concentration of L- rather than d-α-tocopherol. Competition among the fat-soluble vitamins for absorption has been demonstrated. Thus, in diets containing barely adequate levels of vitamins A, D, E and K, a marked increase in the dietary level of vitamin A may cause decrease in growth or egg production. This situation has been attributed to the induced deficiency of one or more of the other fat-soluble vitamins rather than to any toxic effect of vitamin A.

Inside the intestinal epithelium much of the β-carotene is converted into vitamin A by the enzyme β-15, 15' dioxygenase. Most of the retinol and tocopherol are then converted to mixed esters, the nature of which depends to a great extent upon the type of fatty acids being absorbed with these vitamins. Palmitic acid appears to be used preferentially with vitamin A. Vitamins A and E are transported in plasma both as a free alcohol and in the esterified form.

Most water-soluble vitamins require specific enzymes for their conversion from natural forms in feedstuffs into the forms that are ultimately absorbed. For example, biotin is often covalently linked to lysine as biocytin that requires biotinidase that is secreted from the pancreas and mucosal cell for proteolytic release of the free biotin. Pyridoxine and thiamin exist in some feedstuffs as active phosphorylated forms, that need non-specific alkaline phosphatases from intestinal cells for their hydrolysis into free absorbable forms (Linder, 1985). These vitamins exist as dephosphorylated forms in plant feedstuffs that require no digestion. Most folic acid exists in plant feedstuffs naturally attached to a polymer of glutamic acid, which is hydrolysed into the absorbable monoglutamate form at the brush border membrane by the enzyme folate conjugate or pteroryl polyglutamate hydrolase. Unlike fat-soluble vitamins that are absorbed mostly by passive diffusion, absorption of water-soluble vitamins involves different active carrier systems. The mechanism of uptake of vitamin B_{12} is not adequately understood, but it is believed to involve pinocytosis (Castro, 1981). As with fat-soluble vitamins, water-soluble vitamins are mostly absorbed in the proximal small intestine.

Digestibility values

There is very little information available on the digestibility of vitamins in natural feedstuffs. Data that is available often relates to individual feed ingredients and there seems to be no systematic attempt at developing such information. Perhaps this situation is justified on the basis that few nutritionists today rely on the major feed ingredient to supply vitamins. Rather they are supplied as synthetics, but here again we have little reliable information on digestibility under controlled conditions. One assumes the fat-soluble vitamins will be digested and absorbed at rates comparable to that occurring for fat. Assuming no digesta antagonists, then water-soluble vitamins are assumed to be 100% available. Table 1.7 attempts to summarize reported values on vitamin digestibility in feeds and/or common ingredients such as corn and soybean meal. A useful but still limited reference for such information is McDowell (1989).

TABLE 1.7 Digestibility of vitamins in commercial feed ingredients	
"	% Digestibility
Vitamin A	40-70
Vitamin D_3	50-66
Vitamin E (α-tocopherol)	10-25
Vitamin K (phylloquinone)	50%
Thiamin	?
Riboflavin	?
Niacin	85%
Pyridoxine	?
Pantothenate	?
Biotin (corn)	90
Biotin (wheat)	0
folic acid	50
Vitamin B_{12}	?
Choline	60-75%

Factors affecting digestion

Biotin provides a classical situation for variability in digestion across various ingredients. The total biotin content of wheat is comparable to that of other cereals (110 µg/kg), but is almost completely unavailable to the chick (Bryden, 1990). This may relate to differences in susceptibility to the hydrolytic action of biotinidase, which is required for digestion to free biotin. The biotin bioavailability for vegetable protein sources is also quite variable. Groundnut meal has a very high biotin content of about 1630 µg/kg, about 53% of which is available to the chick, while sunflower meal has about 1000 µg/kg biotin with bioavailability of only about 40%. The niacin in cereal grains and their by-products is in a bound form which also has very low bioavailability for chicks (Cunha, 1982). Ionov and Surai (1994) investigated the bioavailability of vitamin E in cereals for laying hens. They calculated the vitamin E availability for wheat, corn and barley to be 17, 14 and 11% respectively.

Stability, and subsequent availability of vitamins is affected by other compounds that are present in the premixes of complete diets and by the conditions occurring during storage. Factors such as length of storage, temperature, pH, humidity, presence of enzymes and exposure to ultraviolet light decrease vitamin stability. The presence of polyunsaturated fatty acids (PUFA) can cause oxidative rancidity, which will lead to destruction of vitamins A, D and E. In diets that are formulated with PUFA, an effective antioxidant is required to prevent oxidative damage. The presence of minerals in the premix or diets, can enhance oxidative destruction of such vitamins and this can be further enhanced by the presence of highly hygroscopic compounds, such as choline chloride.

While pelleting can improve the nutritive value of feeds, it can also decrease the stability and digestibility of heat sensitive vitamins (Jones, 1986). The stability of vitamins A, D, K, C and thiamin for example, is substantially reduced in pelleted feeds (Gadient, 1986). This effect is attributed to the high temperature, moisture and pressure that the feed ingredients are subjected to during pelleting. The bioavailability of certain vitamins like biotin and niacin, that are often present in bound forms, can however, be improved by pelleting (Scott, 1973).

1.6 MINERALS

Normal digestion process

Absorption of minerals occurs throughout the jejunum and ileum. The rate of absorption depends on factors such as pH, carriers, forms of the minerals and presence of other minerals that will influence competition for absorption. Numerous mechanisms of mineral absorption have been elucidated and many minerals, such as iron, sodium and zinc, require active transport systems and absorption is regulated. Absorption of non-metal minerals such as sulfur, and selenium is very efficient, unregulated and depends mainly on the source and presence of other minerals in the gut. Calcium absorption involves both carrier proteins and simple diffusion mechanisms where absorption rate is regulated to maintained blood calcium level by factors such as parathyroid hormone and vitamin D_3. Such regulation means that calcium absorption is usually proportionally lower compared to phosphorus which is unregulated and where absorption efficiency can be as high as 95%.

Digestibility values

As with the vitamins, there has been little research done in determining mineral digestibility in poultry feeds and ingredients. Because of its relative cost, most interest has been given to phosphorus, and the relative bioavailability of available sources. Table 1.8 summarizes some data on digestibility of trace minerals in some feed ingredients.

TABLE 1.8 Digestibility of trace minerals in some common feed ingredients						
	Digestibility (%)					
	Ca	P	Cu	Zn	Mg	Mn
Rapeseed meal	68	75	74	44	62	54
Barley	69	77	69	49	55	55
Wheat	71	68	78	49	53	48
Corn	70	61	87	58	51	60
Adapted from Aw-Yong et al., (1983) and Nwokolo and Bragg (1980)						

As described more fully in Chapter 5, the availability of phosphorus in plant material will depend greatly on the relative contribution of phytic acid. For other trace minerals, digestibility is often of little practical significance, because requirements are most often met with synthetic supplements. In situations of mineral excess, the contribution by cereals and protein ingredients may be of concern.

Factors affecting digestion

Between 50 to 70% of organic phosphorus in poultry diets is present in the form of phytate which is not available to birds, because of the absence of endogenous phytase enzyme (Frapin and Nys, 1994). As detailed in Chapter 6 the addition of microbial phytase to cereal-based diets improves phosphorus utilization and reduces phosphate excretion (Simons *et al.*, 1990). Frapin and Nys (1994) reported that reducing the phosphorus intake and addition of microbial phytase to broiler diets improved phosphorus digestibility, resulting in 40 and 50% decrease in phosphorus excretion in diets that contained 0.55 and 0.47% total phosphorus, respectively. These results are in agreement with that of Simons *et al.*, (1990) which also showed that the use of phytase-supplemented low-phosphorus broiler diets resulted in a 50% reduction in the phosphorus excreted in manure. Synthetic phytase may also improve digestion of other nutrients in the diet, such as energy, nitrogen and amino acids (Namkung and Leeson, 1999).

For trace minerals, their chemical and physical forms are probably the most significant factors affecting digestibility and availability. Table 1.9 summarizes availability of various trace mineral sources, where digestibility is the major variable.

TABLE 1.9 Availability of trace minerals from various sources		
	Mineral Source	**Relative Availability**
Manganese	Sulfate	100
	Carbonate	40
	Oxide	75
Zinc	Sulfate	100
	Oxide	44
Copper	Sulfate	100
	Oxide	75
	Chloride	70
Ferrous	Sulfate	100
	Carbonate	5
	Chloride	95
	Oxide	50
Ferric	Sulfate	100
	Oxide	5
	Chloride	44

The values shown in Table 1.9 show sulfates as 100% digestible and rank other sources relative to this. There is interaction between minerals that can affect digestion and absorption. For example Baker and Halpin (1991) showed a unidirectional interaction between manganese and iron with excess manganese impairing utilization of iron, while iron has little effect on manganese. Excess zinc seems to have the same unidirectional effect on iron and copper, while higher levels of phosphorus reduce manganese availability. High levels of zinc and copper also influence selenium uptake. In many feeding situations these interactions are of little practical significance, since levels necessary to induce the "interaction" are rarely achieved. However, in situations such as high zinc feeding, used to induce molt, there will invariably be mineral interaction occurring in the digesta and at the jejunal mucosa. Physical form of mineral supplements also seems to affect digestibility. For any given product, the finer the grind, the greater the overall availability.

Minerals readily form chelates in the digesta, and again this can influence availability. Chelate formation with sugars, amino acids and other carbohydrates within the digesta are quite common and in fact, few minerals are found unattached. In most instances these chelates will be digested and/or dissociate in the jejunum or ileum when subjected to a pH change. Some mineral chelates are now, in fact, considered as additives (see Chapter 8).

SELECTED REFERENCES

Anderson-Hefermann, J.C., Y. Zhang and C.M. Parsons, 1993. Effects of processing on the nutritional quality of canola meal. Poultry Sci. 72:326-333.

Araba, M. and N.M. Dale, 1990. Evaluation of protein solubility as an indicator of over-processing soybean meal. Poultry Sci. 69:1749-1752.

Araba, M., J. Gos, P. Kerr and D. Dyer, 1994. Identity preserved varieties: High oil corn and low stachyose soybean. pp 135-142. In: Proc. Arkansas Nutr. Conf. Fayetteville, Arkansas.

Atteh, J.O. and S. Leeson, 1983. Effects of dietary fatty acids and calcium levels on performance and mineral metabolism of broiler chickens. Poultry Sci. 62:2412-2419.

Atteh, J.O. and S. Leeson, 1984. Effects of dietary saturated or unsaturated fatty acids and calcium levels on performance and mineral metabolism of broiler chicks. Poultry Sci. 63:2252-2260.

Atteh, J.O. and S. Leeson, 1985. Influence of age, dietary cholic acid and calcium levels on performance, utilization of free fatty acids and bone mineralization in broilers. Poultry Sci. 64:1959-1971.

Aw-Yong, J. Sim and D.B. Bragg, 1983. Mineral availability in corn, barley, wheat and triticale for the chick. Poultry Sci. 62:659-666.

Baker, D.H. and K.M. Halpin, 1991. Manganese and iron interrelationship in the chick. Poultry Sci. 70:146-152.

Bryden, W.L., 1990. Inclusion of low metabolizable energy wheat in broiler diets and the incidence of the fatty liver and kidney syndrome. Res. Vet. Sci. 49:243-244.

Butler, L.G., D.G. Lebryk and H.J. Blytt, 1984. Interaction of proteins with sorghum tannin: Mechanism, specificity, and significance. J. Am. Oil Chem. Soc. 61:916-920.

Carpenter, K.J., 1973. Damage to lysine in food processing its measurement and significance. Nutr. Abstr. Rev. 43:423-451.

Castro, G.A., 1981. Principles of digestion and absorption, pages 95-106. In: Gastrointestinal physiology. Ed. L.R. Johnson. The C.V. Mosby Company, Toronto.

Cherry, J.A. and D.E. Jones, 1982. Dietary cellulose, wheat bran, and fishmeal in relation to hepatic lipids, serum lipids, and lipid excretion in laying hens. Poultry Sci. 61:1973-1980.

Croom, W.J., J. Brake, B.A. Coles, G.B. Havenstein, V.L. Christensen, B. McBride, E.P. Peebles and I.L. Taylor, 1999. Is intestinal absorption capacity rate-limiting for performance in poultry. J. Appl. Poult. Res. 8:242-252.

Cunha, T.J., 1982. Niacin in animal feeding and nutrition. In: Vitamins the life essentials. National Feed Ingredient Association (NFIA), Des Moines, Iowa.

Dale, N., 1992. Pelleting effects on lysine bioavailability in diets containing bakery products. J. Appl. Poultry Res. 1:84-87.

Frapin, D. and Y. Nys, 1994. Growth performance and phosphorus excretion of broiler chicks supplemented with microbial phytase. Proc. 9th European Poult. Conf., Glasgow, UK 1:459-460.

Freeman, C.P., 1969. Low pH reduces micellar solubilization – reason for poor fat diges-tion in rats fed lactic acid. Br. J. Nutr. 23:249-255.

Gadient, M., 1986. Effect of pelleting on nutritional quality of feeds. In: Proc. of Maryland Nutritional Conf. For Feed Manufacturers. College Park, Maryland.

Green, J. and T.F. Kellogg, 1987. Bile acid concentrations in serum, bile, jejunal contents and excreta of male broiler chicks during the first six weeks posthatch. Poultry Sci. 66:535-540.

Groneuer, K.J. and W. Hartfield, 1975. Influence of fat of higher linoleic acid content on the intestinal flora of laying hens. Archiv. Fur Geflugelkunde 3, p 178-182.

Halley, J.T., T.S. Nelson, L.K. Kirby and J.A. York, 1986. The effect of tannin content of sorghum grain in poultry rations on dry matter digestibility and energy utilization. Arkansas Farm Research Agricultural Experiment Station, University of Arkansas, Fayetteville, AR. 35(2):8.

Hanock, J.D., E.R. Peo, Jr., A.J. Lewis and J.D. Crenshaw, 1990. Effect of ethanol extrac-tion and duration of heat treatment of soybean flakes on the utilization of soybean protein by growing rats and pigs. J. Anim. Sci. 68:3233-3243.

Hurrell, R.F, 1990. Influence of the Maillard Reaction on nutritional value of foods, pages 245-358. In: The Maillard Reaction in food processing, human nutrition and physiology. Birkhauser Verlag, Basel, Switzerland.

Ionov, I. and P. Surai, 1994. Vitamin E availability from grains for laying hens. Proc. 9th European Poultry Conf., Glasgow, UK 1:505:506.

Jin, S., A. Corless and J.L. Sell, 1998. Digestive system development in post-hatch poul-try. Wld. Poult. Sci. J. 54:335-345.

Jones, F.T., 1986. Effect of pelleting on vitamin A assay levels of poultry feed. Poultry Sci. 65:1421-1427.

Katongole, J.B.D. and B.E. March, 1979. Fatty acid binding protein in the intestine of the chicken. Poultry Sci. 58:372-375.

Ketels, E. and G. DeGroote, 1989. Effect of ratio of unsaturated fatty acids in the dietary lipid fraction on utilization and metabolizable energy of added fats in young chicks. Poultry Sci. 68:1506-1512.

Krogdahl, A. and J.L. Sell, 1989. Influence of age on lipase, amylase and protease activ-ities in pancreatic tissue and intestinal contents of young turkeys. Poultry Sci. 68:1561-1568.

Langhout, D.J. and J.B. Schutte, 1996. Nutritional implications of pectins in chicks in relation to esterification and origin of pectins. Poultry Sci. 75:1236-1242.

Lewis, D., 1989. Fat improves use of other nutrients in poultry diets. Feedstuffs, Feb. 29, pg 33.

Linder, M.C., 1985. Nutrition and metabolism of vitamins: In: Nutritional biochemistry and metabolism with clinical application. Pages 69-132. Ed. M.C. Linder Elsevier, New York.

Longstaff, M. and J.M. McNab, 1991. The inhibitory effects of hull polysaccharides and tannins of field beans *(Vicia faba L.)* on the digestibility of amino acids, starch and lipid and on digestive enzyme activities in young chicks. Br. J. Nutr. 65:199-216.

Mateos, G.G. and J.L. Sell, 1981. Influence of fat and carbohydrate source on rate of food passage of semipurified diets for laying hens. Poultry Sci. 60:2114-2119.

Mateos, G.G., J.L. Sell and J.A. Eastwood, 1982. Rate of food passage (transit time) as influenced by level of supplemental fat. Poultry Sci. 61:94-100.

Moran, E.T., Jr., J.D. Summers and S.J. Slinger, 1966. Keratins as sources of proteins for the growing chick. I. Amino acid imbalance as the cause for inferior performance of feather meal and the implication of disulfide bonding in raw feathers as the reason for poor digestibility. Poultry Sci. 45:1257-1266.

McDowell, L.R., 1989. Vitamins in animal nutrition. Publ. Academic Press. London, UK.

Namkung, H. and S. Leeson, 1999. Effect of phytase enzyme on dietary AMEn and illeal digestibility of nitrogen and amino acids in broiler chicks. Poultry Sci. 78:1317-1320.

Nitsan, Z., G. Ben-Avraham, Z. Zaref and I. Nir, 1991. Growth and development of the digestive organs and some enzymes in broiler chicks after hatching. Br. Poultry Sci. 32:515-523.

Noy, Y and D. Sklan, 1994. Enzyme secretion and small intestinal passage time in the young chick. Proc. 9th European Poultry Conf., Glasgow, UK 2:451-452.

Nwokolo, N. and D.B. Bragg, 1980. Biological availability of minerals in rapeseed meal. Poultry Sci. 59:155-158.

Parsons, C.M., K. Hashimoto, K.J. Wedeking, Y. Han and D.H. Baker, 1992. Effect of overprocessing on availability of amino acids and energy in soybean meal. Poultry Sci. 71:133-140.

Ritz, C.W., R.M. Hulet, B.C. Self and D.M. Denbow, 1995. Endogenous amylase levels and response to supplemental feed enzyme in male turkeys from hatch to 8 weeks of age. Poultry Sci. 74:1317-1322.

Scott, M.L, 1973. Effect of processing on the availability and nutritional value of vitamins. In: Effect of feed processing on the nutritional value of feeds. Pages 119-128. National Academy Press, Washington D.C.

Sell, J.L., A. Krogdahl and N. Hanyu, 1986. Influence of age on utilization of supplemental fats by young turkeys. Poultry Sci. 65:546-554.

Sewell, J.E., S.K. Davis and P.S. Hargis. 1990 Isolation, characterization and expression of fatty acid binding protein in the liver of Gallus domesticus. Comp. Biochem. Physiol. (B) 92:509-516.

Sibbald, I.R. and M.W. Wolynetz, 1985. The bioavailability of supplemental lysine and its effect on the energy and nitrogen excretion of adult cockerels fed diets diluted with cellulose. Poultry Sci. 64:1972-1975.

Simons, P.C.M., H.A.J. Versteegh, A.W. Jongbloed, P.A. Kamme, P. Slump, K.D. Bos, M.G.E. Wolters, R.F. Beudeker and G.J. Verschoor, 1990. Improvement of phosphorus availability by microbial phytase in broilers and pigs. Br. J. Nutr. 64:525-540.

Sklan, D., N. Cohen and S. Hurwitz, 1996. Intestinal uptake and metabolism of fatty acids in the chick. Poultry Sci. 75:1104-1108.

Sklan, D., 1979. Digestion and absorption of lipids in chicks fed triglycerides or free fatty acids: Synthesis of monoglycerides in the intestine. Poultry Sci. 58:885-889.

Tonroy, B.R. and T.W. Perry, 1975. Effect of roasting corn at different temperature on grain characteristics and in vitro starch digestibility. J. Dairy Sci. 58:566-569.

Wedekind, K.J. and D.H. Baker, 1990. Zinc bioavailability in feed-grade sources of zinc. J. Anim. Sci. 68:684-689.

Whitehead, C.C. and C. Fisher, 1975. The utilization of various fats by turkeys of different ages. Br. Poultry Sci. 16:481-485.

Wiseman, J., 1986. Antinutritional factors associated with dietary fats and oils. IN: Recent advances in animal nutrition. Ed. Haresign and Cole. Butterworths.

Wiseman, J. and F. Salvador, 1991. Influence of free fatty acid content and degree of saturation on the AME of fats fed to broilers. Poultry Sci. 70:573-582.

Zhang Y. and C.M. Parsons, 1993. Effect of extrusion and expelling on the nutritional quality of conventional and kunitz trypsin inhibitor-free soybeans. Poultry Sci. 72:2299-2303.

The term energy is a combination of two Greek words: *en*, meaning "in" and *ergon*, meaning work. There are a variety of definitions and descriptions of energy, depending upon whether energy is being considered in reference to its properties in the physical or in the biological sciences. In the physical sciences, energy is designated broadly to be work or anything that can be converted to work. Work, as usually defined, is only one of several uses of energy in biology, particularly in the living animal.

Energy manifests itself in many ways or forms: (1) mechanical; (2) thermal; (3) electrical; (4) light; (5) nuclear; and (6) molecular (chemical).

Most of the energy on earth comes originally from the sun although molecular energy is the most vital and useful form of energy to animals. The nutritionist deals basically with the conversion of chemical energy stored in the molecules of feed into kinetic energy of chemical reactions of metabolism and of work and heat.

2.1   HEAT AND CHEMICAL REACTIONS

Some reactions proceed with an evolution of heat and are said to be exothermic. Other reactions require an input of heat and so are endothermic. For example, under properly controlled conditions, carbon can be made to react with steam to produce carbon monoxide and hydrogen. This production of hydrogen is an endothermic reaction, requiring addition of 31.4 kcal of heat per mole of reactants:

$$(1)\ C + H_2O + 31.4\ kcal \rightarrow CO + H_2$$

This is an endothermic reaction. However, when the carbon monoxide and hydrogen formed in the above reaction are oxidized to carbon dioxide and water, they give off heat energy, which means an exothermic reaction:

$$(2)\ CO + \tfrac{1}{2}O_2 \rightarrow CO_2 + 67.6\ kcal;\ and$$

$$(3)\ H_2 + \tfrac{1}{2}O_2 \rightarrow H_2O + 57.8\ kcal/mol.$$

These reactions yield a net output of 94 kcal of heat: 67.6 + 57.8 (heat output) − 31.4 (heat input) = 94 kcal. This is the same heat output, which results from the direct oxidation of carbon:

$$(4)\ C + O_2 \rightarrow CO_2 + 94\ kcal.$$

Thus, in reaction (1), 31.4 kcal of energy absorbed was "stored" in the reaction products. This is not a random energy requirement but rather definite and reproducible. It depends on the reactants and products in the reaction. One mole (one gram-molecular weight) of each of these reactants requires this exact amount (31.4 kcal) of energy to rearrange the atoms to form CO and H_2.

The heat effect of a chemical reaction measures the difference between the heat content (stored energy contents) of the products and those of the reactants. Thus, if more energy is stored in the reactants than in the products, heat will be released during the reaction, and conversely, heat will be "absorbed" if more energy is stored in the products than in the reactants.

A mole of each molecular substance contains a characteristic amount of heat, which is the quantitative index of the energy stored in the substance during its formation. For common pure nutrients such as starch, monosaccharides, or amino acids, this stored energy is listed in tables of "Heats of Combustion".

In the thermódynamics of physical chemistry the heat balance of a reaction is the difference between the heat content of the products (H) and the heat content of the reactants (H^1); the heat of reaction is delta-H (ΔH), which represents the change or difference in the heat contents. Using the above reactions of carbon monoxide and hydrogen as an example, according to the equation, $\Delta H = H$ (of products) $- H^1$ (of reactants). The algebraic sum of the ΔH of reactions 1, 2 and 3 is: [(31.4) + (-67.6), + (-57.8)] = -94.0 kcal. This value is the same as that of reaction 4, which represents the overall reaction of 1, 2 and 3.

According to the Law of Additivity of Reaction Heats or the Law of Hess of Constant Heat Sums, as shown in the above reactions, it is not necessary to know the dynamics of all chemical changes (i.e., the heat content of all intermediates in a sequence of reactions). If the initial and final states are known, the desired, overall ΔH value can be determined from these data alone.

2.2   CONSERVATION OF ENERGY AND ADDITIVITY OF REACTION HEATS

The energy of chemical reactants is conserved in the products. As an example, the breakdown of water by electrolysis requires the addition of 68.3 kcal per mole:

(1) H_2O + 68.3 kcal equivalent of electrical work $\rightarrow H_2 + \frac{1}{2} O_2$. During the reaction, the hydrogen and oxygen store potential energy.

The heat of reaction of hydrogen and oxygen (also called the heat of combustion of hydrogen) has been found to be 68.3 kcal of heat: $H_2 + \frac{1}{2} O_2 \rightarrow H_2O$ + 68.3 kcal of heat (H_2 and O_2 release energy).

In the example above, 68.3 kcal of energy were put into the system to degrade 1 mole of H_2O to hydrogen and oxygen; in the recombination of these two elements to form 1 mole of water, 68.3 kcal of energy are recovered as heat. Thus, energy was stored in hydrogen and oxygen as potential energy. This capacity is known as the heat content, also called the chemical energy or the molecular energy. All chemical reactions are known to conform to the Law of Energy Conservation.

In biological systems, however, the total energy content of the reactants (ΔH) is not as useful in predicting whether reactions may occur, as are the changes in free energy (ΔF) that take place in the reactions. Thus, in biological systems where reactions occur at relatively constant temperature and pressure, the fundamental thermodynamic expression becomes $\Delta F = \Delta H - T\Delta S$. In this expression, T represents the absolute temperature, while ΔS is the change in the entropy of the system. Entropy, while difficult to visualize, is a measure of the degree of organization of the reactants in the system. It is a function of the size, configuration, vibrations, resonance, and other energy properties of the molecules. In a spontaneous chemical process occurring at constant temperature and pressure, energy is required to restore the system to its original state. Some of the total energy released during a spontaneous chemical process is not available for work at constant temperature and pressure. This "unavailable" energy represents the entropy of the system.

If the ΔF for a reaction is negative, the reaction may occur without adding energy to the system; reactions with a positive ΔF require energy input to occur. In practical nutrition, where it is not possible to measure the free energy changes in all of the various reactions of bioenergetics, the most useful measure of the potential energy of foods is the total heat produced on complete oxidation. Thus, the ΔH of the complete oxidation of glucose, for example, represents the total potential energy of glucose, which is available to the animal. The portion of this total (gross) energy, which is actually used for maintenance and productive purpose represents the net energy available to the animal.

2.3   CHEMICAL REACTIONS AND SECOND LAW OF THERMODYNAMICS

All chemical reactions tend to follow this law which states that the energy of the universe tends to become less and less useful; nature's reactions move toward the formation of molecules that contain less and less energy in a quest for maximum molecular stability. This is true, whether we are speaking of the burning of coal, or the metabolism of glucose within the body.

Before the carbon of coal can react with oxygen, both must be decomposed into their respective atomic forms. The application of heat to the carbon atoms on the surface of the coal and to the oxygen atoms causes these atoms to vibrate faster and faster. Eventually the vibrations become sufficiently violent for the atoms to separate from their original states and to combine with each other. The heat produced by the initial reaction causes the burning to become self-perpetuating, thereby involving more and more atoms of the elements until one of the reactants is used up. This reaction, therefore, requires an initial application of heat emitted or absorbed during the reaction. The heat produced is measured in kilocalories, joules or watts. By definition, one kilocalorie (kcal) of energy is the amount of heat needed to raise the temperature of 1000 gm of water by 1°C (i.e., from 14.5 to 15.5°C). One calorie = 1/1000 kcal = amount of heat required to raise the temperature of 1 gm of water by 1°C. One megacalorie (megcal) = 1000 kcal. In many countries the Joule is the unit of energy, rather than the calorie, since it lends itself more readily to application in physical sciences for measurements of work etc. For conversion purposes, 1 kcal = 4.184 kJ.

2.4   MEASUREMENT OF REACTION HEAT

The amount of energy locked up by the bonds that hold a molecule together cannot be determined by direct means. However, the amount of heat energy given off or absorbed when a molecule is formed or decomposed during a chemical reaction can be determined in a calorimeter. A common type of calorimeter for use in energetic studies with animals is the so-called oxygen-bomb calorimeter. Such instruments (Fig 2.1) consist of an insulated chamber in which water circulates around a reaction chamber, or bomb. The test material is ignited within the bomb, which is pressurized with oxygen to ensure complete oxidation. As the sample burns, the surrounding mass of water (known weight) is heated. Surrounding this bomb and associated water is yet another enclosed water jacket, the temperature of which is kept at exactly the same level as the water immediately surrounding the bomb. As the sample oxidizes therefore, the outer water jacket is heated to keep step with the rise in temperature of the water surrounding the bomb. This achieves adiabatic conditions, in that there is no loss of temperature (heat) or change in pressure of the oxidizing sample. The rise in temperature is recorded with an integrated computer system and based on sample size and the mass of water surrounding the bomb, the total heat of combustion (gross energy) of the sample calculated. Benzoic acid is usually used as a standard for calibration. One kcal is equivalent to 4.184 kJ (1 Joule = 10^7 ergs = 0.239 cal). The kilocalorie and megacalorie are the most commonly used units in bioenergetics in North America while the Joule is used almost exclusively in Europe. The kilocalorie will be used to express energy values throughout this book.

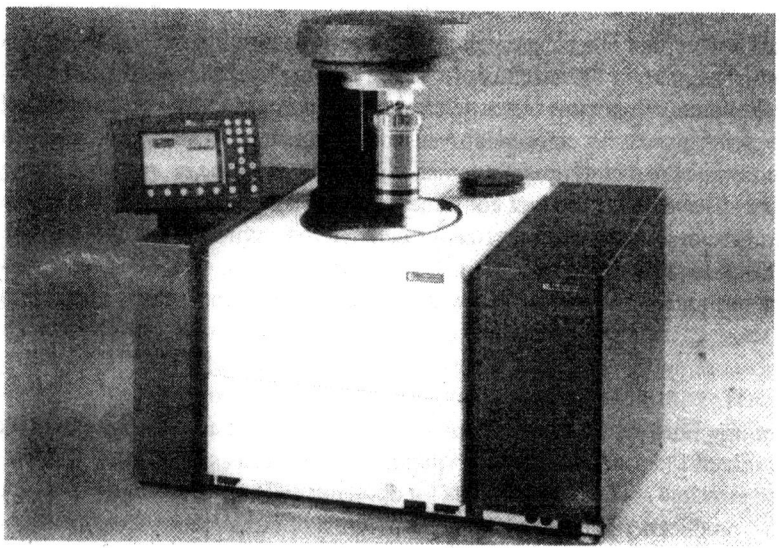

Figure 2.1 IKA C5000 adiabatic bomb calorimeter

2.5 ENERGY METABOLISM IN THE CHICKEN

The energy required by chickens for growth of body tissues, production of eggs, carrying out of vital physical activities and maintenance of normal body temperature, is derived from carbohydrates, fats and proteins in the diet. The dietary energy consumed by an animal can be used in three different ways: it can supply the energy for activity, it can be converted to heat, or it can be stored as body tissue. Dietary energy exceeding that needed for normal growth and metabolism of the bird is usually stored as fat. Excess available energy cannot be excreted by the animal body. Optimum nutrient utilization by the chicken is achieved when the diet contains the proportion of energy to other nutrients needed to produce the desired growth, egg production or body composition.

Energy is described by Kleiber as the fire of life. The major portion of all feed consumed by an animal is used for energy since both anabolic and catabolic reactions create a demand for energy. In the short term, gastric distension has some influence on feed intake, although long term (days) there is involvement of blood glucose. Regions of the hypothalamus are influenced by both high and low levels of glucose, and so this association can serve as a basis for feed intake regulation. More long term (weeks), the levels of adipose tissue may be important while as described in Chapter 3, levels of certain amino acids in the blood can also influence feed intake. Chickens in general have a remarkable ability to control their energy intake when confronted with diets or diet components of varying energy concentration. This important mechanism is the basis for many decisions made during feed formulation.

While the taste of food may have a large influence on the amount of energy consumed by man and certain other mammals, taste appears to play a relatively minor role in feed consumption by the chicken. Energy level of the diet appears to be the overwhelmingly important factor determining feed intake. When an animal such as the growing or laying chicken is given a diet adequate in all nutrients, the animal will consume the diet to obtain a remarkably constant intake of available energy per day. The absolute amount consumed depends upon the needs of the animal which vary depending upon its size, its activity, the environmental temperature, whether it is growing, simply maintaining itself or laying eggs. It is of utmost importance, therefore, that we know the energy requirements of chickens during each stage of their growth and development and that we have precise information concerning the available energy values of the feedstuffs used to formulate their diets. With this information, it is possible to closely predict the feed consumption of any flock of chickens in a particular environment and thus to determine the levels of protein, amino acids, vitamins and minerals such that all nutrients will be provided in adequate amounts for optimum daily growth and performance. Poultry producers often think of energy in terms of those feedstuffs which have been shown to be particularly rich sources, such as corn, wheat, sorghum grains, and animal and vegetable fats and oils. However it must be remembered that all organic components of a diet provide energy and in high protein diets, ingredients such as soybean meal can provide substantial proportions of total energy.

The nutritionist must consider energy in terms of the digestible starch, sugars, fats and proteins in the feedstuff and must consider how processing of the ingredients, balancing of the diet and addition of special supplements such as antioxidants or enzymes may aid in providing the birds with the maximum amount of available energy. This is of utmost importance because in diets containing adequate amounts of all required nutrients, the efficiency of feed utilization depends upon the available energy content of the diet.

Energy is stored in the carbohydrates, fats and proteins of feed ingredients. This energy comes originally from the sun and is initially stored in plant materials as a result of photosynthesis. All materials containing carbon and hydrogen in forms that can be oxidized to carbon dioxide and water represent potential energy for animals. The amount of heat produced when a feed is burned completely in the presence of oxygen can be measured in a bomb calorimeter (Fig 2.1) and is termed the gross energy of the food. The percentage of the gross energy that can be taken into the animal body and used to support the metabolic processes depends upon the ability of the animal to digest the feedstuffs. Digestion represents the physical and chemical processes which take place in the gastro-intestinal tract (Chapter 1) and result in breaking down the complex chemical compounds in feeds into the smaller molecules that can be absorbed and used by the animal. This absorbed energy is termed digestible energy. Further losses of energy occur in the urine in the form of nitrogenous wastes and other compounds not oxidized by the animal body. When the digestible energy is corrected for these losses the resultant energy is called the metabolizable energy value of the food or feedstuff. During metabolism of the nutrient further losses of energy occur (Heat Increment). The remaining energy of feed that is available for the animal to use for maintenance and productive purposes is called net energy. The relationship between the various measures of the energy value of feed are shown in Figure 2.2.

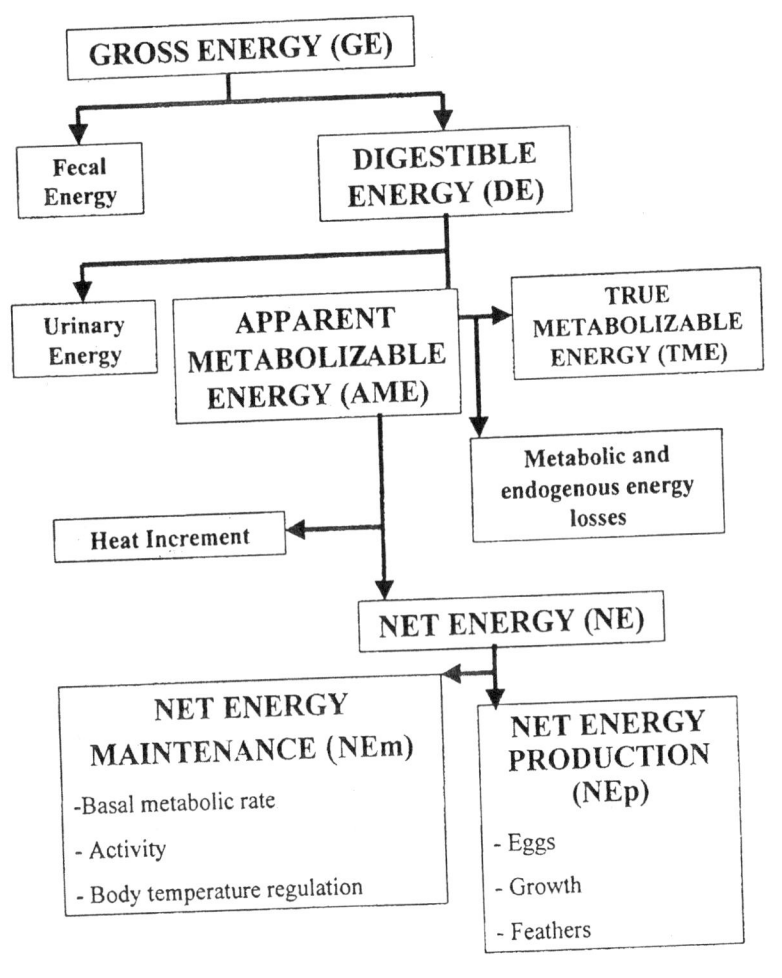

Figure 2.2 Definition and interrelationship of energy measurement systems.

2.6 ENERGY ASSAYS

Gross energy

Gross energy is determined by adiabatic bomb calorimetry as described previously, and is the only simple lab assay for energy. In nutritional studies, gross energy has no meaningful value, other than providing a starting point for other systems of evaluation. Requesting a gross energy value of a feed, from an analytical service, is totally wasteful and a misleading exercise. At best the gross energy will indicate a balance of organic vs. inorganic components. Other measures of energy require the use of live birds involving a classical bioassay procedure. The use of live birds in such protracted assays (3-4d) means high cost and limited locations willing to provide such a service.

Metabolizable energy

It is very difficult to separate the feces and urine of the bird without resorting to surgical modification that exteriorizes the ureters. This seems an unnecessary procedure, since collection of feces and urine together (as excreta) lead directly to estimates of metabolizable energy. Metabolizable energy has become the standard measure of energy availability in chickens and most other farm species. In a metabolizable energy assay (Chapter 9) not all of the excreta energy will originate from the feed. Some excreta will occur, even in a fasted bird, and represents sloughed intestinal cells, hormones, enzymes and endogenous urinary energy. If these non-feed energy losses are measured, and the value subtracted from the AME, then True Metabolizable Energy is derived. The relationship between AME and TME was originally described by Guillaume and Summers (1970). As shown in Fig. 2.3, TME is unaffected by feed intake, while AME will decline dramatically when feed intake is very low. At low feed intakes (approximately 50% maintenance) the metabolic fecal and endogenous urinary energy losses assume a large portion of excreta energy, and hence the low AME value. At maintenance feeding and above (50 g/d for an adult rooster shown in Fig. 2.3) the correction is quite low and in the order of 2-5%.

In most situations, it is also necessary to correct all estimates of metabolizable energy for nitrogen balance. During a bioassay it is impossible to ensure that all animals grow at the same rate or produce the same egg mass etc. The common choice of adult roosters, which are not growing, in these bioassays is partly based on reducing such variance. However even with adult birds at maintenance, there will still be some variation in nitrogen (protein and amino acid) balance of animals. For example, if two birds are used in an assay, and one deposits 5g N and the other 10g N over the balance period, this differential growth will affect AME or TME. Eventually, all such stored protein will be catabolized as part of normal body protein turnover and at that time the retained nitrogen (energy) is excreted.

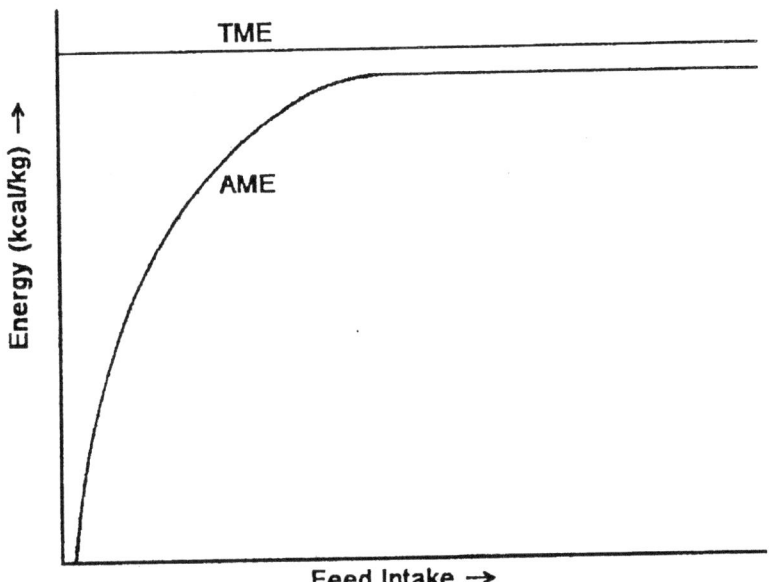

Figure 2.3 Relationship between feed intake, AME and TME
(adapted from Guillaume and Summers, 1970)

In a short-term (3-4d) bioassay, such turnover is far from complete. In the above example, the bird retaining 10g N will have higher ME, because its urinary energy will be less. Mathematically, we can make each bird retain the same amount of nitrogen, so as to standardize energy retention as protein. The correction usually applied is to zero nitrogen retention and the corrected value is termed nitrogen-corrected metabolizable energy (AMEn or TMEn). The usual correction is 8.22 kcal GE/g N retained or excreted, since this is the energy value of uric acid. Assuming birds retain N in the bioassay, the correction is added to excreta energy, so AMEn will be less than AME. If animals are in negative nitrogen balance over the assay period, then the correction factor is subtracted from the excreta energy, and then AMEn will be greater than AME. The same correction scenarios apply to TME.

Net energy

Metabolizable energy provides a useful measure of the gross energy available for production. Unfortunately such retained energy is not used 100% efficiently for growth, egg production etc. During these metabolic processes, some 15% of energy will be 'wasted' as heat, and this is commonly referred to as heat increment or specific dynamic action. Different nutrients are utilized with varying efficiencies, and so net energy becomes a variable dependent on the bird's stage of growth, production or development. It is very difficult to measure NE, because the necessary correction factor, namely heat increment, is difficult to quantify. A measure of heat output can be obtained from estimates of respiratory quotient, which is an estimate of the volume of CO_2 produced, divided by the volume of O_2 consumed. Respiratory quotient is usually between 0.7 – 1.0. When fats are preferentially oxidized, RQ is 0.7 and with carbohydrate the value is 1.0. Because no one nutrient is ever catabolized independently of others, then the composite RQ will fall somewhere within these boundaries. RQ's outside this range sometimes occur with very high values resulting from net synthesis of fat from carbohydrate. Low RQ's can result from synthesis of carbohydrate from fat, and also from the catabolism of proteins. When proteins are catabolized then lower RQ's occur in birds than in mammals which is related to uric acid vs. urea formation. For example in the catabolism of alanine:

Mammals

$2 CH_3 CH NH_2 COOH + 6O_2 (NH_2)_2 CO + 5H_2O + 5CO_2$
                                        (Urea)

$\therefore RQ = 5 \div 6 = 0.83$

Birds

$8CH_3 CHNH_2 COOH + 21O_2 \rightarrow 2C_5H_4N_4O_3 + 24O_2 + 14CO_2$
                                        (uric acid)

$\therefore RQ = 14/21 = 0.67$

By measuring RQ at variable levels of feed intake, an estimate of heat increment can be determined. Subtracting this value from AMEn, produces an estimate of total net energy. This value can be further subdivided into net energy needs for production vs. maintenance. The net energy used for production is sometimes referred to as productive energy.

The NE for production vs. maintenance can also be ascertained by direct estimates of energy deposited in products. The classical work of Fraps and co-workers involved the tedious challenge of estimating "Productive Energy" of feeds by comparative slaughter techniques. The Net Energy System is by far the most accurate and applicable measure of energy utilization in animals. Unfortunately it is very difficult to measure directly, and is a value that represents energy yield for a particular class of bird for a given production of body mass, eggs etc. In reality NE values vary with age of bird, species and level of production, and this poses a logistical problem during formulation. There is current interest in NE and especially where energy systems are modeled. Unfortunately many such values are based on AMEn with appropriate correction or modifier values, and so are of limited value. For practical formulation, AMEn or TMEn values are used.

Nearly all NE systems use AMEn as a starting point in some way and most assume linearity in efficiency of converting AMEn into NE. In reality the partition of metabolized energy into maintenance, activity and fat and protein accretion vary with age, and so prediction coefficients need to accommodate this complexity. Pirgozlieve and Rose (1999) suggest a linear relationship between AMEn and NEp, with 69% conversion efficiency. Although some 93% of variance was accounted for in this prediction, AMEn tends to overestimate NEp for high protein feedstuffs of animal origin. A potentially confounding factor in prediction of NEp is the energy cost of protein deposition. Many years ago Kielanowski (1965) showed that the determined cost of protein deposition was 5-6x higher than estimates based on stoichiometry of ATP use. Because protein synthesis far exceeds protein deposition in most birds, the logical explanation for discrepancies of energy costs is protein turnover. While protein turnover can account for about 50% of the discrepancy in determined vs. calculated cost of protein deposition, another explanation is that many ATP dependent biochemical pathways are stimulated when protein deposition occurs.

NE systems are therefore fraught with complexity especially considering the vast range of ingredients and feeding situations now common in poultry nutrition. However, we cannot dismiss this important concept and as specialization continues in the industry, the potential for NE systems is more appealing. In N. America for example, nutritionists are often faced with a very limited number of ingredients and a limited range of bird types. For example a NE system seems quite feasible for a broiler nutritionist feeding birds to just 56d of age, or a layer nutritionist formulating diets for layers at 80-95% egg production for the majority of their productive cycle.

Effective Energy

Emmans (1994) suggested 'Effective Energy' as a system for defining feed ingredients and diets. This system is analogous to a productive or net energy system in that it attempts to categorize heat increment. Unlike the classical theories of Armsby and co-workers, the effective energy system takes into account differential heat increments dependent on the catabolism of proteins vs. lipids in the body, and the variable efficiency of utilization and deposition of body lipids dependent upon whether or not they are derived from dietary lipids or synthesized from non-lipid material. Emmans suggests that heat increment of feeding is linearly related to five measurable traits:

Heat increment correlates:

- urinary nitrogen
- fecal organic matter
- positive nitrogen retention
- positive lipid retention derived from dietary lipid
- positive lipid retention derived from non-lipid feed ingredients

Taking into account these variables for heat increment, the energy distribution flow can be redefined (Figure 2.4).

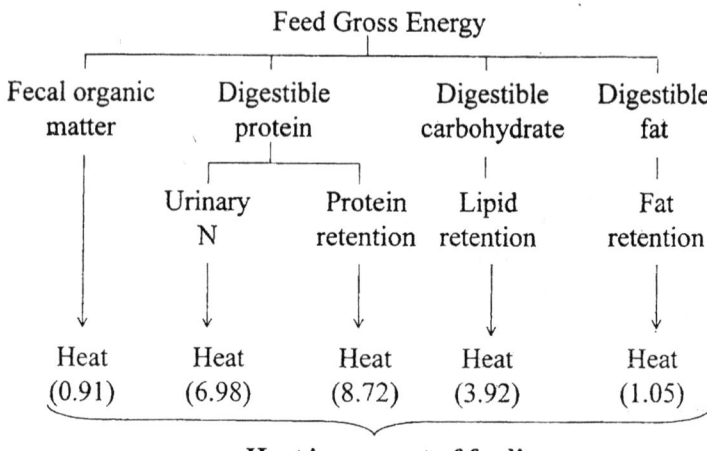

Heat increment of feeding

Figure 2.4 Contributions of heat increment of feeding. Values in parenthesis are estimates of heat increment (kcal/g product) as described by Emmans (1994)

Being able to define the components of heat increment allows for more accurate prediction over a range of dietary situations. For example, effective energy will be increased as dietary body fat accumulation originates from diet fat, rather than de novo synthesis from carbohydrate (Figure 2.4 predicts a reduction in heat increment of approximately 3 kcal/g fat deposited directly from dietary fat vs. carbohydrate). Using such components, Emmans (1994) describes the derivation of a simple equation for estimation of effective energy in monogastrics. Effective Energy (kcal/kg) = 1.17 AMEn – (10 x % crude protein) – 580. Table 2.1 shows calculations of effective energy using this equation, based simply on AMEn and crude protein level.

TABLE 2.1 Calculations of effective energy expressed as % of AMEn				
AMEn (kcal/kg)	Diet Crude protein (%)			
	16	18	20	22
2600	88.4	87.6	86.9	86.1
2800	90.4	89.7	89.1	88.3
3000	92.2	91.6	90.9	90.2
3200	93.8	93.1	92.5	91.9
3400	95.1	94.6	94.0	93.4

A more complex equation to be used in experimental derivation of effective energy is given as: Effective Energy (kcal/kg) =

$$\text{AMEn} - \frac{(1000 \times [(3.8 \times FOM) - (0.16 [29.2 \times DCP]) + (12 \times Z \times DCL)])}{4.184}$$

FOM   = Fecal organic matter (g)

DCP   = Digestible crude protein
DCL   = Digestible crude fat
Z   = proportion of body fat derived directly from dietary fat
4.184   = conversion factor joules to calories

The effective energy system is therefore a refinement of existing systems taking into account anticipated inefficiencies associated with protein catabolism. Since the system is based on AMEn, then errors associated with this value are directly transposed to effective energy values.

2.7   ENERGY BALANCE

T he classical relationship between energy intake and energy retention is described in Figure 2.5.

As energy intake increase, there is an increase in relative energy retention in the body, usually as fat and protein. With a ME intake (MEI) of Z (Figure 2.5), energy retention is zero, and is the point of maintenance energy requirement. At MEI greater than Z, the bird will retain energy in an almost linear manner, up to the point dictated by maximal fat accretion. The energy balance for a growing broiler chicken is shown in Figure 2.6.

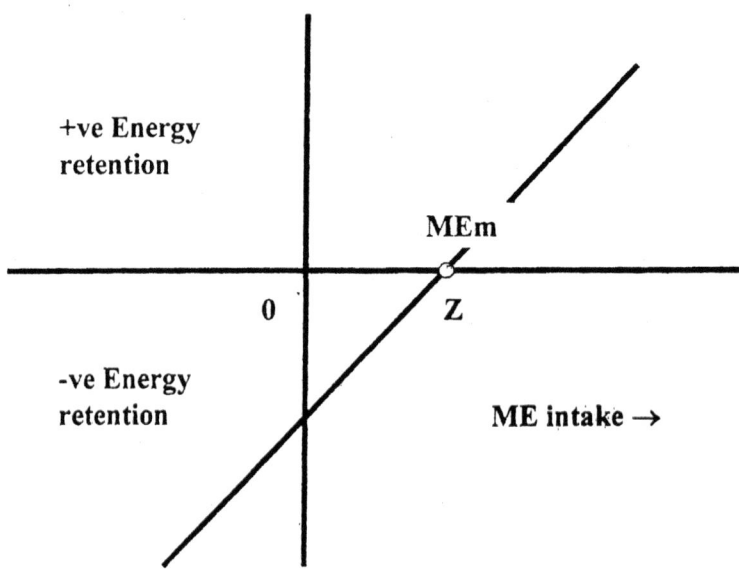

Figure 2.5 Relationship between metabolizable energy intake and retained energy.

Intake	**Output(kcal/kg$^{.75}$)**	
350 kcal ME/kg$^{.75}$	A. Basal metabolic rate	40
	B. Activity	40
	C. Maintenance (A+B)	180
	D. Heat Increment	40
	E. Total Heat Production (C+D)	220
	F. Protein deposition	70
	G. Fat deposition	60
	H. Growth (F +G)	130
	Total	350

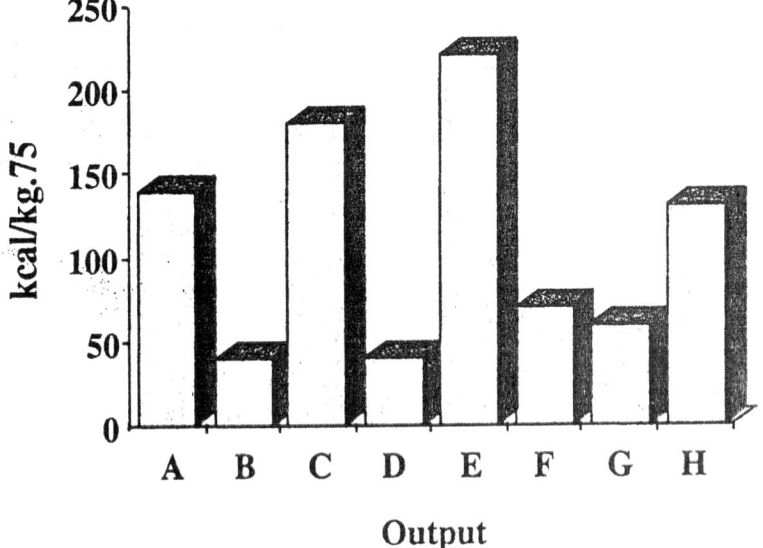

Figure 2.6 Daily energy balance for a 28d old male broiler chicken maintained at 22°C.

To some extent the utilization and balance of metabolizable energy intake will be influenced by diet energy level. Even though broiler chickens, to a marked degree, eat to their energy requirement, there is usually greater energy intake at high diet energy concentrations. If protein/amino acid level is constant under such conditions, then proportionally more energy is diverted to fat deposition. Also because higher energy diets are most easily formulated by including more fat in the diet, heat increment is also reduced proportionally, as energy level of the diet is increased (Figure 2.7).

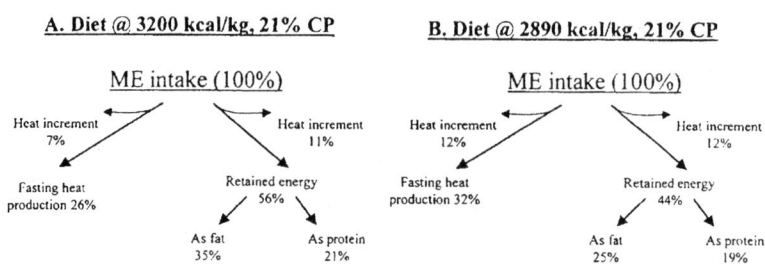

Figure 2.7 Influence of diet energy on energy balance of 21d female broilers. *(Adapted from Macleod, 1990)*

The energy cost of protein deposition is very high in relation to that of fat, and so carcass composition of the growing bird can have a marked influence on efficiency of energy utilization. Both protein and energy require remarkably similar quantities of net energy for their deposition in the body. With fats however, a large proportion of this energy is due to the energy content of fat per se. One gram of protein represents about 5.5 kcal of gross energy, which is only 48% of the 11.5 kcal needed for overall deposition in the body. Fats contain about 9.1 kcal/g and this energy value represents 82% of the overall energy cost of 11.2 kcal needed for deposition of 1 g of fat in the body. Efficiency for protein (Kp) and fat (Kf) deposition are therefore around 48% and 82% respectively.

Energy balance of laying hens is somewhat similar to that of broilers, taking into account metabolic body size and daily egg mass production. There is convincing evidence that the energy requirements of layers is linearly related to body weight over the range 1.2 –2.5 kg. A typical energy balance picture, as shown in Figure 2.8, depicts energy balance for a bird of about 1.5 kg producing 54 g egg mass daily.

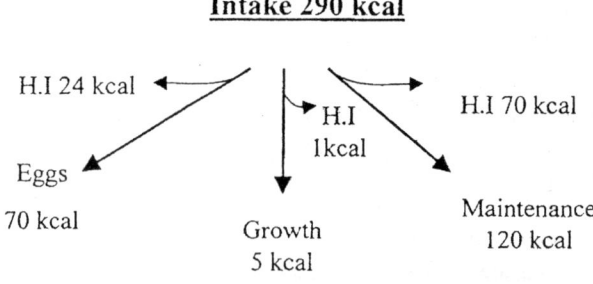

Figure 2.8 Energy balance of 1.5 kg laying hen.

Egg size influences the situation shown in Figure 2.8 because as eggs get larger their energy content increases. As a generalization, small, medium, large and extra large eggs contain about 1.0, 1.3, 1.6 and 1.8 kcal gross energy/g. Egg production per se does not seem to be an energy demanding process, and there is no evidence that energy requirement for egg synthesis is any different to that for body fat or protein accretion. In fact, when an egg is laid or encapsulated in the shell, there is a net loss of 60g of "body mass" and so maintenance requirement should be reduced accordingly.

In quantitating energy balance in individual laying hens, there is sometimes up to 30% variance in feed intake that cannot be accounted for on the basis of body mass, growth or egg mass output. More typically the difference is 10-12g feed per day, and this is often referred to as residual feed consumption. This residual or unaccountable feed consumption is not caused by feed wastage, ability to metabolize diet energy, or variable body composition. The most plausible explanation is differences in activity related to basal metabolism. Geraert et al., (1991) show the characteristics of adult male cockerels selected for comparable body weight but with vastly different feed intake (Table 2.2).

Table 2.2 Characteristics of adult roosters selected for variance in residual feed intake		
	Low residual intake	High residual intake
Body wt. (kg)	3.28	3.35
Feed (g/b/d)	80	112
ME intake (kcal/d/kg^{75})	102	142
TMEn (% GE)	82	80
Heat Production (kcal/kg^{75})		
Fasting	100	117
Fed	136	156
MEm (Maintenance)	125	163
Rectal temperature (°C)	40.8	41.2
Plasma T_3 (ng/ml)	2.19	1.65
		Adapted from Geraert et al., (1991)

Maintenance energy requirement is significantly elevated in the "high intake inefficient" line of birds, and about half of this increase can be accounted for by fasting metabolic rate alone. In chicks, activity can account for 13% of total fasting heat production, or about 4-5% of total energy expenditure. Birds would have to be noticeably very active in order to expend the energy available in 10-12 g feed each day.

2.8   ENVIRONMENTAL INFLUENCES ON ENERGY METABOLISM

Most environmental parameters influence energy metabolism of birds and because birds are homeotherms, temperature has the most noticeable and predictable effect. Most animals have a so-called comfort or thermal neutral zone of environmental temperature, within which there is minimal energy expenditure as basal metabolism. For chickens, this comfort zone changes with age as a consequence of reduction in body surface area per unit of body mass and due to the insulating effect of feathers that develop in the first 3-4 weeks of life. The comfort zone of chickens, depicted by the boundaries of Upper Critical Temperature (UCT) and Lower Critical Temperature (LCT), is shown in Figure 2.9.

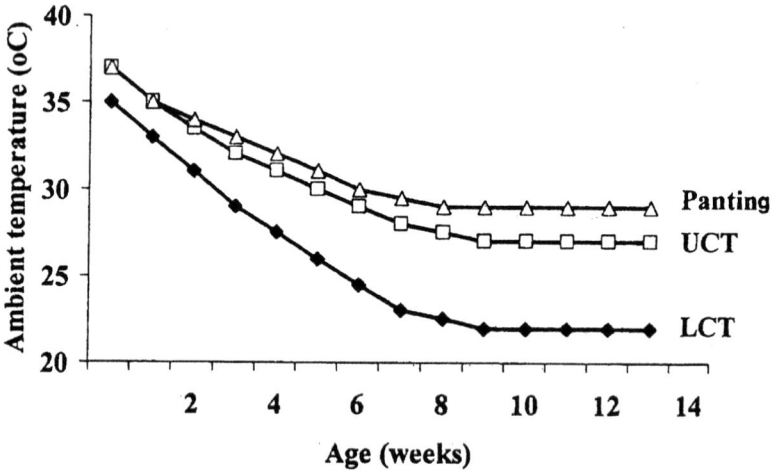

Figure 2.9 Thermoneutral zone for growing White Leghorn chickens.
(Redrawn from Meltzer et al. 1982)

At any one age, the energy balance and performance of birds will be optimized within the comfort zone. At both high and low environmental temperatures, maintenance needs will increase in response to needs for heating or cooling the body respectively. For a laying hen, Figure 2.10 shows a schematic representation of response to change in environmental temperature. Egg production will be maximized at temperatures between the UCT and LCT. Outside of this range, egg production will decline because of a deficiency of energy. At extremes of temperature there will also be insufficient energy available for growth, and at some point birds will rely on weight loss to augment energy supply.

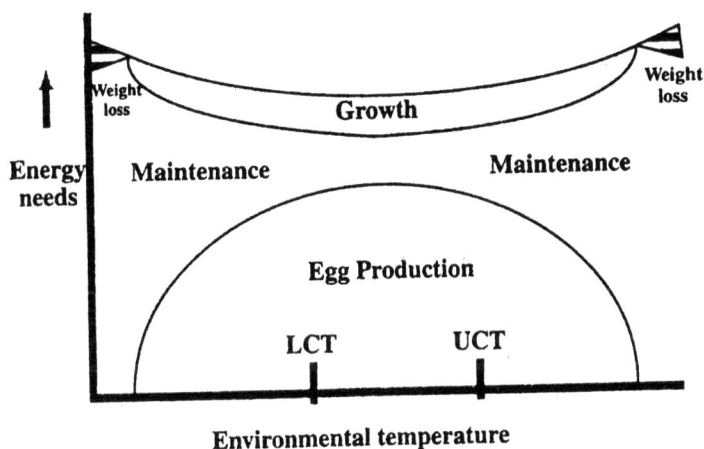

Figure 2.10 Energy balance of layers in response to environmental temperature.

Marsden and Morris (1987) provide a more detailed breakdown of energy balance of layers over the range 10 to 40°C (Figure 2.11).

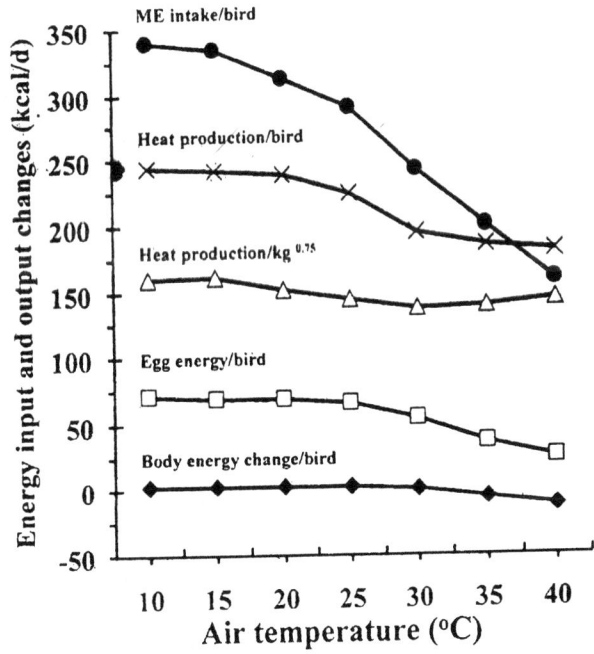

Figure 2.11 Energy balance of White Leghorns
(Adapted from Marsden and Morris, 1987).

From the viewpoint of practical nutrition, the major challenge is ensuring that the bird consumes enough energy at high environmental temperatures. Paradoxically, egg production declines at the elevated temperatures due to a deficiency of energy. There is an indication that the laying hen will consume more energy, at high environmental temperatures in response to an increase in diet AMEn. Pesti *et al.*, (1992) show the potential advantage of moderate increases in diet AMEn on stimulating energy intake (Figure 2.12).

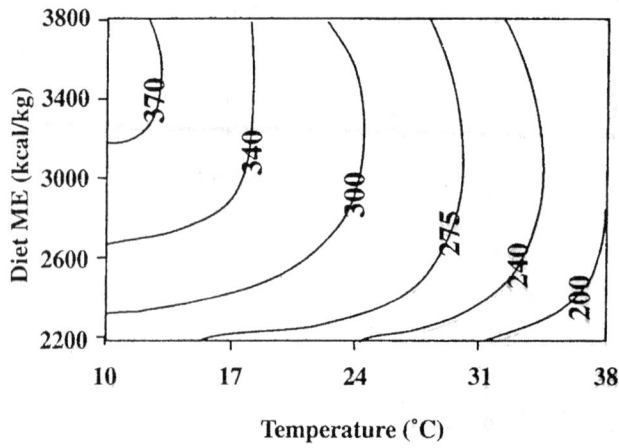

Figure 2.12   Daily metabolizable energy intake (kcal) for White Leghorns fed various diets and kept at 10-38°C.
(Adapted from Pesti et al, 1992)

As a generalization, laying hens will adjust their energy intake by about 3.5 kcal AMEn/°C over the range 10-30°C. This represents just over a 1% change in feed intake per 1°C change, for white egg birds. After the initial brooding period, the growing bird's response to change in environmental temperature is comparable, proportionally, to the changes specified for laying hens. Photoperiod and light intensity can also affect energy metabolism, mainly via their effects on activity. Figure 2.13 shows a typical pattern of heat production for a laying hen subjected to a conventional light schedule. As soon as lights are switched off there is a 30% decline in heat production, likely due to reduced activity. The lighting program also indirectly affects heat production via its control of oviposition. There is a slight increase in heat output of layers for 2 hrs. around the time of oviposition that accounts for about 4 kcal AMEn utilization each day.

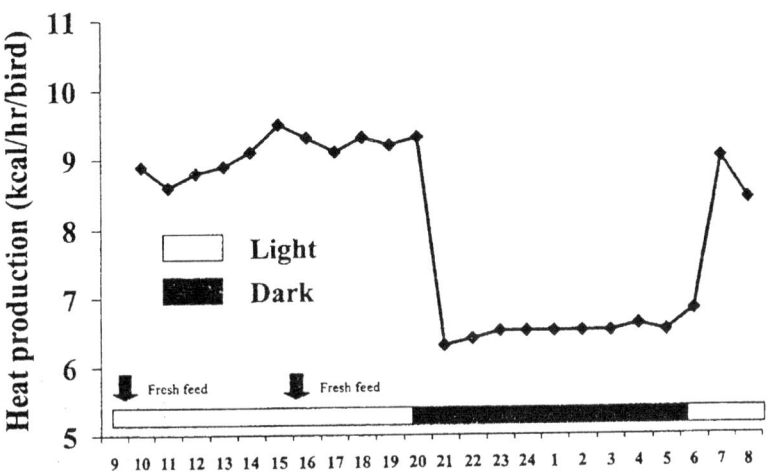

Figure 2.13 Daily heat production of layers in relation to photoperiod.
(Adapted from Li et al., 1991).

Intermittent or biomittent lighting programs that involve periods of darkness within the 'light' phase also lead to reduced activity and so less maintenance energy needs. Using 16 periods of 15 minute light:45 minute dark, compared to a continuous 16 hours of light, reduces the adult layers maintenance energy needs by about 10%. Reducing light intensity can also have similar effects on activity of laying hens, and as long as the light phase has 10x the intensity of the dark phase, the ovulatory cycle is unaffected.

In broiler chickens, use of intermittent light programs such as 1 hr light:3 hr dark repeated 8 times daily is known to improve feed efficiency by up to 10 points. Again this improved energy efficiency is due to reduced activity during the dark phases. In Figure 2.13, a large portion of the activity allowance occurring in the light phase occurs as a result of feeding activity. For breeder pullets and cockerels subjected to periods of feed restriction, there are significant peaks in heat output at the times that feed is available. This situation is most easily observed in skip-a-day vs. daily fed birds (Figure 2.14, Bennett *et al.*, 1990). For daily fed birds there is a peak in heat production associated with feed allocation. With skip-a-day feeding, the effect is greatly magnified with alternate day heat output doubling at this critical time. During times of heat distress, it is important that this peak of heat output does not coincide with time of maximum daily environmental temperature.

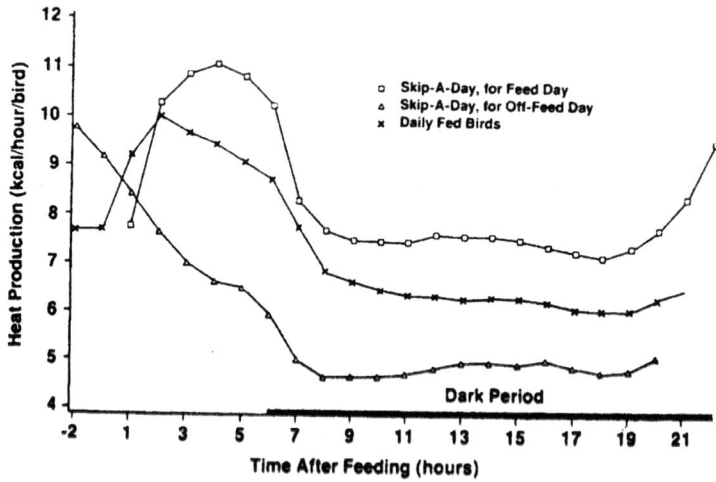

Figure 2.14 Heat production of broiler pullets.

2.9 PREDICTING ENERGY INTAKE

Over the years, a number of regression equations have been developed to be used for prediction of energy intake, especially for laying hens. Most of these equations predict energy needs in joules rather than calories, and it is always cumbersome to convert coefficients to depict caloric needs as sub-components. An easier system is to work with such original equations and then the reader can simply convert any final answer, given in joules, directly to calories if desired. Most equations are based on metabolic body size (Table 2.3).

Table 2.3 Metabolic body size ($W^{.75}$) in relation to regular body size			
Body wt (kg)	$W^{.75}$ (kg)	Body wt (kg)	$W^{.75}$ (kg)
.050	0.106	2.000	1.680
.100	0.178	3.000	2.280
.200	0.300	4.000	2.830
.400	0.504	5.000	3.350
.600	0.682	10.000	5.620
.800	0.845	15.000	7.620
1.000	1.000	20.000	9.460

Other parameters used in predicting feed intake are growth, egg mass, and sometimes environmental temperature. Table 2.4 outlines some of the prediction equations published for prediction of feed or energy intake of laying hens. A comparable equation for broiler chickens of around 2 kg live weight is given by Kirchgesner *et al.*, (1991):

AME intake kJ/d = 753 + 48 (protein gain/d) + 46 (fat gain/d)

Table 2.4 Feed and energy intake prediction equations for layers
Byerly (1941) Feed (g/d) = $0.523W^{.673}$ + 1.126ΔW + 1.135 EM
Emmans (1974) ME (kJ/d) = W(170-2.2T°C) + 2EM + 5ΔW
Chwalibog (1985) ME (kJ/d) = $414W^{.75}$ + 0.86 EB + 1.56 EE
NRC (1994) ME (kJ/d) = $W^{.75}$(724-8.15T°C) + 23ΔW + 8.66 EM
Where W = body weight (kg); T = environmental temperature (°C); ΔW = change in body wt (g); EM = daily egg mass (g); EB = body energy gain; EE = daily egg energy

2.10 SOURCES OF ENERGY

The ultimate source of energy for the chicken is obtained from high-energy phosphate bonds. When adenosine triphosphate (ATP) loses a phosphate group to form adenosine diphosphate (ADP) around 8 kcal/mol are liberated. The turnover of ATP is very high with most molecules reacting within 40 minutes of formation. On any given day a 2.5 kg bird will utilize the equivalent of up to 1 kg ATP. The resynthesis of ATP from ADP occurs as a result of oxidation of various dietary substrates, the most important being carbohydrates, proteins and fats. In most poultry diets, carbohydrates will be the major source of energy.

2.10.1 Carbohydrates

i) *Monosaccharides*

There are four six-carbon monosaccharides of importance, namely D-glucose, D-fructose, D-galactose and D-mannose. D-glucose is by far the most important in the nutrition and metabolism of the chicken since it is the major blood sugar. Its level in the blood of normal animals is controlled within narrow limits by complex physiological mechanisms and it is the basic source of energy within the animal.

The series of chemical reactions by which glucose is broken down to provide energy will be described in detail later in this chapter. Some D-glucose is found in the sap of plants, although the amount of monosaccharide existing free in nature is very small in comparison to that present in polymeric form as units of the polysaccharides and disaccharides. D-glucose (dextrose) is produced on a commercial scale by acid hydrolysis of cornstarch to produce either corn syrup or dried crystalline dextrose. D-glucose may exist in either of the two chemical forms shown in Figure 2.15.

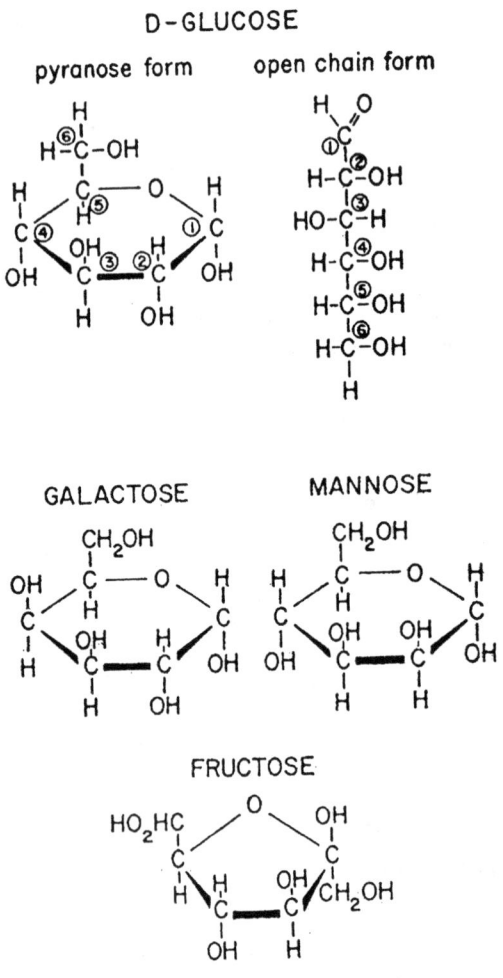

Figure 2.15 Chemical structures of the nutritionally important monosaccharides.

The carbons are numbered from 1 to 6, starting with the active aldehyde group as number 1. Glucose in its open-chain form is a pentahydroxyaldehyde. In solution D-glucose exists largely in the pyranose ring form, in equilibrium with a small amount of the open-chain form. Nutritionally and metabolically, these forms are equivalent. Also shown in Fig. 2.15 are the structures of fructose, galactose and mannose. For an understanding of the complex stereochemistry, the optical rotations and methods of characterizing the monosaccharides and their various isomers, the reader is referred to a modern biochemistry textbook.

ii) Starch

This carbohydrate reserve of plants is stored mainly in grains and other seeds. Like cellulose, starch is a polymer of glucose, the only difference being that in starch the glucose molecules are linked together by a 1,4' α-linkage instead of the 1,4' β-linkage of cellulose. Starch occurs in cereal grains and other feedstuffs as small granules, which may be spherical, oval, lens-shaped or irregular depending upon the source. Cereal starch is arranged in concentric layers, potato starch in eccentric layers. Microscopists can identify the source of starch by examination of granule shape and arrangement. Within the natural feedstuffs, starch exists in a hydrated, polymeric form arranged in a crystalline lattice. Its composition corresponds to the empirical formula $(C_6H_{10}O_5 \cdot H_2O)_n$. When the water of hydration is driven off by heat, the structure becomes amorphous.

Isolated starch granules contain up to 0.05% nitrogen, some fatty acids and some phosphate. The nitrogenous matter can be removed by treatment with hydrochloric acid; the fatty acids and some of their phosphatide phosphorus may be extracted with alkali. These nitrogenous and phospholipid materials in starch have complicated the interpretation of experiments for chickens where starch is used in purified basal diets as the carbohydrate source. Glucose (cerelose) and sucrose, produced commercially in almost pure form, are better sources of carbohydrate for this type of experimental work.

When starch is treated with hot water it separates into two fractions; the more soluble component, amylose, is dissolved, while amylopectin remains as the insoluble fraction. In natural feedstuffs amylose usually represents about 10 to 20% and amylopectin 80 to 90% of the total starch. Amylose, upon treatment with iodine, gives a blue color while amylopectin produces a violet or red-violet color. Like cellulose, amylose has a straight, long-chain molecular structure. Amylopectin is made of the same glucose units as amylose but differs physically by having a branched-chain molecular structure. The main portions of its chains are joined by 1,4' α-glucose linkages which yield maltose as the first digestion product. The branches are joined by 1,6' α-linkages which yield iso-maltose residues prior to final breakdown to D-glucose. The structural unit of amylopectin is shown in Figure 2.16.

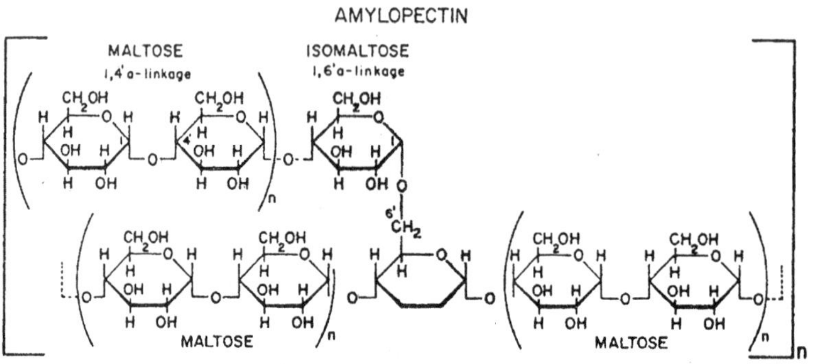

AMYLOPECTIN

Figure 2.16 The structural unit of amylopectin, the principle component of starch.

The storage form of carbohydrate in animals is glycogen, which has a structure similar to that of amylopectin. The enzyme β-amylase, found in plants, splits only the 1,4' α-linkage. It hydrolyzes amylose completely but breaks down only about 60% of the amylopectin structure. The remaining polymeric structure, called dextrin, contains a high proportion of 1,6' α-linkages. Alpha-amylase, the starch-splitting enzyme in the digestive system of animals, can hydrolyze 1,4' α-linkages on both sides of the 1,6' branching points, producing very small, branched oligosaccharides which are further degraded to glucose by oligo-1, 6'-glucosidase from the intestinal mucosa. This enzyme splits the 1,6' linkages of the dextrins, and breaks down the resulting iso-maltose into D-glucose units. The enzyme, α-glucosidase, also called maltase, cleaves maltose into glucose units.

All animals contain an abundance of α-amylases. In mammals, these enter the gastro-intestinal tract via the saliva and as pancreatic secretions. Although the saliva and crop of the chicken contain some α-amylases, little starch digestion has been demonstrated in the crop. In the small intestine of chickens quite good digestion, even of the raw starches of corn, wheat and potatoes, takes place through the action of the pancreatic amylases. In its natural state, starch exists as an insoluble granular form, which physically resists digestion. The cooking of foods markedly aids digestion of starch by breaking down and solubilizing the starch granules. These granules also can be broken down by physical disruption, aided by soaking in water. Thus, in the chicken, it appears likely that good starch digestion is partially due to the initial soaking of feed in the crop and subsequent grinding action of the gizzard which precedes action of the pancreatic amylases. Precooking of feedstuffs may increase their metabolizable energy values, as may the steam and pressure used in pelleting of feeds.

The utilization of barley grown in arid areas is improved for chickens by soaking in water or feeding it together with fungal amylases. This phenomenon may be due to an inefficiency of the chicken's own amylases in digesting the barley starch or to effects upon the hemicellulose or oligosaccharide fractions of the barley of natural enzymes in the moistened grain and in any fungal residues.

iii) Oligosaccharides

The term oligosaccharides, applies to structures containing two or more simple monosaccharide units, but which are smaller than the complex units classed as polysaccharides. Oligosaccharides of major importance in the nutrition of the chicken contain sucrose and maltose. While other disaccharides and oligosaccharides of three and four simple units exist they are of little nutritional importance. In most poultry diets soybean meal is the major source of oligosaccharides some of which are poorly digested.

Sucrose consists of one glucose unit and one fructose unit, wherein the hydroxyl of carbon 1 of D-glucose is linked through the hydroxyl of carbon 2 of D-fructose, thereby blocking the reducing groups of both monosaccharides and resulting in a non-reducing sugar. Mild acid hydrolysis or treatment with sucrase (sometimes called invertase), the sucrose-hydrolysing enzyme, releases the monosaccharides, both of which can be measured by their ability to reduce Fehling's solution (an alkaline solution of copper sulfate and sodium potassium tartrate which yields a red cuprous oxide upon reduction). Maltose, consisting of 2 glucose units in 1,4 linkages, arises mainly from hydrolysis of starch. It is readily converted to glucose by the action of maltase in the brush border of the mucosal cells.

iv) Energy from carbohydrate metabolism

Most of the energy used by chickens for activity and the multitude of chemical reactions which support their metabolism and growth is derived from the high energy phosphate compounds, adenosine phosphates and creatine phosphate, produced by the various steps involved in the metabolism of glucose. These high-energy phosphates yield immediate energy on demand. They can regenerate themselves to their previous high energy state by acquiring energy which is liberated by the oxidation of glucose within the cells. In order to show the complete oxidation of glucose to carbon dioxide and water, it is necessary to follow first the various steps in the breakdown of glucose to pyruvic acid by the Embden-Myerhof-Parnas scheme of carbohydrate utilization (Figure 2.17) and then the entrance of this pyruvic acid into the citric acid cycle, as shown in Figure 2.18.

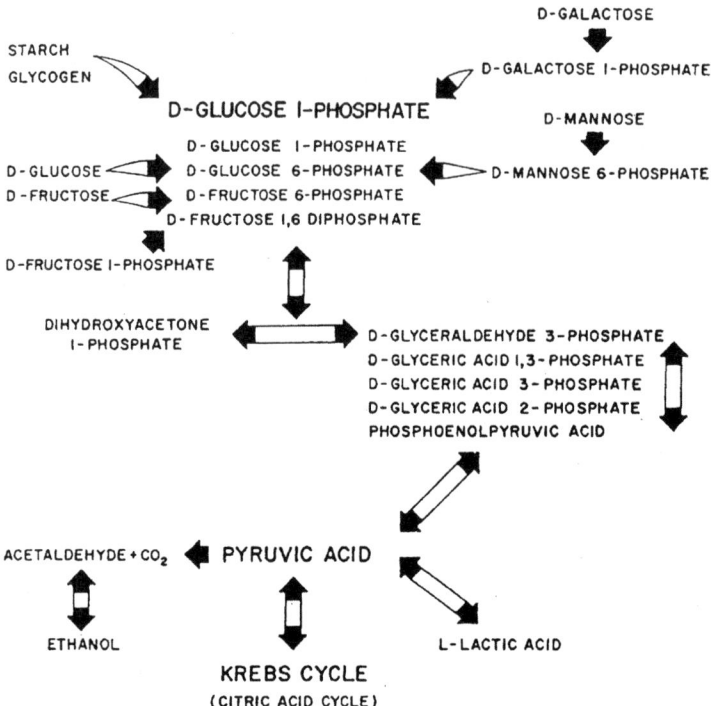

Figure 2.17 Embden-Myerhof-Parnas scheme for the degradion of glucose to pyruvic acid.

The citric acid cycle is the common oxidative pathway for the final breakdown of carbohydrate, fats and proteins. An alternative system for glucose oxidation is the pathway sometimes called the "hexose, monophosphate shunt" which begins with the oxidation of glucose-6-phosphate to yield 6-phosphogluconic acid. Although the D-glucose represents the blood sugar of the initial starting point of the Embden-Myerhof-Parnas scheme, this glucose can be replenished by incoming glucose, fructose, galactose or mannose from the diet, and by glucose synthesized by the body from glycerol or from the glucogenic amino acids. There may also be some breakdown of reserve glycogen stored in the liver and muscle. The amount of glycogen found in these tissues depends somewhat on the nature and availability of the diet and the amount of physical activity being performed by the animal. During continuous muscular exercise, lactic acid is formed in the working muscle which is gradually withdrawn from the blood by the liver and converted back into glycogen. While the skeletal and smooth muscles draw continuously on the glycogen reserves for energy purposes, cardiac muscle is unique in that it tenaciously preserves its glycogen reserves and preferentially uses blood glucose for its energy of maintenance and muscular work.

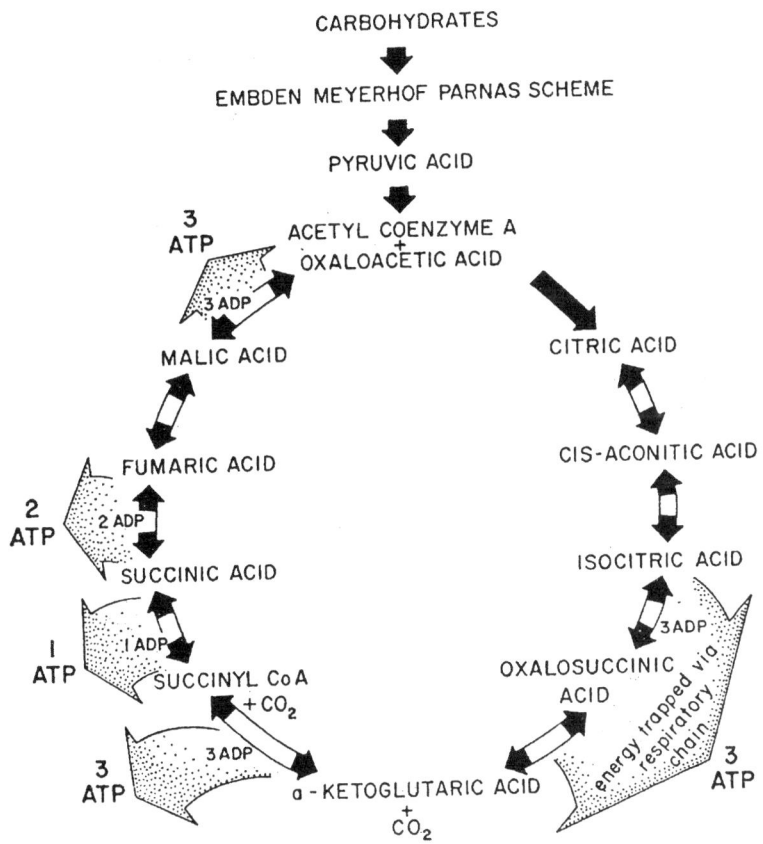

Figure 2.18 The citric acid cycle for the final oxidation of carbohydrates and the release of energy.

Although glucose undergoes the many reactions shown in Figures 2.17 and 2.18, its overall oxidation can be described as follows:

$$C_6H_{12}O_6 + 6O_2 \rightarrow 6CO_2 + 6H_2O + 673 \text{ kcal/mole}$$

Thus, the overall energy from one gram molecular weight of glucose may be expressed as $\Delta H = -673$ kcal/mole, (The ΔH for glucose is given a minus sign indicating that the utilization of glucose is an exothermic reaction.). The molecular weight of glucose is 180.16. Therefore, glucose yields a total energy value of $673 \div 180.16 = 3.74$ kcal/gm.

A considerable portion of the gross energy of glucose and other substrates would be lost as heat if these substances were simply oxidized by the body without going directly through the many physiological steps involving the production of adenosine triphosphate (ATP).

v)   *Importance of ATP*

Adenosine triphosphate is distributed in every cell of the body. It is formed by union of one molecule of phosphoric acid with one molecule of adenosine diphosphate (ADP); this union requires an input of free energy of about 8 kcal/mole. Thus trapping of the energy of glucose and fat degradation not only eliminates a great deal of wasteful heat loss, but furnishes a constant supply of potential energy within all cells at all times. When a chemical reaction within a cell calls for energy, it is derived by coupling with the breakdown of ATP i.e. ATP $\rightarrow$ ADP + Pi + 8 kcal/mole where Pi = high energy phosphate.

2.10.2   Fats.

The terms, fats and oils, usually refer to triglycerides of variable fatty acid profile. Fats are those glycerol esters which are solids while oils are liquids at room temperature. The term lipid is used for all ether-soluble materials.

i)   *Lipid classification*

Simple lipids. These are simple esters of fatty acids and certain alcohols, particularly glycerol and cholesterol. Esters of fatty acids with an alcohol other than glycerol are called waxes and have little nutritional importance.

Compound lipids. Esters of glycerol which contain two fatty acid residues plus another chemical group such as choline (linked through phosphoric acid) are called compound lipids. Most important are the phospholipids such as lecithin, cephalin and sphingomyelin.

Derived lipids. Substances which are derived by hydrolysis from groups 1 and 2: (a) fatty acids; (b) alcohols, such as glycerol, cetanol and lanol; and (c) the sterols such as cholesterol, ergosterol and sitosterol.

From a nutritional point of view, of all lipids, only linoleic acid is an essential nutrient for the chicken. The importance of linoleic acid for chick growth and for maximum egg production and egg size will be dealt with in a later section of this book. All other lipids are important primarily as sources of energy and as "solvents" which aid in absorption of the fat-soluble vitamins. Lipids also reduce the dustiness of feeds and help, by lubrication, the passage of feeds through pellet dies and perhaps help the palatability of some feeds. Of all these properties, the energy value of the lipids is by far the most important.

ii) *Relative energy values of various lipids*

The empirical formula of a typical fat is $(C_{57}H_{105}O_6)$. The chemical structure of such a fat is shown in Figure 2.19. Compared with glucose, with an empirical formula of $(C_6H_{12}O_6)$ fat contains many times more carbon and hydrogen atoms in relation to its oxygen content. In fats C:O = 8.5:1 and H:0 = 16.3:1 while in glucose, C:O = 1:1 and H:O = 2:1. Thus, fat contains a large excess of carbon and hydrogen capable of being oxidized to CO_2 and H_2O. The energy value of fat, therefore, is considerably higher per unit weight than the energy value of glucose or other carbohydrates. Experimentation has shown that the gross energy value of pure fats and oils is about 9.4 kilocalories per gram, approximately 2.25 times that of starch which has a gross energy value of approximately 4.15 kilocalories per gram.

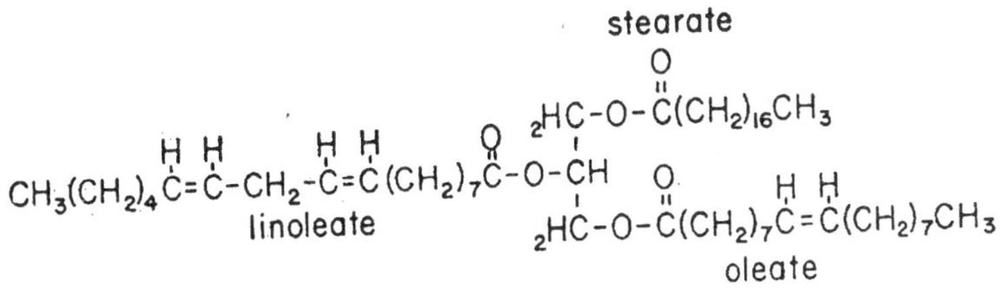

Figure 2.19 Chemical structure of a typical triglyceride, β-linolein α-oleo α'-stearin.

The fatty acid composition of a number of common fats and oils is shown in Table 2.5 while a description of the common fatty acids found in these fats and oils is given in Table 2.6. Titre is a measure of melting point, and as seen in Table 2.5, most animal fats are usually solid at room temperature. Iodine attaches to the unsaturated double bond, and so a high iodine value indicates greater unsaturation of the fat.

iii) *Fat digestion*

The processes of digestion and absorption of fats and fatty acids are detailed in Chapter 1. In summary, fats are cleaved by lipase enzymes, and in the small intestine the formation of mixed micelles composed of lipase, fat and bile are an important prerequisite to digestion and absorption. Unsaturates readily form mixed micelles, while saturates because of their polar characteristics are less inclined to be incorporated. However, unsaturates aid in the uptake of saturates within mixed micelles and this action is part of the concept of fatty acid synergism that is capitalized upon by nutritionists. Once absorbed, fats are metabolized almost exclusively in the liver, unlike the situation in mammals where adipose tissue per se is an important site of de novo synthesis.

Table 2.5 Fatty acid composition (%) and some physical properties of various fats and oils										
	Titre °C	Iodine Value	12:0	14:0	16:0	16:1	18:0	18:1	18:2	18:3
Vegetable oils:										
Coconut oil*	20-23	8-10	47.4	18.0	8.0	-	2.8	5.6	1.6	-
Corn oil	18-20	115-127	-	-	12.0	-	2.7	30.1	54.7	1.4
Olive oil	17.26	79-90	-	-	14.0	1.3	2.6	74.0	8.1	-
Safflower oil	16	145	-	0.2	12.3	-	1.8	11.2	74.3	0.2
Soybean oil	20-21	130-138	-	-	11.5	-	4.3	27.3	49.7	6.9
Animal fats:										
Beef tallow	38-43	35-45	-	3.3	26.2	-	22.4	45.3	1.6	0.5
Lard	36-43	50-65	-	1.5	25.7	-	12.1	49.2	9.6	1.1
Menhaden oil*	31-33	148-172	-	11.9	23.2	16.4	5.6	15.3	2.7	1.9
Poultry fat	35-43	80	0.2	1.4	21.4	6.8	5.9	39.5	23.5	1.0

*In addition to the fatty acids shown, coconut oil also contains 8:0 - 8.8%; 10:0 - 7.2%; menhaden oil also contains 14:1 - 0.4%; 18:4 - 2.4%; 20:4 - 2.0%; 20:5 - 11.5%; 22:5 - 0.7%; 22:6 - 7%.

Table 2.6 Properties of the common fatty acids found in feed fats and oils					
Fatty acid			Molecular weight	Iodine value	Melting point °C
Common name	Systematic name	Designation			
Lauric	Dodecanoic	12:0*	200	0	43.6
Myristic	Tetradecanoic	14:0	228	0	53.8
Palmitic	Hexadecanoic	16:0	256	0	62.9
Stearic	Octadecanoic	18:0	285	0	69.9
Palmitoleic	9-Hexadecenoic	16:1	254	99.8	11.5
Oleic	9-Octadecenoic (cis)	18:1	283	89.9	4.0
Linoleic	9,12-Octadecadienoic (cis, cis)	18:2	281	181.0	-5.0
Linolenic	9,12,15-Octadecatrienoic (cis,cis,cis)	18:3	279	273.5	-14.4
Arachidonic	5,8,11,14-Eicosatetraenoic (cis,cis,cis,cis)	20:4	305	316.2	-49.5
Timnodonic	4,8,12,15,18-Eicosapentaenoic (presuamble all-cis)	20:5	302	335.7	-62.7
Clupanodonic	4,8,12,15,19-Docosapentaenoic (presumably all-cis)	22:5	331	384.5	-78.0

*First number shows number of carbon atoms; number to right of colon shows number of double bonds

iv) Liver fat

The liver not only is the receptor of dietary fat, but also is the site of fat synthesis from excess carbohydrate in the chicken. Thus, any fat eventually stored in the adipose tissues must be transported there via the blood from the liver to these tissues. The newly synthesized lipid is transported mainly as very low-density lipoproteins. Because only free fatty acids can pass through the adipocyte membranes, the triglycerides carried to the adipose site must be hydrolyzed by lipoprotein lipase.

The liver of the non-laying chicken and rooster do not accumulate high levels of fat. The usual fat content of the liver is about 3-5% of wet weight or 10-15% on a dry weight basis. This is primarily neutral fat, together with other lipids, mainly cholesterol esters of fatty acids. After sexual maturity, under the influence of high plasma estrogen in female birds the normal liver will accumulate fat up to 50% on a dry weight basis. A friable, fatty liver is therefore a normal situation in laying hens. Unfortunately this liver fat is prone to oxidation under certain conditions, and so liver hemorrhage, due to membrane dysfunction is not uncommon. Higher than normal levels of vitamin E in the diet (100 IU/kg) may help prevent such liver fat oxidation.

v) Nutritional value of fat

Addition of fats to nutritionally complete diets often produces a slight increase in growth, and always improves efficiency of feed utilization in both broilers and laying hens, due to the higher energy density of a fat-containing diet. However, benefits from fat can only be obtained when the amounts of all other nutrients in the diet are increased in proportion to the increase in energy level. The chicken can use high levels of fat as a source of energy provided that the diet is formulated to supply a constant ratio of all nutrients to total energy. Experiments have shown that chicks and laying hens will grow and produce normally when fed carbohydrate-free diets with triglycerides as the major source of energy. However, growth is depressed when such diets contain more than 20% free fatty acids. Under these conditions, where the glycerol moiety of triglycerides is absent and therefore cannot form glucose, blood glucose levels cannot be maintained from gluconeogenesis of amino acids alone.

vi) Relationship of metabolizable energy value to digestibility

The energy value of fats and oils depends mainly upon the absorbability of the fatty acids from the intestinal tract. Since fatty acids are not excreted in the urine, their metabolizable energy values are directly related to their absorbability. The metabolizable energy value of a fat may be calculated by multiplying the percent absorbability by the gross caloric energy value of the fat as determined in a bomb calorimeter. This latter value is approximately the same for all pure fats namely 9.4 kcal/gm.

vii) The influence of fat on efficiency of energy utilization

When fats are included in diets for growing animals, the efficiency of utilization of energy consumed is improved compared with that of animals fed low fat diets. This phenomenon is sometimes termed the associative dynamic action of fats. The improvement in energetic efficiency can be attributed to a lowered heat increment with diets containing fats. This physiological effect is shown by tallow, lard, corn oil and soybean oil but not by hydrogenerated coconut oil.

viii) Oxidative rancidity of fats and oils

Rancidity of fats and oils is of two types, hydrolytic and oxidative. Hydrolytic rancidity usually results from the action of microorganisms upon the fat or oil, causing simple hydrolysis of the fat into fatty acids, diglycerides, monoglycerides and glycerol. The fact that a fat has undergone hydrolytic rancidity does not influence its nutritional value.

Oxidative rancidity or lipid peroxidation, however can result in a major decrease in the energy value of a fat or oil. With lipid peroxidation, the unsaturated fatty acids first undergo removal of hydrogen, resulting in the formation of a free radical at the site of unsaturation. This reaction is catalyzed by trace minerals in the presence of oxygen. If the feed material in which this reaction is taking place does not contain vitamin E, ethoxyquin or some other effective antioxidant. the free radical is quickly converted by atmospheric oxygen to a fatty acid peroxide free radical and subsequently to a fatty acid hydroperoxide. Products such as vitamin E and ethoxyquin (6-ethoxy-1,2-dihydro-2,2-4-trimethylquinoline) can block this peroxidation by supplying a hydrogen to the first free radical formed, thereby reconverting it to the original fatty acid. If the hydroperoxides are allowed to form, they continue to decompose by breaking down into a variety of aldehydes and ketones, the size of which depends upon the number and position of the double bonds that have undergone peroxidation.

ix) Phospholipids as energy sources

The three most important phospholipids are lecithin, cephalin and sphingomyelin. Studies on the metabolizable energy content of soybean lecithin show that the fatty acid and glycerol moieties are completely utilized by chicks with an energy value of around 6.5 kcal/g. This represents the maximum theoretical energy value of lecithin, since approximately 25% of the molecule is phosphoric acid and choline. The lecithinases or phospholipases very efficiently remove the fatty acids from the lecithin molecule.

Of interest is the so-called lecithinase A (phospholipase A) of rattle-snake and cobra venoms which removes only the fatty acid in the 1-position of the lecithin, yielding a compound called lysolecithin which contains a saturated fatty acid in the 2-position and phosphorylcholine in position 3. This compound has a powerful hemolytic action, destroying the animal's red blood cells resulting in a consequent disturbance of the respiratory functions of the blood. A phospholipase B has been isolated from liver, which is capable of removing both fatty acids from the complete lecithin molecule, or the single residual fatty acid from lysolecithin.

Little work has been done on the energy value of cephalins and sphingomyelins for poultry. However, these compounds are not found in significant amounts in feeds.

x)   *Energy from fat metabolism*

Although the chicken stores small amounts of glycogen in the liver and muscles, the main energy storage of the body is in the form of neutral fats. These lipids are stored in the adipose tissues and other sites throughout the body. The bird obtains its lipid from the diet plus the fats derived from the acetyl CoA obtained during lipogenesis from carbohydrates and certain amino acids. The composition of the fatty acids obtained from the diet may vary considerably in regard to degree of unsaturation and chain length. The process of lipogenesis from carbohydrates and amino acids appears to favor formation of saturated over unsaturated fatty acids in most mammals. In the chick, however, lipogenesis apparently favors the production of oleic acid as well as some saturated fatty acids, particularly palmitic and stearic. From the overall mixture of fatty acids available both from the diet and from lipogenesis, the liver produces a composite fat which is quite characteristic of the species. This operation involves shortening or elongation of the carbon skeleton of some dietary fatty acids as well as the introduction of a double bond in the synthesis of oleic acid. The fatty acid profile of eggs and poultry meat can however, be modified in direct proportion to the fatty acid profile of the diet. The chicken, like other animals, is incapable of synthesizing linoleic acid and arachidonic acid can be synthesized only from linoleic acid.

xi)   *The metabolic products of fat which are used as sources of energy*

The glycerol moiety of fats can be converted by the body either to fructose and then to glucose, which serves as a source of blood sugar, or it can be converted to pyruvic acid. Both products of glycerol metabolism, therefore, are important energy metabolites. The chemical reactions involved in these conversions are shown in Figure 2.20. Glycerol is the only portion of the triglyceride molecule that can be converted to glucose.

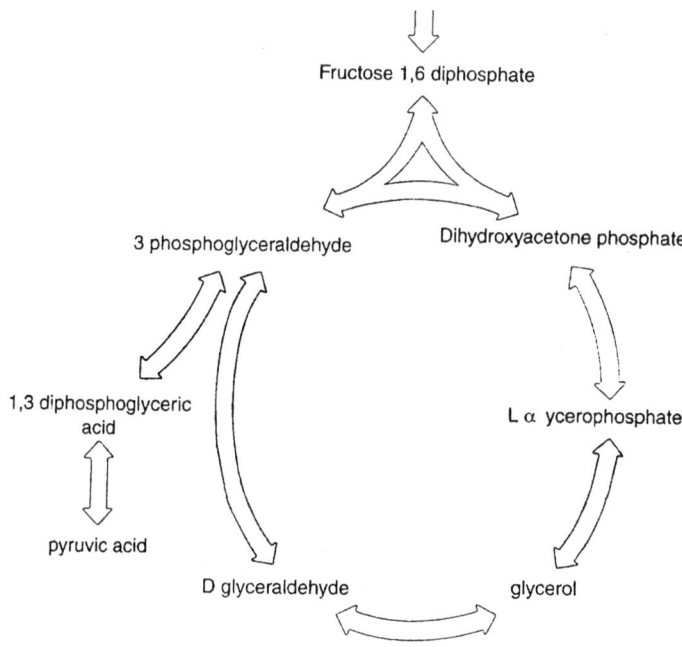

Figure 2.20 Conversion of glycerol to either glucose or pyruvic acid in the body.

xii) β-Oxidation of fatty acids

The metabolism of the fatty acids for production of energy is brought about by degradation of the fatty acids in a stepwise fashion by a series of reactions in which two carbon fragments are removed beginning at the carboxyl end of the fatty acid chain. The first step in the reaction involves combination of the fatty acid with coenzyme A to form the fatty acyl CoA compound (Figure 2.21). The lipid portion then undergoes oxidation according to the reaction shown in Figure 2.22. At least three different enzymes present in the liver mitochondria have been shown to have different specificity ranges in the activation of fatty acids from C_4 to C_{18}. After the fatty acid has reacted with coenzyme A, it undergoes unsaturation at the α–β-position by a dehydrogenase. In β-oxidation of stearic acid, for example, water is then added to the molecule at this position by the enzyme, enoyl hydrase, yielding β-hydroxy stearyl CoA. This is acted upon by another dehydrogenase to produce β-keto stearyl CoA whereupon there is a cleavage at the α–β-position brought about by another molecule of reduced CoA and catalyzed by a cleavage enzyme, yielding palmityl CoA and one molecule of acetyl CoA. The palmityl CoA residue is then sequentially degraded, two carbons at a time, until the molecule is reduced finally to the last molecule of acetyl CoA.

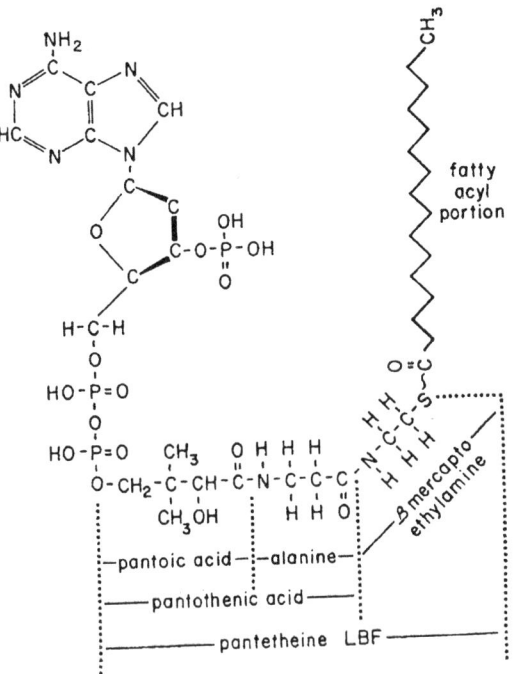

Figure 2.21 Acyl coenzyme A. A structural diagram of palmitoyl-S coenzyme A. The diagram emphasizes the large water-soluble, polar CoA moiety containing pantothenic acid compared with the nonpolar fatty acyl portion.

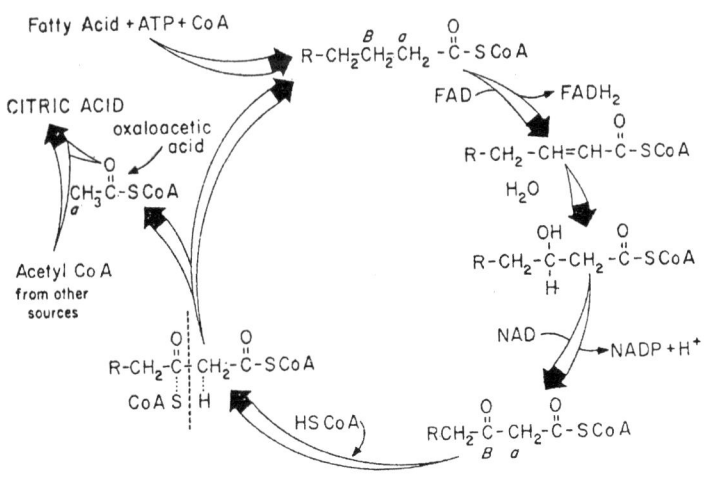

Figure 2.22 The two carbon degradation of fatty acids (beta oxidation) and the relationship to the citric acid cycle.

The acetyl CoA formed by β-oxidation reacts with oxaloacetic acid to form citric acid and then is oxidized to carbon dioxide and water in the citric acid cycle, as discussed earlier. The energy derived from fatty acids results in the formation of ATP synthesized in the course of the reactions involved in the citric acid cycle. Although the β-oxidation of a fatty acid yields many acetyl CoA's and many ATP molecules, the overall reaction can be written as:

$$C_{17}H_{35}COOH + 26O_2 \rightarrow 18CO_2 + 18H_2O + 2711.8 \text{ kcal}$$

For stearic acid, $\Delta H = 2711.8$ kcal/mole. Thus, the overall energy obtained by the body from the β-oxidation of one gram-molecular weight of stearic acid is 2712 kcal. Since the gram-molecular weight of stearic acid is 284.5, this amounts to 9.53 kcal/gm of stearic acid. The fatty acids contain slightly more energy than the triglycerides because of the greater excess of carbon and hydrogen over oxygen in fatty acids as compared with those in glycerol.

Early studies on fat supplementation of chick diets indicated that levels of fat in excess of about 10% are not well tolerated. More recent work has shown that the reason for the earlier poor results with fat was due to a failure to increase the diet protein and amino acids levels in proportion to the increased energy content, thereby allowing the chicks to obtain their energy requirements with such little total feed that they were deficient in amino acids. It has subsequently been shown that chicks can grow and develop almost as well on carbohydrate-free diets containing up to 33.8% triglyceride as they do with normal diets containing carbohydrates, as long as the metabolizable energy:protein ratio (ME/P) is maintained at about 13.2 kcal/gm of ideal protein.

Attempts to use free fatty acids in place of the triglycerides in carbohydrate-free diets have resulted in severe growth retardation, since the glycerol portion of the triglycerides is needed to supplement glucogenesis from amino acids for maintenance of blood glucose levels. A small amount of carbohydrate completely prevents hypoglycemia but does not restore normal growth. The reason for slower growth with pure fatty acids has not been explained.

2.10.3 Proteins and amino acids

Variable portions of the dietary protein can be converted into carbohydrate derivatives or into fatty acid metabolites and can supply the necessary glucose for maintaining blood sugar levels. When the various amino acids are fed individually, some are glucogenic (glycogenic), i.e., give rise to glucose and glycogen (Figure 2.23) while others are ketogenic and give rise to acetone or other ketones. A discussion of the metabolism of amino acids and their conversion to carbohydrate is given in Chapter 3.

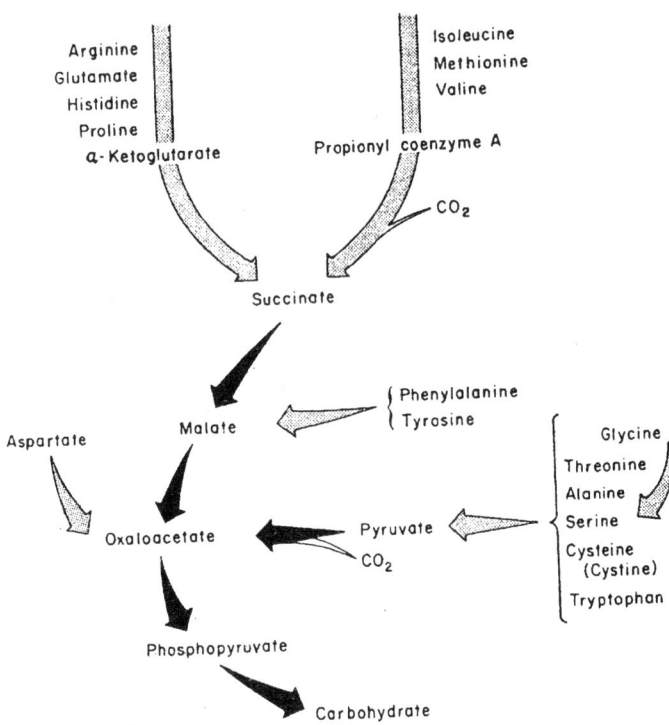

Figure 2.23 Conversion of glucogenic amino acids to carbohydrate.

All non-essential amino acids are glucogenic, indicating that the process of synthesis of these amino acids from carbohydrate is reversible. The ketogenic amino acids are all essential amino acids. Fats and fat metabolites contribute very little to the synthesis of amino acids.

The heat of combustion of alanine is 387.7 kcal per one gram-molecular weight. Since its molecular weight is 89.90, this amounts to 4.35 kcal/gm. Glutamic acid, which contains less carbon and hydrogen in relation to its oxygen content, has a heat of combustion of 542.4 for a gram-molecular weight of 147.13. This amounts to only 3.69 kcal of energy derived per gram of glutamic acid utilized in glucogenesis. The value of 4.1 kcal usually used to represent the metabolizable energy of protein reflects an average of the various amino acids joined in peptide linkages to make up the protein. It also takes into consideration the fact that the nitrogen of proteins is not oxidized under physiological conditions.

2.11 ENERGY CONTENT OF FEED INGREDIENTS

The energy value of feedstuffs for poultry and other animals has been assessed in many different ways. The most common designations of energy values are in terms of gross energy, digestible energy, metabolizable energy or net energy. The relationships between these various energy values have been described previously. Replicate determinations of the metabolizable energy values of feedstuffs have been shown to vary only ± 2-3%, while the variation in productive energy content found for a given feedstuff may vary as much as ± 20%, largely because of the errors inherent in productive energy measurements. The wide variation in productive energy content of an individual feedstuff is due also to the fact that the amount of heat lost by animals consuming feed depends upon the nutritional balance of the diet. Diets adequately balanced in all nutrients produce a minimum heat loss, whereas unbalanced diets, especially those markedly deficient in or containing large excesses of protein, cause very high wastage of energy as lost heat. This heat loss, which occurs following ingestion of the diet, is known as the specific dynamic effect of feed.

In the formulation of diets for poultry, the metabolizable energy content of the feedstuffs is most commonly used in calculating the energy content of the diet. At the same time it is important that the diet is completely balanced so that there will be a minimum loss by the animal of energy as wasted heat. The metabolizable energy contents of the common poultry feedstuffs are presented in Table 8.1. The higher metabolizable energy values of the vegetable oils as compared with the animal fats is due to the higher degree of absorbability of these oils which contain high amounts of oleic and other unsaturated fatty acids.

Fiber, which is largely cellulose and lignins, is almost completely indigestible by poultry. Feedstuffs containing high amounts of fiber possess relatively low energy values for poultry unless they are also high in fat content. The cereal grains, being relatively high in digestible carbohydrate, are regarded as the major energy sources. Corn has become the cereal of choice in many areas of the world, because of its high energy value and content of xanthophylls which impart a yellow color to the skin and yolk.

In some areas of the world sorghum grains and wheat are more plentiful and lower in cost per unit of energy than is corn. These grains may be used as the major carbohydrate source with very satisfactory results if care is taken to balance the diets. Milo and wheat usually contain less energy, less linoleic acid, less methionine and certainly less xanthophyll pigments than does yellow corn.

At times, wheat byproducts and barley become so economically priced in relation to corn that these feedstuffs can be used to advantage to provide a large portion of the carbohydrates in the diet. In some areas rice polishings are an excellent energy source. Although barley and rice bran also are good sources of linoleic acid,

Table 3.14 Essential amino acid composition of the proteins of chicken meat, eggs, corn, soybean and fish meal					
	% of Protein				
Amino acid	Chicken tissue	Egg	Corn	Soybean meal	Fish meal
Arginine	7.3	6.4	5.0	7.5	6.7
Cystine	2.5	2.2	1.3	1.7	1.8
Histidine	4.0	2.3	2.5	2.7	2.7
Isoleucine	3.9	5.0	6.3	5.4	6.8
Leucine	6.5	8.3	12.5	7.7	8.3
Lysine	9.6	7.1	2.5	6.7	8.8
Methionine	1.9	3.2	2.5	1.5	3.0
Phenylalanine	3.6	4.7	6.3	5.2	4.5
Threonine	3.4	5.0	5.0	4.2	4.8
Tryptophan	1.0	1.4	1.3	1.5	1.0
Valine	4.4	6.5	5.0	5.2	6.0

Table 2.17 Response of brown and white egg pullets to diet energy level					
Body weight (g)			**Feed intake (g)**		
Brown egg	42d	82d	126d	0–42d	42-84d	84-126d
2750 kcal/kg	410	1090	1590	1010	2700	3240
3030 kcal/kg	450	1160	1660	1020	2700	3070
White egg	42d	82d	126d	0–42d	42-84d	84-126d
2750 kcal/kg	380	953	1362	940	2490	3100
3030 kcal/kg	360	940	1375	910	2360	2790

As energy level is increased at a fixed protein level (Table 2.17) a reduction in growth rate is sometimes seen because protein and amino acid intake are limited. Brown egg pullets seem to change their feed intake very little under these conditions, and consequently there is an improvement in growth rate. In another study pullets were fed diets at 2750 or 3000 kcal ME/kg. Over the 126d growing period, brown egg pullets consumed 6% more energy when fed the high energy diet (20.6 vs. 19.4 Mcal). Contrary to this increased energy intake, white egg pullets consumed about 18 Mcal ME regardless of energy level in the diet. An alternative scenario in explaining these results is that the heavier brown egg pullet has reduced amino acid needs and so when fed high energy diets there is less effect on amino acid intake relative to energy. The energy balance of white and brown-egg pullets through the period of maturity and early egg production is shown in Table 2.18.

For the mature laying hen energy seems to be the main nutrient controlling egg production. As energy intake increases there is an increase in number of eggs produced independent of protein or amino acid intake (Figure 2.28).

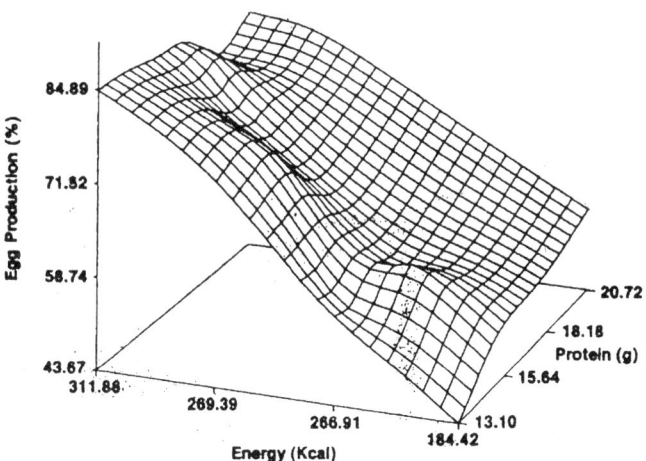

Figure 2.28 Egg production (18-66 weeks) in response to intakes of energy and protein.

	Theoretical Daily Energy Requirement (kcal ME per bird)					Required intake of 17% CP, 2850 ME diet (g/d)
Age (wks)	Maintenance	+20% Activity allowance	Growth	Eggs	Total	
1. White egg strains						
16	111	133	50		183	64
18	118	142	45		187	66
20	125	150	40	5	195	68
22	132	158	40	24	222	78
24	139	167	35	61	263	97
26	142	170	30	85	285	100
28	147	176	25	89	286	102
30	150	180	20	91	291	102
2. Brown egg strains						
16	128	147	80		227	80
18	136	156	80		236	83
20	144	166	80	8	254	89
22	152	175	70	66	309	108
24	160	184	40	94	320	112
26	164	186	40	96	322	113
28	170	196	34	98	328	115
30	172	198	32	100	330	116

Table 2.18 Energy balance of laying hens during early egg production when maintained at around 23°C

As protein/amino acid intake increases, at very low energy intakes there is a slight response in egg output. However, as energy intake reaches about 230 kcal ME/d, there is no response to protein, even at just 13g intake per day. The picture for egg weight is opposite to this (see Figure 3.12) with protein being the controlling nutrient and energy having little effect. However, when the two graphs are superimposed, to predict daily egg mass output, the plane is similar to that shown in Figure 2.28, indicating energy intake as the major determinant. In practical feeding situations, it is often difficult to convince young layers to eat enough feed so as to optimize energy intake and this situation is most critical at high environmental temperatures. Depending upon prior acclimatization, and effect of air speed and humidity, the bird can approach negative energy balance at around 33°C (Figure 2.29).

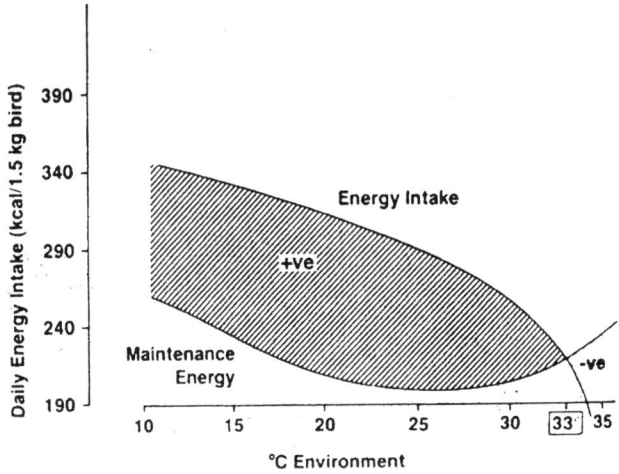

Figure 2.29 Environmental temperature and energy balance

The shaded area shown in Figure 2.29 represents energy available for egg production and growth. If this available energy is plotted against temperature then we can make some predictions about consequences to egg production and liveability (Figure 2.30).

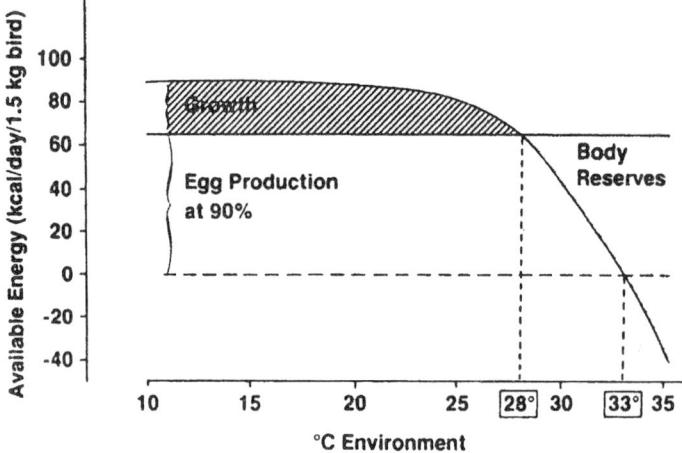

Figure 2.30 Environmental temperature and energy balance.

Up to about 22°C, there is sufficient energy to maintain egg production at 90% (about 54g egg mass/d) and some growth. At 28°C growth will stop and the bird will have to start using some body energy reserves in order to augment the feed supply. At 33°C, egg production is supported by body energy reserves alone. Obviously this scenario can only continue for a short time, and eventually the layer has to reduce her egg output. As previously described the key temperatures shown in Figure 2.30, namely 28° and 33°C will vary depending upon bird acclimatization and for birds normally exposed to 28-30°C corresponding values may be 34°C and 39°C. The actual temperatures where heat distress occurs is characterized by behavioural changes such as excess panting and wing-drooping. Assuming there is no major heat distress then the laying hen will reduce her feed intake by about 2.5 kcal ME for each 1°C increase in effective temperature, over the range 10-33°C.

c)   **Broiler Breeders.** For the heavier broiler breeder hen maintenance assumes the major need for energy and as with the laying hen, egg production is mainly responsive to energy intake. However because of the bird's voracious appetite it is necessary to physically restrict daily intake and so managing energy and nutrient supply becomes an exercise in both feed formulation and feeding management. Even at peak egg output, about 75% of the bird's energy needs are directed towards maintenance (Table 2.19).

Table 2.19 Theoretical energy needs of heavy breeders at 22°C					
Age (wks)	Body wt (kg)	Total maintenance (kcal)	Growth (kcal)	Eggs (kcal)	Total daily energy req. (kcal)
20	2.07	235	85	-	320
21	2.17	245	85	-	330
22	2.27	255	105	-	360
23	2.39	260	105	-	365
24	2.57	280	110	10	400
25	2.82	300	75	40	415
26	2.82	300	75	40	415
27	2.95	305	50	60	415
28	3.05	310	30	80	420

Table 2.20 Predicted energy needs of broiler breeder pullets (kcal/bird/day)						
Age (wks)	Body wt (g)	Egg mass (g/d)	Temperature (°C)			
			18	24	29	35
2	77	-	-	-	95	92
4	417	-	-	134	125	115
6	720	-	170	156	143	131
8	1003	-	188	172	156	140
10	1249	-	204	185	167	148
12	1476	-	216	195	175	155
14	1684	-	227	205	182	160
16	1870	-	236	212	188	165
18	2084	-	243	218	193	168
20	2190	-	250	224	198	171
22	2320	-	256	229	201	175
24	2450	3.5	272	254	215	187
26	2565	18.0	320	290	260	235
28	2665	44.3	409	379	348	320
30	2758	53.7	444	413	382	352
40	3100	53.6	456	423	390	357
50	3310	48.0	445	411	376	341
60	3425	41.0	428	393	357	322
70	3500	34.0	410	373	337	302

Adapted from Waldroup et al., (1976)

Because of this major energy need for maintenance and the fact that this need is influenced by environmental temperature, the bird is very sensitive to fluctuations in her environment. Theoretical energy needs, across a range of temperatures, can be calculated according to the model of Combs (1968) as used by Waldroup et al., (1976), and such values are shown in Table 2.20.

Change in environmental temperature of about 12°C has as much effect as does the production or not, of a single egg. Spratt and Leeson (1987) partitioned the energy balance of caged breeders during the first half of the normal production cycle (Table 2.21).

Table 2.21 Energy balance of broiler breeders (24-40 weeks)			
	Daily energy intake (kcal/bird)		
	450	385	325
Input:Feed (kcal)	60,000	51,000	32,000
Output: Body fat (kcal) Body protein (kcal) Eggs (kcal)	21,300 0 11,000	14,700 1,900 10,000	12,100 2,400 8.000
% ME into growth	36	32	33
% ME into eggs	18	20	18
		Adapted from Spratt and Leeson (1987)	

Offering a wide range of energy intake, breeders produced a remarkably consistent proportion of retained energy, as eggs. With intakes of from 325-450 kcal/d, breeders directed about 18% of energy into eggs. The most notable effect of reduced energy intake was reduction in energy as body fat and increase in energy deposited as body protein. Presumably when energy intake is insufficient to fuel adequate egg production, a more quiescent ovary means a greater proportion of digested protein is available for growth. With high protein intakes for adult breeders (at constant energy and amino acids) we also find greater growth and so the bird is able to capitalize on 'unused' protein/amino acids beyond that needed for maintenance and egg production. Since egg production is correlated with energy intake (Table 2.21) then it would seem logical to attain as high an energy intake as possible. Unfortunately the breeder hen reacts adversely to excess energy intake in terms of both multiple ovulations and fat accretion. The two situations are likely linked and reflect a change in hormonal control of ovulation. While high energy intakes are necessary, it is still essential to control intake, usually by physical feed restriction. The daily maintenance energy need of the breeder is around 100 kcal ME/kg body mass. For a 3.2 kg breeder at peak production we therefore can justify an optimum energy intake of around 450 kcal/bird/day. Data from Burke and Jensen (1994) support this assumption (Table 2.22)

Table 2.22 Effect of energy allotment on breeder performance (21-61 wks)			
	Peak energy allotment (29-34 wks, kcal/day)		
	450	424	396
Eggs per hen	165	149	141
Fertility (%)	92.6	89.8	87.2
Chicks per hen	123	116	102
Egg weight (g)	66.1	66.5	66.7
			Adapted from Burke and Jensen (1994)

There is very little information published on the energy needs of male breeders. Because most male breeders are fed through separate equipment, it is now possible to tailor diets and feed allocation to more adequately suit their needs for maintenance and growth. Environmental temperature has an even larger effect on male breeders because some 95% of energy needs are directed towards maintenance. Table 2.23 shows estimates of daily energy needs of mature adult broiler breeder males.

Table 2.23 Energy needs of adult broiler breeder males (kcal ME/bird/day)		
Age (wks)	20-28°C	<15°C
20	319	348
22	334	362
24	342	377
26	363	390
28	377	406
30	392	435
32	406	450
34	392	440
36	377	430
40	370	420
50	365	410
60	365	410

A minor complication of attempting to meet heavy breeder energy requirements is the fact that these birds metabolize some 2% less energy from feed than do Leghorn birds. The Leghorn bird has been used most frequently in AMEn and TMEn studies and so published ingredient energy values usually reflect the needs of this strain. In attempting to fine tune breeder energy nutrition, it may be important to confirm validity of ingredient energy values in the formulation matrix.

SELECTED REFERENCES

Bennett, C.D., S. Leeson and H.S. Bayley, 1990. Heat production of skip-a-day and daily fed broiler breeder pullets. Can. J. Anim. Sci. 70:667-671.

Burke, W. and L.S. Jensen, 1994. Energy restriction of breeder hens affects performance. Arbor Acres Review 37 (1).

Byerly, T.C., 1941. Feed and other costs of producing market eggs. Technical Bulletin A-1. Mayland Agric. Exp. Stn. College Park MD.

Choct, M., 1999. Soluble non-starch polysaccharides affect net utilization of energy by chickens. Recent Advances in Animal Nutrition. Univ. Armidale, NSW. P 31-35.

Chwalibog, A., 1985. Studies on energy metabolism in laying hens. Report #578. National Inst. An. Sci. Copenhagen, Denmark.

Dale, N. and A. Villacres, 1986. Nutrition influences ascites in broilers. World Poultry Misset. April, pp. 40.

Emmans, G.C., 1974. The effect of temperature on the performance of laying hens. In: Energy Requirements of Poultry. p79-90. Br. Poult. Sci. Ltd..

Emmans, G.C., 1994. Effective energy: A concept of energy utilization applied across species. Br. J. Nutr. 71:801-821.

Geraert, P.A., S. Guillaumin, A. Bordas and P. Merat, 1991. Evidence of genetic control of diet induced thermogenesis in poultry. Proc. European Energy Symposium. p 380-382.

Guillaume, J. and J.D. Summers, 1970. Maintenance energy requirement of the rooster and influence of plane of nutrition on metabolizable energy. Can. J. Anim. Sci. 50:363-369.

Hruby, M., M.L. Hamre and C.N. Coon, 1995. Predicting amino acid requirements for broilers at 21.1°C. J. Appl. Poultry Res. 4:395-401.

Iji, P.A. and D.R. Tivey, 1998. Natural and synthetic oligosaccharides in broiler chicken diets. Wld. Poultry Sci. J. 54:129-143.

Kielanowski, J., 1965. In: Proc. 3rd Symposium on Energy Metabolism of Farm Animals. P. 13-20. Academic Press.

Kirchgesner, M., E.M. Maurus-Kukral and F.X. Rott, 1991. Energy utilization of broilers between 1500 and 3000g liveweight. Proc. European Energy Symposium p. 5-8.

Leeson, S., L. Caston and J.D. Summers, 1996. Broiler response to energy or protein dilution in the finisher diet. Poultry Sci. 75:522-528.

Leske, K.L. and C.N. Coon, 1999. Nutrient content and protein and energy digestibilities of ethanol extracted low α-galactoside soybean meal as compared to intact soybean meal. Poultry Sci. 78:1177-1183.

Li, Y., T. Ho and S. Yamamota, 1991. Diurnal variation in heat production related to some physical activities in laying hens. Br. Poultry Sci. 32:821-827.

MacLeod, M.G., 1990. Energy and nitrogen intake, expenditure and retention at 20° in growing fowl given diets with a wide range of energy and protein contents. Br. J. Nutr. 64:625-637.

Marsden, A. and T.R. Morris, 1987. Quantitative review of the effects of environmental temperature on food intake, egg output and energy balance in laying pullets. Br. Poultry Sci. 28:693-704.

Meltzer, A., G. Goodwan and J. Fistool. 1982. Thermoneutral zone and resting metabolic rate of growing WL chickens. Br. Poultry Sci. 23:383-392.

National Research Council (NRC), 1994. Nutrient Requirements of Poultry. 9th Rev. Ed. NAS-NRC. Washington D.C.

Parsons, C.M., R.H. Zimmerman, K.W. Koelkebeck and Y. Zhang, 1994. Effect of abrupt dietary energy changes on daily caloric intake and performance of young laying hens. J. Appl. Poultry Res. 3:133-140.

Payne, C.G., 1967. In: Environmental Control of Poultry Production. pp 40-54. Ed. T.C. Carter, Publ. Longmans, London.

Pesti, G.M., J.H. Dorfman and M.J. Gonzalez-A., 1992. Model for predicting egg output and metabolizable energy intake of laying pullets. Br. Poultry Sci. 33:543-552.

Pirgozlieve, V. and S.P. Rose, 1999. Net energy systems for poultry: A quantitative review. Wld. Poult. Sci. J. 55:23-36.

Smits, C.H.M. and G. Annison, 1996. Non-starch polysaccharides in broiler nutrition – towards a physiologically valid approach to their determinations. Wld. Poultry Sci. J. 52:203-221.

Spratt, R.S. and S. Leeson, 1987. Broiler breeder performance in response to diet protein and energy. Poult. Sci. 66:683-693.

Waldroup, P.W. A., Z. Johnson and W. Bussell, 1976. Estimating daily nutrient requirements for broiler breeder hens. Feedstuffs. 48 (28).

Wilson, P.N. and D.F. Osbourn, 1960. Compensatory growth after undernutrition in mammals and birds. Biol. Rev. 35:325-363.

Proteins
And Amino Acids

Although all of the proteins in a feedstuff are often referred to collectively as "protein", they do differ in individual composition. It is the specific sequence of amino acids and the manner in which the amino acids strands are connected to each other that determine the physical and chemical properties of each individual protein, and thereby its biological function and need by the bird.

Proteins form important structural parts of the soft tissues of the body such as muscle, connective tissue, collagen, skin, feathers, toenails and the horny portion of the beak. The blood proteins, albumin and globulins, help to maintain homeostasis, regulate osmotic pressure, and act somewhat as a reserve supply of amino acids, together with numerous other anabolic functions. Fibrinogen, thromboplastin and several other proteins are involved in blood clotting. Also found in the blood is the conjugated protein, hemoglobin, which carries oxygen to the cells, and lipoproteins which transport fat-soluble vitamins and other fatty metabolites. Lipoproteins also occur in the cell membranes where they comprise essential structural features. Other conjugated proteins found throughout the body are nucleoproteins, glycoproteins, enzymes and some hormones while the vitellin of egg yolk is a phosphoprotein. Young (1996) provides an extensive and comprehensive overview of biochemical aspects of protein and amino acid metabolism

3.1   CLASSIFICATION OF PROTEINS

Although all proteins contain amino acids, their sequential arrangement in the multitude of proteins that exist in nature differs considerably, and these differences have specific influences upon the properties of each individual protein. However, general classification can be made based largely upon the solubilities of the various proteins in water, salt solution, acids, bases and ethanol.

3.1.1   Globular proteins

a. Albumins: Proteins which are soluble in water and coagulated by heat, such as egg and serum albumin. Although classically included with the simple proteins these serum albumins contain as much as 4% carbohydrate as hexosamine and, so can also be described as conjugated proteins (glycoproteins).

b. Globulins: Proteins insoluble or sparingly soluble in water but soluble in dilute neutral solutions of salts such as sodium chloride and are also heat labile. Globulins may be extracted from plant or animal tissue by 5-10% NaCl solutions and then precipitated by dilution of the extracts with pure water. Examples are serum globulin (also a glycoprotein), fibrinogen, myosinogen, and legumin of peas, and concanavalin of the jack bean.

c. Glutelins: Insoluble in water and all neutral solvents but may be readily dissolved in dilute acids or bases. Examples are the glutelin of wheat and corn.

d. Prolamines or Gliadins: Simple proteins which are soluble in 70-80% ethanol but insoluble in water, alcohol or neutral solvents. Examples are zein of corn and wheat, gliadins of wheat and rye and hordein of barley.

e. Histones: Basic proteins, soluble in water, but insoluble in dilute ammonia. Histones can be used to precipitate other soluble proteins which are then soluble in dilute acids. The histones are characterized by a large excess of basic amino acids and most are combined with nucleic acids. An example of histones is globin of hemoglobin.

3.1.2   Fibrous proteins

a. Collagens: Being the major protein of skeletal connective tissues, collagens represent more than 50% of the total protein in the body. They are insoluble in water and are resistant to endogenous digestive enzymes, but are readily changed into soluble, easily digestible gelatins by boiling in water or in dilute acids or bases. The collagens have a unique amino acid structure characterized by large amounts of hydroxyproline and some hydroxylysine and a complete absence of cysteine, cystine and tryptophan.

b. Elastins: These are the proteins of the elastic tissues such as tendons and arteries. Although similar in makeup to collagens, the elastins cannot be converted to gelatins. The fibrils of elastin are bound together by the compound desmosine, derived by conjugation of lysine molecules.

c. Keratins: The proteins of feathers, hair, claws and beak are very insoluble and indigestible and contain as much as 14-15% cystine. Digestibility of ground feather meal and hog hair has been shown to be raised to 70-80% by appropriate treatment with heat and pressure. Such treatment reduces the cystine content to 5-6%, but concurrent increase in digestibility relates to there being fewer -S-S- bonds within the keratins that contribute in large part to the insolubility and indigestibility of these proteins. There is now interest in pretreating raw feathers with keratinase enzymes in order to improve amino acid digestion and/or to enable the use of less stringent and potentially damaging physical cooking. In addition to the keratins in feathers, there are also neurokeratins of the gray matter of the brain, spinal cord and the retina of the eye.

3.1.3   Conjugated proteins

These proteins contain amino acids bound to some type of non-amino group which dictates their functionality and often their distribution in body tissues.

a. Nucleoproteins: One or more molecules of protein combined with nucleic acids. These are present in cells as deoxyribonucleoproteins, and as ribonucleoprotein within the ribosomes.

b. Mucoids or Mucoproteins: The carbohydrate portions of these proteins are mucopolysaccharides containing a N-acetyl-hexosamine such as glucosamine or galactosamine in combination with a uronic acid such as galacturonic or glucuronic acids. Many also contain sialic acid.

c. Glycoproteins: Proteins containing less than 4% carbohydrate, often as a simple hexose such as mannose found in egg albumin.

d. Lipoproteins: Water-soluble proteins conjugated with lecithin, cephalin, cholesterol, or other lipids or phospholipids.

e. Chromoproteins: A group of compounds characterized by the union of a simple protein with a colored prosthetic group. Chromoproteins include hemoglobin, the cytochromes and flavoproteins, the visual purple of the retina of the eye and the enzyme catalase.

Plants are the primary initial source of all proteins.   Each portion of every plant (seed, leaf, stem) contains specific proteins. Green plants synthesize these characteristic proteins, utilizing the carbon skeletons derived from photosynthesis and incorporating the amino group from inorganic ammonia or nitrate salts in the water supplied to the plant. All of the twenty-two amino acids known to be involved in building all plant and animal proteins are readily synthesized by plants. Animals however, can synthesize only twelve amino acids, thereby relying on the plant for the initial synthesis of the amino acids, which are known as the nutritionally essential amino acids.

Some bacteria residing in the soil and in the root nodules of certain legumes and other plants can convert atmospheric nitrogen to nitrogenous compounds, which may supply plants with the nitrates needed to form the amino and other organic nitrogenous compounds. Plants synthesize many different kinds of proteins and store varying amounts in the different parts of the plant. Some plants synthesize far more protein than do others, often in association with extra lipid. The dicotyledonous seeds such as most oil seeds are much richer sources of proteins than are the cereal seeds. For example, the dry weight of the soybean seed contains approximately 43% protein, while the dry weight of the corn seed contains only about 9% protein. Within the green portion of plants, the young, tender grasses and leaves contain more protein (in the neighborhood of 20-25% of the dry weight) as compared with the stalks or older leaves, which are higher in cellulose and much lower in total protein, and much lower in digestible protein.

Even within a single seed such as the soybean, many different proteins are found. The proteins in the cereal grains are largely prolamines and glutelins whereas in the oilseeds approximately 80% are in the globulin fraction. In each fraction there are many individual specific proteins. In soybean, the major globulin is a specific protein called glycinin. The glutenin and gliadin of corn have long been considered to be single proteins. Protein chromatography, however, has shown that each of these protein fractions consists of several individual proteins.

3.2   CLASSIFICATION OF AMINO ACIDS

Animals, like plants, synthesize proteins containing twenty-two amino acids. However, unlike plants, animals cannot synthesize all of the amino acids. Amino acids which cannot be synthesized by animals and therefore must be supplied in the diet are classified as the essential or indispensable amino acids. Those amino

Table 3.1 Nutritional Classification of Amino Acids		
Not synthesized in chickens (Essential, Indispensable)	Synthesized from limited substrates*	Readily synthesized in chickens from simple substrates (Nonessential, Dispensable)
Arginine Lysine Histidine Leucine Isoleucine Valine Methionine Threonine Tryptophan Phenylalanine	Tyrosine Cystine Hydroxylysine	Alanine Aspartic acid Asparagine Glutamic acid Glutamine Hydroxyproline Glycine** Serine** Proline***

*   Tyrosine is synthesized from phenylalanine, cystine from methionine, hydroxylysine from lysine.
**   Under some conditions glycine or serine synthesis may not be sufficient for very rapid growth; either serine or glycine may need to be supplied in the diet.
*** When diets composed of crystalline amino acids are used, proline may be necessary to achieve maximum growth.

acids that can be synthesized by the animal are termed non-essential or dispensable amino acids. Of these, a few cannot be synthesized at a rate fast enough for maximum growth and therefore should be supplied in the diet. The essential and non-essential amino acids involved in protein synthesis are shown in Table 3.1.

The chemical structure of most of these amino acids are shown in Figures 3.1 and 3.2.

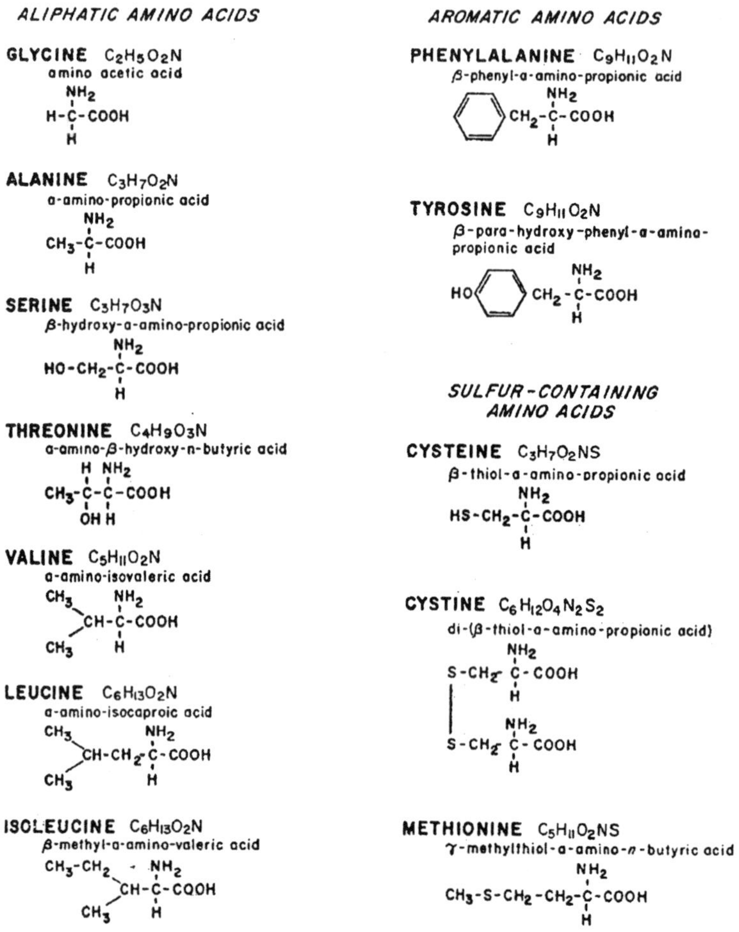

ALIPHATIC AMINO ACIDS

GLYCINE $C_2H_5O_2N$
amino acetic acid

$$\underset{\underset{H}{|}}{\overset{\overset{NH_2}{|}}{H-C-COOH}}$$

ALANINE $C_3H_7O_2N$
a-amino-propionic acid

$$\underset{\underset{H}{|}}{\overset{\overset{NH_2}{|}}{CH_3-C-COOH}}$$

SERINE $C_3H_7O_3N$
β-hydroxy-a-amino-propionic acid

$$\underset{\underset{H}{|}}{\overset{\overset{NH_2}{|}}{HO-CH_2-C-COOH}}$$

THREONINE $C_4H_9O_3N$
a-amino-β-hydroxy-n-butyric acid

$$\overset{\overset{H\ \ NH_2}{|\ \ \ |}}{\underset{\underset{OH\ H}{|\ \ |}}{CH_3-C-C-COOH}}$$

VALINE $C_5H_{11}O_2N$
a-amino-isovaleric acid

$$\overset{CH_3}{\underset{CH_3}{>}}CH-\overset{\overset{NH_2}{|}}{\underset{\underset{H}{|}}{C}}-COOH$$

LEUCINE $C_6H_{13}O_2N$
a-amino-isocaproic acid

$$\overset{CH_3}{\underset{CH_3}{>}}CH-CH_2-\overset{\overset{NH_2}{|}}{\underset{\underset{H}{|}}{C}}-COOH$$

ISOLEUCINE $C_6H_{13}O_2N$
β-methyl-a-amino-valeric acid

$$\overset{CH_3-CH_2}{\underset{CH_3}{>}}CH-\overset{\overset{NH_2}{|}}{\underset{\underset{H}{|}}{C}}-COOH$$

AROMATIC AMINO ACIDS

PHENYLALANINE $C_9H_{11}O_2N$
β-phenyl-a-amino-propionic acid

$$\bigcirc CH_2-\overset{\overset{NH_2}{|}}{\underset{\underset{H}{|}}{C}}-COOH$$

TYROSINE $C_9H_{11}O_2N$
β-para-hydroxy-phenyl-a-amino-propionic acid

$$HO-\bigcirc CH_2-\overset{\overset{NH_2}{|}}{\underset{\underset{H}{|}}{C}}-COOH$$

SULFUR-CONTAINING AMINO ACIDS

CYSTEINE $C_3H_7O_2NS$
β-thiol-a-amino-propionic acid

$$HS-CH_2-\overset{\overset{NH_2}{|}}{\underset{\underset{H}{|}}{C}}-COOH$$

CYSTINE $C_6H_{12}O_4N_2S_2$
di-(β-thiol-a-amino-propionic acid)

$$S-CH_2-\overset{\overset{NH_2}{|}}{\underset{\underset{H}{|}}{C}}-COOH$$
$$S-CH_2-\overset{\overset{NH_2}{|}}{\underset{\underset{H}{|}}{C}}-COOH$$

METHIONINE $C_5H_{11}O_2NS$
γ-methylthiol-a-amino-n-butyric acid

$$CH_3-S-CH_2-CH_2-\overset{\overset{NH_2}{|}}{\underset{\underset{H}{|}}{C}}-COOH$$

Figure 3.1 Nomenclature and chemical structure of amino acids.

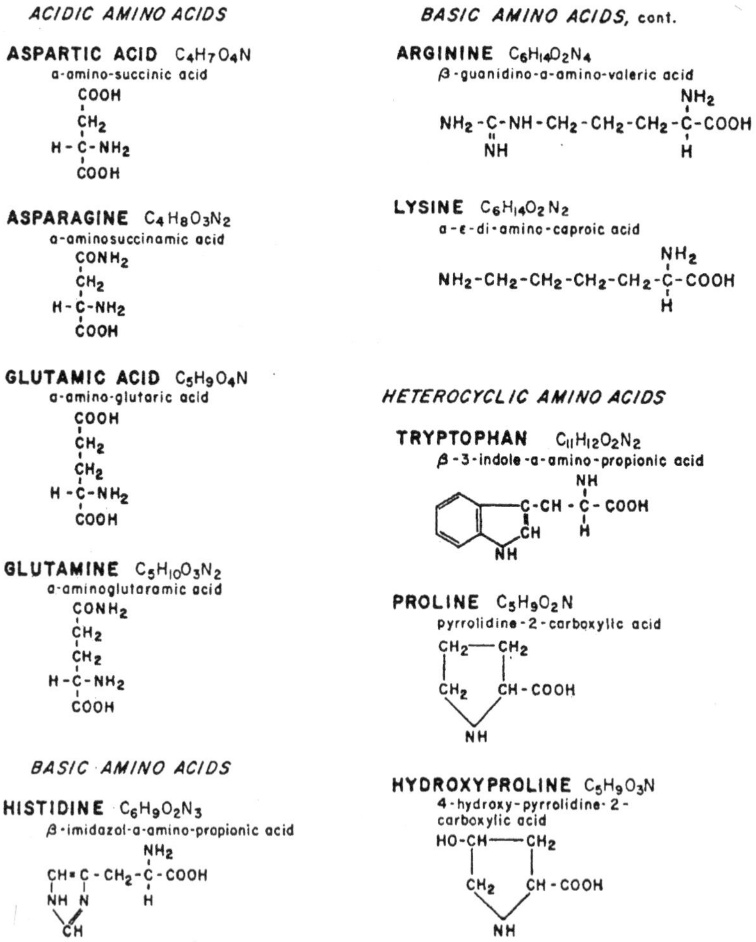

ACIDIC AMINO ACIDS

ASPARTIC ACID $C_4H_7O_4N$
a-amino-succinic acid

$$
\begin{array}{c}
COOH \\
| \\
CH_2 \\
| \\
H-C-NH_2 \\
| \\
COOH
\end{array}
$$

ASPARAGINE $C_4H_8O_3N_2$
a-aminosuccinamic acid

$$
\begin{array}{c}
CONH_2 \\
| \\
CH_2 \\
| \\
H-C-NH_2 \\
| \\
COOH
\end{array}
$$

GLUTAMIC ACID $C_5H_9O_4N$
a-amino-glutaric acid

$$
\begin{array}{c}
COOH \\
| \\
CH_2 \\
| \\
CH_2 \\
| \\
H-C-NH_2 \\
| \\
COOH
\end{array}
$$

GLUTAMINE $C_5H_{10}O_3N_2$
a-aminoglutaramic acid

$$
\begin{array}{c}
CONH_2 \\
| \\
CH_2 \\
| \\
CH_2 \\
| \\
H-C-NH_2 \\
| \\
COOH
\end{array}
$$

BASIC AMINO ACIDS

HISTIDINE $C_6H_9O_2N_3$
β-imidazol-a-amino-propionic acid

$$
\begin{array}{c}
NH_2 \\
| \\
CH=C-CH_2-C-COOH \\
|\ \ | \qquad\quad | \\
NH\ \ N \qquad\quad H \\
\ \ \backslash\!\swarrow \\
\ \ CH
\end{array}
$$

BASIC AMINO ACIDS, cont.

ARGININE $C_6H_{14}O_2N_4$
β-guanidino-a-amino-valeric acid

$$
\begin{array}{c}
\qquad\qquad\qquad\qquad\qquad NH_2 \\
\qquad\qquad\qquad\qquad\qquad | \\
NH_2-C-NH-CH_2-CH_2-CH_2-C-COOH \\
\ \ \ \ \ \| \qquad\qquad\qquad\qquad\qquad | \\
\ \ \ \ NH \qquad\qquad\qquad\qquad\qquad H
\end{array}
$$

LYSINE $C_6H_{14}O_2N_2$
a-ε-di-amino-caproic acid

$$
\begin{array}{c}
\qquad\qquad\qquad\qquad\qquad NH_2 \\
\qquad\qquad\qquad\qquad\qquad | \\
NH_2-CH_2-CH_2-CH_2-CH_2-C-COOH \\
\qquad\qquad\qquad\qquad\qquad\quad H
\end{array}
$$

HETEROCYCLIC AMINO ACIDS

TRYPTOPHAN $C_{11}H_{12}O_2N_2$
β-3-indole-a-amino-propionic acid

$$
\begin{array}{c}
\qquad\qquad\quad NH \\
\qquad\qquad\quad | \\
C-CH-C-COOH \\
|\qquad\quad H \\
CH \\
| \\
NH
\end{array}
$$

PROLINE $C_5H_9O_2N$
pyrrolidine-2-carboxylic acid

$$
\begin{array}{c}
CH_2\!-\!\!-\!\!-CH_2 \\
|\qquad\quad | \\
CH_2\quad CH-COOH \\
\ \ \ \backslash\ \ \ / \\
\ \ \ \ NH
\end{array}
$$

HYDROXYPROLINE $C_5H_9O_3N$
4-hydroxy-pyrrolidine-2-
carboxylic acid

$$
\begin{array}{c}
HO-CH\!-\!\!-\!\!-CH_2 \\
|\qquad\qquad | \\
CH_2\quad\ \ CH-COOH \\
\ \ \ \backslash\ \ \ \ \ / \\
\ \ \ \ \ NH
\end{array}
$$

Figure 3.2 Nomenclature and chemical structure of amino acids.

The essential amino acids can be classified into one of three categories, dependent upon the bird's ability to achieve limited synthesis or not.

a.   Lysine and threonine have no intermediary precursors, and so 100% of need must be supplied by the diet.

b.   Leucine, isoleucine and valine can be synthesized from precursor intermediary metabolites. However, the production is very limited and may supply at best 2-5% of requirement.

c.   Arginine and histidine can also be synthesized from intermediates during general metabolism. Again synthesis will be limited although under unusual circumstances may yield 5-8% of requirement.

The semi-essential amino acids (Table 3.1) can be synthesized from another essential amino acid. Cysteine is derived for methionine and tyrosine is metabolized from phenylalanine. Methionine is converted into adenosyl methionine and then homocysteine and eventually cysteine. Tyrosine can be synthesized directly from hydroxylation of phenylalanine.

The major non-essential amino acids found in tissue and feedstuffs are glycine, serine, alanine, glutamic acid and aspartic acid. Glycine is synthesized from choline or serine, and in addition to glycine normally supplied in the diet, this usually provides adequate glycine for metabolism. However because glycine plays an integral role in uric acid synthesis, there have been reports of a chick response to supplemental diet glycine under somewhat atypical feeding situations. Regardless of the need for dietary supply, the need for uric acid synthesis accounts for the relatively high chick requirement for glycine.

During synthesis of protein in the cell, these amino acids join together in long chains in a definite, characteristic sequence and then the chains may interlock in specific characteristic ways to form individual proteins. The linkages within the chains are termed peptide bonds. These are strong, covalent bondings between the carboxyl (acid) group of one amino acid and the amino group of another amino acid. Other bonds which serve to hold two or more protein chains together to form the final three dimensional protein are hydrogen bonds, disulfide bonds, ionic bonds or hydrophobic bonds.

Most proteins are depicted as existing in an α-helix (spiral) form, in which there are 3.7 amino acid residues for each coil, the shape being maintained largely by hydrogen bonding between the CO and NH group of adjacent coils. However, not all proteins exist in helix form. Some are bent and intertwined like a complicated pretzel or perhaps resembling a stiff roll of ribbon confetti that has been stretched and then released to take the shape of less stress. In all cases, the ultimate shape depends upon the attractions, which exist in certain atoms or groups of atoms or groups within the same chain (thereby causing twisting), or in a near-by chain (thereby holding two or more chains together).

The disulfide bonds occur between one cysteine molecule in a chain and another cysteine molecule in the same chain or in another chain, thus forming a cystine molecule which holds the two parts together. This disulfide bond can be broken by coming in contact with a "reducing agent" that is strong enough to force two atoms of hydrogen between the two sulfur atoms of the disulfide linkage or alternatively, by further oxidation of the sulfur.

Ionic bonds may occur between such groups as the epsilon amino group of lysine (which may be present in certain cases as an NH_3^+ ion) and a free carboxyl group such as the γ-carboxyl of glutamic or δ-carboxyl of aspartic acid (which may exist in ionic form as -COO- groups). Theoretically, these bonds would be decomposed when a protein containing such bonds is exposed to water, since water would tend to hydrate both ions.

Hydrophobic bonds may occur when the nonpolar side portions of certain amino acids come into contact with each other. Thus the chains or other hydrophobic portions of phenylalanine, tyrosine, leucine, isoleucine, valine and other amino acids may join together as hydrophobic centres in a manner somewhat similar to that described in Chapter 2 for the formation of lipid-bile salt micelles. These various types of bondings are not only important in determining the exact structure of each individual protein but probably are even more important in providing the means by which proteins can enter into all of the many enzymic, hormonal, chromosomal etc. functions, which are so vital to metabolism.

The molecular weights of proteins range from about 1,000 for oxytocin to the very high value of 2,800,000 for octupus hemocyanin. The molecular weights of most proteins however, range in the area of 35,000 to 500,000. Since the average molecular weight of an amino acid is about 115, the number of amino acid residues present in most protein molecules ranges from about 300 to about 5,000. A few proteins such as insulin and adrenal corticotropic hormone (ACTH) are relatively small, having molecular weights of only 5,733 and 4,540 with 51 and 39 amino acid residues, respectively. These proteins and several others including lysozyme from eggs, have been completely characterized as to amino acid sequence, type and number of cross-bond linkages.

The amino acid composition of some individual egg proteins is presented in Table 3.2 while protein components are shown in Fig 3.3. It is apparent from this table that individual proteins differ in the percentages of the various amino acids which they contain. Review of these data makes one wonder, for example, how the oviduct manages to concentrate the tryptophan, as supplied by the blood supply, sufficiently to synthesize lysozyme and whether or not lysozyme synthesis could be improved by increasing the tryptophan content of the diet,

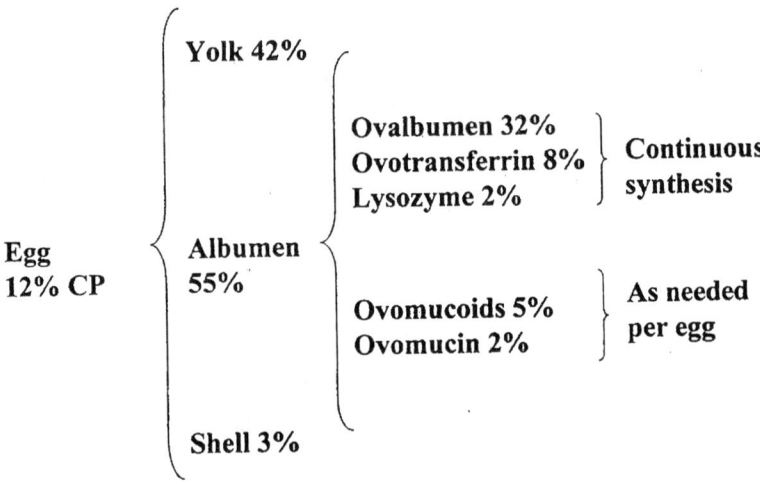

Figure 3.3 Egg protein components.

Table 3.2 Amino acid profile of egg and egg components (% of protein)							
	Egg	Yolk	Ovalbumen	Ovotransferrin	Ovomucoids	Ovomucin	Lysozyme
Arginine	6.4	7.2	4.2	4.0	3.0	4.2	10.2
Histidine	2.3	1.9	1.8	1.4	2.2	2.8	1.3
Isoleucine	5.0	6.5	6.2	3.4	1.5	4.0	5.0
Leucine	8.3	8.2	7.8	7.2	6.0	6.2	7.1
Lysine	7.1	5.8	5.8	8.0	7.2	7.0	5.8
Methionine	3.2	2.9	4.1	1.5	1.0	2.5	2.4
Cystine	2.2	2.0	1.6	4.0	7.0	6.5	8.2
Phenylalanine	4.7	4.5	5.0	3.9	2.8	5.0	3.6
Tryptophan	1.4	1.5	1.5	1.7	0.6	1.4	5.8
Threonine	5.0	5.3	5.5	5.6	7.0	7.8	6.9
Valine	6.5	7.0	6.8	7.8	7.2	5.2	5.0

3.3 PROTEIN AND AMINO ACID STRUCTURE AND SYNTHESIS

Protein synthesis in plant and animal cells is controlled by the deoxyribonu-cleic acid (DNA) present in the nucleus of the cell in which that particular protein synthesis occurs. The DNA of that cell carries genetic information which determines the exact structure of the protein being synthesized, and transmits this as an inherited characteristic from generation to generation. DNA controls the devel-opment of the proteins in the cell by controlling the formation of the ribonucleic acids (RNA) present in the cytoplasm of the cell. Three different types of RNA in cells are involved in the biosynthesis of proteins. Ribosomal RNA is an integral part of the structure of the ribosome (a specific portion of the cell particle fraction known as the microsome). The ribosomal RNA acts as the final template upon which the proteins are formed. Transfer RNA (tRNA) carries the specific amino acids to the ribosome. In the well-nourished animal, a constant supply of all amino acids is available to all cells. These have been obtained by hydrolysis of dietary protein and have been transported to the cells via the blood either as free amino acids or as blood proteins, which were synthesized in the liver. The messenger RNA (mRNA) determines the sequence of amino acids in the protein being formed. Thus a different messenger RNA is formed from each DNA template and controls the formation of each protein. Protein synthesis involves a complex series of biochemical steps involving RNA and ribosomes. Messenger RNA essentially determines the order that amino acids are linked and so the type of protein being constructed. Transfer DNA is responsible for supplying mRNA with a constant supply of amino acids. The actual process of protein synthesis starts as an initiation phase at the amino group, progresses through elongation under the action of mRNA and tRNA and culminates in a so called termination site where the RNA entities are released. Ribosomal RNA forms ribosomes and dictates the steriotaxic alignment of peptides within the forming protein. The properties of proteins are based upon those of their individual amino acids. Some of these properties include: the numbers of basic or acidic amino acids; the ionic groupings they contain; the number and relative size of their hydrophobic centres; the presence or absence of carbohydrate, lipid or phosphate and; whether or not the proteins are ligands, which are capable of forming chelates with one or more polyvalent mineral elements.

Because amino acids have both a basic group (the amino group) and an acidic group (the carboxyl group) they are amphoteric (they are called ampholytes i.e., they will react with both acids and bases). The relative acidic vs. basic properties of each individual amino acid are quite unique. The monoamino, monocarboxylic acids in aqueous solution are termed zwitterions, meaning "both way" ions. Each amino acid has a characteristic pH at which it is present in aqueous solution in a form whereby its carboxyl group is exactly balanced by its amino group. At this pH the dipolar ion will not migrate to either pole in an electrical field. This pH therefore, is termed the isoelectric point of the amino acid. Amino acids are weak acids and weak bases and so are excellent buffering agents.

Because proteins contain terminal carboxyl and amino groups in their peptide chains and also free carboxyl and amino groups which are present in the dicarboxylic and diamino amino acids, proteins have a characteristic isolectric point. Proteins serve as excellent buffers and because of their large molecular size and low degree of dissociation they contribute in a major degree to the osmotic pressure of cell contents and plasma. These buffering and osmotic properties are of primary importance in the maintenance of homeostasis by the blood proteins.

Many enzymatic and other properties of protein stem from the ability of specific proteins to act as ligands for certain polyvalent cations. Chelation with minerals may also account for the biological properties of many non-enzyme proteins. For example, mucin, which acts to protect the mucous membrane of the respiratory and gastro-intestinal tracts is a chelate containing calcium. When the calcium is removed from the protein, the mucin loses its protective properties. The ability of hemoglobin to transport oxygen resides in the oxygen attracting forces of the iron molecule chelated within the heme molecule that is conjugated within the protein.

Certain proteins contain special groupings which react spontaneously with specific foreign materials that may gain entrance into the body. These proteins are termed antibodies, while the foreign materials are called antigens. Most proteins stimulate the formation of specific antibodies when injected into test animals. If the protein is pure, it will result in the formation of a single specific antibody. A mixture of proteins will produce a corresponding number of antibodies. This reaction can be used as the basis of a method for identification of certain proteins. Functional proteins such as enzymes, hormones and hemoglobin can be checked for purity by determining the minimum amount required to perform the specific biological function and comparing this with previously standardized data.

When amino acids are catabolized, the amino group can be used for synthesis of other amino acids or incorporated into uric acid. Transamination involves the transfer of the amino group to an α-keto acid generating a new amino acid. This principal is involved in synthesis of methionine from methionine analogues such as Alimet® and in the synthesis of many non-essential amino acids. Vitamin B_6 is the usual co-factor in these reactions, which are most often reversible, and all involve specific transaminase enzyme systems. During oxidative deamination the amino acid is converted into the corresponding α-keto derivative which is usually further catabolized to yield energy.

3.4   FORMS OF AMINO ACIDS

Amino acids can exist as D-, or L- isomers or mixtures of the two products. The isomers are mirror images of each other and at first glance the structures seem to be quite similar (Figure 3.4).

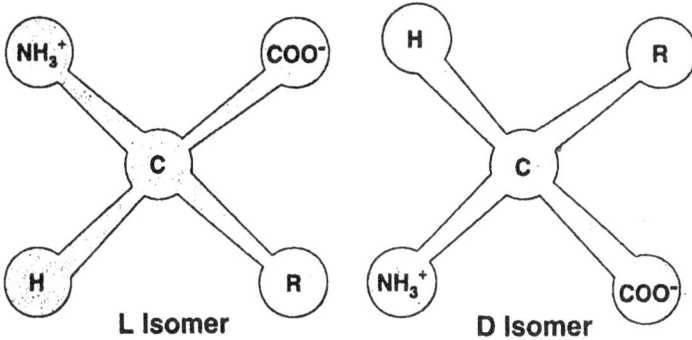

Figure 3.4 Schematic representation of L- and D-amino acids.

All amino acids occurring in animal tissues however are L-isomers, since D-isomers have no biological function. The exception to this is methionine, where the bird is able to use D- or L- forms, or as occurs most frequently, a DL racemic mixture. All other amino acids must therefore be provided as L-isomers. There is an indication that D-methionine is less efficacious when diet protein and/or amino acid levels are low. Theoretically a racemic mixture of threonine should be at least 50% as efficacious as L-threonine. However studies show efficacy of DL-threonine at about 25% compared to L-threonine. Some amino acids are sold as salts usually chlorides and so estimates of potency must take this dilution into account (Table 3.3).

Table 3.3 Relative potency of amino acids and protein equivalents		
Amino Acid	Relative Activity	Crude Protein (%)
DL-Methionine	100	59
L-Lysine	100	120
L-Lysine HCl	79	96
L-Arginine	100	200
L-Arginine HCl	83	166
L-Tryptophan	100	86
L-Threonine	100	74
Glycine	100	117
Glutamic acid	100	177
Methionine hydroxy analogue	88	0

Most essential amino acids can be replaced by the corresponding α-keto acid, sometimes called an analogue. This α-keto acid is then converted into the active amino acid by transamination involving the addition of an NH_2 group. This process is active for most amino acids other than lysine and threonine. A somewhat unusual feature of amino acid analogues is that they have zero protein equivalency (Table 3.3) because they do not contain nitrogen. Analogues are routinely used to replace methionine (Table 3.4), although there is no commercial application at this time for other amino acids.

Table 3.4 Structure of methionine sources			
DL-methionine	**DL-methionine Na**	**Methionine hydroxy analogue**	**Methionine hydroxy analogue-Ca**
CH_3	CH_3	CH_3	CH_3
$\mid$	$\mid$	$\mid$	$\mid$
S	S	S	S
$\mid$	$\mid$	$\mid$	$\mid$
CH_2	CH_2	CH_2	CH_2
$\mid$	$\mid$	$\mid$	$\mid$
CH_2	CH_2	CH_2	CH_2
$\mid$	$\mid$	$\mid$	$\mid$
$H\text{-}C\text{-}NH_2$	$H\text{-}C\text{-}NH_2$	$H\text{-}C\text{-}OH_2$	$H\text{-}C\text{-}OH_2$
$\mid$	$\mid$	$\mid$	$\mid$
COOH	$COONa^+$	COOH	$COOCa^+$
Powder	Liquid	Liquid	Powder

There has been considerable controversy surrounding the efficacy of analogues such as Alimet® , fueled mostly by the manufacturers of both DL-methionine and the analogues. Early work using crystalline amino acids in purified diets showed DL-methionine to be vastly superior to the hydroxy analogue. Baker and Boebel (1998) suggested this reduced efficacy was due to inefficiency of conversion of D- and L-isomers of the analogue possibly due to some missing factor such as a peptide in this type of diet. However, there are virtually no differences in utilization of hydroxy isomers when diets contain intact protein and under such feeding conditions equimolar concentrations of DL methionine and products such as Alimet® seem comparable. The majority of commercial poultry in North America are now fed on the liquid methionine hydroxy analogue.

3.5 TRANSPORT OF AMINO ACIDS

When the absorbed amino acids reach the liver some of them are used for the synthesis of liver tissue proteins or blood proteins. The bulk of amino acids however pass through the liver in free amino acid form. Thus a considerable portion of the amino acids needed by the cells of the body may be derived from free amino acids present in the plasma. However, since the metabolic needs of the cells for amino acids are continuous while the influx of amino acids from the intestine is sporadic, the body needs a storage place in which to hold surplus amino acids in times of excess for use by the cells during times of deficit. Free amino acids can be taken up by the muscles and other tissues and held for a period of a few hours without being chemically changed. If under experimental conditions, free amino acids are given intravenously, muscle, liver, intestine and other organs will retain some 30-60 mg/100 g tissue. Because of the much larger mass of the muscles compared to other organs, then it is obvious that most transient amino acid storage occurs here. Muscles and other organs can only store amino acids for 2-4 hours. If amino acids are fed some 12 hours out of phase with energy and other diet nutrients, bird performance is suboptimal, showing that birds cannot store sufficient amino acids over a 12 hour period. Amino acid transport across the barrier of the cell wall is probably similar to the absorption process. It appears that two distinct mediating sites are present at the cell wall, and while there is definite competition between many pairs of amino acids, certain combinations tend to help or mediate the transport of both amino acids. It is believed that methionine, for example, can mediate the passage of other amino acids such as leucine and similar neutral amino acids. It is well known that several of the amino acids form chelates with polyvalent cations. There is strong evidence that these chelates aid in the passage of the metal ions across cell membranes.

3.6 BIOSYNTHESIS OF NON-ESSENTIAL AMINO ACIDS

To synthesize proteins, all component amino acids must be present in adequate and relatively balanced amounts. The dietary essentials, which are those amino acids not synthesized by the body must come from ingested proteins. The body can synthesize many amino acids provided an appropriate source of nitrogen is available.

The carbon skeletons of amino acids synthesized by the chicken come from intermediates of carbohydrate metabolism. Serine and glycine arise from 3-phosphoglyceric acid and alanine is derived from pyruvic acid, both being intermediates of anaerobic glycolysis. Oxaloacetate and α-ketoglutarate, intermediates of the citric acid cycle, give rise to aspartic acid and glutamic acid, respectively. Glutamic acid, in turn, acts as the precursor of proline and hydroxyproline. The biosynthesis of proline from glutamic acid is not sufficiently rapid to support maximum growth when diets contain predominantly free amino acids. Under these circumstances, a dietary source of proline is required.

Transamination is a critical process in the efficient utilization of dietary nitrogen. If, for example, the diet contains an excess of phenylalanine, the amino group from this amino acid is transferred by a transamination reaction to form glutamic acid. This amino group can then be transferred from glutamic acid to pyruvic acid to form alanine. In this way, nitrogen from amino acids present in excess can be used to synthesize some of the non-essential amino acids. Glutamic acid and alanine transaminases are especially important in the transamination process. While glutamate or α-ketoglutarate must be present as one of the substrates for glutamic transaminase, many other amino acids or their keto analogs will act as a substrate for this enzyme. Similar broad specificity is found for alanine transaminase. These reactions, together with an active glutamic acid-alanine transaminase, provide a means for redistributing amino acid nitrogen, both in the biosynthesis of the non-essential amino acids and in amino acid catabolism.

It is possible to formulate a diet that contains adequate amounts of all essential amino acids but is deficient in the nitrogen needed for synthesis of the non-essential amino acids. This diet can be made nutritionally complete by: (1) addition of one or more non-essential amino acid (e.g. glutamic, aspartic etc.) or; (2) by use of an ammonium source such as diammonium citrate or even urea in small amounts. However there are limits to the use of ammonia or urea by the bird since performance usually declines when, regardless of amino acid balance, these products represent more than 2% crude protein equivalency.

3.7   GLUCONEOGENESIS AND AMINO ACID DEGRADATION

When a chicken is fasted, or when very low levels of dietary carbohydrate are fed, glycogen stored in the liver and muscle cannot provide enough glucose to both maintain blood glucose level and fill the specific needs for glucose in tissues such as the brain or erythrocytes. Under these circumstances, amino acids must be degraded to provide carbon skeletons that can be converted to glucose. This process is called gluconeogenesis. Reactions resulting in gluconeogenesis are under complex metabolic control. In particular, glucocorticoids produced in the adrenal gland can stimulate gluconeogenesis and artificial administration of these hormones elevate the levels of many enzymes responsible for amino acid degradation.

Not all amino acids can be glucose precursors, because the end products of their degradation cannot be converted to glucose. The major end products of amino acid degradation are shown in Table 3.5.

Table 3.5 Major end products from degradation of carbon skeletons of amino acids	
Amino Acid	End Product
Glucogenic amino acids	
Alanine, serine, glycine, threonine, tryptophan	Pyruvic acid
Arginine, proline, histidine, glutamic acid	α-Ketoglutaric acid
Methionine, isoleucine, valine	Succinic acid (Coenzyme A ester)
Phenylalanine, tyrosine	Fumaric acid
Aspartic acid	Oxaloacetic acid
Ketogenic amino acids	
Tryptophan	Acetoacetic acid
Leucine	Acetyl coenzyme A
Phenylalanine, tyrosine, leucine, lysine	Acetoacetic acid (or CoA ester)

Some amino acids are metabolized in a manner whereby only a portion of their carbon skeletons are converted to glucose precursors. These amino acids may be either glucogenic or ketogenic and this is particularly true of phenylalanine, tyrosine and tryptophan. Products of amino acid catabolism also give rise to other important compounds needed by the body (Table 3.6).

Table 3.6 Some degradation products of selected amino acids	
Amino acid	Products of metabolism
Methionine	Homocysteine, cysteine, cystine and the methyl group of compounds such as creatine, choline and carnitine
Cysteine	Glutathione, taurine and the sulfate present in chondroitin sulfate and other mucopolysaccharides
Arginine	Ornithine (used by the chick in certain detoxification reactions), creatine, and urea
Histidine	Histamine
Lysine	Carnitine, desmosine
Phenylalanine and tyrosine	Thyroxine, adrenalin, noradrenalin, dopamine, melanin pigments

In some instances, feeding these metabolites will spare the dietary need for the amino acid from which they are derived. When creatine is added to a diet for chicks that is deficient in arginine, a growth improvement can generally be demonstrated. Alternatively, excesses of arginine added to diets marginally deficient in methionine causes a growth depression apparently because the arginine causes a greater biosynthesis of creatine, which also requires a methyl group from methionine.

Inorganic sulfate can replace a portion of dietary cystine under appropriate conditions. When chicks receive diets containing adequate amounts of methionine and suboptimal amounts of cystine, growth rate can be improved by addition of sodium or potassium sulfate to the diet, if this diet does not already contain 150 ppm or more of inorganic sulfate. Apparently sulfate spares cystine for the synthesis of taurine or sulfated mucopolysaccharides. The sulfate sulfur is not used to synthesize cystine *per se*.

Excess of amino acids beyond the metabolic needs for protein synthesis are degraded. The nitrogen of degraded amino acids is incorporated into uric acid while the carbon skeleton can be used for: (1) glucose synthesis; (2) fat synthesis or; (3) degraded directly to $CO_2 + H_2O$ and energy. Some amino acid degradation occurs constantly and there is a linear relationship between diet CP and the quantity of amino acids degraded. This is one reason why the utilization of dietary protein is never 100% efficient. Each amino acid has a specific pathway of degradation that may be modified according to levels of amino acid in the diet. When the dietary level of an amino acid is low, the enzymes of its degradative pathway are present at low levels while high dietary amino acids induce production of the enzymes responsible for degradation of those amino acids. This adaptation to level of protein intake helps to conserve amino acids when they are at low levels in the diet. In chickens, degradation of most amino acids occurs in the liver and kidney but leucine, isoleucine and valine are primarily degraded in muscle.

Because birds do not have a functioning urea cycle, arginine is not synthesized in the course of urea formation, and therefore is an essential amino acid for chickens. At least two separate enzymes required for arginine synthesis are lacking in avian kidney and nearly all enzymes of the urea cycle are absent from avian liver. Ornithine in chickens is not produced from glutamic acid as in most mammals. Citrulline can be converted to arginine by the chicken kidney and can be substituted for a limited amount of arginine in diets for chicks.

Chickens have a peculiar detoxifying process for excreting aromatic acids such as benzoic acid. This compound is conjugated with ornithine to form dibenzoylornithine prior to excretion in the urine. Since ornithine can arise only from the degradation of arginine, it is possible to produce an arginine deficiency in chicks by feeding excess benzoic acid under experimental conditions.

The essential enzyme for arginine degradation in chickens is arginase, which catalyzes the formation of urea and ornithine from arginine. This enzyme is found in the kidney mitochondria. The level of this enzyme can be increased when chicks are fed dietary excesses of arginine, lysine or several other amino acids such as histidine, isoleucine, tyrosine or ornithine. Small excesses of lysine in a diet can cause marked elevation of kidney arginase activity and increased arginine degradation. This results in a lysine-arginine antagonism in which dietary excess of lysine can cause a growth depression, which can be prevented by increasing the arginine level of the diet. For this reason the lysine content of a diet for growing chicks should be balanced against that of arginine. Dietary excesses of other amino acids that cause increased arginase activity in avian kidney also cause an increased arginine requirement of chicks. However, compared to lysine, much higher levels of these amino acids are necessary to have an influence on arginine requirement.

Avian kidney arginase activity also can be greatly decreased by certain amino acids in the diet. The amino acid α-aminoisobutyric acid (AIB) causes a striking reduction in avian kidney arginase activity when it is fed to chicks at as little as 0.5% of the diet. Under these circumstances arginine breakdown is greatly reduced and chicks fed arginine deficient diets may show improved growth when AIB is added to their diet. Higher levels of threonine and glycine have an effect similar to AIB. The complete picture of the lysine-arginine antagonism seems to be multifaceted. Arginine and lysine share transport systems in kidney tubules and excesses of one can cause reduced efficiency of reabsorption in the kidney and some urinary losses can occur. Reduced food intake, resulting from excess lysine, seems to be a factor in the interaction and high levels of dietary chloride seem to increase the effects of excess lysine on arginine requirement (see Section 3.14).

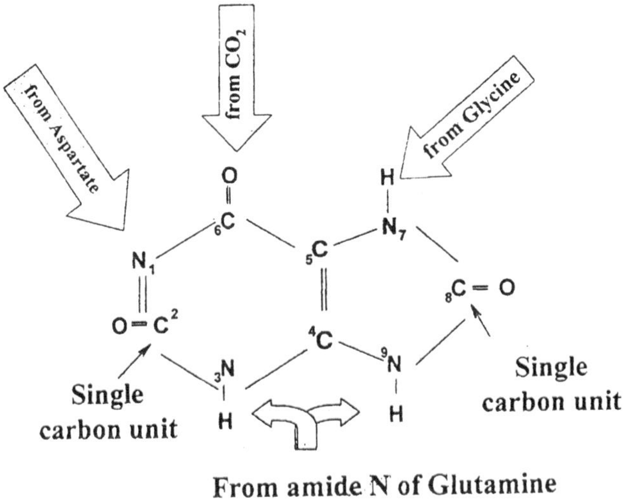

Figure 3.5 Uric acid synthesis

3.8   URIC ACID SYNTHESIS

Unlike mammals, birds secrete waste or excess nitrogen as uric acid rather than as urea. Uric acid is a purine synthesized by a series of reactions that also are used for synthesis of other purines such as adenine and guanine, which are components of DNA. The final step in uric acid synthesis is controlled by the enzyme xanthine oxidase, a molybdenum-containing enzyme. The level of xanthine oxidase in chick liver changes with protein level in the diet. The origin of the carbon and nitrogen atoms in uric acid is shown in Figure 3.5.

Avian kidney tubules actively secrete uric acid into the urine and the removal of uric acid from the blood is normally quite efficient. Blood uric acid levels rarely exceed 5-10 mg per 100 ml of chicken blood, even though adults may excrete 4-5 grams of uric acid per day. This is necessary in chickens since uric acid is extremely insoluble (0.4 mmol/litre) and when blood levels are elevated, uric acid may precipitate in joints, under the skin and in the kidney, producing severe gout. Similarly, kidney damage as sometimes occurs with infectious bronchitis infection may hamper uric acid excretion and cause uric acid to accumulate in the body. There have been descriptions of genetic strains of bird that have difficulty in clearing uric acid from the kidney tubules, and so are prone to gout. Birds carrying the dw dwarf gene seem to have higher rates of amino acid catabolism and urate synthesis. All these bird types are therefore susceptible to diets high in crude protein and/or amino acids.

Glycine is an integral part of the uric acid molecule. Each time a molecule of uric acid is excreted, a molecule of glycine is lost. This is the reason that chickens have a very high requirement for glycine. Although glycine is readily synthesized by chickens, this synthesis may not be rapid enough to satisfy needs for tissue growth and nitrogen excretion during periods of rapid growth. Serine is an intermediate in glycine biosynthesis and can substitute for dietary glycine under these conditions.

3.9   ENDOGENOUS NITROGEN AND AMINO ACID LOSSES

In measuring ileal digestibility values of AA's there is always the confounding effect of endogenous AA secretion into the lumen. This is substantial and is sometimes corrected by having reference animals that are not fed any diet, or given a protein-free diet. This does not totally resolve the problem, because protein metabolism *per se* is not the only factor influencing such endogenous losses. When feeding a protein-free diet endogenous AA secretions into the lumen are reduced, but still influenced by diet fiber and even level of feed intake. It has also been suggested that real digestibility values as opposed to TAA (true available amino acids) are specific to particular ingredients, and so must be measured with these ingredients.

Guanidation of lysine to homoarginine offers a potential means of measuring endogenous losses for individual animals under specific feeding scenarios. Lysine in proteins is converted to homoarginine (HA) by treatment with O-methylisourea under alkaline conditions. HA is not recycled in the gut because it is not incorporated into tissues. After intravenous infusion, HA is not found in the gut. Any lysine appearing in the digesta, must be of endogenous origin. Assuming the endogenous flow of amino acids into the gut lumen have a consistent profile, then measuring the appearance of lysine allows for estimates of endogenous secretion of the other amino acids. Such studies are necessarily short term because of the imposed lysine deficiency. When adult birds are fed a protein-free diet, the endogenous urinary nitrogen loss is around 140 mg/kg$^{.75}$/d. Metabolic fecal losses are about 40 mg/kg$^{.75}$/d depending on the fiber content of such a diet, and so 'maintenance' endogenous nitrogen losses total about 180 mg/ kg$^{.75}$/d. Estimates of total endogenous nitrogen losses in growing broiler chickens range from 200-300 mg/kg/d.

3.10 RATES OF PROTEIN SYNTHESIS

Protein accretion occurs as a result of protein synthesis, which is an ongoing process in all birds. Protein degradation also occurs, sometimes referred to as protein turnover. If protein synthesis (Ks) is larger than protein degradation (Kd) then protein accretion occurs. Such accretion is usually proportionally greater in younger birds, and also in birds consuming more protein/amino acids. However, even in a young, fast-growing broiler chicken fed adequate quantities of balanced protein, Kd can approach 30-40% of Ks. In order to improve efficiency of protein deposition Ks must be maximized and/or Kd minimized. From an energetic point of view it is always more efficient to ensure minimum Kd. It appears as though broiler strains have inadvertently been selected for increased Ks per unit of nucleus DNA. Also the fractional growth rate of broilers is about 50% higher than in Leghorn birds, while the fractional rate of protein deposition (Ks-Kd) is about 10% higher mainly due to reduced Kd.

Different organs and muscles exhibit different rates of protein synthesis. In the liver almost 10% of the labile protein is turned over each day and so Ks is close to 90%. On the other hand Ks in muscle of laying hens is only around 15% indicating a less dynamic system (Fig 3.6). If the mass of each organ is also taken into account in the laying hen, the liver and digestive tract account for about 25% of overall protein synthesis, and the oviduct around 15%.

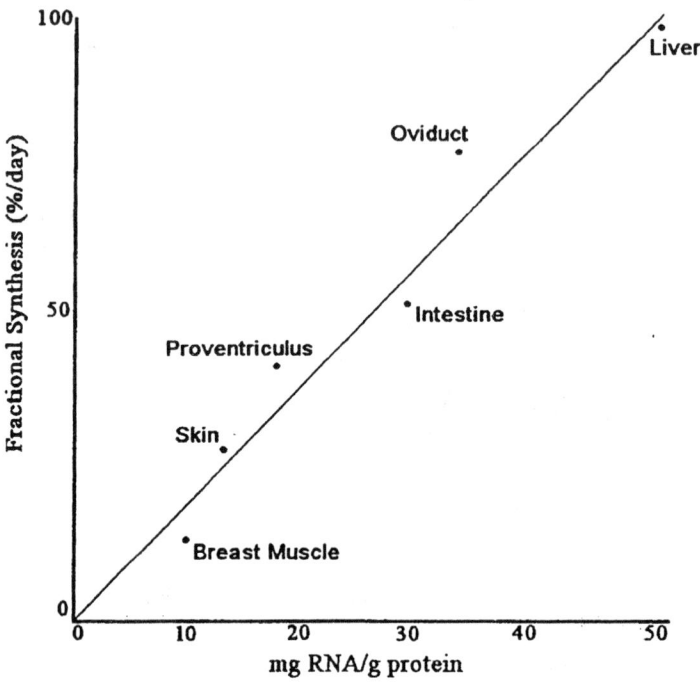

Figure 3.6 Fractional protein synthesis of layers
(Adapted from Hiramoto et al, 1989.)

The ability of a bird to deposit protein is obviously influenced by energy avail-ability. At intakes close to maintenance, little net protein accretion occurs under these situations. Even when birds are in negative nitrogen retention, Ks may still be occurring, but obviously Kd > Ks. As energy intake increases, then both protein and fat deposition occur. There are genetic limits to Ks, unlike fat accretion, and so as energy intake continues to increase, there will be more fat deposited in the carcass. The aim in supplying energy is to fuel maximum Ks while concomitantly placing arbitrary limits related to adipose hypertrophy and hyperplasia.

For the White Leghorn chicken consuming a diet of adequate protein and amino acids, protein synthesis at 3 weeks of age is around 10g/bird/day. With protein degradation at around 8g/bird/day, there is a resultant body protein accretion of about 2g/bird/day. Kang *et al.*, (1985) reported fractional rates of protein synthe-sis and protein degradation in broiler breast muscle.(Table 3.7).

Table 3.7 Protein synthesis and degradation rates in broiler breast meat				
	7d	**14d**	**28d**	**42d**
% Fractional protein synthesis (Ks)	48	24	17	16
% Fractional protein degradation (Kd)	16	11	9	12
%Δ (Kg)	32	13	8	4
Ks (mg/d)	700	1190	2500	5100
Kd (mg/d)	225	570	1340	3900
Kg (mg/d)	475	620	1160	1200
Adapted from Kang *et al.*, (1985)				

After 28d, it seems as though breast muscle is being deposited at about 8g/d (assuming muscle is around 12% protein). The study shown in Table 3.7 was conducted 20 years ago and since that time higher rates of breast meat deposition have occurred as a result of genetic selection. Nieto *et al.*, (1994) showed that fractional rates of protein synthesis are less affected than expected by amino acid balance of the diet. For example synthesis rates were similar for broilers fed corn-soy diets with or without methionine supplementation. However birds grew faster on the more balanced protein, suggesting that with marginal levels of amino acid supply, it is Kd rather than Ks that is affected. Higher rates of growth in this situation are presumably due to lower Kd since there is less need to supply the limiting amino acid(s)

3.11   ENERGY COST OF PROTEIN METABOLISM

Both the synthesis and degradation of protein and amino acids are energy demanding processes and these costs are necessarily included in model predictions of energy balance. Uric acid synthesis is much more energy demanding than is urea synthesis, and so birds inherit an energy cost for excreting an insoluble nitrogenous product. Buttery and Boorman (1976) estimate energy cost of uric acid synthesis at about 330 kcal/mole, compared to just 85 kcal/mole for urea production. These same workers suggest the energy cost of protein deposition to be around 0.7 kcal/g protein deposition. For a 900g chick Buttery *et al.*, (1973) calculate total costs of protein anabolism, turnover and uric acid synthesis to represent about 11% of ME intake (Table 3.8).

Table 3.8 Estimates of the energy cost of protein metabolism in 900g birds	
Muscle accretion (3.9g)	= 23 kcal/d
Muscle turnover (6.8g)	= 5 kcal/d
Uric acid synthesis (1gN)	= 6 kcal/d
Total	34 kcal/d
Intake	= 300 kcal/d
∴ Cost protein metabolism	10%
Buttery *et al.,* (1973)	

In other studies it has been shown that feeding diets devoid of supplemental methionine, which effectively gives a methionine deficient diet, increases energy cost by an extra 1%. This latter cost is presumably related to increased synthesis of uric acid and perhaps increased protein catabolism necessary to maintain blood amino acid profiles.

3.12   DIET PROTEIN VS. SYNTHETIC AMINO ACIDS

Nutritionists currently use synthetic sources of methionine and lysine and in certain situations threonine and tryptophan may be considered as dietary ingredients. Such synthetic amino acids are assumed to be utilized 100% since there is no loss due to ineffective digestion. The same amino acids in intact proteins, such as soybean meal, may be only 90% digestible, and so free amino acids seem to have distinct advantages as ingredients. However, not all amino acids within intact proteins need to be released as such during digestion, because there is some absorption of peptides. In fact, uptake of amino acids as peptides may be advantageous to the bird, relative to processing of free amino acids from within the gut lumen. Boorman and Ellis (1996) suggest that one advantage of a bird utilizing peptides is that there will be less bacterial degradation within the digesta and that this activity should not be underestimated.

It has been shown that when pigs eat their feed as one (restricted) meal, utilization of synthetic lysine is only about 60% of expectation, due not to impaired absorption, but to the sudden overwhelming supply of free lysine exceeding immediate metabolic needs. We are unaware of comparable studies conducted in poultry. Sudden influxes of feed are not normal in poultry, and in broiler breeder pullets that are severely restricted in feed, use of synthetic amino acids as a proportion of total amino acids is quite small. Apart from the suggestion about interference by bacterial degradation, it is assumed that synthetic amino acids are utilized as efficiently as are those in digestible intact proteins, in most practical feeding situations.

If the diet contains a preponderance of synthetic amino acids, there could be a limitation on supply of non-essential nitrogen, either as intact protein or free amino acids. In a normal diet the supply of non-essential nitrogen arises from dietary non-essential amino acids plus any excess of essential amino acids. When more synthetic amino acids are used, not only is crude protein supply reduced but excess of limiting amino acids is usually minimized. Limiting supplies of non-essential nitrogen is often quoted as a cause for poorer performance of birds fed low protein-amino acid fortified diets, although this concept has never been adequately quantitated. There are about equal numbers of well-conducted studies by eminent researchers showing normal or sub-optimal growth, when protein content of the diet is reduced. Such differential results may occur from overestimation of amino acid supply in intact proteins, failure to maintain supply of some other nutrients that influence amino acid utilization, strain differences in amino acid needs (most unlikely scenario) or failure of growth *per se* to fully quantitate the complex reaction of birds to amino acid supply. For young broiler chickens at least, caution is necessary when using diets with crude protein equivalents of much less than 16-17% assuming optimum growth rate is desired. Likewise, the growth rate of birds is often inferior when regardless of amino acid balance, the ratio of crude protein:synthetic amino acids is much less than 16:1.

3.13   CRUDE PROTEIN AFFECTS AMINO ACID NEEDS

Theoretically, protein quality or amino acid balance should not affect bird performance as long as all amino acids are at requirement and there is no overt antagonism. For example, supplying a diet higher in crude protein but with poor amino acid balance should elicit the same growth response as a diet formulated to exactly meet the birds requirements, assuming both provide the same level of the limiting amino acid. In practice, the poorly balanced diet usually results in inferior performance. This situation suggests that in "poor quality" diets, the amino acids are in such disproportion as to impair the utilization of the first limiting amino acid. Boorman and Ellis (1996) studied this phenomena in diets formulated to total amino acid levels. These workers concluded that the limiting amino acid is used with the same efficiency in so called 'good' or 'poor' quality protein diets, and that impaired growth with the latter cannot be explained on reduced utilization of the first limiting amino acid. Boorman and Ellis (1996) suggest a more likely cause of impaired growth with poor quality - amino acid adequate diets, is reduced net energy resulting from an increase in gluconeogenesis. Alternately there may be increased catabolism of the limiting amino acid from muscle in order to maintain homeostasis of plasma amino acid levels. These data suggest that it is not always economical to arbitrarily increase the crude protein level of a diet in order to meet the 'requirement' level of the limiting amino acid.

Poorer than expected results may be a consequence of the requirement for the limiting amino acid actually increasing with increments of crude protein. If this concept is correct, then it makes it very difficult to adequately feed birds in regions where protein ingredient supply is limited and of inferior quality. Morris *et al.*, (1999) suggest that amino acid requirements, expressed as a percentage of the diet, will increase with increase in protein level of the diet. Considering all possible reasons for such an effect, Morris *et al.*, (1999) conclude that the only reasonable explanation is a form of generalized amino acid imbalance. Distinct from specific imbalances (lysine:argine etc.) this situation arises due to impairment of the first limiting amino acid resulting from loading the diet with protein *per se*, which perhaps causes a change in efficiency of protein utilization for muscle deposition or for maintenance needs. Reviewing available data, Morris *et al.*, (1999) applied regression analysis to derive a prediction for change in amino acid need relative to protein level of the diet:

$$\% \text{ lysine} \quad = \quad 0.057\% \text{ CP}$$

$$\% \text{ tryptophan} \quad = \quad 0.012\% \text{ CP}$$

$$\% \text{ methionine} \quad = \quad 0.025\% \text{ CP}$$

By deduction, we can likewise assume the coefficient for methionine + cystine to be 0.05% CP. Using these values, Table 3.9 was developed using standard amino acid requirement values for a 22% CP broiler starter and then varying protein by increments of 2% for a range of 18-26% CP. Simply changing crude protein in the diet regardless of amino acid balance, means that lysine needs, for example, change from 1.02 to 1.47% of the diet, as diet CP increases from 18 to 26%. Surisdiarto and Farrell (1991) show a similar change in lysine needs of broilers as crude protein level changes from 15 to 22% (Fig 3.7).

Table 3.9 Prediction of percentage amino acid requirements based on change in amino acid need due to change in crude protein as suggested by Morris et al., (1999)					
	Prediction		Standard	Prediction	
	18%	20% CP	22% CP	24% CP	26% CP
Lysine	1.02	1.13	1.25	1.36	1.47
Methionine	0.40	0.45	0.50	0.55	0.60
Methionine + Cystine	0.70	0.80	0.90	1.00	1.10
Tryptophan	0.20	0.22	0.24	0.26	0.28

It is more common today to feed lower protein diets in order to limit early growth of broilers and so it is reasonable to use lower amino acid levels. More problematic perhaps is the increased amino acid supply necessary to optimize growth when higher crude protein levels are used. This situation can occur where poorer quality feed ingredients are used which is often a situation that does not coincide with the economic ability to supply such generous levels of synthetic amino

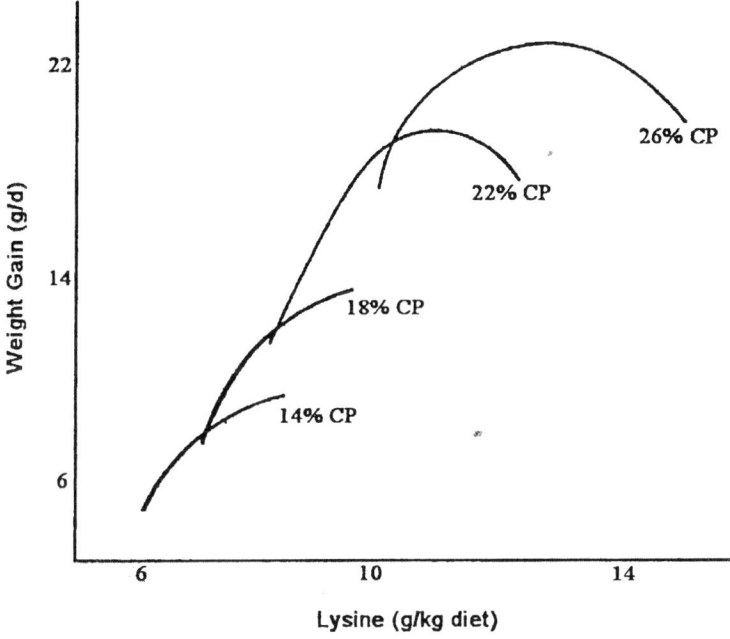

Figure 3.7 Change in lysine needs relative to diet crude protein
(Adapted from Surisdiarto and Farrell, 1991)

acids. If diets high in crude protein are necessary, as often occur in developing countries; and if the assumption of Morris *et al.*, (1999) is confirmed, then it would be wise to accept lower nutrient dense diets rather than attempting to maintain arbitrary standards for say, lysine or methionine, a situation, which often dictates these protein levels. The poor quality of a protein source cannot be accommodated by simply providing more of the ingredient.

3.14 AMINO ACID INTERACTIONS

In certain situations the levels of amino acids in a diet cannot be considered independently of the concentrations of other amino acids and nutrients. The classical situation is exemplified by interdependence of lysine with arginine, lysine with some electrolytes and between the branched chain amino acids leucine, isoleucine and valine. Four states of amino acid adequacy are often described, although all are not true interactions involving interdependence:

Deficiency - one or a number of amino acids do not meet the bird's need. All amino acids could be within an ideal balance, but fed at inadequate levels.

Imbalance - a situation where at least one amino acid is below requirement level.

The effective protein/amino acid content of the diet is dictated by the concentration of the limiting amino acid.

Antagonism - the classical situation in which the level of (usually) one amino acid influences the metabolism of another amino acid. All amino acids are often at or above theoretical requirement level, yet because of an induced metabolic deficiency, performance is sub-optimal.

Toxicity - when a very high level of an amino acid (often > 2x requirement) causes poor growth, which usually cannot be corrected by supplementing with other amino acids to re-set the balance.

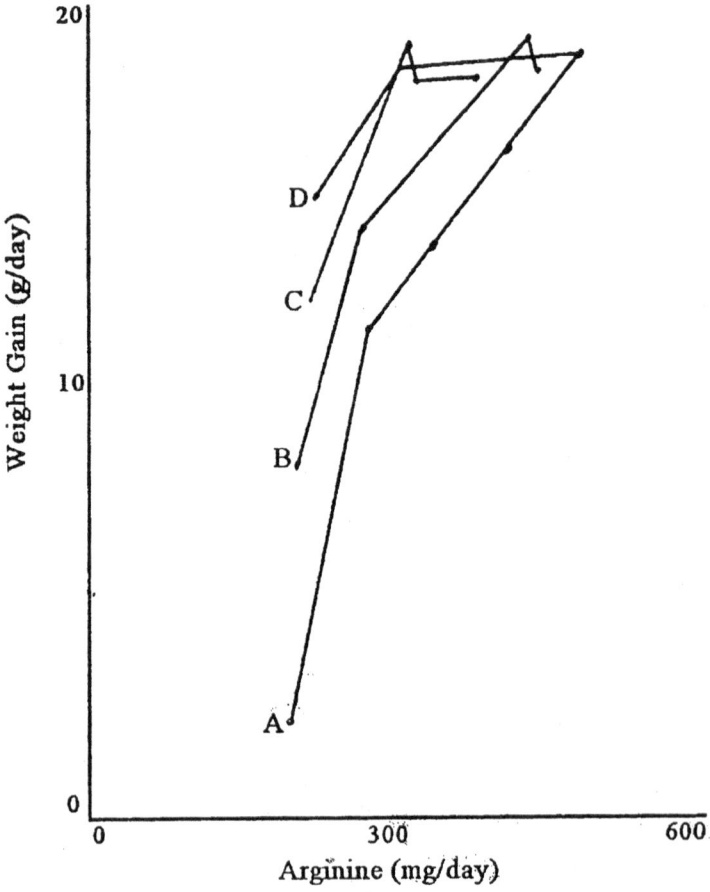

Figure 3.8 Growth response to arginine of chicks fed variable lysine levels; A=18.0g/kg; B=16.0g/kg; C=13.5g/kg; D=11.0·g/kg (Adapted from D'Mello & Lewis, 1970)

It is often difficult to differentiate cause and effect with such derangements of amino acid levels, although decline in feed intake is invariably a prelude to reduced growth rate. In fact, chicks respond very quickly to major deficiencies, imbalances, and antagonism etc. of dietary amino acids, with decline in feed intake sometimes noticed within hours of offering such diets. Imbalance of amino acids also cause change in amino acid transport systems or reduction in protein synthesis and increase in protein degradation, and there is usually increased catabolism of excess amino acids. The antagonism between lysine and arginine has been well documented in young chicks (Fig 3.8).

These two amino acids share common cell membrane transport systems, and so excess of one amino acid will lead to increased competition with cell transport. More specifically, lysine impairs the resorption of arginine in the kidney, and also stimulates the production of arginase enzyme, also in the kidney, leading to arginine breakdown and formation of ornithine and some urea. If moderately high levels of lysine (1.6% for the young chick) are fed in combination with marginal levels of arginine (0.8%) then up to 25% of arginine can be degraded leading to a severe reduction in growth rate. Austic (1978) suggested that performance is somewhat improved under these conditions when arginase inhibitors are fed, but since growth rate is still abnormal, then the antagonism may have a negative effect on feed intake. It is possible that the induced imbalance of amino acids has a direct effect on hypothalamic receptors. Infusing imbalanced amino acid mixtures into the carotid artery causes almost immediate reduction in the feed intake of rats. Infusing the same mixture into the jugular vein has a less profound effect, presumably because the liver intervenes prior to the blood reaching the brain. Most animals will, in fact, preferentially select a protein-free diet over an amino acid imbalanced diet when given a choice-feeding situation. In this later situation, force feeding the imbalanced diet will partially correct growth depression, a situation that obviously will never occur with a protein-free diet.

The antagonism between lysine and arginine may also be influenced by dietary levels of other amino acids. For example histidine and leucine seem to stimulate argininase production while threonine has the opposite effect. Presumably diets high in lysine, histidine, and leucine will have the most deleterious effect on the bird's arginine status. At this time it is unclear if moderately high levels of threonine would counteract the deleterious effect of high dietary lysine with diets marginal in arginine. Virtually all experimentation involving lysine-arginine have been conducted with young birds. There is anecdotal evidence that the antagonism is much less noticeable in mature birds. Muramatsu *et al.*, (1991) attempted to quantitate the relationship between lysine and arginine, suggesting that arginine utilization will decline linearly as lysine level increases:

% arginine efficiency = 140.82 - 4.916 (Lysine g/kg diet).

Arginine efficiency is therefore 100% at a lysine level of 8 g/kg. At 1.25% dietary lysine as is now common for young broiler chicks, arginine potency declines to 80%. If a lysine:arginine ratio of 100:105 is to be maintained, as suggested by ideal protein then the arginine level needs to be 1.31% and assuming an efficiency of 80%, this suggests a diet concentration of 1.64%. This level may be difficult to achieve under practical feeding situations since it is uneconomical to consider synthetic arginine at this time.

The metabolism of lysine, and hence its potential interaction with arginine can be influenced by electrolyte balance of the diet. Scott and Austic (1978) were one of the first to show that high levels of potassium (1.8%) have an ameliorating effect on growth depression caused by high lysine intakes. Potassium seems to stimulate lysine-α-ketoglutarate reductase, an enzyme involved in lysine catabolism. If, because of ingredient selection, diets are necessarily very high in lysine, then growth rate can be normalized by feeding potassium carbonate. In subsequent studies Calvert and Austic (1981) showed that comparable high levels of chloride can exacerbate the lysine-arginine antagonism. There have also been concerns about the level of ionophore anticoccidials affecting lysine-arginine balance, although work with monensin fails to support the concern.

A further complication to the involvement of lysine in arginine metabolism, is the effect of environmental temperature. Brake et al., (1998) suggest that at high temperature, then in the presence of equimolar concentrations of lysine, the uptake of arginine by the intestinal epithelium is reduced during heat stress conditions. Environmental temperature may therefore exacerbate the lysine-arginine interaction by simply reducing arginine absorption from the diet. There are also interactions between the branch-chained amino acids. An increase in the dietary level of leucine leads to increased need for both valine and isoleucine. A corresponding increase in isoleucine leads to increased need for valine and leucine. These interactions manifest themselves through impaired growth rate and/or abnormal feathering. Muramatsu et al., (1991) suggest that efficacy of valine and isoleucine can be described in relation to dietary leucine:

$$\% \text{ efficacy valine} = 111.4 - (1.115 \times \text{Leucine, g/kg}) + (0.00813 \times \text{Leucine}^2 \text{g/kg})$$

$$\% \text{ efficacy isoleucine} = 104.4 - (0.564 \times \text{Leucine g/kg}).$$

Feed intake may again be the major factor influenced by antagonisms within these three amino acids. With mild antagonism, the depression in feed intake may be almost totally normalized within 48 hrs, although with more severe antagonism feed intake remains depressed and growth rate declines. A moderate excess of leucine does seem to increase the catabolism of isoleucine.

Toxicities of amino acids seem quite rare, because very high levels are needed to elicit a response. Koelkebeck et al., (1991) reported that laying hens performed normally when either 1% of lysine, methionine, threonine or tryptophan were added to a diet already adequate in all amino acids. Theoretically adding 1% lysine should have predisposed an antagonism with arginine, and so this reinforces the statement made earlier that older birds seem less susceptible to situations of apparent amino acid antagonism.

Some amino acids can be converted to, or be part of, the structure of specific vitamins. Choline can be synthesized from monomethyethanolamine or dimethylethanolamine, as long as methyl groups are contributed by methionine (or betaine). Compared to the synthesis of choline in mammals, the process is very inefficient in birds and only under extreme dietary situations would such choline synthesis be meaningful to the bird. Choline can also donate methyl groups for the biosynthesis of methionine from homocysteine, although again the process is very inefficient relative to the birds need for larger quantities of methionine.

Tryptophan can also be converted to niacin (see Chapter 4). The conversion, which requires pyridoxine as a co-factor is quite inefficient in birds because of relatively low inherent concentrations of a key enzyme, picolinic acid carboxylase.

3.15   DIGESTIBLE AMINO ACIDS

Amino acids in most ingredients will not be totally digested, and knowledge of such efficiency is important in formulating diets. Many essential amino acids in common ingredients such as corn and soybean meal are digested with about 90% efficiency, although there are some differences among individual amino acids. For some vegetable protein ingredients, amino acid digestibility can be much lower, while for animal proteins there is more variance associated with severity of heat processing. Digestibility is essentially a function of endogenous enzyme secretion as digesta traverses through to the ileum. However, inspection and analyses of excreta is complicated by cecal activity, endogenous amino acid loss and potential loss in the urine (Figure 3.9).

Measuring digestible or metabolizable amino acid supply is somewhat more complex than comparable studies described in Chapter 2 for estimates of energy availability. Digestible amino acids will be assimilated in the liver and, depending upon dietary balance, most will appear as eggs or body tissue including feathers. Some amino acids will be unusable and most will be deaminated to form uric acid. There will be virtually no amino acid loss in the urine for normal healthy birds and so the mixing of urine with feces is not problematic for estimates of amino acid digestibility. Determination of digestible protein or nitrogen is obviously more complex because it is very difficult to separate urine and fecal sources of nitrogen without resorting to surgical intervention.

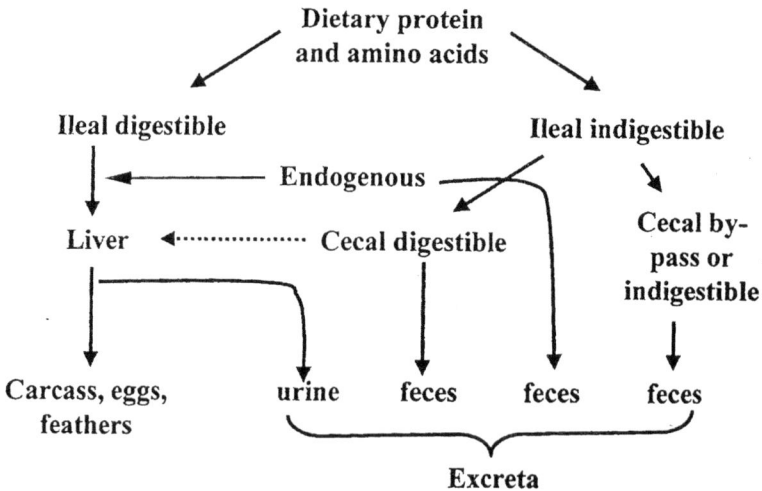

Figure 3.9 Schematic of amino acid and protein digestion.

If digesta could be sampled at the ileum, as is common in swine nutrition studies, then it would be quite straight forward to determine amino acid digestibility. Birds, and especially young birds, are difficult to surgically modify with ileal fistulas. Determination of ileal digestibility can therefore only be carried out by sacrificing the bird, sampling the ileal digesta for amino acids and an inert marker, and relating these to diet concentrations. More commonly amino acid digestibility (availability) is determined by assay of the excreta using a procedure similar to that developed for TME.

True digestibility of amino acids can only be determined if a correction for endogenous losses is accommodated. While most amino acids appearing in the excreta originate from the diet, some will be endogenous in origin, and represent amino acids secreted into the gut lumen as enzymes, hormones, sloughed epithelial cells and free amino acids. The correction for endogenous amino acid losses is quite small (2-4%) for birds fed within 20-30% of ad libitum intake, but can represent 15-20% of amino acid secretions for birds given very small quantities of feed that are below maintenance requirement. However there is still considerable controversy surrounding methodology for estimating endogenous amino acid losses in the fed bird. Simply starving the bird (or related birds) for a time period equivalent to the collection for fed birds was a technique originally proposed for estimating endogenous losses. It quickly became apparent that such estimates were low because the physical presence of feed in the tract induces more endogenous losses. Johnson (1992) quotes values of around 300, 600 and 780 mg/bird/48h for endogenous amino acids in adult cockerels that were fasted or fed a protein-free diet either low or high in fiber respectively. Parsons *et al.*, (1983) also showed that the amino acid profile of such endogenous losses can be influenced by the composition of such protein-free diets. Increasing the fiber content of the diet increases the endogenous loss of most essential amino acids, presumably because they are contained in epithelial cells lost from the digestive tract. Using moderate levels (4-5%) of pure cellulose in a protein-free diet seems to provide a reliably consistent, and hopefully representative, estimate of endogenous amino acid losses over a 24-48h period. Another complexity in determining digestibility of amino acids, is the role of the ceca. Some, but not all digesta will enter the paired ceca where proteins can be digested and some amino acids degraded. The major unknown factor in cecal digestion is the usefulness of products of anaerobic digestion for the bird. The ceca are not well supplied with blood vessels and even for wild birds such as grouse, it is unclear just what role the active ceca play in the bird's nutrition. In the wild, there is undoubtedly some coprophagy, which can be useful to the bird, although this action is minimal in a caged bird. Early studies on amino acid digestibility indicated that the cecal microflora had little influence on results. If cecectomized birds are used in the assay, then there are minor effects for cereals and most vegetable proteins, although quite large differences are seen with animal proteins (Green and Kiener, 1989, Table 3.10).

Table 3.10 Effect of cecectomy on true amino acid digestibility (%)			
	Bird type	Soybean meal	Meat meal
Lysine	Regular	91	85
	Cecectomized	92	79
Methionine	Regular	87	89
	Cecectomized	91	85
All amino acids	Regular	92	85
	Cecectomized	91	75
			Adapted from Green and Kiener (1989)

There is up to a 10% increase in true digestibility of amino acids in products such as meat meal due to the microbial activity of the ceca. Presumably the cecal microbes digest any intact undigested proteins entering from the large intestine, although it seems certain that most products of digestion are then excreted, rather than being picked up by the venous system. It appears that the cecal microbes are most influential in affecting the digestibility of products with inherently low digestibility.

Another problem caused by the cecal microbes, is their influence on endogenous amino acid losses. When protein-free diets are fed to measure such output, then cecectomized birds will have a much higher output, again due to less breakdown of amino acids by the microbes. In most amino acid digestibility studies today, it is advisable to use cecectomized birds. Table 3.11 shows estimates of true amino acid digestibility compiled by NRC (1994).

Table 3.11 True digestibility coefficients (%)					
	Methionine	Cystine	Lysine	Arginine	Threonine
Corn	91	85	81	89	84
Wheat	87	87	81	88	83
Soybean meal	92	82	91	92	88
Corn gluten meal	97	86	88	96	92
Meat meal	85	58	79	85	79
Wheat shorts	80	69	81	86	79
Feather meal	76	59	66	83	73
					NRC (1994)

There is little advantage to using digestible amino acid values when diets are composed of ingredients such as corn and soybean meal. However when ingredients of lower amino acid digestibility are used, then there are distinct advantages to formulation based on available or digestible amino acids. Rostagno *et al.*, (1995) show such an advantage when corn-soybean meal diets are compared to more complex diets containing some poultry by-product meal, meat meal and 1% feather meal (Table 3.12). In the complex diet levels of available amino acids were adjusted by including synthetics to equate the available amino acids supplied by the corn-soy diet.

Table 3.12 Performance of broilers fed diets formulated to total or available amino acids			
Diet type Amino acid formulation	Corn-Soy Total	Complex Total	Complex Available
42d body weight gain (g)	2333a	2241b	2330a
1-42d Feed:Gain	1.79a	1.85b	1.80a
		Adapted from Rostagno *et al.*, (1995)	

3.16 IDEAL PROTEIN

The concept of an ideal protein was first described by Mitchell (1964) who attempted to produce a diet that met the chick's requirements using purified ingredients. Simulating the amino acid profile of such 'ideal' proteins as egg white and casein was however, only partly successful in attempting to optimize growth and feed efficiency. Likewise, subsequent formulation of amino acids linked to body composition of the bird also failed to optimize growth. It was only after modeling the amino acid needs for maintenance, growth and feather production that formulations resulted in a more consistent and optimum growth. The Agricultural Research Council in the United Kingdom, was the first to propose an ideal protein for pigs in which lysine was used as the reference amino acid. Giving lysine a value of 100%, the other amino acids are ranked accordingly with, for example, methionine + cystine at 50% and tryptophan at 15%. Regardless of protein or energy level, the balance of all amino acids will remain constant. The reasoning behind using an ideal amino acid profile with lysine as a standard is based on the premise that adequate information is not available on requirement values for all amino acids under all conditions. Likewise it is difficult to obtain precise information on the profile of all amino acids in ingredients. On the other hand, there is a vast wealth of data on lysine requirements and digestible lysine content of ingredients. Lysine is also relatively easy to assay. A limitation of these early estimates was an assumption that the optimal concentration of lysine in protein is 7% for pigs, regardless of age or body size. Also the estimate relied heavily on the profile of the pig carcass with less emphasis on maintenance needs.

Only about 30-40% of amino acids needed for growth and metabolism originate directly from the diet with the largest proportion coming from on-going tissue catabolism. Because each amino acid has different rates of catabolism, then this situation influences calculation of need, and infers a different profile relative to analyses of body composition at any one point in time. This is especially true for lysine, which has a relatively low oxidation rate and this leads to overestimation of lysine needs (or lysine relative to actively catabolized amino acids such as methionine) when the basis of calculation is solely on carcass or body composition. Wang and Fuller (1989) again working with pigs, attempted to improve the ideal protein estimates for pigs by including a proportional maintenance component.

Table 3.13 Comparison of ideal protein, with relative amino acid estimates of NRC (1994) and commercial broiler diet formulations

	0-21d			21-42d		
	Ideal[1]	NRC[2]	Commercial[3]	Ideal	NRC	Commercial
Lysine	100	100	100	100	100	100
Meth+Cys	72	82	68	75	72	66
Methionine	36	45	40	36	38	40
Cystine	36	36	28	·39	34	26
Arginine	105	114	100	108	110	100
Valine	77	82	67	80	82	60 ·
Threonine	67	73	58	70	74	55
Tryptophan	16	18	17	17	18	15
Isoleucine	67	73	63	69	73	50
Histidine	32	32	33	32	32	29
Phe+Tyr	105	122	117	105	122	100
Leucine	109	109	117	109	109	100

Han and Baker (1994); [2]NRC (1994); [3]Leeson and Summers (1997)

The University of Illinois has seen considerable research in this area and most recently Baker and co-workers (1998) have developed an ideal protein for young broilers. The main difference between the chicken data and that originally proposed for the pig, is greater relative need for arginine and methionine with less need for tryptophan. Table 3.13, compares the ideal protein as proposed by Han and Baker (1994) from Illinois with relative values shown by NRC (1994) and commercial diet estimates of Leeson and Summers (1997). The ideal protein is often a compromise between research estimates (NRC, 1994) and commercial diet specifications as suggested by Leeson and Summers (1997). All estimates of nutrient requirements have some biases inherent in their system of calculation and development. For ideal protein, the major current limitation perhaps relates to change in carcass composition of modern broilers, where there is greater emphasis on lean meat yield. A leaner animal, or one with greater proportional muscle yield, will likely have different amino acid needs. For breast meat yield most emphasis has been placed on lysine, which is obviously the most critical amino acid in ideal protein. Also, as broilers are grown to heavier weights, the early estimates may need adjustment to account for proportionally greater maintenance. Undoubtedly these factors will be accounted for as newer estimates of ideal protein evolve.

Mack *et al.*, (1999) recently developed ideal protein values, based on true fecal amino acid digestibility with results very similar to the Illinois data shown in Table 3.13. Because all estimates of ideal protein use lysine as a standard, it is obvious that estimates of lysine requirements must be very exact. Baker and co-workers at Illinois (Edwards *et al.*, 1999), in fact, question some of their own previous assumptions about lysine needs. As previously described, the requirement for any amino acid is based on model predicted needs for maintenance and growth. Lysine estimates for maintenance usually show relatively low values per unit of body mass compared to other amino acids such as methionine. Lysine is therefore regarded as a more 'inert' amino acid, with low rates of degradation (Kd). Most estimates of lysine requirements for maintenance are calculated using zero nitrogen retention as the main criterion. Using a lysine deficient diet, the bird will be in negative nitrogen balance while adding lysine will reduce this deficit. At some point, nitrogen equilibrium is achieved and this is the estimate of lysine need for maintenance. Edwards *et al.*, (1999) suggest that a more relevant criteria, is zero lysine balance, rather than zero nitrogen balance. These workers suggest lysine maintenance requirement at around 7 mg/kg$^{.75}$ /d using zero nitrogen balance studies. If zero lysine balance is used, then maintenance estimate increases dramatically to 89 mg/kg$^{.75}$. This apparent dicotomy is based on the premise that at zero nitrogen balance, the bird is still loosing lysine due to catabolism of muscle. Because the bird is in zero nitrogen balance, this situation infers that other amino acids are actually accreting, (at the expense of lysine). For example, higher levels of proline and glycine are seen in the protein of chicks fed low protein diets, which is probably a reflection of collagen synthesis. If this situation is substantiated, then it questions our estimates of lysine needs, especially for older broilers because they have ever increasing maintenance needs and ideal protein estimates, for such birds, may need to be adjusted relative to current standards.

Formulating diets based on estimates of ideal protein has proven successful in terms of optimizing growth and feed utilization, although results are not always economically attractive. Also using ideal protein to formulate low protein diets supplemented with synthetic amino acids still results in inferior broiler performance.

3.17   PROTEIN QUALITY

Individual proteins are characterized by having a definite amino acid makeup which is exactly reproducible from the parent to its progeny. Some single proteins are good sources of all essential amino acids, while others are very deficient or devoid of one or more of the essential amino acids. The biological value of a protein, which is defined and discussed later in this chapter, is high if it contains all of the essential amino acids in the proper ratio for birds. However, if even a single essential amino acid is missing, the biological value of the protein is zero. The overall amino acid makeup of a product depends upon the relative combination of the various individual constituent proteins. The biological value of corn can be improved by changing the relative levels of the various individual proteins within the corn seed. Normal hybrid corn, for example, is generally recognized not only as having a low protein content, but also as having a protein of poor biological value for animals because of deficiencies in several of the nutritionally essential amino acids, particularly lysine. Lysine deficiency of hybrid corn is known to be due to its high content of the individual protein zein, which is very low in both lysine and tryptophan. Through genetic selection, there have been attempts in isolating a variety of corn which contains a lower amount of zein and a much higher percentage of glutelin. Since glutelin is higher in lysine and tryptophan than is zein, the resultant Opaque-2 corn has a much higher biological value for poultry and other animals because it contains lysine and the other essential amino acids in approximately the proper amounts to meet the bird's requirements.

Not all proteins in plant materials are beneficial for animals. For example, soybean, which is the most plentiful protein source for use in animal feeds in the world has certain drawbacks. In addition to a high amount of protein, which has an excellent amino acid balance except for a deficiency of methionine, the soybean also contains several proteins that are detrimental for chicks. These inhibit growth, interfere with trypsin digestion of proteins in the gastro-intestinal tract of the bird, cause enlargement of the pancreas and interfere with the absorption of dietary fats in the young chick. Fortunately, these proteins are destroyed when flaked soybeans or soybean meal are heat treated.

In addition to specific proteins, plants contain free glutamine, free asparagine, other free amino acids, some peptides, inorganic nitrates, ammonium salts, and many other nitrogenous compounds. The amounts of nitrates and ammonia vary considerably depending upon the intensity of fertilizer application to the soil in which the plants are grown. The lignins of the cell walls of green plants contain nitrogen, but wood lignins are practically nitrogen-free. Of the non-protein nitrogenous substances in plants, glutamine and asparagine represent the major portion. These amino acid amides are believed to serve in the transport of nitrogen to the various cells throughout the plant.

In the 1930-40s it was shown that when animal protein sources such as fish meal, meat scrap and dried skimmed milk, were added to poultry diets, results were vastly superior to those obtained with similar diets containing only plant proteins. The mysterious extra values previously ascribed to proteins of animal origin have been elucidated. It is now generally accepted that highly digestible plant proteins, heat-treated to remove inhibitors, and properly supplemented with essential amino acids where needed, will produce results equivalent or sometimes superior to those obtained with the animal protein supplements. The factors responsible for the early superiority of animal proteins as compared with plant proteins were: (1) the calcium and phosphorus supplied by the bone in animal protein supplements; (2) B-complex vitamins, particularly riboflavin, in dried skimmed milk and whey; (3) vitamin B_{12}, which is present in all animal materials, but not in plants; and finally (4) the amino acids methionine and lysine, which are present in the proteins of fish, eggs and milk at much higher levels than in the common protein supplements of plant origin.

The essential amino acid composition of the mixed proteins of poultry meat and eggs compared with that of the proteins of corn, soy and fish meal is presented in Table 3.14. It is apparent that poultry meat and eggs are relatively high in many of the essential amino acids. These amino acids also are present in approximately the optimum proportions for good chick growth, and this situation is true of most animal proteins. This is why animal proteins have long been recognized to have a higher biological value than do most plant proteins.

Table 3.14 Essential amino acid composition of the proteins of chicken meat, eggs, corn, soybean and fish meal

Amino acid	% of Protein				
	Chicken tissue	Egg	Corn	Soybean meal	Fish meal
Arginine	7.3	6.4	5.0	7.5	6.7
Cystine	2.5	2.2	1.3	1.7	1.8
Histidine	4.0	2.3	2.5	2.7	2.7
Isoleucine	3.9	5.0	6.3	5.4	6.8
Leucine	6.5	8.3	12.5	7.7	8.3
Lysine	9.6	7.1	2.5	6.7	8.8
Methionine	1.9	3.2	2.5	1.5	3.0
Phenylalanine	3.6	4.7	6.3	5.2	4.5
Threonine	3.4	5.0	5.0	4.2	4.8
Tryptophan	1.0	1.4	1.3	1.5	1.0
Valine	4.4	6.5	5.0	5.2	6.0

3.18   ASSESSING PROTEIN QUALITY

Throughout the study of animal nutrition, researchers have attempted to develop improved methods for determining the relative effectiveness of dietary proteins in meeting the bird's protein and amino acid requirements.

3.18.1 Nitrogen balance

In experiments conducted during the 1850's it was noted that a dog weighing 35 kilograms excreted 12 g of urea in 24 hours, and that the same dog after receiving 2,500 g of meat excreted 184 g of urea. In the late 1800's Voit showed that if the quantity of protein administered corresponded exactly to that oxidized during starvation, nitrogen equilibrium was not established because some of the body's tissue also was metabolized. The amount of body tissue lost decreased steadily as the amount of protein in the diet was gradually increased, until finally a point of nitrogen equilibrium was reached at which point the amount of protein ingested was exactly equal to the amount catabolised in the body. This method is still used to determine the effectiveness of a given diet to maintain birds in nitrogen balance. However, as previously described in Section 3.16 zero balance of a particular amino acid may occur at a higher intake than does zero nitrogen balance.

3.18.2 Biological value

This measure is defined as the percentage of digested and absorbed protein that is retained by the bird. Egg white protein is usually used as a standard and given an arbitrary value of 100. Standard conditions for measurement of biological value involve the use of low protein diets (approximately 9-10% protein) and measurement of true digestibility and net nitrogen retention.

The measurements of biological value have represented attempts to determine biologically how closely the pattern of amino acids in a particular feed protein will satisfy the needs of the growing bird. Whole egg protein under these conditions has been found to have a biological value of about 100, animal proteins, 72 to 79 and cereal proteins, 50 to 65. Biological value measurements are useful in giving relative values to individual proteins and in assessing the influence of factors such as processing on the nutritive value of an individual protein, but are of limited value in formulating diets adequate in amino acids for practical animal production.

Biological value depends to a considerable extent on the protein content of the diet. Thus whole egg may have a biological value of 100 for young chicks when fed at 12% of the diet. When using the same assay with diet protein levels approaching that required for maximum growth rate, the biological value will decline. A protein which shows a relatively poor biological value when fed at a very low level may perform quite well as a source of essential amino acids when fed at or slightly above the optimum protein requirement level, since borderline deficiencies of limiting amino acids may be overcome as the dietary protein level is increased.

3.18.3 Net protein utilization

The use of the biological value technique for evaluating specific proteins in chickens is difficult because of the problems associated with separate collection of urine and feces. To overcome these limitations, Net Protein Utilization (NPU) has been suggested for poultry nutrition studies. This procedure is based on carcass analysis rather than on balance techniques.

Net protein utilization is defined by the following equation:

$$NPU = \frac{B_f - B_k}{I_f} \times 100$$

Where:

Bf is the carcass nitrogen of birds fed the test diet

If is nitrogen intake of birds fed the test diet

Bk represent carcass nitrogen of groups of comparable chicks fed a nitrogen-free diet.

Thus the NPU is the difference between the carcass nitrogen content of groups of chicks fed a diet containing a test protein, and the carcass nitrogen content of a group on a nitrogen-free diet, expressed as a percentage of nitrogen intake. This measure of protein quality correlates well with classical nitrogen retention methods based on balance studies. NPU falls as the protein content of the diet is increased and so all proteins must be studied at the same dietary protein level. Using this method, the NPU of soybean meal is around 55 and when supplemented with methionine, the value increases to 68; whole egg has a value of 66, peanut meal, 39 and sesame meal around 56.

Methods of reducing the number of analytical procedures required for measuring NPU have been suggested. Within a single species, the amount of water is closely related to carcass nitrogen content over a variety of feeding conditions. Once this relationship is known, nitrogen content of a dry carcass may be estimated by determining only the carcass moisture content.

3.18.4 Protein Retention Efficiency

Net protein utilization has also been estimated by another method, which involves determination of the Protein Retention Efficiency (PRE). This is obtained simply from body weight gains by the equation:

PRE = $\dfrac{G_f - G_k}{P_f}$ x 18.0

Where G_f and G_k represent gain or loss in weight with the experimental and nitrogen-free diets, respectively, and P_f is the protein intake from the experimental diet. The value 18 represents the mean percentage carcass protein content of the chicken. Thus, this method substitutes body weight changes for the directly measured carcass nitrogen changes used in the determination of NPU.

3.18.5 Protein efficiency ratio (PER)

One of the oldest measures of protein quality is the protein efficiency ratio, which is simply the weight gain of an animal divided by protein intake.

PER = $\dfrac{\text{weight gain (g)}}{\text{protein intake (g)}}$

Ingredients are normally compared at a suboptimal diet protein level. The standard AOAC method for protein evaluation by means of PER provides for a level of 9% crude protein in a diet for rats. A high quality protein will promote more weight gain per unit of protein consumed than will a low quality protein. Usually PER assays include a standard sample of casein as a reference protein to determine if the assay results are valid and consistent. Scott and co-workers at Cornell devised a chick growth assay procedure for comparing relative values of various proteins. As in other growth assay procedures, a low level of protein is fed to accentuate differences in protein quality. In this work, it was found that the chicks were most sensitive to differences in protein quality when fed diets at 10% protein. At higher protein levels some of the differences among various protein sources could not be detected. In this assay, the various protein sources were scored based on how well chicks grew on the test protein compared with growth on the reference protein which was given a value of 100.

3.18.6 Protein quality measures not additive

The procedures outlined above have found wide application for evaluation of individual protein sources for animal feeding. These procedures may be particularly useful for comparing the values of several sources of a single type of protein - such as assessment of various fish meals that have undergone different treatments during processing that may have resulted in more or less damage to the protein. These methods of protein evaluation provide a biological test for the amino acids which are most limiting for growth or nitrogen utilization. However, these methods do not furnish a set of protein values that can be used in the same manner as the metabolizable energy values of feedstuffs. Also the protein quality values of the individual protein sources to be used in a diet cannot be used to estimate the value of a mixture of such ingredients.

Although many protein balance studies are still being conducted, many new methods have been developed in recent years to aid in determining the protein requirements of animals through more precise measurements of optimum amino acid nutrition.

3.19 EFFECTS OF INGREDIENT AND FEED PROCESSING ON AVAILABILITY OF PROTEIN AND AMINO ACIDS

Most proteins used as supplementary sources of essential amino acids in poultry diets must undergo some processing prior to use. Autoxidation of fats may cause excessive heating in fish meals during drying while many plant sources of protein usually undergo oil extraction and heat treatment for destruction of inhibitors. Unless properly applied, these processing conditions may cause damage to protein quality.

Most plant proteins contain reducing carbohydrates which readily react with the free amino groups of the proteins. Lysine is particularly subject to attack, but arginine, histidine and tryptophan can also be affected. Such carbohydrate-amino acid reactions, often termed the browning or Maillard reaction, result in the formation of linkages that are resistant to hydrolysis by endogenous digestive enzymes. If the reaction proceeds far enough the amino acids may become so firmly bound that they are not recovered by acid hydrolysis of the protein. Heat treatment accelerates these carbohydrate-protein interactions.

Other reactions occurring between groups within a protein molecule, such as between free carboxyl groups of glutamic and aspartic acid and free amino groups on the protein, also may be affected by heat treatment. These produce some linkages which may be resistant to enzymatic hydrolysis. If such reactions occur, digestibility and subsequent availability of the amino acids involved are reduced.

Good in vitro laboratory methods for measuring amino acid availability are not yet in general use. Perhaps the most useful method developed thus far is the available lysine method devised by Carpenter. This method determines the available lysine by reaction of 1-fluoro-4,4-dinitrobenzene (FDNB) with the free epsilon amino groups in the intact protein prior to hydrolysis of the protein, thereby allowing colorimetric determination of the epsilon dinitrophenyl lysine in the hydrolysate. The difference between total lysine and that which has reacted with FDNB shows the extent to which the lysine may have been rendered unavailable through previous reactions with reducing sugars under the influence of excessive heat treatment. The basic principle of Carpenter's method has been used with modification by many other investigators who have attempted to measure lysine availability by chemical means. These studies have been reviewed by Carpenter (1973). More recently Dale and Araba (1987) describe a protein solubility assay for soybean meal (see Chapter 10).

Several attempts have been made to simulate conditions of digestion *in vitro* in order to estimate availability of amino acids in proteins. Rate of appearance of free amino acids in pepsin, trypsin or papain digests have been used as indicators of amino acid availability. Usually, solubility in 0.002% pepsin under acid conditions has been attempted and does provide some basis for ranking ingredients. In such *in vitro* assays, fineness of grind of samples seems to have a major effect on protein digestibility, with particles < 400µ showing the highest and most consistent results. Growth of microbes, such as *Streptococcus zymogenes*, has also been used to assess protein quality and amino acid availability. Microbes require certain amino acids for growth, and as with chickens, their growth (and multiplication) is proportional to the supply of nutrients. The sample to be assayed is treated with papain prior to assay and the enzymes of the organism are allowed to complete the hydrolysis. The microorganism requires 8 amino acids for growth. If all but the amino acid in question are added to the basal medium, the growth of the organism is proportional to the release of the amino acid being determined. The organism has proved useful in detecting processing damage to proteins. Available methionine assays in fish meal using this method have correlated well with animal growth assays.

Numerous growth assays for available amino acids also have been developed. In these methods, an assay diet is used which is deficient only in the amino acid to be studied. The relative growth of chicks fed pure supplements of the limiting amino acid is compared with the response obtained from test proteins. These methods represent the major standard with which chemical or microbiological methods for amino acid availability are compared.

3.20   SYNERGISM BETWEEN PROTEIN INGREDIENTS

Some 40 years ago it was common practice to always include at least two protein rich ingredients in a poultry diet. Bird performance was invariably improved compared to use of a single protein ingredient and the cause of such effects was not always clear. Providing a better balance of amino acids, especially levels of available or digestible amino acids in relation to requirement, was likely the reason for improved performance. Today, single protein-rich sources, such as soybean meal, are commonly used and there seems no benefit to using additional sources of protein or amino acids other than methionine for any reason other than economics.

However, it is interesting to review some older studies that seem to show synergism between protein ingredients that cannot readily be explained even with today's knowledge about amino acid balance, imbalance and digestibility of ingredients. Woodham and Deans (1977) conducted a study involving mixtures of protein sources, and their paper provides interesting reading for those studying aspects of protein quality. Using Total Protein Efficiency (g weight gain/g protein consumed) these workers show clear synergy between mixtures of such ingredients as sunflower and groundnut, and sunflower and fish meal for example. Results cannot be explained on the basis of chemical score of the diets (limiting amino acid relative to chick's requirement) or the so called essential amino acid index (summation of amino acid supply relative to requirement). A cursory re-evaluation of their data to accommodate digestible amino acid values still leaves room for unexplained synergism between pairs of protein rich ingredients. It would be interesting to repeat such studies using pairs of protein ingredients, with formulations based on determined digestible amino acid content of these ingredients.

3.21 MODEL PREDICTED AMINO ACID CONTENT OF INGREDIENTS

Determination of total amino acid content of ingredients is time consuming and relatively expensive. Few ingredients are routinely assayed for amino acids, and certainly not prior to delivery and acceptance at the feed mill. At best, laboratory analyses are used to develop historic data files that can be used to establish seasonal fluctuations in amino acid profile. The feed manufacturing industry relies heavily on the suppliers of synthetic amino acids for their quality control assays. Consequently, these organizations have collected vast libraries of samples with amino acid analyses, and have subsequently used such data to develop prediction equations. The amino acid content of soybean meal for example, can be predicted with reasonable accuracy, based on such inputs as crude protein, fiber and fat content of the samples.

3.22 MODEL PREDICTED AMINO ACID REQUIREMENTS

Numerous mathematical models have been developed aimed at predicting the amino acid needs of laying hens and growing birds. As a generalization these models summarize amino acid needs for component aspects of production. For laying hens these include maintenance, growth and egg production. Maintenance amino acid needs attempt to account for protein synthesis (Ks) and protein degradation (Kd) in various tissues and organs with particular attention paid to feather regeneration and size of musculature, liver and the gastro-intestinal tract. The amino acids of the egg are found in both the yolk and albumen and so their continuous or discontinuous rates of synthesis are sometimes accommodated in more detailed models.

Combs (1960) was one of the first to predict amino acid requirements of laying hens. This and earlier models did not take into account digestibility of amino acids.

Amino acid (mg/bird/day) = aW + bΔW + cE

W	= Body weight
ΔW	= Growth
E	= Egg mass

There have been various refinements of this model over the years, although most are still based on this simple model. Fisher *et al.*, (1973) suggested a model that takes into account variance in response of birds. This so-called 'Reading Model' takes into account variance associated with body weight and maximum egg mass output, and so has stochastic elements of prediction. A classical response curve is developed, based on egg mass, body weight and the correlation that exists between these variables (Fisher *et al.*, 1973, Fig 3.10).

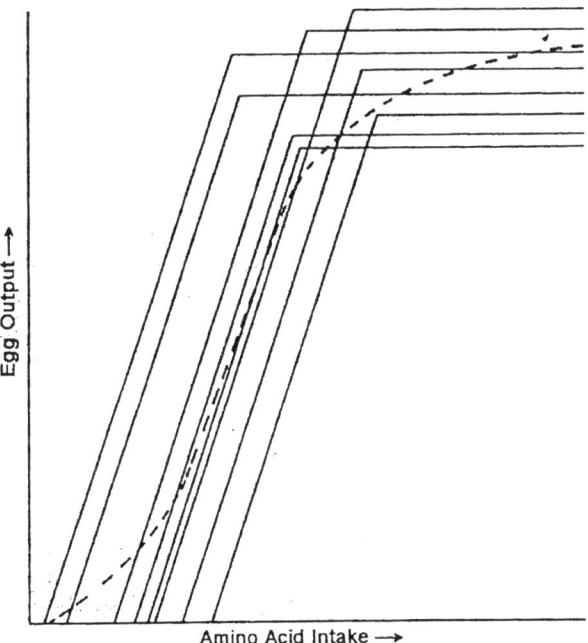

Figure 3.10 Model prediction of the response of layers to graded inputs of amino acids.
(Redrawn from Fisher et al 1973)

McDonald and Morris (1985) used this model to predict amino acid needs of young pullets, deriving the following selected data:

Lysine	=	9.99E + 73W
Methionine	=	4.77E + 31W
Tryptophan	=	2.62E + 11W

The specific amino acid is predicted in mg/bird/day and E = daily egg mass (g) and W = body weight (kg).

Hurwitz and Bornstein (1973) proposed two models for predicting amino acid requirements based on differential estimates of rates of egg protein synthesis. So-called models A and B both assumed similar requirements for maintenance and growth and that yolk proteins were synthesized continuously. In Model A, albumen and shell membrane proteins are assumed to be synthesized at the time of secretion, while in Model B, all oviduct proteins are assumed to be continuously secreted, while ovomucoid and shell membrane synthesis is discrete and occurs only at the time of secretion. Model B of Hurwitz and Bornstein (1973) has often been used as a reference standard for prediction models.

Smith (1978) used a similar model base, and likewise suggested two models based on assumptions about the source of egg proteins. In Model 1 (Table 3.15) only ovomucoids are derived from serum albumin, whereas in Model 2, it is assumed that albumin also supplies amino acids for the shell and associated membranes. Predicted values for a 1.35 kg layer, with growth of 0.7 g/d and daily egg mass of 55 g/d are shown in Table 3.15 using Model B of Hurwitz and Bornstein (1973) and the two models of Smith (1978).

Table 3.15 Model predicted daily amino acid requirements (mg/bird/day) for 1.35 kg layers, growing at 0.7 g/day and producing 55g egg mass daily

Amino Acid	Model designation		
	B	1	2
Arginine	813	620	725
Histidine	195	173	217
Isoleucine	686	549	571
Leucine	958	842	1007
Lysine	664	548	730
Methionine	408	342	347
Methionine+Cystine	617	545	578
Phenylalanine	544	428	544
Phenylalanine+Tyrosine	969	798	985
Threonine	540	490	551
Tryptophan	149	144	144
Valine	812	675	735

Model B - Hurwitz and Bornstein (1973)
Models 1 and 2 - Smith (1978)

Morris and Blackburn (1982) suggested that we disregard the concept of fixed amino acid requirements, because in populations of birds there is always variance and this should be accommodated in any prediction. These authors suggested prediction of optimum economic doses of amino acids and for a laying hen such values are around 600 mg/d for methionine + cystine and 222 mg/d for tryptophan.

Hurwitz et al., (1978) also developed prediction equations for amino acid needs of broilers chickens. The major component inputs relate to growth and maintenance with the latter based on the classical data of Leveille and Fisher (1958) determined with adult roosters. The growth component is based on amino acid profile of carcass and feathers. Table 3.16 shows prediction values for 7d and 56d broilers, with a diet energy base of 3000 kcal ME/kg and assuming 85% digestibility of all amino acids.

Table 3.16 Model predicted amino acid needs of broiler chickens (adapted from Hurwitz et al., 1978)		
	Amino acid (% diet)[1]	
	7d age	56d age
Arginine	1.25	0.98
Histidine	0.29	0.20
Lysine	1.10	0.79
Tryptophan	0.15	0.12
Methionine	0.37	0.28
Methionine+Cystine	0.79	0.67
Threonine	0.75	0.60
Valine	1.19	0.95
Leucine	1.26	1.01
Isoleucine	0.80	0.65
Phenylalanine	0.70	0.56
		[1]3000 kcal ME/kg

Hruby et al., (1995) more recently devised prediction estimates of amino acid requirements of broiler chickens. These workers applied the Gompertz growth function to estimates of body protein obtained from weekly observations of male broilers. Estimates of amino acid levels in carcass and feathers were extrapolated from other work and used as a basis for predictions based relative to TME energy values. Table 3.17 shows estimates of amino acid needs of male broilers, expressed as % of diet and converted to AMEn based on the data of Hruby et al., (1995).

Wk	Arg	His	Iso	Leu	Lys	Met	Met+ Cys	Phe	Thr	Try	Val
1	1.29	0.46	0.76	1.33	1.32	0.44	0.78	0.78	0.82	0.18	0.87
2	1.16	0.41	0.69	1.20	1.13	0.39	0.74	0.71	0.78	0.16	0.80
3	0.98	0.33	0.57	1.01	0.94	0.31	0.64	0.60	0.60	0.14	0.68
4	1.01	0.33	0.60	1.04	0.93	0.31	0.70	0.62	0.65	0.13	0.72
5	0.96	0.31	0.57	0.99	0.91	0.29	0.68	0.60	0.63	0.13	0.69
6	0.97	0.32	0.57	0.99	0.90	0.30	0.67	0.60	0.61	0.13	0.68
7	0.90	0.31	0.53	0.92	0.90	0.29	0.61	0.56	0.60	0.13	0.63
8	0.87	0.30	0.51	0.88	0.88	0.29	0.59	0.54	0.58	0.12	0.60

Table 3.17 Predicted requirements of amino acids for male broilers (adapted from Hruby *et al.*, 1995)

Amino acid (% diet)

Week 1-3 @ 3000 kcal AMEn/kg
Week 4-6 @ 3050 kcal AMEn/kg
Week 7-8 @ 3150 kcal AMEn/kg

Figure 3.11 shows estimates of amino acid requirements expressed as a percent of the diet, adapted from the report of Emmert and Baker (1997) who based their prediction on ideal ileal amino acid levels. In these revised estimates, amino acids are assumed 88% digestible.

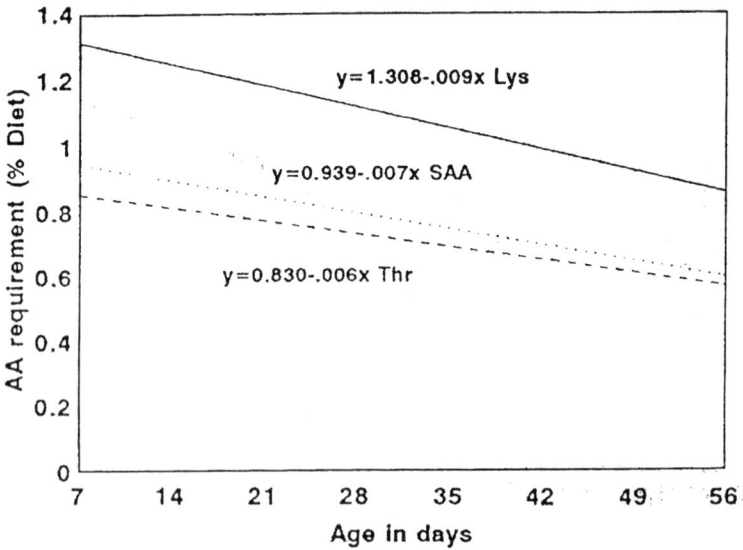

Figure 3.11 Estimates of total diet % amino acids, derived from estimates of Illinois ideal Protein.
(Adapted from Emmert & Baker 1997)

3.23   CARCASS AMINO ACIDS

There is a remarkably consistent pattern of amino acids in the carcass of most avian species, and these values are similar to those found in mammals. (Table 3.18).

The close agreement found between amino acid requirements calculated from carcass composition data and the requirements determined by nutritional studies support the conclusion that carcass analysis is a valid method for evaluating the growth requirements for most, if not all, of the essential amino acids. The essential amino acid requirements expressed as percentages of the dietary protein for growth of chickens, bear a remarkable similarity to the percentages of these amino acids in the chicken carcass proteins. A similar relationship can be shown between the amino acid composition of the egg and the laying hen's requirement for essential amino acids.

Table 3.18 Carcass amino acid content (% of protein)								
Amino Acid	Chicken		Pheasant	Quail	Turkey	Pig	Rat	Avg. all Species
	Leghorn	Broiler						
Arginine	7.8	6.8	7.8	7.4	7.6	7.1	5.9	7.2
Cystine	2.6	2.4	2.8	2.8	2.4	2.0	1.5	2.4
Histidine	3.9	4.1	4.5	3.9	3.9	2.7	2.2	3.6
Isoleucine	3.9	3.9	4.0	3.9	4.2	3.8	3.5	4.0
Leucine	6.4	6.5	6.3	6.7	6.7	7.1	6.5	6.7
Lysine	9.4	9.9	10.1	10.0	10.2	8.6	7.6	9.3
Methionine	1.8	1.9	1.8	2.0	1.9	1.8	1.7	1.9
Phenylalanine	3.5	3.6	3.5	3.5	3.6	3.8	3.7	3.6
Threonine	3.4	3.4	3.4	3.5	3.5	3.8	3.9	3.6
Tryptophan	1.2	1.1	0.9	0.9	1.3	0.8	0.8	1.0
Tyrosine	2.9	3.1	3.1	3.0	2.9	2.6	2.9	2.9
Valine	4.4	4.4	4.3	4.3	4.3	6.0	5.5	4.7

In comparing the essential amino acid composition of the proteins of typical commercial broiler or layer diets with the essential amino acid composition of the proteins of the tissues of the chicken or the proteins of the egg, the most outstanding deficiency in the feed proteins is of methionine. Biological studies with practical diets based largely upon corn or milo and soybean meal have shown that methionine supplementation of both broiler and layer diets produces noticeable improvements in growth, production and especially in efficiency of feed utilization.

3.24   ESTIMATING AMINO ACID REQUIREMENTS

There are many possible ways of expressing amino acid requirements. For example, they might be expressed as: (1) mg of each amino acid per bird per day; (2) mg of each amino acid per kcal metabolizable energy; (3) percentages of the diet, or (4) percentages of the dietary protein. Method (1) is certainly the most precise way to express the amino acid requirements but relies on knowledge of daily feed intake. Method (3) is unsatisfactory because feed intake of the chicken depends to a large extent upon the energy content of the diet and, therefore, the percentage of each amino acid present in the diet must be increased when the dietary energy is increased and the birds consume less feed. Thus, it would seem best to use Method (2), which ties the amino acid requirements to the energy content of the diet. However Method (3) is still used extensively, and in these situations there obviously needs to be a statement about diet energy level.

In most instances, it is considered best practice to determine the protein level which will provide most of the essential amino acids and the non-essential amino acid nitrogen requirements of the chicken at any given energy level. This protein is then adjusted with ingredients such as meat meal or synthetic amino acids in such a way that each essential amino acid as nearly as possible meets the requirement expressed as a percentage of the dietary protein (Method 4).

Knowing the amino acid requirements of poultry and the amino acid content of the feedstuffs, it would seem to be a relatively simple matter to 1) calculate the amino acid composition of a feed, 2) compare this with the known amino acid requirements of the animal, 3) if necessary supplement the feed with synthetic amino acids or with other protein sources, and in this manner always be sure that the combination of proteins in a given feed is of optimum amino acid balance. This procedure is commonly used in formulations of feed, but it does not in itself necessarily ensure adequate amino acid nutrition for the following reasons:

(1)   Amino acid values of feedstuffs determined by chemical procedures provide no information concerning the digestibility of the protein and release in the digestive tract of all of the essential amino acids.

(2)   Even when digestibility of the protein and amino acid is known under standard conditions, it is still possible that heat treatment or other treatments to which the protein has been subjected may bind some of the essential amino acids in such a way that they are unavailable to the bird.

(3)   Amino acid requirements will vary during different stages of the bird's life, depending upon the amino acid composition of the tissues being formed. For example, amino acid needs will be different during rapid feather development, or during, or immediately after a severe molt. Also when young pullets begin to produce

eggs, which have an amino acid pattern that is much different from chicken body tissues, the dietary amino acid needs will be quite different.

(4) Amino acid requirement may differ depending upon the balance (excesses as well as deficiencies) of other essential amino acids in the proteins being fed.

3.25   PROTEIN AND AMINO ACID NUTRITION OF GROWING PULLETS AND LAYING HENS

The protein and amino acid requirements of pullets and layers have been fairly well established. For the immature bird, growth rate, feathering and skeletal development are the major criteria, while for the laying hen the emphasis changes to egg mass production and maintenance.

3.25.1 Growing birds up to maturity

Appetite of the immature pullet is often limited, and so ensuring adequate earlier growth rate is a key to optimizing subsequent adult performance. The pullet is very responsive to energy intake (see Chapter 2) but obviously a minimal intake of balanced protein is essential for orderly growth and development. We can model the pullet's protein requirements, based on needs for growth, maintenance and feather development. Since the carcass of the chicken contains approximately 18% protein, daily protein requirements for tissue growth may be calculated by multiplying the daily gain in body weight (in grams) by 0.18 (18% protein in tissues) and dividing by 0.61 (61% efficiency of utilization of feed protein).

The daily endogenous nitrogen loss in younger chickens has been determined to be approximately 250 mg of nitrogen per kg of body weight. Multiplying the nitrogen x 6.25 indicates that almost 1600 mg of protein is lost per kg body weight per day. The dietary protein requirement for maintenance, therefore is around 2.6 g/kg body weight, assuming 61% efficiency of protein utilization.

At three weeks of age, the feathers represent about 4% of the body weight. This increases to approximately 7% at 4 weeks of age, and remains relatively constant thereafter. The protein content of feathers is about 82%. Thus, the daily protein requirement for feather production can be determined by multiplying the percentage feather weight (0.04 to 0.07) times the daily gain in body weight in grams, and then multiplying this figure by 0.82 (the percentage protein in feathers) and dividing by 0.61.

The following formula may be used to compute the daily protein needs of growing White Leghorn chickens:

Daily protein requirement (gms) $= \dfrac{\text{Daily gain (g) X 0.18}}{0.61}$

$+ \dfrac{0.0016 \text{ X body weight (g)}}{0.61}$

$+ \dfrac{(0.07) \text{ X daily gain (g) X 0.82}}{0.61}$

Using the formula, calculated protein needs are shown in Table 3.19 for pullets up to 18 weeks of age. The protein requirements, expressed as a percentage of the diet, are very low in relation to commercial application, especially as the pullet gets older. Estimated amino acid requirements, expressed as % of diet per 1,000 kcal ME are shown in Table 3.20.

Table 3.19 Model predicted protein requirements of immature Leghorn pullets					
Age (wks)	Body Weight (g)	Body Weight Gain/day (g)	Feed Intake/day (g)	Protein Required/bird/ day (g)	Diet Protein (%)
1	70	5.0	10	2.1	21.3
2	110	6.0	15	2.6	17.5
3	190	11.0	20	4.8	23.9
4	270	11.0	30	5.0	16.6
5	350	11.0	36	5.2	14.4
6	440	13.0	42	6.2	14.8
7	540	14.0	53	6.9	13.0
8	650	16.0	55	7.9	14.4
9	750	14.0	57	7.4	13.0
10	830	12.0	58	6.8	11.8
11	900	10.0	59	6.3	10.6
12	970	10.0	61	6.4	10.6
13	1030	10.0	63	6.6	10.5
14	1090	8.5	66	6.2	9.3
15	1150	8.5	68	6.3	9.3
16	1210	8.5	71	6.5	9.1
17	1270	8.5	72	6.6	9.2
18	1330	8.5	74	6.8	9.2

Table 3.20 Estimated amino acid requirements of immature Leghorn pullets (%/1000 kcal ME)			
	Chick Starter	Chick Grower	Prelay
Approximate age	0-6 wk	6-18 wk	16-18 wk
Protein equivalent (%)	20	17	17
Amino Acid			
Arginine	0.36	0.31	0.28
Lysine	0.34	0.29	0.24
Methionine	0.16	0.14	0.12
Methionine+Cystine	0.25	0.22	0.21
Tryptophan	0.07	0.06	0.05
Histidine	0.12	0.11	0.10
Leucine	0.44	0.38	0.34
Isoleucine	0.23	0.21	0.19
Phenylalanine	0.22	0.20	0.18
Phenyl.+Tyrosine	0.43	0.38	0.34
Threonine	0.21	0.19	0.17
Valine	0.26	0.23	0.21

Because pullets tend to eat to their energy requirement, then it is essential to balance protein and amino acids according to energy level of the diet. There is an indication that growth rate can be maximized with high energy diets, and so there has been a trend in this direction. However pullets will eat less of these high energy diets, even though energy intake will increase slightly, and so amino acid levels must be adjusted accordingly. There seems to be no advantage to the pullet consuming much more than 800 g of balanced protein to 18 weeks of age. Intakes of protein below this will cause reduced growth (and/or fatter pullets) while higher intakes are wasteful and in extreme cases may also result in increased fat deposition, because of increased energy supply through gluconeogenesis.

The protein and amino acid requirements of immature brown egg pullets are comparable to those described for Leghorns, with appropriate adjustments made to accommodate the slightly heavier body weight. Brown egg pullets have larger appetites, and there is less need to encourage intake in order to stimulate growth. In moderate climates, it may in fact be necessary to practice restricted feeding after 12-14 weeks of age, and under such conditions it is necessary to calculate amino acid needs in terms of mg/bird/day and ensure such intakes relative to restricted feeding.

There do not seem to be any special amino acid needs during the so-called pre-lay period. Depending upon lighting program, there will be an increase in size of the liver, ovary and oviduct starting at around 16 weeks of age. However, there is no evidence that nutrient needs for such development are any different to those of growth *per se*. Even at this time, daily weight gain will be less than that occurring earlier, and so amino acid specifications in specialized pre-lay diets can be the same as, or even lower than, grower diets used up to this time. The main nutrient change in pre-lay diets relates to calcium and phosphorus metabolism.

3.25.2 Mature layers

Many factors may influence feed consumption and protein requirements of mature laying hens. Among these are: (1) size and breed of hen; (2) environmental temperature; (3) daily egg mass production; (4) housing (cage or floor pens); (5) feeding space per hen; (6) depth of feed in automatic feeders; (7) whether or not the hens are properly beak-trimmed; (8) stocking density; (9) availability and composition of drinking water; (10) disease status in the flock; and (11) energy content of the diet.

a)   Major factors affecting protein needs.

If one assumes that all management factors are controlled satisfactorily, feed consumption depends to a major degree upon size and breed of hens, environmental temperature, egg mass output and energy content of diet.

Size and breed of hen. Heavy breeds of poultry consume considerably more feed than do light weight breeds because heavier chickens require more energy for maintenance. The heavy breeds also require more protein per day for maintenance and so need a somewhat higher overall daily protein intake than do White Leghorns. Assuming that a heavy breed hen consumes approximately 115 grams of feed per day, a level of 18% protein in the diet provides about 21 grams of protein per hen per day. However, a modern strain of small White Leghorn receiving a feed containing the same energy level under the same environmental conditions would consume only about 95 grams of feed per hen per day and therefore would require 19% protein in the diet to obtain 18 grams of protein per hen per day. The protein and amino acid level in diets for heavy vs. light weight birds can vary by as much as 10%, a value similar to that for the most popular white vs. brown egg strains of bird.

Effect of environmental temperature. Experiments indicate that with conventional corn-soybean type diets providing approximately 2900 kcal metabolizable energy per kg, White Leghorn hens consume about 105 grams of feed per hen per day during the winter months when temperature is around 13°C. During the summer months at 30°C the same birds may consume as little as 90 grams of feed per hen per day. Thus, in winter, a protein level of 16% would provide 16.8 g protein daily, while in summer a protein level of 18.6% is required to provide the same daily protein intake. In practice the crude protein level of the diet may not be increased, because this increases the SDA (heat increment) of the diet so contributing to potential heat stress. It is more important to maintain the intake of critical amino acids, and so the same type of calculation is applied to these nutrients, as previously described for protein, such that daily intake is maintained.

Stage of production. Egg production commences at about 18 weeks of age, rises sharply, reaching a peak at about 25 weeks of age, and then gradually declines to a level of approximately 75% after 60 weeks of lay when the hens are about 78 weeks of age.

The production cycle may be conveniently divided into two phases:

Phase I. At onset of lay (18-19 weeks of age), the average White Leghorn pullet weighs approximately 1350 grams and is consuming about 75 grams of feed daily. During the period from 19 to 42 weeks of age, this pullet is expected to (1) increase egg production from zero to a peak of approximately 95% production; (2) increase in body weight from 1350 grams to approximately 1650 grams; (3) produce eggs of gradually increasing size from about 43 grams per egg at 20 weeks of age to over 61 grams per egg at 42 weeks of age. Thus the Phase I period is the most critical in the productive life of the pullet. The necessity for providing adequate protein, amino acids, vitamins and minerals for optimum egg mass production and for normal growth to physiological maturity, is not only important for maximum economic returns during Phase I, but also is necessary to provide the mature hen with the health and tissue reserves needed for maximum production throughout the subsequent stages of her productive life.

Phase II is the period after 42 weeks of age when the hens have attained mature body weight (empirically, Phase II encompasses the period from 42 to 72 weeks of age). Egg production declines more slowly at this time, and there is minimal weight gain.

b)   Daily protein needs of a hen during production Phases I and II.

During peak egg production the daily protein needs of a pullet can be divided into three components: (1) protein required for production of an egg; (2) protein needed for maintenance; and (3) protein required for growth of body tissues and feathers. The approximate amounts of protein needed for these functions for Phases I and II are shown in Table 3.21.

Table 3.21 Daily protein needs of White Leghorn hens during two phases of egg production		
Protein needed for:	Protein need (g/d)	
	Phase I	Phase II
Production of an egg	12.2	13.5
Maintenance of body protein for one day	3.0	3.4
Growth per day	1.4	0
Feather growth per day	0.4	0.1
Totals	17.0	17.0

The data presented in Table 3.22 show the absolute requirements for methionine, lysine and isoleucine for 100% production during Phases I and II. These requirements remain the same for both phases of egg production for those hens that are laying eggs almost continuously over prolonged periods of time. However, most hens do not lay at 100% for very long periods, but lay clutches of nine to ten eggs and then pause for a day or so before laying another similar clutch of eggs. Because of this pause between clutches of eggs, the protein and amino acid requirements determined experimentally have been shown to be somewhat lower than those needed for 100% production. This is true because hens have the ability to borrow protein and essential amino acids from tissues, and to subsequently repay this nutrient demand on days that ovulation does not occur. Although the average produc-

Table 3.22 Model predicted daily needs for methionine, lysine and isoleucine (mg)		
	Phase I	Phase II
Methionine:		
Daily deposition in egg	228	251
Daily deposition in tissue growth	13	-
Used each day for maintenance	30	33
Daily feather growth	2	0.5
Total	273	285
Lysine:		
Daily deposition in egg	482	532
Daily deposition in tissue growth	57	-
Used each day for maintenance	127	140
Daily feather growth	6	2
Total	672	674
Isoleucine:		
Daily deposition in egg	536	592
Daily deposition in tissue growth	31	-
Used each day for maintenance	70	76
Daily feather growth	25	6
Total	662	674

tion during Phase I may be only 78%, and during Phase II only 80%, many of the hens may be laying close to 100% production for extended periods of time. To encourage this rate of lay, it is necessary to provide sufficient protein for the production of one egg per day. Although the average egg size may be only approximately 55 grams during Phase I, it is economically advisable to feed diets which will allow egg size to increase to the large size category as rapidly as possible.

A fresh egg contains 66% water, 12% protein, 10% fat, 1% carbohydrate and 11% ash. Thus a 56 gram egg contains 6.7 grams of protein, and during Phase II, 7.4 grams of protein are required for production of the larger egg of this older bird. With an efficiency of protein utilization of 61%, hens must consume 6.7 x 0.61 = 10.9 g protein/day during Phase I and 12.1 grams during Phase II in order to supply the protein needed for one egg each day.

Protein is also required for maintenance. The daily total endogenous nitrogen excretion of layers (including normal feather loss) is around 200 mg per kg.[75] body weight. Thus, for a laying hen during Phase I (19-42 weeks of age), the endogenous nitrogen excretion may be calculated as:

200×1.4 kg.[75] = 257 mg/day

Using the standard factor (6.25) for conversion of nitrogen to protein, we find that the amount of protein which is degraded to provide this endogenous nitrogen excretion is (0.257 g x 6.25) or 1.6 g of protein/day. Since the hen is approximately 61% efficient in converting dietary protein to body proteins, the hen during Phase I will need to consume 2.6 grams of protein per day to meet her daily protein requirements of body maintenance. During Phase II, the hen has reached mature body weight and the maintenance requirement increases to 2.8 grams per day.

Protein is also required for some growth during Phase I. At 21 weeks of age, most modern White Leghorn pullets weigh about 1350 grams. During the early part of Phase I (21 to 36 weeks of age), they gain in weight by approximately 450 grams. Assuming that 18% of this gain is protein, then the pullet must deposit a total of 0.18 x 450 = 81 g protein in 105 days, or 0.77 g protein/day. At an efficiency of 61%, this relates to a requirement of 1.3 grams of protein per day.

c)   Experimental determinations of protein requirements.

Numerous studies on the protein requirements of laying hens have indicated that for 90% egg production and for best efficiency of feed utilization with corn-soya laying diets, mature White Leghorn hens require about 17.5 - 18.5 grams of protein per day. It appears that the hen is about 61% efficient in converting the protein of commercial diets into egg protein and into the protein and other nitrogenous compounds required for maintenance. There are some discrepancies in reported values for protein requirements of layers and this may relate to differences in digestibility of ingredients. It is recognized that the proteins of feedstuffs are not completely digestible. The crude protein of most feedstuffs used in poultry diets ranges in digestibility from 75 to 90% with an average of about 85%. There will also be variability in assessment of protein requirements caused by variation in amino acid balance of diets. Wastage of feed proteins occurs in the course of producing the balance of essential amino acids in the ovary and oviduct necessary for the formation of egg protein. For example, twice as much methionine is present in egg protein as in a corn-soya diet. Assuming that this discrepancy is alleviated by the addition of synthetic methionine to the diet, the hen will still require about 10 grams of feed protein to obtain the amounts of lysine, isoleucine and valine needed for 6-7 grams of egg protein. By adding methionine to a corn-soya laying diet, the hen no longer must consume 18 grams of feed protein in order to obtain the methionine required to produce a large egg. The large number of experiments conducted have shown that with methionine supplementation, the usual cereal-soya diets provide adequate levels of all essential amino acids for both Phase I and Phase II when consumed at a level providing 17 grams of protein per hen per day.

This level of 17 grams of protein is needed for 100% production and to maintain large egg size. As indicated previously, many hens are laying at near 100% levels, even during Phase II. Confusion has arisen over protein recommendations because many experiments have shown that diets which provided as little as 15 grams of protein per hen per day were capable of supporting production levels of 85-90%. This is readily possible since hens laying only at this stage of production have the ability to store some protein on the day that no egg is laid and to use this protein to supplement a daily protein intake which, in itself, would not be sufficient for all of the protein needs of that day.

d)   Level of protein in diet in relation to feed consumption.

Because it is not possible to individually hand-feed laying hens a specified quantity of protein per hen per day, it is necessary to understand the relationship between the minimum protein needs of laying hens and their daily feed consumption. With this knowledge it is possible to adjust the energy content of the diet such that in a specific environment a reasonable prediction of daily feed consumption can be made. The approximate minimum protein requirements as percentages of the diet in relation to feed consumption, are shown in Table 3.23. Protein levels below 14.5% are not indicated because at these lower levels cereal protein represents such a large proportion of the total protein that the amino acid levels are adversely affected.

Table 3.23 Protein requirements of White Leghorns for egg production	
Feed Intake (g/bird/day)	Protein (% of diet)
80	21.2
85	20.0
90	18.9
95	17.9
100	17.0
105	16.2
110	15.5
115	14.8
120	14.5

e)   Adjusting the dietary protein level in relation to the energy content of the diet.

Layers can adjust their feed consumption in order to obtain adequate energy when receiving laying diets ranging in energy from approximately 2500 to 3300 kcal ME per kg of diet. Since a greater quantity of feed is consumed when the energy level is decreased and a lesser amount when the energy is increased, it is necessary to adjust the protein content of the diet in relation to such changing energy level. The metabolizable energy to protein ratio (ME/P) should be around 165 (determined by dividing the kilocalories of metabolizable energy per kg of diet by the percentage of dietary protein). In hot climates, the ME/P ratios should be reduced about 10%. These ratios should still provide a hen with 17 grams of protein per day.

As energy level of the diet increases, then there should theoretically be a major increase in crude protein (and amino acids) to accommodate the reduced feed intake. For example, moving from 2600 to 3000 kcal ME/kg should be balanced by an increase in crude protein from about 15 to 17% assuming the bird eats exactly to its energy requirement. Modern laying strains do not eat exactly to energy requirements, tending to consume more energy with moderately high energy diets (> 2800 kcal/kg) and having difficulty eating enough feed when bulky low energy diets (< 2700 kcal/kg) are offered. These adaptations tend to temper the change in intake expected in response to change in diet energy, and so protein and amino acid levels do not change dramatically over a fairly wide range of diet energy levels (Table 3.24).

Table 3.24 Percentage dietary protein levels necessary to ensure 17g CP intake daily						
Diet ME (kcal/kg)	At 15-20°C			At 27-32°C		
	ME/day	Feed/day	% CP	ME/day	Feed/day	% CP
2600	265	102	16.7	250	96	17.7
2700	270	100	17.0	255	94	18.1
2800	275	98	17.3	260	93	18.3
2900	282	97	17.5	265	91	18.7
3000	285	95	17.9	270	90	18.8

Protein and amino acid requirement values for White Leghorn layers are shown in Table 3.25. The values are dependent on level of feed intake, which is mainly influenced by bird size and environmental temperature. In diets based on soybean meal as the major protein-rich ingredient, then methionine + cystine, sometimes referred to as total sulfur amino acids (TSAA) are usually the first limiting amino acids. It is unusual to have to consider any synthetic amino acids other than methionine and lysine, although where major emphasis is placed on ingredients other than soybean meal, threonine and tryptophan levels may become more marginal. Knowledge of feed intake is therefore essential today for efficient nutrition of laying hens.

Table 3.25 Amino acid requirements of White Leghorn hens @ 95% egg production (% of the diet)						
	Feed intake/day (g)					
	120	110	100	90	80	70
Approximate protein level (%)	14.0	15.5	17.0	19.0	20.5	22.1
Amino acids (% of diet):						
Arginine	0.60	0.68	0.75	0.82	0.90	0.98
Lysine	0.56	0.63	0.70	0.77	0.84	0.91
Methionine	0.31	0.34	0.37	0.41	0.47	0.56
Methionine+Cystine	0.53	0.58	0.64	0.71	0.80	0.91
Tryptophan	0.12	0.14	0.15	0.17	0.18	0.20
Histidine	0.14	0.15	0.17	0.19	0.22	0.25
Leucine	0.73	0.82	0.91	1.00	1.09	1.18
Isoleucine	0.50	0.57	0.63	0.69	0.73	0.82
Phenylalanine	0.38	0.42	0.47	0.52	0.57	0.61
Phenylalanine+Tryosine	0.65	0.75	0.83	0.91	0.99	1.08
Threonine	0.50	0.57	0.63	0.69	0.73	0.82
Valine	0.56	0.63	0.70	0.77	0.82	0.91
Metabolizable energy (kcal/kg)	2700	2700	2800	2850	2850	2900

f)   **Environmental conditions.**

Environmental temperature has a large effect on feed intake, and under so-called heat stress conditions, it is common practice to change protein and amino acid levels in the diet. In the past, it has been common practice to increase protein levels during heat stress conditions. This has been done on the basis of reduced feed intake, and hence protein levels have been adjusted upwards in attempting to maintain intakes of around 17 g crude protein/bird/day. It is now realized that such adjustments may be harmful. When any nutrient is metabolized in the body, the processes are not 100% efficient and as a result some heat is produced. Unfortunately, protein is the most inefficiently utilized nutrient in this regard and so proportionately more heat is evolved during metabolism of protein and amino acids. The last thing that a heat stressed bird needs is additional waste heat being generated in the body. This extra heat production may well overload heat dissipation mechanisms (panting, blood circulation). Nutritionists are therefore faced with a difficult problem of attempting to maintain protein intake in situations of reduced feed intake, yet we know that more crude protein may be detrimental. The answer to the problem is not to increase crude protein, but rather to increase the levels of essential amino acids. By feeding additional synthetic amino acids, we can therefore maintain the intake of these essential nutrients without loading up the body systems with excess crude protein (nitrogen). General recommendations are, therefore, to increase the use of synthetic methionine and lysine so as to maintain daily intakes of approximately 360 and 720 mg respectively regardless of feed intake while concomitantly reducing crude protein level.

g)   Protein and egg size.

Protein and amino acids, and especially methionine, have a large influence on egg size. Assuming there are no deficiencies, then protein and amino acid levels in the diet have relatively little influence on egg numbers. However, these nutrients are perhaps the major nutrients controlling egg size. Egg size is greatly influenced by genetics and body size of the bird, while Fig. 3.12 shows the relative significance of energy and protein as they influence egg weight. At each protein level used in this study, methionine and lysine were balanced at 2 and 5% of protein respectively. At low protein intakes, an increase in energy intake actually has a negative effect on egg size. At more normal levels of intake, then energy level has no meaningful effect on egg size. Protein intake, regardless of energy intake, seems linearly related to egg size. However it is not always clear if the responses recorded to crude protein *per se* can be totally attributed to intake of component amino acids. Table 3.26 provides a summary of 6 experiments reported by Waldroup and Hellwig , (1995) where a range of methionine levels were tested, at 0.2% cystine, for various ages of birds.

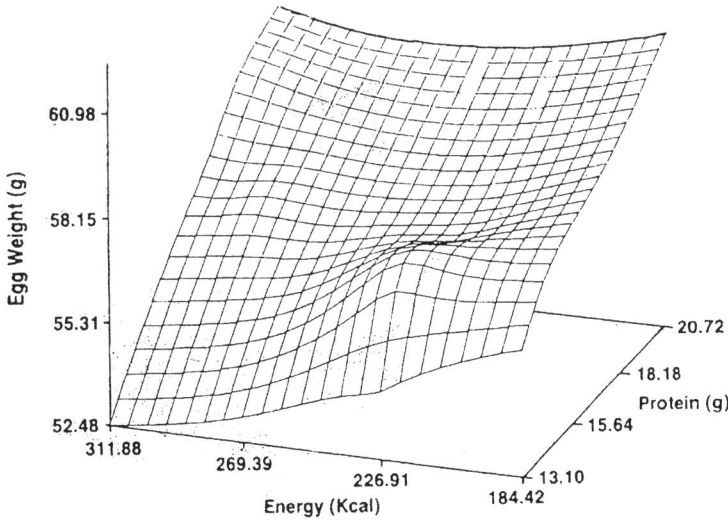

Figure 3.12 Egg weight (18-66 weeks) in response to intakes of energy and protein.

Table 3.26 Effect of dietary methionine levels on egg weight (g)						
Bird age (wks)	% Diet Methionine[1]					
	0.23	0.26	0.29	0.32	0.35	0.38
25-32	49.8	51.0	51.9	52.1	52.0	52.6
38-44	53.2	55.0	56.4	56.3	56.3	57.1
51-58	56.2	57.9	59.6	59.2	59.2	60.0
64-71	56.8	59.4	59.5	59.5	59.5	60.2

[1]@0.2% cystine   Adapted from Waldroup *et al.,* (1995)

These data show that as methionine level of the diet is increased, there is an almost linear increase in egg size.   As the bird progresses through a production cycle, the egg weight response to methionine changes slightly. In the first period, between 25-32 weeks, using 0.38 vs. 0.23% methionine results in a 5.6% increase in egg size (Table 3.26). Comparable calculations for the other age periods show 7.3% improvement from 38-44 weeks, and 6.7% and 6.0% at 51-58 and 64-71 weeks respectively. The egg weight response to methionine, therefore closely follows the normal daily egg mass output of the laying hen. In another study, Calderon and Jensen (1990) show a generalized curvilinear response in egg weight to graded levels of methionine (Fig. 3.13).

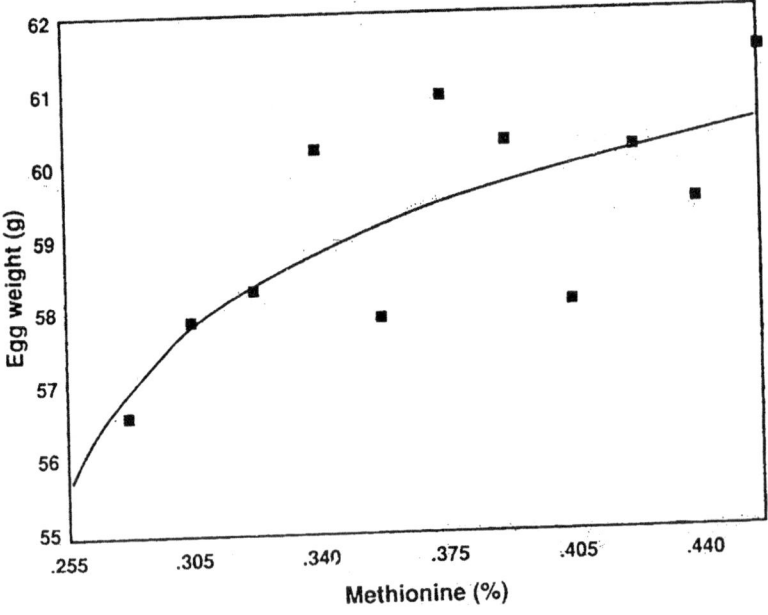

Figure 3.13 Egg weight response to methionine
(Adapted from Calderon & Jensen, 1990)

Over the last few years there has been considerable research involving the source of methionine as it affects egg size. When comparing DL-methionine with Alimet®, a methionine hydroxy analogue Harms and Russell (1994) show the classical response of egg weight to both methionine sources (Table 3.27).

Talbe 3.27 Effect of methionine source on egg weight				
Diet methionine (%)	Egg weight (g)			
	Experiment 1		Experiment 2	
	DL-Methionine	Alimet®	DL-Methionine	Alimet®
0.228	54.5	54.5	51.5	51.5
0.256	56.2	55.3	53.2	52.7
0.284	56.8	56.8	55.1	56.2
0.311	57.6	57.2	55.9	55.7
0.366	58.0	57.5	57.0	56.8
[1]Mean 80% egg production				
			Adapted from Harms and Russell (1994)	

There has been a suggestion that L-methionine may, in fact, be superior to any other source. This product is not usually produced commercially because routine manufacture of methionine produces a racemic mixture of D- and L-methionine. However most research data indicates no difference in potency of L- vs. DL-methionine sources in terms of egg size.

One role of methionine is as a methyl donor, and so the efficacy of methionine vs. choline in influencing egg size often arises. While choline can spare some methionine in a diet, it is obvious that there are severe limitations to this process, and this becomes most obvious when egg size rather than simply egg production, is a consideration. Data from Parsons and Leeper (1984) clearly show the advantage of using methionine over choline in terms of egg size, and that this effect becomes most critical as diet crude protein level is reduced (Table 3.28).

Table 3.28 Egg size in response to dietary methionine or choline (23-35 wks)			
Diet protein	Supplement	Egg production (%)	Egg weight (g)
16.0%	None	82.8	53.2
	0.1% methionine	84.0	56.6
	0.1% choline	82.4	54.0
14.0%	None	72.8	52.5
	0.1% methionine	84.5	54.9
	0.1% choline	78.9	51.9
		Adapted from Parsons and Leeper (1984)	

As layers get older, their egg size increases. In most markets, it is uneconomical to produce eggs much larger than the lower limit for the large grade category and the larger the egg size, the weaker the shell. At around 50 weeks of age therefore, it is often necessary to try and temper the gradual increase in egg size. Again protein and methionine contents of the layer diet are often scrutinized. However, there are limits to just how much and how quickly these nutrients can be removed from the diet, and not affect egg production. Table 3.29 shows the effect of feeding reduced protein (methionine at 2% of protein and methionine + cystine at 4.8% protein) to 60 week old layers.

Table 3.29 Effect of reducing dietary protein level on egg size of 60-68 week old layers					
Dietary protein level (%)	Avg. intake per day (g)		Egg		
	Feed	Protein	Production (%)	Weight (g)	Daily Mass (g)
17	114	19.4	78.8	64.8	51.0
15	109	16.4	77.5	64.3	49.7
13	107	13.9	78.3	62.2	49.1
11	108	11.9	72.7	61.7	45.1
9	99	8.9	54.3	58.2	36.1
					All diets 2800 kcal ME/kg

In this and other studies, the response to reduced crude protein is likely a response to methionine. However such results are often difficult to achieve under commercial conditions because reduction in diet methionine levels often leads to loss in egg numbers and body weight. Phase feeding of amino acids must, therefore, be monitored very closely. As stated at the beginning of this section, mature body weight is the main determinant of egg size, and this applies particularly to late cycle performance. The best way to control late cycle egg size is through manipulation of body weight at time of light stimulation. Larger birds at maturity will produce much larger late cycle eggs and vice versa. There is obviously a balance necessary between trying to reduce late cycle egg size without unduly reducing early cycle egg size.

Waldroup and Hellwig (1995) outlined estimates of methionine and methionine + cystine requirements for both egg production and for egg weight/mass at various stages of the production cycle (Table 3.30). During peak egg mass output (38-45 weeks) the methionine requirement for egg weight is greater than for egg numbers, while the latter requirement peaks at 51-58 weeks of age. If these data are verified in subsequent studies, it suggests that we should be very careful in reducing methionine levels much before 60 weeks of age. As protein and amino acid level of the diet are reduced, there is also a tendency for greater fat deposition in the body. Feeding 15 vs. 17% CP diets can result in 3-5% increase in liver fat, and so predispose layers to Fatty Liver Syndrome.

Table 3.30 Estimated methionine and methionine + cystine requirements (mg/bird/day)				
	Bird age (wks)	Egg Criteria		
		Number	Weight (g)	Mass (g)
Methionine	25-32	364b	356b	369b
	38-45	362b	380a	373b
	51-58	384a	364a	402a
	64-71	374ab	357b	378b
Methionine + cystine	25-32	608b	610ab	617b
	38-45	619b	636a	627b
	51-58	680a	621ab	691a
	64-71	690a	601b	676a
			Adapted from Waldroup and Hellwig (1995)	

h)   Manure nitrogen loading

Reducing the crude protein content of a diet, regardless of amino acid nutrition, does have an influence on excreta nitrogen content. For this reason, there is renewed interest in considering diet protein levels rather than merely amino acids, since concerns over environmental pollution are dictating strategies to limit nutrient loading in feces and urine. Poultry manure has always been a valuable source of fertilizer for pasture land and arable crops. However, large scale intensive units have led to the physical concentration of manure in relatively small areas. Because layer manure contains so much water, it is expensive to transport and there are severe limits on economical distance for disposal. A farm with 1 million layers yearly produces manure containing about 750 tonnes of nitrogen and 150 tonnes of phosphorus which are the main nutrients of concern for effective land use relative to potential for environmental contamination. Land used for corn production requires about 60 kg nitrogen and 25 kg P_2O_5 equivalents each year. This means that to effectively utilize the manure from a 1 million bird unit, it should be spread over 5,000 hectares in order to effectively use the nitrogen in the manure.

Most of the nitrogen in manure originates from crude protein, and to a lesser extent free amino acids and non-protein nitrogen. Many layer diets are formulated to a crude protein specification, simply in order to supply component amino acids. If diets are formulated solely on the basis of essential amino acids, with no crude protein minimum, then diets will usually contain less protein, and consequently less nitrogen. As protein/nitrogen level of the diet is reduced, there are resultant declines in nitrogen intake and nitrogen excretion. For example, in a recent study at Guelph, we fed diets varying in crude protein level from 19% down to a low of 9%, while maintaining levels of critical amino acids (Fig. 3.14).

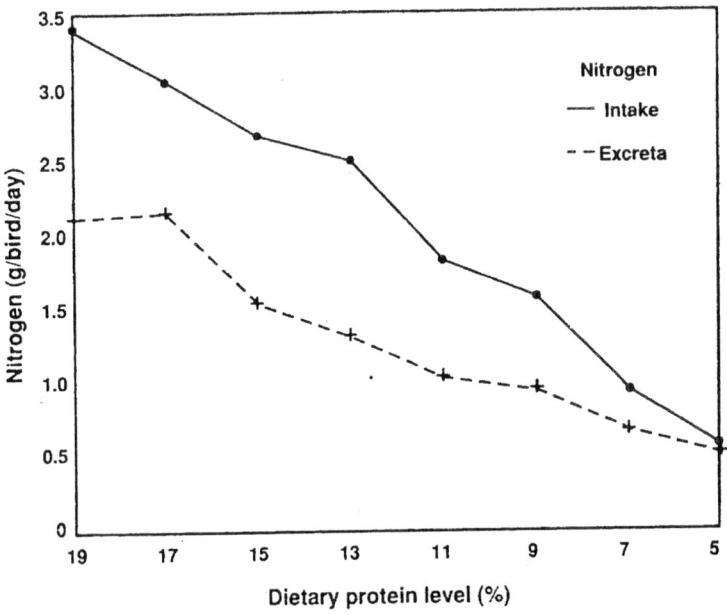

Figure 3.14 Nitrogen intake and excretion of layers in relation to diet protein level.

Layers do not seem to adjust their feed intake as the crude protein level of the diet is reduced, suggesting no appetite for protein *per se*. This is to be expected because any such appetite would likely be related to specific amino acids rather than protein *per se*. As protein intake declines, so does excreta nitrogen output (Fig. 3.14). For example if the crude protein level of the diet is reduced from 17% down to 14%, then nitrogen excretion declines from around 2 g/bird/day to about 1.5 g/bird/day. For the 1 million bird unit referred to earlier, this means a reduction in manure nitrogen of about 200 tonnes per year, and in turn 1300 hectares less land is needed for manure disposal. However the overall economic picture is not quite as straightforward as depicted by land use alone. Unfortunately, as meaningful reductions in crude protein level occur there is often a reduction in daily egg mass output. This latter situation may be due to incorrect assessment of amino acid needs and/or amino acid availability, or perhaps that the layer has need for some non-protein nitrogen in addition to amino acids. This loss in egg mass is often a consequence of reduced egg size, rather than reduced egg production. For the study depicted in Fig. 3.14, reducing crude protein from 17 to 13% resulted in a 2.3 g loss in average egg size.

3.26 PROTEIN AND AMINO ACID NUTRITION OF BROILER CHICKENS

Dietary levels of amino acids for broilers are shown in Table 3.31, including approximate crude protein equivalents and a corresponding metabolizable energy level.

Table 3.31 Dietary amino acid levels for broiler chickens (% of diet)							
	Pre-Starter	Starter		Grower		Finisher/Withdrawal	
Approximate protein level (%)	23	22	20	20	18	18	16
Amino acids							
Arginine	1.40	1.20	1.10	1.05	0.95	0.90	0.85
Lysine	1.35	1.20	1.05	1.10	0.90	0.90	0.80
Methionine	0.52	0.48	0.42	0.44	0.38	0.37	0.36
Methionine+Cystine	0.95	0.82	0.75	0.73	0.65	0.64	0.61
Tryptophan	0.22	0.20	0.18	0.17	0.15	0.14	0.13
Histidine	0.42	0.40	0.35	0.32	0.30	0.28	0.27
Leucine	1.50	1.40	1.20	1.10	1.00	1.00	0.90
Isoleucine	0.85	0.75	0.60	0.55	0.50	0.47	0.45
Phenylalanine	0.80	0.75	0.65	0.60	0.55	0.53	0.50
Phenylalanine+tyrosine	1.50	1.40	1.20	1.10	1.00	1.00	0.90
Threonine	0.75	0.70	0.62	0.60	0.55	0.55	0.50
Valine	0.90	0.80	0.70	0.65	0.60	0.58	0.55
Metabolizable energy (kcal/kg)	3050	3050	2900	3150	3000	3200	3050

Depending upon the complexity of ingredient usage, it is advisable to consider digestible amino acid requirements. Such values have not been clearly defined, but in many instances values will be close to 90% of total levels shown in Table 3.31. The balance of all amino acids to lysine, often called Ideal Protein (See Section 3.16) can also be considered to construct tabulated values for available amino acid requirements. For the starter, grower and finisher periods, requirements for available (digestible) lysine have been established at around 1.15%, 1.00% and 0.90% respectively. As previously indicated (Section 3.13) the lysine needs of the bird may change according to dietary crude protein level (Morris, et al., 1999). In previous studies these researchers suggested that lysine need was 54 g/kg crude protein, over a wide range of protein concentrations. Rose and Uddin (1997) indicate optimum lysine concentration for growth rate, expressed as a proportion of crude protein, to be curvilinear with optimum at around 60-70 g/kg. However the response is affected by environmental temperature, with much less response to lysine concentration at higher temperatures (Fig 3.15).

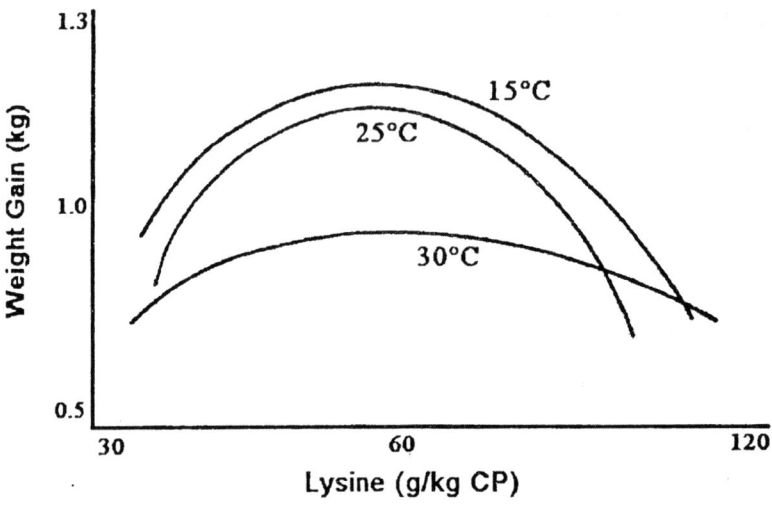

Figure 3.15 Effect of environmental temperature on broiler response to lysine (Adapted from Rose and Uddin, 1997)

An area of recent research interest has been the establishment of lysine require-ments for breast meat yield. In North America, breast meat contributes about 60% of total revenue and so small changes in yield are of economic significance. It is quite difficult to influence muscle deposition in birds via nutrition, other than the obvious effect of a deficiency situation (Tessaraud et al., (1999). However, assuming birds are growing at maximum genetic potential, it is not totally clear the role that amino acid intake plays in muscle accretion. Since all muscles are of remarkably similar amino acid profile, it is difficult to appreciate that diet can influence the growth of one muscle over another. However, many nutritionists are convinced that requirements for lysine needed for breast meat yield are greater than requirements needed to optimize growth rate and feed utilization. Bilgili et al., (1992) for example suggest that the lysine requirement of 42-53 d broiler chick-ens is higher than standard recommendations, if breast meat yield is a major criterion. Likewise, Kidd et al., (1998) suggest that lysine requirement for breast meat yield is higher than the requirement for maximizing growth rate. In their study maxi-mum breast yield was obtained with 1.25% lysine to 42 d and 1.06% lysine in the finisher period to 49 d.

Diet crude protein *per se* can, however, have a marked influence on fat deposi-tion in the body. As diet crude protein level increases, then there is less fat deposited (Table 3.32). There are proportional changes in carcass protein, in response to increased diet protein but there is virtually no effect on grams of protein or muscle in the carcass. The proportional changes in protein are of course a consequence of proportional changes in carcass fatness.

Table 3.32 Proportional and absolute changes in 42d broiler carcass components in response to diet protein level when diet energy remains constant				
	Carcass fat		Carcass Protein	
Diet protein level (%)	Grams	%	Grams	%
16	252d	50.0d	202a	40.7a
20	237c	46.2c	227b	44.9b
24	210b	42.4b	233b	47.7c
28	189a	39.4a	233b	49.2cd
32	185a	39.2a	233b	50.3d
36	179a	38.3a	234b	50.7d

Protein and amino acid intake can influence feather growth and development in the growing bird. Feathers are composed of about 90% crude protein, of which 60% are as amino acids, with cystine representing some 7% of protein. Most of the feather structure is keratin protein that is synthesized in the feather forming cells of the epidermis. The keratin structure is very rich in cystine, with each molecule containing around 8 half-cystine residues, and this is why methionine/TSAA levels are important for good feather structure. Marginal levels of methionine + cystine will cause abnormal feather growth and/or reduced feathering, although deficiencies of other amino acids will also cause feathering problems. With general amino acid inadequacy, the primary feathers have a characteristic spoonlike appearance that is caused by retention of an abnormally long sheath that covers the first 50% of the feather shaft. Deficiencies of many essential amino acids also cause abnormal curling of feathers away from the body. Interestingly, these same characteristics are seen with deficiencies of some of the B vitamins. However, methionine and especially methionine + cystine levels come under close scrutiny when abnormal feathering occurs. About 2% of the dietary methionine and 25% of the dietary cystine are needed for feather development. Because of the importance of methionine in maintaining normal growth and development, this amino acid is not likely to be deficient in situations where growth is adequate and feathering is abnormal. More likely, if feathering problems relate to TSAA metabolism, then overestimation of digestibility/availability of cystine in feedstuffs is usually the major problem. A number of years ago there was concern about feathering in broilers fed various ionophore anticoccidials. However subsequent research failed to show any definitive relationship between these compounds and metabolism of sulfur containing amino acids. Feathering is however, usually worse when ionophores are included in low protein diets (<18%CP equivalent) for young broilers.

Amino acid nutrition is sometimes questioned in relation to skin structure in broilers. About 5% of downgraded carcasses are due to tearing, and almost 1% of broilers are condemned due to cellulitis where skin tearing is a prerequisite. Skin strength is highly correlated with its collagen content, and so skin with greater collagen content is less prone to tearing. Any nutritional factor that influences skin collagen content will therefore indirectly affect susceptibility to tearing. The amino acid proline is a component of hydroxyproline, which itself is responsible for the stability and rigidity of collagen. Zinc, copper and vitamin C all play a role in collagen synthesis and so deficiencies of any one of these nutrients results in less skin collagen production. However, gross deficiencies of these nutrients also cause poor growth rate, a characteristic that is not usually seen in situations of excessive skin tearing. Unfortunately there seems to be little benefit to increasing the dietary levels of these nutrients, or even increasing the level of proline in the diet.

A specific dietary situation involves the anticoccidial, halofuginone. When this product is fed at normal recommended levels, there is significant loss in skin thickness and skin strength, especially in female birds. In one study, using halofuginone at 3 ppm of the diet resulted in a 50% reduction in skin collagen content and 50% increase in the incidence of skin tears. Halofuginone seems to affect skin strength in female birds, more than it does with males, and because the female has an inherently weaker skin, this leads to the greater incidence of tearing. It has been shown that halofuginone interferes with conversion of proline to hydroxyproline in the skin cells, and that this adverse effect cannot be corrected by adding more proline to the diet. When skin tearing is a problem, assuming that processing conditions have been scrutinized, the only potential nutritional factors appear to be halofuginone and levels of zinc, copper and vitamin C. Skin tearing is more problematic in hot weather. This situation leads to recommendations of supplemental vitamin C, although birds under these conditions almost always carry more subcutaneous fat. Feeding higher levels of crude protein has also been shown to increase skin strength although the reason for this is not clear. More crude protein may provide more of the non-essential amino acid glycine, which accounts for about 30% of the amino acids in collagen, or alternatively more protein *per se* may simply reduce carcass fatness.

3.27   PROTEIN AND AMINO ACID NUTRITION OF BROILER BREEDERS

Protein and amino acid requirements of juvenile and mature heavy breeders are shown in Table 3.33. Breeders will likely be subjected to quantitative feed restriction after 2-3 weeks of age. Juvenile breeders can be fed lower protein diets as a means of tempering growth rate. There has been research conducted on use of amino acid imbalanced diets for growing birds as a means of reducing growth rate. Unfortunately such formulation results in excessive variation in bird size which likely reflects genetic variance in requirement for certain amino acids, and particularly for lysine. Mature breeders are usually fed 150-170 g feed daily, depending upon environmental temperature. If such breeders are fed 16% CP diets, protein intake is around 25 g daily. Such an intake is difficult to rationalize based

Table 3.33 Dietary protein and amino acid levels for broiler breeders						
	Juvenile		♀ Adult Breeder (g peak feed/bird/day)			♂ Adult Breeder
	0-6wk	6-20 wk	165	155	140	
Approximate protein level (%)	18.0	16.0	15.5	16.0	16.5	12.0
Amino acids (% of diet):						
Arginine	.72	.62	.53	.58	.62	.48
Lysine	.90	.72	.60	.64	.68	.50
Methionine	.42	.38	.30	.33	.35	.23
Methionine+Cystine	.74	.63	.53	.57	.60	.40
Tryptophan	.18	.14	.11	.12	.13	.10
Histidine	.19	.17	.14	.15	.16	.12
Leucine	.92	.84	.71	.75	.80	.60
Isoleucine	.75	.67	.51	.58	.62	.40
Phenylalanine	.62	.55	.41	.46	.49	.30
Phenylalanine+Tryosine	.95	.90	.65	.70	.79	.50
Threonine	.75	.70	.52	.59	.63	.40
Valine	.80	.70	.60	.62	.65	.50
Metabolizable energy (kcal/kg)	2850	2800	2850	2900	2950	2700

on a peak daily egg mass of around 47 g and a body weight of 2.5 kg. In theory, breeder diets should provide proportionally less protein, and Lopez and Leeson (1995) showed the ability of breeders to perform adequately when fed diets as low as 10% CP that were fortified with methionine and lysine (Fig 3.16).

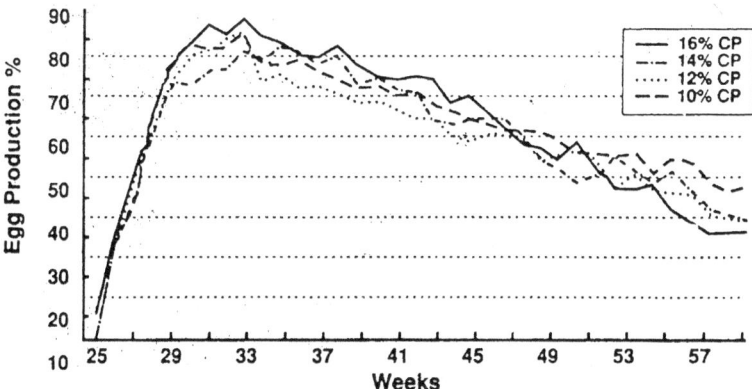

Figure 3.16 Egg Production of Broiler Breeder Hens From 25 to 60 Weeks of Age.   *(From Lopez and Leeson, 1993)*

In this same study, there was dramatic increase in fertility for breeders fed the lower protein diet (95.4 vs. 91.6%) a factor associated with the smaller body size of birds fed 10% rather than 16% CP. These data suggest that conventional protein and amino acid supply to adult breeder hens is in excess of requirement for reproduction, and that such excess nutrients fuel increased growth. There are also distinct advantages to feeding breeder males diets low in crude protein (Fig 3.17). Such improved fertility is correlated with increased semen volume and sperm numbers as a direct consequence of greater control over body weight.

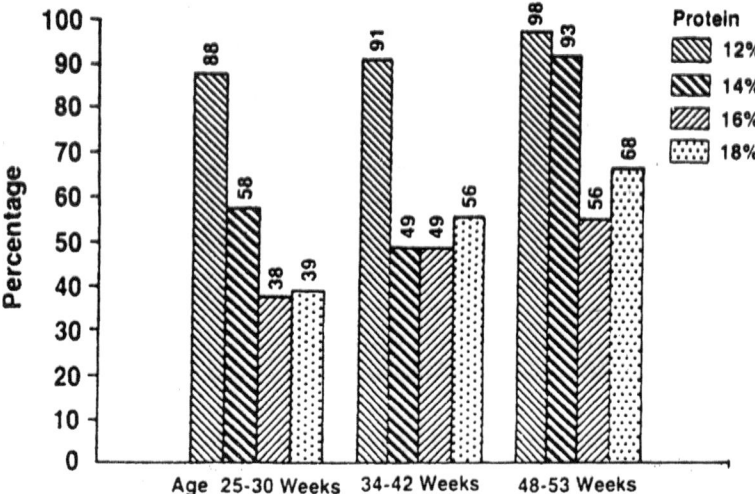

Figure 3.17 Diet protein level and percentage of roosters producing semen.
(From McDaniel, 1986)

SELECTED REFERENCES

Austic, R.E., 1978. Nutritional interactions of amino acids. Feedstuffs 50 (29) p 24-26.

Baker, D.H. and K.P. Boebel, 1998. Utilization of the D and L isomers of methionine and MHA as determined by chick bioassay. J. Nutr. 110:959-964.

Bilgili, S.F, E.T. Moran and N. Acar, 1992. Strain-cross response of heavy male broilers to dietary lysine in the finisher period. Poultry Sci. 71:850-858.

Boorman, K.N. and G.M. Ellis, 1996. Maximum nutritional response to poor quality protein and amino acid utilization. Br. Poultry Sci. 37:145-156.

Brake, J., D. Balnave and J.J. Dibner, 1998. Optimum dietary arginine:lysine ratio for broiler chickens is altered during heat stress in association with changes in intestinal uptake and dietary sodium chloride. Br. Poultry Sci. 39:639-647.

Buttery, P.J. and K.N. Boorman, 1976. The energetic efficiency of amino acid metabolism. In Protein Metabolism and Nutrition. Ed. Cole *et al.* Publ. Butterworths, UK.

Buttery, P.J., K.N. Boorman and E. Barratt, 1973. Proceedings of the Nutrition Society, UK. Vol. 32, p80A.

Calderon, V.M. and L.S. Jensen, 1990. The requirement for sulfur amino acids by laying hens influenced by protein concentration. Poultry Sci. 69: 934-944.

Calvert, C.C. and R.E. Austic, 1981. Lysine-chloride interactions in the growing chick. Poultry Sci. 60:1468-1472.

Carpenter, K.J., 1960. The estimation of the available lysine in animal protein foods. Biochem. J. 77:604-609.

Carpenter, K.J., 1973. Damage to lysine in food processing. Its measurement and its significance. Nutr. Abs & Rev. 43:423-429.

Combs, G.F. 1960. A method for calculating the methionine requirement of the laying hen. Feedstuffs. May 7, p 18.

Dale, N. and M. Araba, 1987. Protein solubility as an indicator of over-processing of soybean meal. Poultry Sci. 66. Suppl. 10-11.

D'Mello, J.P.F. and D. Lewis, 1970. Amino acid interaction in chick nutrition. Br. Poultry Sci. 11:367-385.

Edwards, H.M., S.R. Fernandez and D.H. Baker, 1999. Maintenance lysine requirement and efficiency of using lysine for accretion of whole body lysine and protein in young chicks. Poultry Sci. 78: 1407-1411.

Emmert, J.L. and D.H. Baker, 1997. Use of the ideal protein concept for precision formulation of amino acid levels in broiler diets. J. Appl. Poultry Res. 6:462-470.

Fisher, C., T.R. Morris and R.C. Jennings, 1973. A model for the description and prediction of the response of laying hens to amino acid intake. Br. Poult. Sci. 14:469-484.

Green, S. and T. Kiener, 1989. Digestibilities of nitrogen and amino acids in soybean, sunflower meal and rapeseed meals measured with pigs and poultry. Animal Prod. 48:157-179.

Han, Y. and D.H. Baker, 1994. Lysine requirement of male and female broiler chicks during the period three to six weeks post hatching. Poultry Sci. 73:1739-1745.

Harms, R.H. and G.B. Russell, 1994. A comparison of the bioavailability of DL-methionine and MHA for the commercial laying hen. J. Appl. Poult. Res. 3:1-6.

Hiramoto, K., T. Muramatsu and J. Okumura, 1989. Protein synthesis in several tissues of laying hens. Jpn. Poultry Sci 26: 340-347.

Hruby, M., M.L. Itamre and C.N. Coon, 1995. Predicting amino acid requirements of broilers at 21.1°C and 32.2°C. J. App. Poultry Res. 4:395-401.

Hurwitz, S. and S. Bornstein, 1973. The protein and amino acid requirements of laying hens: Suggested models for calculation. Poultry Sci. 52:1124-1130.

Hurwitz, S., D. Sklan and I. Bartov, 1978. New formal approaches to determination of energy and amino acid requirements of chicks. Poultry Sci. 57:197-206.

Johnson, R.J., 1992. Principles, problems and application of amino acid digestibility in poultry. World Poultry Sci. J. 48:232-246.

Kang, C.W., M.L. Sunde and R.W. Swick, 1985. Growth and protein turnover in the skeletal muscle of broiler chicks. Poultry Sci. 64:370-379.

Kidd, M.T., B.J. Kerr, K.M. Halpin, G.W. McWard and C.L. Quarles, 1998. Lysine levels in starter and grower -finisher diets affect broiler performance and carcass traits. J. Appl. Poultry Res. 7:351-358.

Koelkebeck, K.W., D.H. Baker and Y. Han, 1991. Effect of excess lysine, methionine, threonine or tryptophan on production performance of laying hens. Poultry Sci. 70:1651-1653.

Leeson, S. and J.D. Summers, 1997. Commercial Poultry nutrition. 2nd Ed. Publ. Univ. Books, Guelph, Ontario.

Leveille, G. and H. Fisher, 1958. The amino acid requirements for maintenance in the adult rooster. J. Nutr. 66:441-450.

Lopez, G. and S. Leeson, 1995. Response of broiler breeders to low-protein diets. Poultry Sci. 74:685-695.

Mack, S., D. Bercovici, G. DeGroote, B. Leclercq, M. Lippens, M. Pack, J.B. Schutte and S. Canwenberghe, 1999. Ideal amino acid profile and dietary lysine specification for broiler chickens of 20-40 d. Br. Poultry Sci. 40:257-265.

McDaniel, G.R., 1986. Feeding systems found to improve breeder performance. Feedstuffs, 58(49).

McDonald, M.W. and T.R. Morris, 1985. Quantitative review of optimum amino acid intakes for young laying pullets. Br. Poultry Sci. 26:253-264.

Mitchell, H.H., 1964. Comparative Nutrition of Man and Domestic Animals. Academic Press. NY. NY.

Morris, T.R. and H.A. Blackburn, 1982. Shape of the response curve relating protein intake to egg formation cycle of unanesthetized laying hens. Br. Poultry Sci. 23:405-424.

Morris, T.R., R.M. Gous and C. Fisher, 1999. An analysis of the hypothesis that amino acid requirement for chicks should be stated as a proportion of dietary protein. Wld. Poultry Sci. J. 55:7-22.

Muramatsu, T., H. Ohshima, M. Goto, S. Mori and J. Okumura, 1991. Growth prediction of young chicks. Do equal deficiencies of different essential amino acids produce equal growth responses? Br. Poultry Sci. 32:139-149.

National Research Council, 1994. Nutrient Requirements of Poultry, 9th Rev. Ed. NAS-NRC, Washington, D.C.

Nieto, R., R.M. Palmer, I. Fernandez, I. Perez and C. Prieto, 1994. Effect of protein quality, feed restriction and short term fasting on protein synthesis and turnover in tissues of the growing chicken. Br. J. Nutr. 72:499-507.

Parsons, C.M. and R.W. Leeper, 1984. Choline and methionine supplementation of layer diets varying in protein content. Poultry Sci. 63:1604-1609.

Parsons, C.M, L.M. Potter and R.D. Brown, 1983. Effect of dietary carbohydrate and of intestinal microflora on excretion of endogenous amino acids by poultry. Poultry Sci. 62:483-489.

Rose, S.P. and M.S. Uddin, 1997. Effect of temperature on the response of broiler chickens to dietary lysine balance. Br. Poultry Sci. 3(S) S36-37.

Rostagno, H.S., J. M.R. Pupa and M. Pack, 1995. Diet formulation for broilers based on total versus digestible amino acids. J. Appl. Poultry Res. 4:293-299.

Scott, R.L. and R.E. Austic, 1978. Influence of dietary potassium on lysine metabolism in the chick. J. Nutr. 108:137-144.

Smith, W.K., 1978. The amino acid requirement of laying hens. Models for calculation 2. Practical application. Wld. Poultry Sci. J. 34:129-136.

Surisdiarto, P. and D.J. Farrell, 1991. The relationship between dietary crude protein and dietary lysine requirement by broiler chicks on diets with and without the ideal amino acid balance. Poultry Sci. 70:830-836.

Tessaraud, S., E. Bihan-Dural, R. Peresson, J. Michel and A.M. Chagueau, 1999. Response of chick lines selected on carcass quality to dietary lysine supply. Poultry Sci. 78:80-84.

Waldroup, P.W. and H.M. Hellwig, 1995. Methionine and total sulfur amino acid requirements induced by stage of production. J. Appl. Poultry Res. 4:283-292.

Wang, T.C. and M.F. Fuller, 1989. The optimum dietary amino acid pattern for growing pigs. 1. Experiments by amino acid deletion. Br. J. Nutr. 62:77-89.

Woodhan, A.A. and P.S. Deans, 1977. Nutritive value of mixed proteins 1. In cereal based diets for poultry. Br. J. Nutr. 37:289-308.

Young, V.R., 1996. Protein and amino acid metabolism and nutrition. Proc 7th Int. Symposium Protein Metabolism and Nutrition. EAAP Publ. #81. Portugal.

V itamin is adapted from the term "vitamine", derived from "vital amines" by Casimir Funk, to describe "accessory food factors", which he thought contained amino nitrogen. It is now known that only a few of the vitamins contain amino nitrogen. However, the word has been shortened to "vitamin" which has been universally accepted as a group name for these essential nutrients.

Although discovery of the vitamins dates back to the beginning of the 20th century, certain diseases associated with dietary deficiencies had been recognized much earlier. What we now recognize as signs of vitamin deficiency have been documented for many years. Scurvy (deficiency of vitamin C) was a way of life for seafarers in the 1600-1700's, the effects being attributed to putrid drinking water. Sailors miraculously recovered once they reached land, but again the fresh water supply was given credit. Lund in 1753, a British naval doctor, published a paper on scurvy in which he reported that the disease could be prevented in humans by consuming diets containing salads and summer fruits. Indeed the action of lemon juice in preventing scurvy had been known since the beginning of the 17th century. The use of cod liver oil in preventing rickets had also been known, while Eijkman in 1897 reported on the essential food factor in brown rice which prevented beriberi. Interestingly, beriberi (thiamin deficiency) was most prevalent in the Chinese aristocracy, who always ate polished rice. Beriberi was less problematic to the Chinese peasants, since they ate the thiamin-rich hull portions.

In the mid 1800's Pasteur and Liebig observed that certain yeasts could grow on a medium of sugar, ammonium salts and the ash of yeast, while others grew very slowly and still others did not grow at all. In 1901, Wildiers confirmed earlier findings by demonstrating that transferring a large inoculum from a growing yeast culture to a sterile medium, resulted in good yeast growth. However, when he transferred only a small amount of the yeast culture to the sterile medium, the yeast invariably failed to grow. Wildiers claimed that the large inoculum was carrying to the medium some unknown factor necessary for life, while the small amount of inoculent transferred failed to carry this substance. He called this particular substance "bios". This term was used for many years to refer to unknown factors required by microorganism to sustain growth. In later years, many of these factors were shown to be identical to the vitamins required by man and animals.

Four years before the discovery of bios by Wildiers, Christian Eijkman was investigating the cause of beriberi on the island of Java. He noted that chickens receiving polished rice, similar to that fed to his hospital patients, developed outbreaks of poylneuritis, which resembled the nervous symptoms of his patients with beriberi. The discovery that this condition was nutritional in origin was accidental, and was based on the chance finding that chickens receiving unpolished rice had no disease symptoms. Later, Grijns working in Eijkman's laboratory, showed that polyneuritis gallinarum was due to a deficiency of a substance in the silver layer of rice bran and that this substance was easily destroyed by moist heat. During the ensuing years, Funk determined the amine-like nature of the substance, thiamin, which cured polyneuritis in birds.

Throughout the discovery, isolation and identification of the vitamins, the chicken has played a prominent role. The Wisconsin workers used chicks in their classic studies of vitamin A and D, while Cornell workers used chickens in studies which helped lead to the discovery and development of pantothenic acid, riboflavin, folic acid, and vitamin B_{12}. Work carried out at Guelph and Davis with chicks, helped lead to the discovery and synthesis of vitamin K.

Since the term "vitamin" was adopted, other terms have been used to describe these vital nutrients. Some of these terms were; advitant, bios, biocatalyst, cataline, ergen, ergon, exogenous hormone, and nutrilite. Of these, only the terms, biocatalyst, bios, and nutrilite are still sometimes used in the literature. The term vitamin is now universally used when referring to the nutrition of animals while the term bios is used in relation to microorganisms, and nutrilite when referring to factors required specifically by microorganisms, but not by animals.

4.1 DEFINITION OF A VITAMIN

A "vitamin" is generally accepted to be an organic compound which : (a) is a component of natural food but distinct from carbohydrate, protein, fat or water; (b) present in foods in minute amounts; (c) is essential for growth, maintenance, health and well being of an animal; (d) when absent from a diet, or poorly absorbed or utilized, results in a specific deficiency disease or syndrome, and (e) cannot be synthesized by an animal and must therefore be obtained from the diet. There are some exceptions among the vitamins. For example, vitamin D can be synthesized on the surface of the skin by ultraviolet light, and nicotinic acid can be synthesized, to some extent, from tryptophan.

Vitamins act as catalysts for many reactions in the body, and so are required in very small quantities. They can occur as vitamins *per se* or as precursors (provitamins).

4.2 VITAMIN NOMENCLATURE

The International Union of Pure and Applied Chemistry established a commission on the nomenclature of biological chemistry in 1957. They established definite rules for the nomenclature of the vitamins. The "Generic descriptors and trivial names of vitamins and related compounds recommendations" of the International Union of Nutrition Science's Committee on Nomenclature are consistent with the recommendations of the IUPAC and the Committee on Nomenclature of the American Institute of Nutrition (1981). This nomenclature is used throughout this publication. Thiamin is still spelled with an "e" in many nutrition journals. Table 4.1 shows the commonly accepted names for vitamins, together with terms that have been used in the past, but today are mostly obsolete.

Table 4.1 Vitamin Nomenclature

Vitamin	Accepted name	Alternate designations in earlier use (some obsolete)	Recognized clinical activities	Remarks
Vitamin A	Retinol (all-trans), 9-cis-Retinol, 13-cis-Retinol, 9.13-disis-Retinol	Vitamin A$_1$, Axerophthol, Axerol	Prevents xerophthalmia, nyctalopia and hemeralopia. Also essential for normal epithelial tissue development and growth. Prevents ataxias and bone abnormalities in certain animals. Required for normal reproduction in poultry.	A group of closely related carotenoids nutritionally active because they serve as precursors.
	Retinaldehyde (six stereo-isomers at 9, 11 & 13 positions)	Vitamin A aldehyde, Retinal, Retinene$_1$, Isoretinene$_{a,b}$, Neoretinene$_{a,b,c}$		Summation of biological activities of all forms should be expressed as "retinol equivalent" (in μg).
	Retinoic acid (Four cis-isomers known)	Vitamin A acid		Has not been found to occur in nature, but may be an instantaneous intermediate in animal metabolism.
	Dehydrotretinol, Dehydrotretinaldehyde, Dehydroretinoic acid	Vitamin A$_2$		Present in livers of fresh water fish.
Vitamin D	Ergocalciferol	Vitamin D$_2$, Oleovitamin D$_2$, Activated ergosterol, Viosterol	Prevents rickets in man and mammals.	Active metabolite is 1,25 dihydroxycholecalciferol, formed from vitamin D$_3$ in liver and kidney.
	Cholecalciferol	Vitamin D$_3$, Activated 7-dehydrocholesterol, Oleovitamin D$_3$	Required for growth, bone and eggshell formation and for normal reproduction in poultry. Also, for normal feather pigmentation in some breeds of poultry. Only cholecalciferol is effective for poultry.	For summation, use cholecalciferol equivalent.

Table 4.1 Vitamin Nomenclature

Vitamin	Accepted name	Alternate designations in earlier use (some obsolete)	Recognized clinical activities	Remarks
Vitamin E	RRR-α-tocopherol	d-α-Tocopherol	Necessary for prevention of reproductive failure, nutritional muscular dystrophy, erythrocyte hemolysis, steatitis in a number of animals, encephalomalacia and exudative diathesis in chicks, necrotic liver degeneration in rats. Activity requivalent to RRR-α-tocopherol on a unit for unit basis.	Activity shared by approximately 7 other chromenols, differing in terms of substituent groups on benzene ring and degree of unsaturation of phytyl side chain. The other naturally occurring vitamins E are β-, γ-, and δ-tochopherols; α-, β-, γ- and δ-tocotrienols.
	All-RAC-α-tocopherol	Anti-sterility vitamin		
Vitamin K	Phylloquione	Vitamin K_1 Phytylmenaquinone PMQ Koagulations vitamin Anti-hemorrhagic vitamin Prothrombin factor	Necessary to prevent hypoprothrombinemic hemorrhage.	Natural form of the vitamin synthesized by plants. Phylloquinone and Menaquinone-4 are metabolically active forms.
	Menaquinone-4	Vitamin $K_{2(20)}$ Prenylmenaquinone-4 MK-4 MQ-4		Menaquinone-4 synthesized in animals from medanione. All other menaquinones arise from microbial synthesis.
	Menaquinone-6	Vitamin $K_{2(30)}$ (Famoquinone) Prenylmenaquinone-6 MK-6 MQ-6		
	Menadione	Vitamin K_3 Menaquinone		Synthetic, may occur in nature as intermediate in animal synthesis of menaquinone-4.

Table 4.1 Vitamin Nomenclature

Vitamin	Accepted name	Alternate designations in earlier use (some obsolete)	Recognized clinical activities	Remarks
Vitamin B$_1$	Thiamin	Thiamine Aneurin(e) Polyneuramin Oryzamin Betabion Vitamin F	Prevents polyneuritis in young animals; beriberi in man. Required for prevention of extreme anorexia.	
Vitamin B$_2$	Riboflavin	Riboflavine Lactoflavin Ovoflavin Uroflavin Hepatoflavin Lyochrome Vitamin G	Stimulates growth; prevents certain ocular and orolingual disturbances in humans; curled-toe paralysis in chicks and poults.	
Niacin Niacinamide	Nicotinic acid Nicotinamide	Pellagra-preventing factor Vitamin PP Pellagramine Vitamin B$_3$	Prevents abnormal hock enlargement in chicks, and especially in turkeys and ducks; pellagra in humans and pigs; black-tongue in dogs. Required for normal feathering in poultry. Nicotinic acid has pharmacological use as vasodilator.	Nicotinamide does not cause flushing or vasodilation.
Vitamin B6	Vitamin B6 group consisting of: Pyridoxine Pyridoxal Pyridoxamine	Yeast eluate factor Adermin Pyridoxol	Necessary for growth and prevention of acrodynia, anemia, epileptic-like convulsions.	

Table 4.1 Vitamin Nomenclature

Vitamin	Accepted name	Alternate designations in earlier use (some obsolete)	Recognized clinical activities	Remarks
Pantothenic acid	Pantothenic acid	Chick anti-pellagra factor Liver filtrate factor Yeast filtrate factor Vitamin B_3	Prevents dermatitis in chicks and rats, achromotrichia in rats, convulsion, coma and death in dogs. Required for hatchability of chicken and turkey eggs, and normal viability of newly-hatched chicks and for normal feathering.	
Biotin	Biotin	Egg white injury-preventing factor Bios IIB Vitamin H Factor X Coenzyme R	Required for growth and prevention of dermatitis and perosis.	Biocytin is (+)-epilson-N-biotinyl-L-lysine.
Folacin	Folic acid	Pteroylmonoglutamic Acid Norit eluate factor L. casei factor Vitamin M Factor U Factor R Vitamin B Vitamin B_{10} PGA	Required for prevention of macrocytic anemias, perosis and feathering in chicks, cervical paralysis in poults, achromotrichia in chickens and dogs, anemia, gingivitis and steatitis in monkeys.	Several other derivatives of pteroylmonoglutamic aid, and the tetra-hydro and N formyl compounds exist.
	5-methyltetera-hydrofolic acid	N^5-M-PHAH$_4$		Appears to be the form of folic acid normally found in blood stream.

		Table 4.1 Vitamin Nomenclature		
Vitamin	Accepted name	Alternate designations in earlier use (some obsolete)	Recognized clinical activities	Remarks
Vitamin B$_{12}$	Cyanocobalamin Hydroxocobalamin Aquocobalamin	Animal protein factor L. lactis Dorner factor Erythrotin Extrinsic factor Anti-pernicious anemia principle Vitamin B$_{12a}$ Vitamin B$_{12b}$	Required for normal growth and hatchability of eggs. Prevents pernicious anemia in man.	Other forms of vitamin B$_{12}$ exist wherein the cyanide group is replaced by such groups as nitrite-, chlorine-, thiocyanate- and cyanate-.
Choline	Choline	Amantine Bilineurine Gossypine Vidine	Prevents perosis (slipped Achilles tendon) in chicks and especially in poults.	Interrelated with Mn, Zn, nicotinic acid, folic acid, and biotin in prevention of perosis; with methionine in transmethylation.
Vitamin C	Ascorbic acid or L-Ascorbic acid	Hexuronic acid Antiscorbutic vitamin Cevitamic acid	Prevents scurvy - not required by the chicken under most environmental conditions.	Required only by humans, other primates, guinea pigs, and fish; most other species biosynthesize it in adequate amounts.

4.3 NATURE OF THE VITAMINS

Vitamins differ markedly in their chemical composition and also their metabolic function. They are found in widely varying concentrations in feedstuffs but no single feedstuff contains all the vitamins in optimal amounts for chickens or other animals. Hence, the contribution of all ingredients in a diet must be assessed, and any deficiencies in the diet made up by synthetic or high potency supplements. Most vitamins are derived initially from plants and their occurrence in animals is only the result of consumption of plants. However, animals contain microorganisms that are capable of synthesizing the water-soluble vitamins. Also provitamin A (β-carotene) and the menaquinones (vitamin K_2) can be synthesized by microorganisms. Indeed vitamin B_{12} (cyanocobalamin) cannot be synthesized by plants or animals, but only by certain microorganisms.

While vitamins naturally occurring in plant and animal based feed ingredients can supply a reasonable proportion of the birds daily needs, their contribution is rarely considered during formulation. This situation arises due to variability, especially in cereals and vegetable proteins, for both total and digestible levels of vitamins. For example, the vitamin E content of corn can vary from 10 to 40 IU/kg. Variable crop location, soil type, fertilizer use, variety, stage of maturity at harvest, and drying and storage conditions all contribute to the concentration of vitamins in most crops. Likewise mold infestation usually results in less fat soluble vitamins in corn and other cereals because molds and fungi invariably invade the germ portion of the grain, where most fat is concentrated. During feed manufacture, some vitamins are unstable during heat treatment (especially A, D_3, E, K, C and thiamin) while bioavailable levels of all vitamins decline over time in stored grains and mixed feeds. The bioavailability of vitamins also varies across ingredients, the classical example being biotin in corn vs wheat. Natural biotin in corn is often 60% available to the young chick, whereas less than 10% is available from wheat. All of these factors lead to uncertainty in the natural supply of vitamins within a feed, and for this reason, they are rarely considered in poultry nutrition. The bird's vitamin supply is therefore met by the addition of synthetic vitamins, usually in the form of a so called "premix", that contains all vitamins and perhaps some other micronutrients and feed additives.

Most synthetic vitamins are produced by chemical processes, the exception being vitamin B_{12} which is manufactured by fermentation. Riboflavin, biotin and vitamin C can also be produced by fermentation, where genetic engineering has recently resulted in much more efficient yield of vitamins from microbes during fermentation.

The B vitamins and vitamins K_3 and C are expressed as mg/kg of diet. Vitamins B_{12} and biotin are often expressed in μg/kg, because of their very low inclusion rate. Vitamins A, D_3 and E are usually expressed in terms of International Units (IU)/kg diet.

Table 4.2 shows common units of vitamin potency, equivalency of various common forms, and the chemical form and appearance of commercial products.

Table 4.2 Vitamin units, equivalency and chemical forms

Vitamin	Unit	Equivalency	Chemical Form	Appearance
A	1 IU	0.344 μg retinly acetate 0.55 μg retinly palmitate	Ester of acetate, palmitate	Yellow-brown oil solid at room temperature.
D_3	1 IU	0.25 μg D_3	Alcohol	Yellow-white resin
E	1 IU	1 mg DL α-tocopherol acetate	Acetate	Yellow-brown oil
K_3	1 mg Menadione	500 μg MSB 350 μg MSBC	Menadione	Yellow oil
Thiamin	1 mg Thiamin HCl	0.89 mg thiamin	Hydrochloride	White powder
Riboflavin	1 mg	–	–	Yellow powder
Niacin	1 mg nicotinic acid 1 mg nicotinamide	–	Nicotinic acid or Nicotinamide	White powder
Pantothenic acid	1 mg	0.92 mg Ca-Pantothenate	Ca-Pantothenate	White powder
Pyridoxine	1 mg pyridoxine HCl	0.82 mg pyridoxine	Hydrochloride	White powder
Folic acid	1 mg		–	Yellow powder
Biotin	1 μg		–	White powder
B_{12}	1 μg		Cyanocobalamin	Red powder
C	1 mg	0.89 mg sodium ascorbate	Sodium salt, polyphosphate	White-yellow powder
Choline	1 mg choline chloride	0.75 mg choline	Chloride	White-yellow powder or liquid

4.4 CLASSIFICATION OF THE VITAMINS

The vitamins have been divided into two groups based upon their solubility in either fats and fat solvents, or water. The fat-soluble vitamins A, D, E, and K, are found in feedstuffs in association with lipids and are thus digested and absorbed along with dietary fats by mechanisms similar to those involved with fats. Conditions favourable to fat absorption also favour fat-soluble vitamin absorption while the reverse is true for factors that are unfavourable to fat absorption. The water soluble vitamins required by the chicken are B_1, B_2, B_6, B_{12}, nicotinic acid, pantothenic acid, folic acid, biotin, and choline. Fat-soluble vitamins are stored in appreciable amounts while water soluble vitamins are not stored to any extent, and excesses are excreted via the urine. Thus, a constant dietary supply of water-soluble vitamins is necessary to avoid deficiency symptoms. The major metabolic activities and functions of the vitamins are listed in Table 4.3.

Table 4.3 Metabolic function of Vitamins	
Vitamin	**Metabolic Function**
A	Protein metabolism, especially in mucosal surfaces. Involved in formation of rhodopsin in the retina.
D_3	Regulation of calcium and phosphate balance. Influences calcium uptake from intestine, uptake and release from bone, and efficiency of recirculation via the kidney.
E	Biologic antioxidant, acting as an electron acceptor especially in cellular membranes. Prevents peroxide formation.
K	Necessary for synthesis of prothrombin and factors involved in blood clotting. Also electron transport in energy systems.
Thiamin	Co-enzyme of pyruvate decarboxylase and trans ketolase enzymes.
Riboflavin	Part of flavin enzymes (FMD and FAD) which act as hydrogen acceptors in NAD, NADH metabolism.
Niacin	Co-enzyme of various dehydrogenase pathways such as NADPH.
Pyridoxine	Co-enzyme of amino decarboxylases and amino-transferases, and so important in protein metabolism.
Pantothenic acid	Involved in acyl transferring enzyme systems such as pyruvate→oxaloacetate. Also β oxidation and synthesis of long-chain fatty acids.
Biotin	Part of carboxylase enzyme systems such as Acety CoA carboxylase, involved in fatty acid synthesis, gluconeogenesis and amino acid catabolism.
Folic acid	Methylation enzyme systems, such as conversion of homocystine into methionine and DNA synthesis.
Vitamin B_{12}	Involved in transmethylation and part of enzyme methyl malonyl-CoA-isomerase.
Choline	Transmethylation and donation of methyl groups.
C	Transfer of hydrogen ions and electrons and hydroxylation processes.

4.5 VITAMIN REQUIREMENTS

Chickens are particularly susceptible to vitamin deficiencies for the following reasons: (1) chickens derive little or no benefit from microbial synthesis of vitamins in their gastro-intestinal tract; (2) chickens have high requirements for vitamins as they are the "catalysts" for vital metabolic body functions; (3) due to modern management conditions many stresses are placed upon the birds, which can increase their vitamin requirement as detailed by NRC (1994) as shown in Table 4.4. These values are generally regarded as absolute minimum requirements, when under ideal conditions, birds will grow or perform quite adequately and not show overt signs of deficiency. Because poultry under commercial conditions are subject to environmental, behavioural and disease stress, vitamin needs are increased. There is also need to increase dietary vitamin levels above minimum requirements, so as to account for loss of potency between the time of feed preparation and tissue metabolism. Consequently, commercial vitamin recommendations are accordingly increased above minimum requirements (Leeson and Summers 1997) and such values are shown alongside minimum NRC (1994) data in Table 4.4.

Table 4.4 Vitamin requirements (NRC, 1994) and suggested commercial diet specifications (Leeson and Summers, 1997)

Vitamin (per kg diet)	Broiler starter		Laying hen	
	NRC	Commercial	NRC	Commercial
A (IU)	1500	6500	3000	7500
D₃ (IU)	200	3000	300	2500
E (IU)	10	30	5	25
K (Mg)	0.5	2.0	0.5	2.0
Thiamin (mg)	1.8	4.0	0.7	2.0
Riboflavin (mg)	3.6	5.5	2.5	4.5
Niacin (mg)	35	40	10	40
Pantothenic acid (mg)	10	14	2	10
Pyridoxine (mg)	3.5	4.0	2.5	3.0
Folic acid (mg)	0.55	1.0	0.25	0.75
Biotin (µg)	150	200	100	150
B₁₂ (µg)	10	13	4	10
Choline (mg)	1300	800	1050	1200

Since the chick has a high requirement for vitamins they show classical deficiency symptoms with low dietary levels. Thus, they have been used extensively as experimental animals in research which led to the isolation and identification of the vitamins. As a result, many of the vitamin requirements for poultry are more precise than those given for other animals. An example of increased vitamin requirements for modern commercial poultry, is demonstrated by comparing the vitamins required in a practical diet over the past several decades. Vitamins such as B_1, B_6, biotin and folic acid, were adequately supplied from feed ingredients in the regular diet some 30 years ago. However, today they must be supplemented in diets for optimum performance.

Vitamins, unlike energy or protein which are consumed in definite amounts per day, are usually supplied in poultry diets in excess of minimum requirements. Thus, the requirements are not stated in amounts per day, but usually as amounts per kg of diet. These levels are set high enough to ensure adequacy in spite of any changes in feed intake due to environment, energy level of the diet, disease stress or any other factor which might influence feed intake or vitamin requirements of the bird (Table 4.4).

4.6   VITAMIN STABILITY

Vitamins can be deactivated due to chemical and physical changes within the premix, in the mixed feed or even in the body of the chicken. When chemical degradation occurs, then such effects can be determined by chemical or microbiological assay. The role of antimetabolites is more difficult to detect because the vitamin is still structurally sound, and so readily detectable during conventional assay procedures. Many "anti-vitamins" are structurally very similar to the target vitamin. All B vitamins are very molecular specific, and slight changes to their structure renders them inactive. Analogues, therefore, have no place in B vitamin metabolism and are in fact often anti-vitamins.

Perhaps the most classical anti-vitamin is avidin which is actually found in raw eggs. One molecule of avidin binds 3 molecules of biotin, one each by the three constituent polypeptide side chains of avidin. Avidin is one part of the antibacterial agents found in eggs, competing with any microbes for biotin, and so depriving them of this important co-enzyme. How avidin influences the biotin status of the developing embryo has never been fully elucidated. Another antivitamin is thiaminase which is found in underheated fish meals. More common 20-30 years ago, with 4-6% improperly processed fish (and sometimes meat meals), there were classical neural disorders seen with thiamin deficiency. Flaxseed also contains an antivitamin known as 1-amino-D-proline, which forms a stable complex with pyridoxine. Of more general concern to nutritionists is the susceptibility of vitamins to oxidation reduction and such factors as temperature, ultraviolet light and pH. Table 4.5 summarizes the general concerns about stability of vitamins.

Table 4.5 General vitamin stability	
Vitamin	Stability characteristics
A	Oxidation, especially with Fe and Cu.
D₃	Moderately stable to oxidation.
E	Stable as acetate. Alcohol very unstable.
K	Very unstable.
Thiamin	Oxidation and pH sensitive.
Pyridoxine, Riboflavin	Moderately stable.
Pantothenate	Susceptible to hydrolysis.
Niacin	Fairly stable.
B₁₂	Highly stable, few losses over time.
Biotin	Fairly stable.
Folic acid	Moderately stable, susceptible to oxidation and reduction.
Vitamin C	Very unstable in natural forms.

Such variability in vitamin oxidation accounts for most of the variance between "requirement" and "commercial" recommendations for the various vitamins. Vitamins K and C are the most susceptible to loss, although the stability of all vitamins declines almost linearly with an increase in temperature, oxidative stress, storage time etc. Coelho (1994) shows the change in assayed vitamins starting with a premix, and then after pelleting, and for the most extreme situation, expanding of feed followed by pelleting (Table 4.6).

Table 4.6 Comparison of vitamin levels in premix and finished broiler feed after 2 weeks storage (units/kg/feed)			
Vitamin	Premix	Pelleting	Expander + Pelleting
A (IU)	10,000	8,000	7,800
D₃ (IU)	3,000	2,400	2,300
E (IU)	20	17.5	17.2
Menadione (mg)	2	1.1	0.8
Thiamin (mg)	2	1.7	1.6
Riboflavin (mg)	9	7.5	7.0
Pyridoxine (mg)	2.5	2.0	1.9
B₁₂ (μg)	30	27	27
Pantothenate (mg)	12	10	9.8
Folic acid (mg)	1.0	0.83	0.81
Biotin (μg)	100	80	78
Niacin (mg)	50	40	37

4.7 VITAMIN INTERDEPENDENCE

There is some indication of interaction between fat soluble vitamins, although it is far from clear if such effects are meaningful at normal levels of inclusion. When very high levels of vitamin A are fed (>60,000 IU/kg), there is a reduction in plasma vitamin E, which could compromise the bird's antioxidant systems. With very high levels of vitamin E, there is an increased accumulation of liver vitamin E, and toxic effects of high levels of vitamin A are reduced. With higher inclusion levels of vitamins E or A, there is an indication of increased requirement for vitamins D_3 and K_3. However these effects have not been demonstrated with more moderate levels of vitamins. For example feeding from 6-20,000 IU vitamin A/kg has no effect on vitamin E status, while feeding as much as 1,000 IU vitamin E/kg, seems to have no influence on vitamin A status. The so-called interdependence of these vitamins could therefore be considered a type of toxicity, since exceptionally high dietary levels are needed to elicit any adverse response.

4.8 VITAMIN DEFICIENCIES

If vitamins are below requirement levels for any length of time, classical deficiency signs will be seen. In general, the onset of deficiency signs is more rapid in young chicks, and the developing embryo is perhaps the most sensitive model. Problems with B vitamins appear fairly quickly, sometimes in 5-7d, because there is little storage of these in the body. Deficiencies of the fat soluble vitamins can take considerably longer to develop, because of storage in fat depots and especially the liver of older birds. In order to induce a classical deficiency of vitamin A in a layer for example, it may be necessary to feed a deficient diet for 6-8 weeks. This does not mean to say that layers can be fed diets devoid of vitamin A for extensive periods because while birds may appear normal with such diets, there will likely be loss in growth, egg production, egg size and/or hatchability with breeders.

Deficiency is therefore a relative term, depending upon the expectation of bird survival, growth and development. The following categories are often used to describe vitamin adequacy, and by definition, failure to meet such specifications can be regarded as a deficiency:

a) **Deficiency** - inadequate supply and clinical signs develop over time.

b) **Minimal supply** - Prevents clinical signs with dietary levels comparable to those established by NRC. Provide adequate growth under ideal conditions.

c) **Optimum supply** - meets all needs for optimum growth and performance taking into account stability losses.

d) **Specialized supply** - meets all conventional metabolic needs under certain special (stress) situations eg. vitamin E for enhanced immune status.

The classical deficiency signs will be described in subsequent sections dealing with individual specific vitamins. Table 4.7 provides a guideline for diagnoses of vitamin deficiencies according to such factors as general bird appearance, neurological disorders etc. Table 4.7 also indicates other factors that can elicit signs and abnormalities similar to those of vitamin deficiencies. Today, because of the

Table 4.7 General signs of deficiency		
1. General Appearance	Vitamins	Other Potential Factors
Rough feathers	Niacin, Pantothenace, Folate, Choline, Biotin	Amino acids, Mycotoxins, Brooding temperature
Dermatitis	Niacin, Vitamin A, Folate, Pantothenate	Zinc, external parasites
Blindness	Vitamin A	Light intensity, Newcastle disease
Mouth lesions	Pantothenate	Mycotoxins
Footpad lesions	Biotin	Litter ammonia
2. Internal organs		
Fatty liver	Vitamin A, Thiamin, Pyridoxine, Vitamin E, Choline	Fat saturation, Mycotoxins
Fatty kidney	Biotin	—
3. Nervous system		
Ataxia	Vitamin A	—
Lameness	Vitamin D_3	Mineral metabolism, Mycotoxins
Convulsions	Thiamin, Pyridoxine	—
Polyneuritis	Thiamin	—
Encephalomalacia	Vitamin E	
Curled-toes	Riboflavin	Genetics
Neck retraction	Thiamin	Tryptophan-embryo
4. Vascular system		
Anemia	Vitamin K, B_{12}	Iron
Cyanosis	Thiamin	Carbon Monoxide
Poor blood clotting	Vitamin K, C	
Delayed healing	Vitamin C	Bacterial infection
Hemorrhage	Vitamin K, C	Mycotoxins
5. Skeletal		
Rickets	Vitamin D_3	Calcium, Phosphorus
Soft bones	Vitamin D_3	Calcium, Phosphorus
Enlarged hocks	Vitamin A, Niacin, Choline	Bacterial
Perosis	Choline, B_{12}, Folic Acid	Manganese

common practice of adding vitamins as composite premixes, one is less likely to see deficiencies of individual vitamins. This situation can obviously occur if a vitamin is excluded from a premix, or some antimetabolite is present in the feed. More common today is the situation where the entire premix is inadvertently excluded from a diet, and in such situations, a complex array of signs develop. In these latter occurrences, a deficiency of riboflavin is often the first sign of a nutritional problem.

As previously described, the developing embryo is particularly sensitive to vitamin deficiencies, and either the embryo will die, or be malformed, or atypical in some way. Table 4.8 describes the common signs of vitamin deficiencies in developing chicken embryos. Such deficiencies are most likely a consequence of inadequate breeder vitamin nutrition although some pre-incubation egg treatment processes can influence embryo vitamin metabolism.

Table 4.8 Embryo vitamin deficiency signs	
Vitamin	**Deficiency signs**
Vitamin A	Early embro mortality (48 hours) with failure to develop circulatory system.
Vitamin D$_3$	Depending on reserves in dams, stunted chicks and soft bones. Usually associated with shell defects and hence changes in porosity of the shell.
Vitamin E	Early embryo mortality at 1-3d. Encephalomalacia may be seen in the embryo and exudative diathesis is common.
Riboflavin	Excessive embryo mortality 9-14 or 17-21d. Embryos show edema and/or clubbed down. Chicks may show a curling of the toes in extreme situations.
Pantothenic acid	Subcutaneous hemorrhages in unhatched embryos.
Biotin	Reduced hatch without reduced egg production. Peak in embryo mortality during first week and last 3 days of incubation. May see skeletal deformities and crooked beaks.
Vitamin B$_{12}$	Embryo mortality around 8-14 days, with possibly edema curled toes and shortening of the beak.
Thiamin	There are two stages of embryo mortality - one very early and the other at 19-21d. Many dead chicks appear on the trays although there are few, if any, deformed chicks. Mortality can be high for 10-14 days for those chickens that do hatch. Injecting the chicks with thiamin results in an almost instantaneous recovery. Certain types of disinfectants, anticoccidials and poor quality fish meal have been implemented in thiamin deficiencies. There is also recent evidence to suggest that thiamin requirements are incresed in the presence of some Fusarium molds.
Vitamin K	Hemorrhage and bleeding in chicks as they hatch. Excess bleeding also seen at day-old beak trimming etc.

4.9 VITAMIN TOXICITY

Vitamins can become toxic if fed at sufficiently high levels. As a generalization, the fat soluble vitamins are likely to be the most toxic, because their effects are seen at 3-30x normal inclusion levels. For the B vitamins, it often takes at least 100x normal feeding level, to initiate a toxic effect (Table 4.9).

Table 4.9 Toxicity of vitamins		
Vitamin	Safe upper feed levels (units/kg feed)	Safe upper level ÷ normal level
A	80,000 IU/kg	10
D_3	10,000 IU/kg > 60d 50,000 IU/kg < 20d	3-4 20-30
E	1,000 IU/kg	20-30
K	2,000 mg/kg	1000
C	5,000 mg/kg	20
Thiamin	3,000 mg/kg	700
Niacin	3,000 mg/kg < 20d	100
Riboflavin	1,000 mg/kg	200
Pyridoxine	4,000 mg/kg	1000
Folic acid	5,000 mg/kg	5000
Pantothenic acid	2,000 mg/kg	150
Biotin	2.5 mg/kg	15
B_{12}	5 mg/kg	350
Choline	20,000 mg/kg	20

In certain situations, toxicity may relate to the form of vitamin, where for example problems with high levels of choline may in fact be caused by the associated chloride molecule. Pyridoxine and thiamin are also commonly used as chloride salts (Table 4.2).

In regular feeding situations, the greatest potential for toxicity arises with vitamins A, D_3 and choline. With toxicity of vitamin A, there will be nervous dysfunction, while for high levels of D_3, calcification of soft tissue, and especially the kidneys will occur. High levels of choline cause depressed growth. mainly as a consequence of electrolyte imbalance, related to its 25% chloride content. Vitamin C, E and biotin are moderately toxic, potentially causing problems at 20-30x normal inclusion levels. The remaining B vitamins are toxic only at levels of at least 100x normal inclusion levels. Toxicity of vitamins administered in the drinking water is quite rare, since birds are reluctant to drink such highly fortified water.

4.10 VITAMIN A

Vitamin A was discovered in 1913 by McCollum and Davis, when they noted that rats fed lard as a source of fat ceased to grow. However, adequate growth was obtained when butter or fat extracted from the egg yolk were used as a source of dietary fat. The same year Osborne and Mendel also reported that something in butter appeared essential for sustaining life in rats.

By 1915, McCollum and Davis had substantiated the earlier findings and proposed that an adequate diet for the rat must provide, in addition to known nutrients, two unidentified factors: "fat-soluble A" and "water-soluble B". In subsequent studies by a number of workers, it was shown that the best source of vitamin A was cod liver oil and other fish oils. However, the initial source of the vitamin in animal products, is the provitamin A, synthesized by plants as a group of yellow pigments called carotenoids. Plants do not synthesize vitamin A *per se*, but all animals possess enzymes in the intestinal mucosa which are capable of converting the provitamin A carotenoids into vitamin A.

Three compounds, vitamin A alcohol (retinol), vitamin A aldehyde (retinal), and vitamin A acid (retinoic acid), and some of their sterioisomers, possess vitamin A activity for the chicken and other animals.

Vitamin A is involved in several body processes: (1) sterioisomers of retinal, termed retinene, play a primary role in vision; (2) vitamin A is required for prevention of severe ataxia in chicks; (3) there is a requirement for normal growth; (4) for maintenance of the normal integrity of the mucous membrane; (5) for reproduction; (6) proper growth of the cartilage matrix upon which bone is deposited; and (7) for maintaining normal cerebrospinal fluid pressure.

4.10.1 Structure and synthesis of vitamin A

The structure of retinol was determined in 1931 by Karrer, *et al.*, on preparations obtained from the unsaponifiable portion of halibut and pike oils. There are several excellent reviews on the structure and syntheses of the various vitamin A compounds, (Wagner and Folkers, 1964). The chemical structures of the important isomers of retinol and retinal are shown in Figure 4.1. The structures of important carotenoid pigments, with indications as to which are provitamins A, and which are inactive, are shown in Figure 4.2. Relative biological activities of the various forms of vitamin A and of the provitamins A for the chick and rat are also shown in these figures. One International Unit (IU) of vitamin A is equivalent to the activity of 0.3g of retinol (or 0.344 g of retinyl acetate), thus the potencies of the various other forms of vitamin A and provitamins can be calculated from these figures.

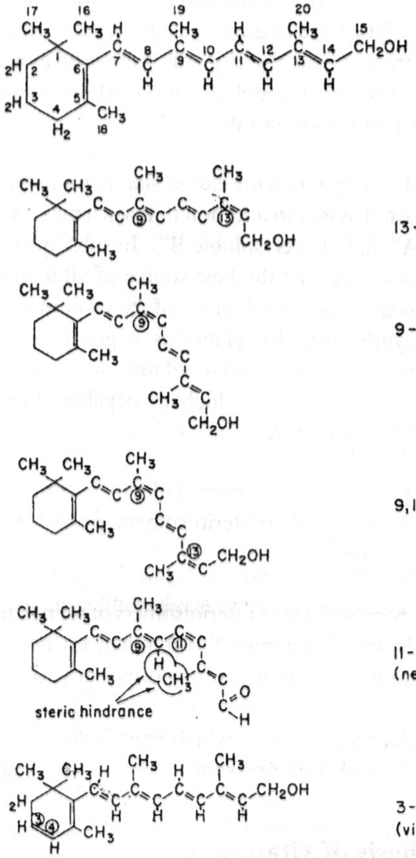

	Relative Biological Activity	
	CHICKS	RATS
Trans-Retinol	100	100
13-*cis* Retinol	50	75
9-*cis* Retinol	?	21
9,13-*cis* Retinol	?	24
11-*cis* Retinal (neo-b-retinene)	?	47
3-Dehydro-retinol (vitamin A_2, retinol$_2$)	?	40

Figure 4.1 Isomeric forms of vitamin A.

4.10.2 Properties of vitamin A

Retinol is a highly unsaturated, fat-soluble compound made-up of isoprene units with alternate double bonds, starting with one in the basic β-ionine ring, which is in conjugation with those in the side chain. The resonance of the conjugated double bonds causes the retinol molecule to have a very pale yellow color and to exhibit a characteristic green fluorescence when exposed to ultraviolet light. However exposure to ultraviolet light also disrupts the bonds and destroys the vitamin. The additional double bond in the carbonyl group of retinal causes this compound to

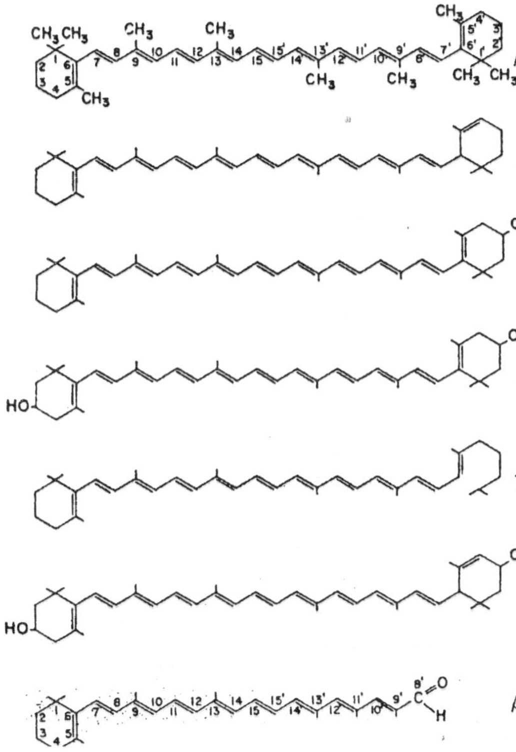

	Relative Biological Activity*	
	CHICKS	RATS
β-Carotene	10	50
α-Carotene	?	25
Cryptoxanthin	?	29
Zeaxanthin	0	0
γ Carotene	?	14
Lutein (Xanthophyll)	0	0
β-apo-8'-Carotenal		

Figure 4.2 The yellow carotenoids (trans form)

* Biological activity is related to trans retinol assigned a value of 100.

have a yellowish orange color. Retinol crystallizes into yellow prisms from petroleum ether or into solvated crystals from methanol or similar molar solvents. Retinol and retinal are insoluble in water but are soluble in absolute ethanol, chloroform, cyclohexane, ether, petroleum ether, fats and oils. Retinol and retinal are readily destroyed by oxidation, especially under hot moist conditions and when in contact with trace minerals or rancid fats and oils. Retinol is stable in the dark in the absence of oxygen and can be kept indefinitely in evacuated ampules in a dark freezer. It is also quite stable in fish oils stored in sealed containers, especially in the presence of suitable antioxidants. Acetate and palmitate esters are more stable to oxidation than are the alcohol or aldehyde forms of the vitamin.

Certain legumes, particularly soybeans and alfalfa, contain an enzyme, lipoxygenase, which readily destroys the carotenes and xanthophylls, and probably also vitamin A, through a coupled oxidation with polyunsaturated fatty acids. However, proper heat treatment of these products will destroy this enzyme.

The four double bonds of the vitamin A side chain are responsible for its instability. Together with the hydroxyl group on the β-ionine ring, these double bonds are prone to oxidation. The OH group can be esterified to acetate, propionate etc., and this process greatly improves stability. The acetate ester is most commonly used in the feed industry as a dry feed additive. This spray-dried product was initially mixed with sugar and antioxidants. In the last few years, further addition of gelatin to this mixture has resulted in spray-dried beadlets that are quite stable. Ethoxyquin seems to be the most effective antioxidant in such vitamin A products.

Table 4.10 Retinol content of natural sources	
Vitamin A source	**Retinol content* (IU/g)**
Whale liver oil	400,000
Herring liver oil	211,000
Tuna liver oil	150,000
Shark liver oil	150,000
Seal liver oil	10,000
Cod liver oil	4,000
Sardine body oil	750
Menhaden body oil	340
As Provitamin A	
Alfalfa meal, leaves and stems, dehydrated	330
Alfalfa meal, leaves and stems, sun-cured	150
Pasture grasses, dried	150
Carrots	120
Corn gluten meal, 60% protein	50
Corn gluten feed, 41% protein	28
Hominy feed	12
Corn	8
Other cereal grains	0

*Values given are maximum levels found; at times the retinol content may be much lower depending upon the recent previous food pattern of the fish or other animal.

4.10.3 Sources of vitamin A

Vitamin A is naturally derived from fish oils where it occurs in the esterified form. It is also produced from chemical synthesis, usually as the all-trans retinyl palmitate or acetate. The retinol content of the most important natural sources are shown in Table 4.10 as well as similar sources of the provitamin A carotenoids.

4.10.4 Absorption and transport of vitamin A

Vitamin A and β-carotene become dispersed in micellar form prior to absorption from the intestine. These micelles are composed of mixtures of bile salts, monoglycerides, and long chain fatty acids, together with vitamins D, E, and K, all of which facilitate transfer of vitamin A and β-carotene to the intestinal cell. Here most of the β-carotene is converted to vitamin A, which in turn, is converted to various esters depending to a great extent upon the type of fatty acid being absorbed with the vitamin A. However, palmitic acid would appear to be preferentially used for the esterification. In plasma, vitamin A can be transported both as the free alcohol as well as in the esterified form. The esters are transported to the liver with the chylomicrons which are derived from absorbed lipids. Physiologically active vitamin A is mobilized from the liver as retinol which is bound to a specific transport protein termed the retinol binding protein (RBP). It is believed the delivery of vitamin A to tissues is controlled by processes which control the production and secretion of RBP by the liver. RBP contains a single polypeptide chain with a molecular weight of 21,000, which forms a 1:1 molar complex with retinol. It is estimated that 90% of the plasma RBP is complexed to thyroxine binding prealbumin. The RBP, prealbumin complex is transported to target tissues where it binds to the cell surface receptor and the retinol is transported into the cells of the target tissue. Cellular retinol binding proteins have also been identified, which may be involved in translocation of retinol within the cell and perhaps its biological action.

4.10.5 Conversion of β-carotene to retinaldehyde and retinol

β-carotene and other provitamins are converted to retinol, retinal, and retinyl esters in the mucosal lining. There is some question as to how efficient this conversion is in the young chick as compared to older birds. In theory one molecule of β-carotene should form, on hydrolysis, two molecules of vitamin A. However, seldom is the efficiency of conversion 100%. Also carotenes are not as efficiently absorbed from the gut as is vitamin A. For poultry, the estimates of the quantity of dietary β-carotene, equal to 1 μg of vitamin A, varies from 4 to 1. Thus, for practical purposes, a value of 3 has been suggested as the efficiency for poultry, suggesting 3 molecules of carotene would equal 1 molecule of vitamin A. The vitamin A content of foods is usually stated in International Units (IU) with one IU of vitamin A being defined as the activity of 0.3 μg of crystalline vitamin A alcohol. It is believed that the conversion of carotene to vitamin follows the pathways shown in Figure 4.3

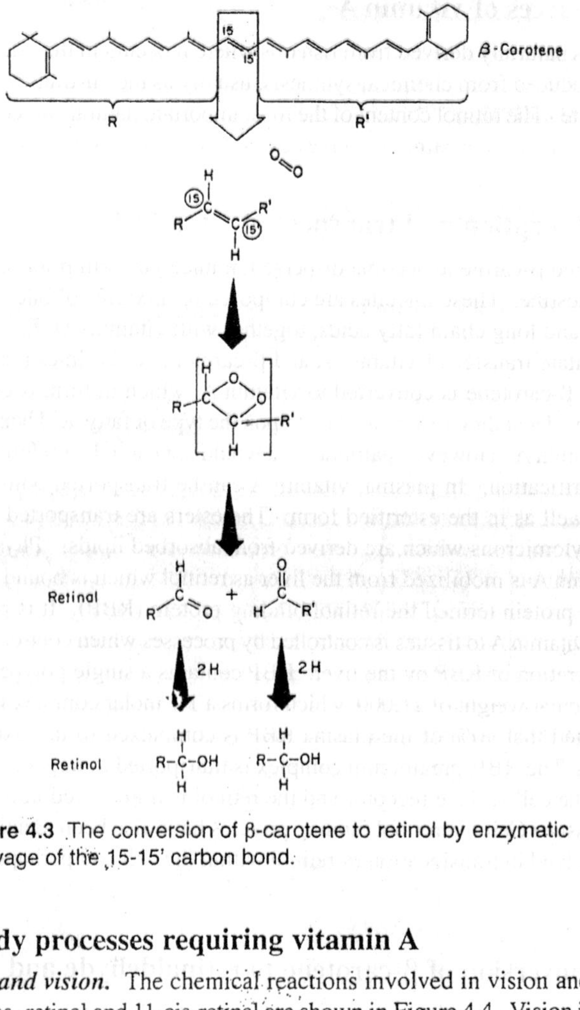

Figure 4.3 The conversion of β-carotene to retinol by enzymatic cleavage of the 15-15' carbon bond.

4.10.6 Body processes requiring vitamin A

i) Vitamin A and vision. The chemical reactions involved in vision and the part played by trans- retinal and 11-cis-retinal are shown in Figure 4.4. Vision is brought about by the energy trapped in 11-cis-retinal, which is produced by retinene isomerase from trans-retinal and its spontaneous reaction in the dark with a protein component called scotopsin to form rhodopsin. Exposing rhodopsin to light, results in the energy derived from light to react with the unstable 11-cis structure to be reduced to trans-retinal and free scotopsin. The instability of the 11-cis structure is due to the stearic hindrance of the cis molecule as shown in Figure 4.1. Energy derived from this reaction is transported to the brain via the optic nerve, and recorded in various intensities depending upon the amount of light received by the eye. Alcohol dehydrogenase plays a role in the conversion of trans-retinol to trans-retinal, and perhaps also the conversion of 11-cis-retinol to 11-cis-retinal.

THE VITAMINS   137

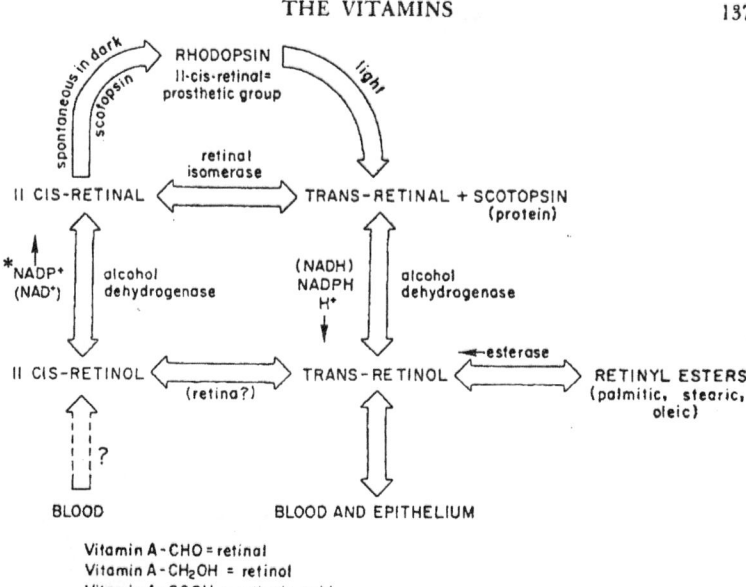

Figure 4.4 Vitamin A and its role in the chemical reactions involved in vision.

*Recent evidence show NADP to be the most active coenzyme.

ii) Vitamin A and reproduction. Retinoic acid carries out all the functions of vitamin A in the body with the exception of vision and reproduction. Hence, by supplementing retinoic acid to a basal diet, it is possible to study the effects of retinol and retinal on vision and reproduction without any complicating effects of other vitamin A deficiencies. Feeding chicks a diet containing adequate levels of all known nutrients, but with vitamin A supplied in the form of retinoic acid, results in normal growth and development, but they gradually become blind. Figure 4.5 shows a picture of a hen which received retinoic acid as a source of vitamin A and also a normal hen. A darkening of the pigment of the eye of the retinoic-fed hen can be noted. If the blind pullet is in a familiar environment, where it can consume the retinoic supplemented diet and adequate water, she will mature and lay eggs. Rate of production, egg size, and all other criteria will appear normal except that her eggs will contain no vitamin A, as retinoic acid is not deposited in the egg. Upon artificially inseminating the hen, normal fertility is observed after 2 to 3 days incubation, however, at this time all the embyros will die and almost all at the same stage of development. Figure 4.6 shows a deficient, 3 day old embryo compared with a normal vitamin A enriched embryo.

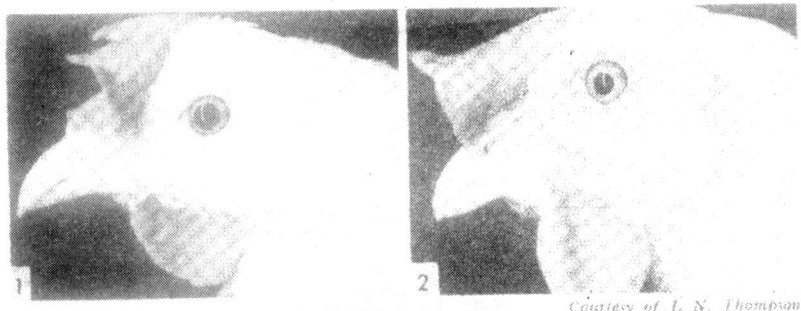

Courtesy of J. N. Thompson

Figure 4.5 The appearance of the eye of a blind hen (1) fed retinoic acid, compared with the normal eye (2) of a hen fed retinol.

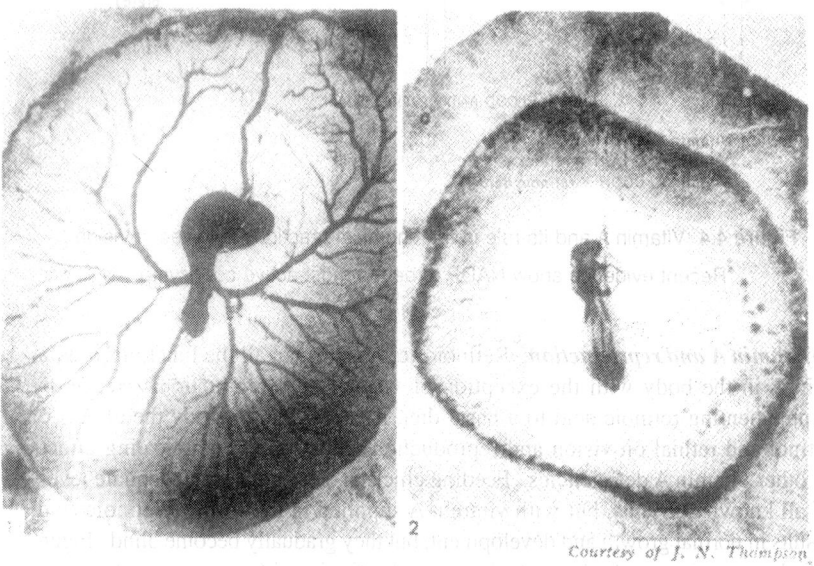

Courtesy of J. N. Thompson

Figure 4.6 Chick embryos after 72 hrs incubation,
1. From hen fed retinyl acetate as the only source of vitamin A. Embryo is normal and extensive extra-embryonic circulation has developed.
2. From hen fed retinoic acid as the only source of vitamin A. Embryo is malformed. The area of vasculosa has expanded but still lacks major blood vessels.

Evidence that feeding retinoic acid affects just the production of retinene and storage of vitamin A in the egg, is apparent from the finding that after months of blindness, sight can be restored within two days by feeding the hen an adequate dietary level of retinol. Hatchability of the eggs is almost immediately restored by feeding the vitamin A adequate diet. Indeed, it has been demonstrated that eggs from hens fed retinoic acid will hatch, if prior to incubation, retinol is injected into the egg.

iii) Vitamin A in maintenance of mucous membranes. Vitamin A is required for maintenance of the epithelial lining of all the external cavities of the body which communicate with the outside air. These include the respiratory tract, the urinary tract, the corneal epithelial and the soft tissues around the eyes. Lesions of vitamin A deficiency may be detected grossly or histologically in these areas depending on the degree of dietary deficiency. Thus, a vitamin A deficiency can not only cause blindness but also structural damage to the eye. The effect of vitamin A in maintaining the integrity of mucous membranes is so well established that vaginal cornification in rats has been used as an assay method for the vitamin. Addition of retinol to vitamin deficient animals results in a rapid return to normal mucous membranes. Impaired fertility in male birds fed vitamin A deficient diets is associated with derangement of epithelial tissue in the semineferous tubules.

Further evidence that vitamin A is directly concerned with the differentiation of the mucous membrane was obtained from studies showing that explants of chicken ectoderm, when grown in a tissue culture supplemented with a high level of vitamin A, failed to develop into typical keratinized epithelium. Instead, the cells differentiated into mucous-secreting, often ciliated columnar epithelial cells, resembling those of the nasal mucosa.

Intestinal mucosa does not however become keratinized in vitamin A deficient animals. Instead, marked reduction in the number of goblet cells occurs and the synthesis of the specific mucous containing glycopeptides normally present in goblet cells decrease. Vitamin A is involved directly in glycosylation reactions that occur during the synthesis of the carbohydrate component of specific glycoproteins. Retinyl phosphate is formed in animal tissues and mannosyl-retinyl phosphate has also been identified. The transfer of mannose residues from retinyl phosphate to membrane glycoproteins can be shown *in vitro*. There is some question as to the significance of these reactions *in vivo* since dolichol phosphate also is known to participate in glycosyl transfer reactions in glycoprotein synthesis and the relative significance of vitamin A in these reactions has not been unequivocally established. This proposed function of vitamin A is an attractive one, however, in view of the physiological effects of vitamin A deficiency in mucous membranes.

Vitamin A deficiency causes the normal columnar epithelium of the cloaca, the bursa of Fabricius, the ureters and the vaginal portion of the oviduct to be replaced by stratified squamous, keratinizing epithelium. Furthermore, the parathyroid glands of vitamin A deficient chickens show marked cellular changes, and if chickens are deficient in both vitamin A and vitamin D_3, the parathyroids, instead of hypertrophying as they normally do in vitamin D_3 deficiency, undergo almost complete degeneration into a keratinized mass, incapable of producing parathyroid hormone.

iv) Vitamin A in cellular and subcellular membranes. In vitro studies with mammalian erythrocytes show that an excess of vitamin A results in hemolysis, with the cells assuming peculiar shapes, vacuoles appear, pinocytosis is evident, with hemoglobin eventually emerging from rupture of the cell membranes. Such conditions are only seen with severe hypervitaminosis. Vitamin A penetrates lipoprotein membranes and at optimum levels may act as a cross-linkage agent between the lipid and protein, thus stabilizing the membrane. Such physiological actions of retinol in the control of membrane structure is consistent with many of the observed biological effects of hypo and hypervitaminosis A.

v) Vitamin A and bone development. Vitamin A deficiency in ducks causes a marked retardation and suppression of endochondral bone growth, while excess vitamin A results in an acceleration of this bone development (Wolbach and Hegsted 1952). Incubation of cultured chick bone cartilage, in the presence of excess retinol, resulted in a loss of amino sugar, nucleic acids and protein. This occurrence has been explained by the release of the protease, cathepsin, from the lysosomes, which acts on the mucoprotein of the bone cartilage releasing protein and mucopolysaccharide derivatives.

vi) Vitamin A and cerebrospinal fluid pressure. A severe ataxia (Figure 4.7) is the first sign of an acute vitamin A deficiency noted with the young growing chick. Since lesions are not usually seen in the cerebellum or cerebrum in the early stages, it is assumed that the ataxis is caused by excess pressure on the brain stem. Woollam and Millen (1955), have shown such a marked elevation in the cerebrospinal fluid pressure.

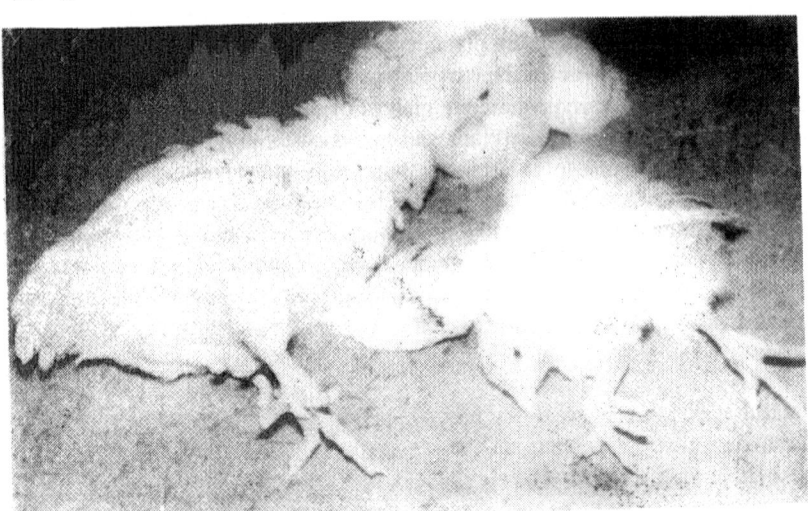

Figure 4.7 Ataxia in chicks due to dietary deficiency of vitamin A.

vii) Vitamin A and cortisone synthesis. A deficiency of vitamin A in rats has been shown to result in atrophy of the adrenal gland and seriously reduced glyconeogenesis. However, Stoewsand and Scott (1964), reported that a high protein diet resulted in stressed chicks as evident by enlarged adrenals and increased corticosterone output, while at the same time vitamin A storage was depleted. Retinol deficiency in chicks did not cause adrenal atrophy or decreased *in vivo* corticoid production. However, addition of retinol to incubating excised adrenals from vitamin A deficient chicks caused *in vitro* production of corticosterone.

viii) Vitamin A and cancer. Involvement of vitamin A in reproduction, and in epithelial tissues, indicates that it plays a role in cell differentiation. Vitamin A deficient animals have been shown to be more susceptible to chemical carcinogens, while high levels of some retinoids have been able to reduce or prevent cancer caused by chemical carcinogens. Synthetic retinoids, such as 13-cis-retinoic acid, show less toxicity than do natural retinoids, and have been investigated for their activity against certain cancers. There is also data to indicate that carotene intake may have a positive affect in regressing certain human cancers.

4.10.7 Vitamin A requirements of chickens

Minimum requirements for vitamin A, as set out by NRC (1994) are shown in Table 4.4, together with commercial recommendations. In establishing a satisfactory level for vitamin A in practical diets, it is necessary to consider a number of factors. The minimum levels shown are an estimate of the levels required to produce optimum performance with chicks and hens under ideal environmental and health conditions. However, in setting the practical requirements one should consider: (1) possible genetic differences which may affect requirements; (2) possible variations in carry over from dam to the chick; (3) variations in potency of vitamin A supplements; (4) possible destruction of vitamin A through oxidation, high temperatures of feed processing, catalytic effects of trace minerals and peroxidizing effects of oxidizing polyunsaturated fats; (5) possible destruction of vitamin A in the gut by various factors; (6) variation in absorption through damage to the intestinal wall by internal parasites, or a fat level in the diet which is too low to optimize fat-soluble vitamin absorption or any other factors which could interfere with mechanisms involved in vitamin A absorption; (7) protein or lipid levels inadequate for optimum formation of β-lipoproteins and/or retinol binding protein for vitamin A transport; (8) an increased vitamin A requirement due to a disease or any other stress.

For the above reasons, the vitamin A requirement shown for practical diets is considerably higher than that shown for minimum requirements. It is important to have reserves of vitamin A stored in the liver, in the event that a dietary deficiency or a disease such as coccidiosis occurs, which can damage the microvilli of the intestinal wall, thus resulting in lower feed intake as well as reduced nutrient absorption.

Not only is it advisable to provide a high level of vitamin A in the chick diet but also in the diet of breeding hens, in order that a good supply is passed on to the hatched chick. The effect of vitamin A content of the hen's diet, on that of egg yolk, is shown in Table 4.11. There is obviously transfer from the hen to the egg, but subsequent transfer to the chick is less efficient. There is no indication that increasing the vitamin A level in the breeder diet has any meaningful effect on vitamin A content of the hatchling. Vitamin A nutrition of breeders has no effect on immune status of chicks, in terms of maternal antibodies or priming of lymphoid tissues. Breeders fed deficient levels of vitamin A will obviously transfer less vitamin A to the egg and chick, and growth and development of the neonate can be compromised. Breeders need to have low plasma retinol (<0.7 μmol/L) in order to produce vitamin A deficient hatchlings. Likewise there needs to be about 2.4 IU vitamin A/g yolk for adequate embryo development and hatchability. Sklan *et al.* (1994) suggest that plasma vitamin A levels in unstressed chicks are maximized with around 6,000 IU vitamin A/kg diet. There seems to be no plateau with liver levels of vitamin A since they keep increasing as diet levels increase. These same workers show T-lymphocyte proliferation to also be maximum with 6,000 IU/kg diet, and that a decline occurs with dietary levels of 14,000 IU/kg.

Table 4.11 Effect of dietary vitamin A on the vitamin A content of egg yolk

Dietary vitamin A level	Vitamin A in yolk
IU/kg	IU/g
1,760	0.9
2,640	3.7
3,520	4.2
4,400	6.3
11,000	12.7
22,000	16.3
	From Hill *et al.*, (1961)

While xanthophyll, zeaxanthin and cryptoxanthin have little vitamin A activity for birds, they can be important in influencing the color of egg yolks, body fat and skin. In markets that demand pigmented poultry products, dietary carotenoid levels can be tailored to commercial needs.

The xanthophylls are quite common in many feed ingredients, with moderately high levels in yellow corn. Carotene has little pigmenting value, whereas zeaxanthin and cryptoxanthin impart an orange/red color dependent on concentration. Only about 1% of dietary β-carotene is deposited in the egg, compared with up to 30% for some synthetic pigments such as β-apo-8-carotenoic acid ethyl ester. The bird accumulates xanthophylls, the most apparent being in the beak and shank. As laying hens progress through a laying cycle, the xanthophyll content in these regions is gradually depleted, regardless of diet pigment supply. This gradual loss of pigmentation can in fact be used to judge the age and stage of egg production of laying hens.

A number of factors can influence the digestion and absorption of carotenoids, and so the degree of body pigmentation. Parasites such as worms and coccidia impair absorption, and birds with these infections are invariably of paler color on the shanks and in the fat depots. Mycotoxins such as aflatoxin also reduce pigmentation, as does the presence of rancid fat. The carotenoids are best protected by judicious use of antioxidants such as ethoxyquin.

The color of poultry products, and especially egg yolks, are most often quantitated on the so called Roche Scale. Ranging from 1-15, the scale provides color gradations from pale yellow to orange-red (15). The pigments impart no real benefit for the bird or humans consuming their products, and so their use is merely cosmetic in accordance with consumer demands.

4.10.8 General signs of vitamin A deficiency

Adult birds, depending on liver storage, could be fed a vitamin A deficient diet for two to five months before signs of any deficiency develops. As the deficiency progresses, the bird becomes emaciated, weak, and feathers become ruffled. During this time, a marked drop in egg production is noted, hatchability is decreased, and there is an increase in embryonic mortality with incubated eggs. As egg production declines, there will likely be atretic follicles in the ovary, some of which show signs of hemorrhage. A watery discharge from the eyes may also be noted. As the deficiency continues, an accumulation of milky white cheesy like material forms in the eyes, which can make it impossible for the bird to see. The eye, in many cases, may be destroyed. This sign of vitamin A deficiency is common for most animals and man, and is referred to as xerophthalmia.

Depending on the quantity of vitamin A passed on from the breeder hen, day old chicks reared on a vitamin A deficient diet may show signs within a week. However, chicks with a good reserve of vitamin A, passed on from breeders fed a well fortified diet, may take up to 7 weeks before signs of a deficiency are noted.

Gross symptoms in the chick are characterized by anorexia, growth retardation, drowsiness, weakness, incoordination, emaciation and ruffled feathers. If the deficiency is severe, the chicks may exhibit an ataxia, similar to that noted with a vitamin E deficiency. The yellow pigment in the shanks and beaks is usually lost and the comb and wattles are pale in color. A cheesy-like material may be noted in the eyes, but xerophthalmia as noted with adults, is seldom seen because with a severe deficiency of dietary vitamin A, the chick usually dies before the eyes become affected. It has been observed that rats fed a vitamin A deficient diet, in a germ free environment, lived up to 272 days, while in a normal environment, fed the same diet, they died within 54 days. This has led to the suggestion that infection plays a role in many of the deaths noted with acute vitamin A deficiency. Lessard et al. (1997) describe different immune responses in chicks related to vitamin A status. With low levels of dietary vitamin A (400 IU/kg), chicks have a smaller

spleen and Bursa, although the antibody mediated immune system is elevated. With
· high levels of vitamin A (15,000 IU/kg), the cell mediated immune system is enhanced.

4.10.9 Pathology of vitamin A deficiency

The first lesion usually noted with a vitamin A deficiency with adult birds is in
the mucous glands of the alimentary tract. The normal epithelium of the glands
becomes replaced by a stratified squamous, keratinized layer, which blocks the
ducts of the mucous glands resulting in them becoming distended with necrotic
secretions. Small, white pustules may be found in the nasal passages, mouth, esophagus and pharynx, and mȧy extend into the crop. Figure 4.8 shows an example
of such a condition. Due to the breakdown of the mucous membrane, pathogenic microorganisms may invade these tissues and enter the body, thus leading to
infections, which are secondary to the original vitamin A deficiency symptoms.

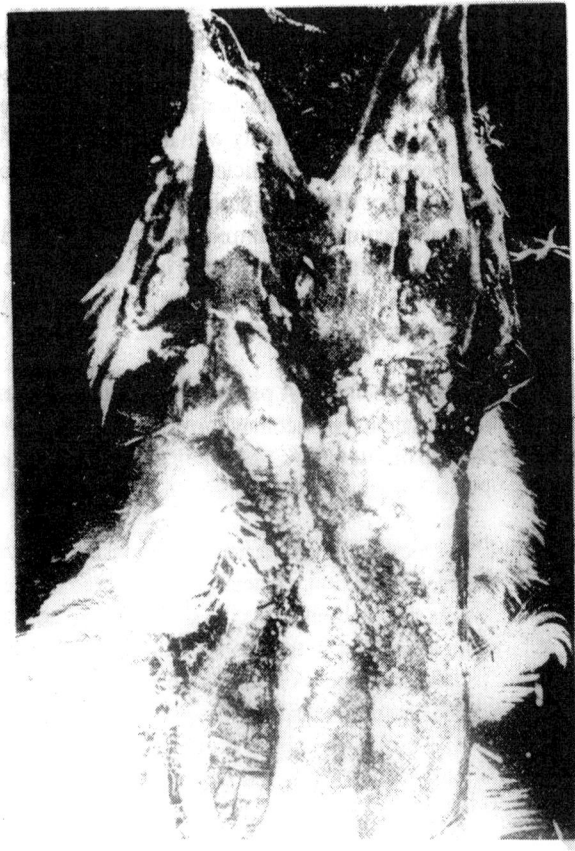

Figure 4.8 Pustules in the pharynx and esophagus resulting from vitamin A deficiency in the chicken.

Young chicks with a chronic vitamin A deficiency may also show pustules in the mucous membrane of the esophagus, and these may extend down the respiratory tract. Kidneys may be pale, and the tubules distended due to uric acid deposits, and in extreme cases, the ureters may be filled with urates (Figure 4.9). Blood levels of uric acid can rise from a norm of around 5 mg to as high as 40 mg per 100 ml of blood. Vitamin A deficiency does not interfere with uric acid metabolism but rather acts in such a manner to prevent normal excretion of uric acid from the kidney.

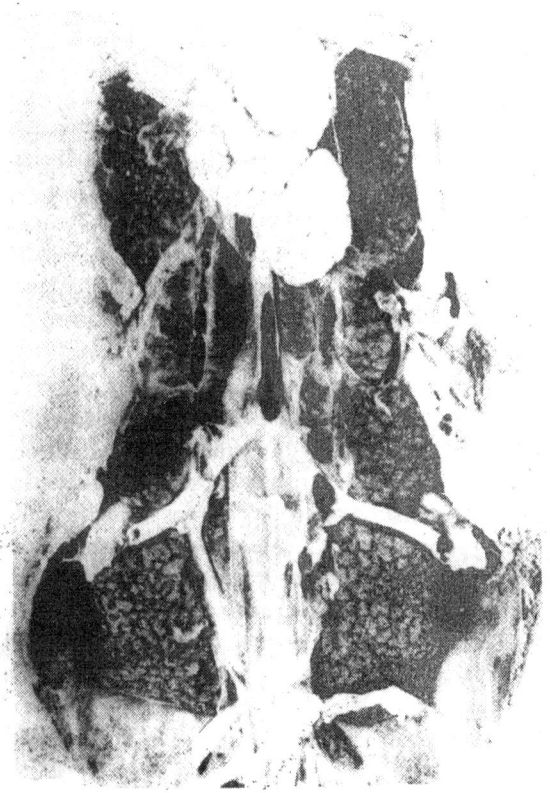

Figure 4.9 Distended kidney of a chicken fed vitamin A deficient diet. Urate deposits are visible.

Histological findings with a vitamin A deficiency is an atrophy of the cytoplasm and a loss of the cilia in the columnar, ciliated epithelium. Cell bodies become less defined and finally the ciliated lining of the trachea, bronchi, and submucous glands become transformed in a squamous stratified, keratinizing epithelium.

While vitamin A deficient chicks can show ataxia, similar to that noted with a vitamin E deficiency, no gross lesions are found in the brain of the vitamin A deficient chicks as compared to degeneration of the Purkinje cells in the cerebellum of vita min E deficient chicks. Also, the livers of ataxic vitamin A deficient chicks, contain little or no vitamin A. Histology of the brain in vitamin E deficiency is described in the section on that vitamin.

4.10.10 Hypervitaminosis A in the chicken

Retinol and its esters are not toxic to chickens up to a level of around 1,000,000 to 1,500,000 IU per kg of diet, or approximately 500 times the minimum requirement. Retinal is somewhat more toxic perhaps due to its ease of conversion into retinoic acid in the body. There is good evidence that retinoic acid becomes toxic around 50 to 100 times the minimum vitamin A requirement.

Symptoms of hypervitaminosis are: (1) weight loss; (2) decreased feed intake; (3) swelling and crusting of the eye lids: (4) inflammatory lesions of the nares, mouth, adjacent skin and skin on the feet; (5) decreased bone strength and increased bone abnormalities; (6) increased mortality. With a dietary level of 1,500,000 IU per kg, blood levels can increase to 1300 IU per 100 ml, with 20,000 IU per gram of liver. In contrast to retinol, even very high dietary levels of retinoic acid do not result in liver storage of vitamin A. Competition has been noted in the absorption of fat soluble vitamins. Thus, with diets borderline in levels of vitamins D, E, and K, a large increase in dietary vitamin A can result in decreases in growth or egg production, due to an induced deficiency of one or more of the other fat soluble vitamins rather than a toxic effect of vitamin A *per se*. Similarly, a marked increase in dietary vitamin A can result in reduced absorption of carotenoid pigment, resulting in decreased pigmentation of eggs or tissues. *In vitro* studies, referred to earlier, indicate that hypervitaminosis A causes (1) production of mucous epithelium in place of the normally cornified epithelium in incubating ectoderm, and (2) rupture of lipoprotein membranes, such as *in vitro* hemolysis of erythrocytes, rupture of lysosomes and swelling of mitochondria. Except for prevention of cornified epithelium in the vagina of rats during certain periods of estrus, none of these effects occur in the living animal. There is work to suggest that the bird possesses mechanisms which guard against hypervitaminosis A. These are 1) a relatively poor conversion of carotene to vitamin A; 2) a plateauing of storage of excess retinal, and 3) a low conversion of retinol to retinoic acid.

4.11 VITAMIN D₃

Vitamin D is thought of as the "sunshine vitamin" as it can be synthesized by most animals when they are exposed to ultraviolet light. Historical aspects covering the discovery of vitamin D have been reviewed by DeLuca (1980) and Loosli (1988). The classical deficiency sign is rickets which results in characteristic bending of the backbone, and bowing or twisting of legs in humans. Since the middle ages, it has been known that sunlight was beneficial in alleviating or preventing the condition. In England, during the industrial revolution, there was a mass migration of people from the country into the industrial centers. This resulted in a marked increase in children with severe bone-deforming diseases because they were deprived of sunlight for extended periods, and often permanently so in winter months.

In 1822, Sniadecki observed that children in the inner part of Warsaw, had a high incidence of rickets while those from the country did not. Thus, he suggested that lack of sunlight was the cause of rickets. Almost 70 years later, Palm concluded from an epidemiological study, that the common denominator in children suffering from rickets was absence of sunlight. He encouraged systematic sun bathing as a means of preventing rickets, but unfortunately the majority of scientists and medical people of the day did not believe in his treatment.

In the early twentieth century, rickets had reached epidemic proportions in England and research was initiated to study the condition. Mellanby initiated nutritional studies, in an attempt to reproduce the condition in laboratory animals. In 1922, he was successful in producing the disease in dogs fed oatmeal. Although not a conscious part of the experimental design, the study was conducted in a room with no windows. Although he was wrong in his assumption that the condition was due to a deficiency of the fat soluble vitamin A, his demonstration that it could be produced in a laboratory animal was a major step forward in finding a cure for the disease.

McCollum, who had discovered vitamin A, realized that the antirachitic activity discovered by Mellanby in cod liver oil was different from the vitamin A activity present in the oil. McCollum bubbled oxygen through heated cod liver oil, to destroy its vitamin A, and found that the treated oil would still cure rickets. In 1922, he concluded that there was a unknown substance present, which represented a new fat soluble vitamin, which he called vitamin D.

Although it was known that ultraviolet light and vitamin D from cod liver oil would cure rickets, the close interdependence of these two factors was not realized at this time. Goldblatt and Soames (1923), irradiated rachitic rats with ultraviolet light, and demonstrated that their livers contained the antirachitic substances, while non-irradiated rats did have the substance. Steebock and Black, (1924) realized that ultraviolet irradiation was causing the alteration of some substance in the animal and demonstrated that irradiating their food could also heal or prevent the condition. A limitation to year-round egg production in northern climates, was an appreciation of the role of vitamin D_3 in replacing summer sunlight. Discovery of vitamin D was one of the factors that subsequently led to year-round egg production.

4.11.1 Properties and function of vitamin D_3

Vitamin D refers to a group of closely related compounds that poses antirachitic activity. While a number of forms of vitamin D are known, all do not occur naturally, the two most important forms are ergocalciferol (vitamin D_2) and cholecalciferol (vitamin D_3). The term vitamin D_1, was originally used to refer to an activated sterol, which was later found to be impure and to consist mainly of ergo-calciferol, which had already been designated vitamin D_2, and so the D_1 term was abolished. Vitamins D_2 and D_3 have virtually the same potency for cattle, sheep and pigs but D_2 has only 3% of the potency of D_3 for poultry.

Vitamin D_2 was first isolated in crystalline form by Linsert in 1931. The provitamin of D_3, (7- dehydrocholesterol) was synthesized by Windaus *et al.,* in 1935, and crystalline D_3, cholecalciferol, was obtained by Schenk two years later.

There are a number of fat-soluble sterol derivatives which are active in preventing rickets in animals. However, only one form, cholecalciferol or vitamin D_3, will act as the nutritional precursor of the hormone, 1, 25-dihydroxycholecalciferol, which is effective in promoting calcium absorption, and bone and egg shell formation in poultry.

Cholecalciferol is produced by irradiation of 7-dehydrocholesterol, which is produced within the body and travels to the outer skin layers, where, by exposure to ultraviolet light, either from the sun or an artificial source, it is synthesized. According to Koch and Koch (1941) the legs and feet of the chicken contain about 8 times more 7-dehydrocholesterol than does body skin. The synthesized cholecalciferol, formed in the skin, is absorbed and transported via the blood to the lipids throughout the body. In contrast to aquatic species, chickens and other land animals, do not store appreciable quantities of vitamin D in the liver. While fish liver oils were the major source of vitamin D for quite some time, they have been replaced by highly potent concentrates prepared commercially by the irradiation of animal sterols or other chemical synthesis.

The cholecalciferol content of some natural ingredients is shown in Table 4.12. Many fish oils contain mixtures of antirachitic sterols, and since ergocalciferol has a low availability for poultry, these oils are usually not as active for chickens as commercially prepared vitamin D_3

Table 4.12 Cholecalciferol content of foods and feedstuffs	
Food or feedstuff	Cholecalciferol (IU/100g)
Cod liver oil	10,000
Halibut liver oil	120,000
Herring, entire body oil	10,000
Sardine, entire body oil	8,000
Menhaden, entire body oil	5,000
Eggs	100
Milk, cow's whole	4
Irradiated 7- dehydrocholesterol	up to 2 billion*

*This is 50% of the theoretically possible yield of cholecaleiferol from irradiation of 7-dehydro-cholesterol, since 1 g of pure vitamin D_3= 40,000,000 IU.

4.11.2 Vitamin D₃ chemistry

The chemical structures of ergocalciferol, cholecalciferol, and their precursors ergosterol and 7-dehydrocholesterol, are shown in Figure 4.10. All sterols possessing vitamin D activity have the same steroid nucleus, but differ in the nature of the side-chain attached to carbon 17.

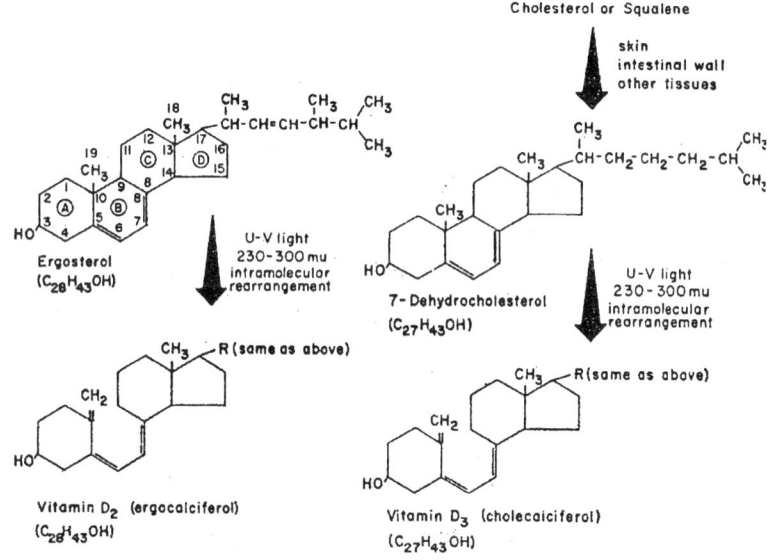

Figure 4.10 Synthesis of Vitamin D₂ and Vitamin D₃.

Cholesterol is converted to 7-dehydrocholesterol in the body, which in turn, results in cholecalciferol when acted on by ultra violet light falling on the skin of an animal. The precursors have no antirachitic activity until the B-ring is opened between the 9 and 10 positions of the steroids. This occurs with ultraviolet irradiation, forming a double bond between the carbon atoms at the 10 and 19 positions of the new compounds. The resulting triene is the vitamin D nucleus. Over-irradiation of ergocalciferol or cholecalciferol produces numerous irradiation products such as tachysterols, supra-sterol₁, supra-sterol₂, and others. Some of these compounds have partial D-activity, some are toxic, and some may be potent antagonists of vitamin D₃.

4.11.3 Properties of vitamin D$_3$

Cholecalciferol is insoluble in water, but soluble in organic solvents and oils. It crystallizes as tiny white needles from diluted acetone. It melts at 84-85°C, and has maximum absorption at 264.5 mµ in alcohol or hexane. It can be removed from oils by molecular distillation or by chromatography following saponification of the oils.

Cholecalciferol can be destroyed by over treatment with ultraviolet light, and by peroxidation in the presence of rancidifying polyunsaturated fatty acids, especially when finely dispersed in the presence of trace minerals. Most commercial feeds usually contain enough vitamin E and other antioxidants to prevent the destruction of cholecalciferol.

One IU or U.S.P. unit of vitamin D activity is defined as the activity of 0.025 µg of vitamin D$_3$. In converting the older AOAC chick unit to IU, the AOAC unit must be reduced by 25%.

4.11.4 Absorption and transport of vtiamin D$_3$

Cholecalciferol is absorbed from the intestinal tract primarily in the duodenum. Like vitamin A, its absorption is facilitated by the presence of fat and bile salts and micelle formation is an important prerequisite. It is poorly absorbed in the absence of bile, the secretion of which is limited in young chicks.

Vitamin D passes into the bloodstream after absorption and is distributed throughout the body within 24 hours, with the highest concentrations found in the intestinal wall, liver, kidneys, spleen, gall bladder, and serum. While concentrations in muscle, bone, pancreas and skin, are low, these tissues account for a large portion of the stored vitamin D. Recent studies suggest that most of the vitamin D is transported in the chylomicron fraction of the blood where it is readily transported across cell membranes. Recent research indicates that one of the metabolites (either 25-OH-D$_3$) or 1,25(OH)$_2$D$_3$ rather than vitamin D$_3$ itself, is transported from the hen to the egg.

Vitamin D$_3$ absorption is enhanced by certain organic acids, especially lactic acid. However, the effect of organic acids in improving calcium absorption may be independent of vitamin D.

4.11.5 Conversion of vitamin D$_3$, into the metabolically active forms, 25 hydroxycholecalciferol (25(OH)D$_3$) and 1α,25 dihydroxycholecalciferol (1α,25(OH)$_2$D$_3$)

A new phase of vitamin D research began in the late 1960's which has resulted in a complete change in the thinking of how this nutrient functions in the body. The discovery that the biological actions of vitamin D can be explained by a hormone-like function, marked a change in the era of vitamin D research. It is now recognized that vitamin D is simply the precursor of the hormone 1,25-dihydroxyvitamin D (1,25-$(OH)_2D_3$). Lund and DeLuca (1966), showed the disappearance of vitamin D_3 following administration, and the appearance of several metabolites that possessed more potent antirachitic activity. The first of these, found in the liver, was 25-hydroxyvitamin D_3, 25$(OH)D_3$, which was chemically synthesized by Blunt and co-workers in 1968. This metabolite is normally the major form of vitamin D circulating in the body. Further studies, by the above workers, showed that 25$(OH)D_3$ was transported to the kidney and metabolically altered to a number of dihydroxy compounds, the most important being 1,25-$(OH)_2D_3$, with the kidney being the main site of production.

Existence in the intestine of a further metabolite of vitamin D_3 became evident from work by a number of investigators. This vitamin D metabolite is transported from the kidney to the intestine, bone or elsewhere in the body where it is involved in the metabolism of calcium and phosphorus.

The studies undertaken on vitamin D metabolism demonstrated that vitamin D_3 functions as a hormone with 1,25-$(OH)_2D_3$ being the active form that functions in intestine and bone, whereas vitamin D_3 does not function at these sites.

Production of 1,25-$(OH)_2$ D_3, is carefully regulated by the parathyroid hormone (PTH) in response to blood calcium and phosphorus levels. Holick, *et al.* (1971) identified this metabolite as 1,25- dihydroxycholecalciferol and showed that the reaction of 25-OH-D_3 in intestinal calcium transport could be prevented by prior administration of actinomycin D, whereas 1,25$(OH)_2$ D_3, stimulated intestinal calcium transport even in the presence of actinomycin D. Henry and Norman (1978) reported that hatchability of eggs was markedly depressed from vitamin D deficient hens, even though they were fed 1,25$(OH)_2$ D_3. Apparently 1,25-$(OH)_2$ D_3, is effective in maintaining blood calcium levels, so that egg production and shell thickness remain normal, however, with vitamin D_3 the upper mandible of the chicks fails to develop and consequently the chick cannot crack the shell, to hatch. Unlike the situation in fish, land animals store very little vitamin D_3 in their tissues.

It is now clear that vitamin D_3, either from the diet or from the skin, is transported to the liver where it is converted to 25 $(OH)D_3$. This metabolite is then transported via the blood stream to the kidney, where it is converted either into the steroid "hormone" 1,25$(OH)_2D_3$, or into one of two other metabolites, 24,25 dihydroxyvitamin D_3, or 1,24,25 trihydroxyvitmain D_3. The metabolic transformations of vitamin D are shown in Figure 4.11.

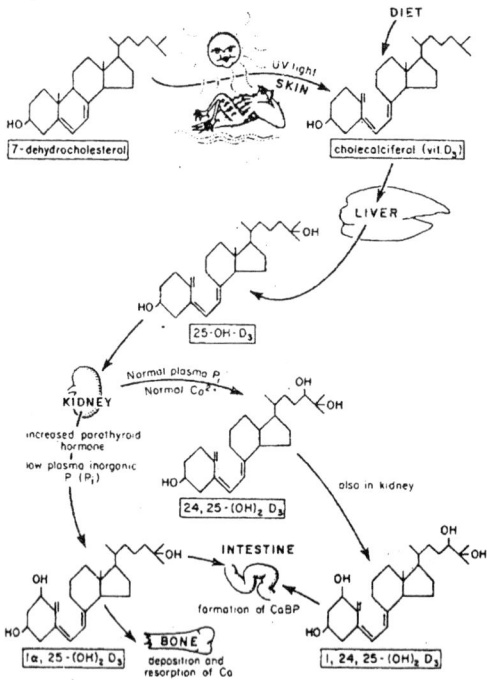

Figure 4.11 Metabolic transformation of vitamin D$_3$.

It has been postulated that parathyroid hormone (secreted because of low blood calcium level), causes phosphorus to be secreted from the kidney, which lowers kidney phosphate levels, and this metabolic change stimulates the kidney to produce 1,25(OH)$_2$ D$_3$. When kidney levels of calcium and phosphorus are normal, and thus no PTH is secreted, the kidney converts 25-hydroxy to 24,25 dihydroxy and then to 1,24,25 trihydroxy D$_3$. These findings help to explain the mechanisms whereby the animal's body regulates calcium absorption and maintains its blood calcium level. The major control of calcium absorption appears to be in the feedback mechanism which stops the conversion by the kidney of 25-OH-D$_3$ to 1,25(OH)$_2$ D$_3$. This conversion is stimulated by a low blood calcium level and the presence of PTH. It is inhibited when blood calcium level becomes normal and the PTH concentration in the kidney drops. A number of workers in the field have suggested that these findings, lend support to the conclusion that the active metabolite 1,25(OH)$_2$ -D$_3$ is in fact a hormone.

According to Norman and Henry (1974), the relative effectiveness of vitamin D$_3$,25-OH-D$_3$ and 1,25 (OH)$_2$ D$_3$ in chicks varies depending upon the biological response being used as the criterion of measurement. These relative biological activities are shown in Table 4.13. Soares, et al. (1978) estimated that 25-OH-D$_3$, is 2.5 to 4.5 times as active as cholecalciferol for the young chick.

Table 4.13 Relative biological effectiveness of cholecalciferol, 25-Hydroxycholecalciferol and 1α, 25-Dihydroxycholecalciferol in the chick		
Biological response	Activity relative to vitamin D_3	
	25-OH-D_3	1α,25(OH)$_2$D$_3$
Intestinal Ca^{2+} absorption	200	1300-1500
Bone Ca^2 Mobilization	150	500-600
Bone ash, %	160	200
Body weight gain	100	300

The half-life of vitamin D_3 in the bird's body is around 25 days, while that of 25(OH)D_3 is closer to 20 days. The half life of 24,25(OH)$_2$ D_3 is only around 2d, and for 1,25(OH)$_2$ D_3 the clearance is as rapid as 6 hours.

4.11.6 Metabolic functions of vitamin D_3

The general function of vitamin D is to elevate Ca and P levels in the plasma necessary to support normal body functions. There is also some evidence that vitamin D_3 may play a regulatory role in immune cell function (Reinhardt and Hustmyer, 1987). Aslam *et al.* (1998) suggest that a deficiency of vitamin D_3 causes a reduction in the cellular immune response, although humoral systems are not affected. Another possible use of vitamin D analogues, is to bring about cell differentiation of myelocytic-type leukemias (DeLuca, 1988).

There are two hormones, thyrocalcitonin (calcitonin) and PTH, that influence release of 1,25(OH)$_2$ D_3 needed to control levels of blood Ca and P. The role of calcitonin appears most important in controling high serum Ca levels by depressing gut absorption, halting bone demineralization and depressing Ca absorption in the kidney. Vitamin D_3 on the other hand brings about an elevation of plasma Ca and P by stimulating specific pump mechanisms in the intestine, kidney and bone, thus maintaining blood levels of Ca and P, from these body reserves.

Vitamin D stimulates active transport of Ca and P across the gut epithelium. This does not involve PTH directly but does involve the active form of vitamin D_3. As early as 1937, Nicolaysen showed that Ca was better absorbed, regardless of dietary inclusion level compared to the situation when diets are deficient in vitamin D_3. Using ^{45}Ca, Keane *et al.* (1956) confirmed these observations, with supplemented and unsupplemented vitamin D diets for chicks. These workers also demonstrated that injected ^{45}Ca was deposited in the bones of vitamin D deficient chicks at a rate similar to that seen in vitamin D_3 supplemented birds, indicating that vitamin D is required for absorption of calcium from the gut, but not for deposition of calcium in the body. Vitamin D_3 is now known to also influence the absorption of phosphorus and Soares and Ottinger (1988) suggest greater release of P from phytic acid in the presence of luminal $1,25(OH)_2 D_3$.

While the mechanism whereby calcium and phosphorus absorption is stimulated by vitamin D is not fully understood, Wasserman, (1981) suggest that $1,25(OH)_2D_3$ is transferred to the nucleus of the intestinal cell. In response to the $1,25(OH)_2 D_3$, specific RNA's are secreted by the nucleus, which in turn are translated into specific proteins by ribosomes, thus leading to the enhancement of calcium and phosphorus absorption.

While it appears there are several proteins in the intestinal wall, which are dependent on vitamin D for absorption, the most studied of these is calcium binding protein (CaBP) as described by Wasserman *et al.* (1966). Although CaBP is involved in calcium absorption, calcium transport appears to be a complex process and probably involves other factors acting along with CaBP. Calcium seems to be absorbed from the intestine into the mucosal cell by both an active transport system as well as a non-saturable mechanism that may operate by facilitated diffusion. Both mechanisms appear to be vitamin D_3 dependent. Calcium is also pumped out of the mucosal cell by an active process. A calcium dependent ATPase is present in the brush border of the cell, as well as the membranes, and this has been suggested as the molecular site of the active calcium pump.

Phosphate absorption appears to be an active process which is highly dependent on the sodium ion. It is believed that sodium and phosphate are interacting with a common component on the brush border membrane. Sodium movement into the cell, across a concentration gradient, provides energy for phosphate transport in the same direction. The sodium gradient is maintained by the sodium pump that keeps the intracellular concentration in balance.

Components of both the calcium and phosphate transport systems are affected by vitamin D_3 status of the bird. The calcium dependent ATPase and alkaline phosphatase activity are increased when vitamin D_3 is present. Several other proteins whose synthesis depends on vitamin D_3 have also been reported. Phosphorus absorption has been reported to be 3-4 times greater for chickens given cholecalciferol compared to rachitic chicks. Further work is necessary to completely clarify the transport systems for calcium and phosphorus and the role vitamin D plays in this process. The role of CaBP is not confined to the intestinal mucosa because it is found in several other tissues, being high in the avian shell gland, and also present in kidney, brain, blood, pancreas, and bone.

In young animals, during bone formation, minerals are deposited on the bone matrix, giving rise to trabecular bone and in the process, bones elongate. With a vitamin D_3 deficiency, the organic matrix fails to mineralize, thus resulting in rickets in the young bird and osteomalacia in the adult bird. One of the roles of $1,25-(OH)_2D_3$ is to bring about matrix mineralization. A possible role for $24,-25-(OH)_2 D_3$ and

25-(OH)D$_3$ in bone metabolism has also been suggested (Bar *et al.*, 1982). Vitamin D$_3$ also plays a role, along with PTH in mobilizing Ca from bone to the extra-cellular fluid. It is an active process requiring metabolic energy and presumably transports Ca and phosphate ions across the bone tissue by acting on osteocytes and osteoclasts, (Garabedian *et al.*, 1974). Another role that has been proposed for vitamin D$_3$ is in its involvement in the biosynthesis of collagen in preparation for mineralization (Gonnerman *et al.*, 1976). Vitamin D$_3$ appears to function in the distal renal tubules to improve Ca reabsorption. While it is known that 99% of the filtered Ca load is reabsorbed in the absence of vitamin D$_3$ and PTH, the remaining 1% is under the control of these two hormones (Sutton and Dirks, 1978).

4.11.7 Vitamin D$_3$ requirements of poultry

So many factors can influence the vitamin D$_3$ requirement of the chicken that it is difficult to quantitate precise estimates of requirement. Such values depend upon the source of phosphorus in the diet, the ratio of calcium to phosphorus and the extent of exposure of the animal to sunlight. There are a number of reports indicating that from 11 to 45 minutes exposure to sunlight per day is sufficient to prevent rickets in growing chickens.

Baker *et al.* (1998) suggest the vitamin D$_3$ requirement of the young broiler chicken to be around 5µg/kg diet. This value is identical to that reported by NRC (1994). Vitamin D$_3$ is needed by the hen for optimum egg production and also for good eggshell quality. For breeding hens, it is important, not only for good hatchability but also in providing a carryover to the chick. It has been reported that the chick does not have an optimum supply of the enzyme cholecalciferol-25-hydroxylase until about two weeks of age. Hence, chicks hatching from eggs where the breeders have been fed a diet low in vitamin D$_3$, may show rickets even though the chick's diet contains sufficient levels of the vitamin. Similarly, chicks hatched from dams fed low vitamin D$_3$ levels and receiving 25-OH-D$_3$, grew normally, as did chicks hatched from eggs with good vitamin D$_3$ reserves, even though both groups of chicks received a vitamin D$_3$ deficient diet for the first two weeks of age.

Competitive interactions between vitamins A and D$_3$, and between E and D$_3$ have been reported. Poults fed a diet containing adequate vitamin D$_3$ and a high level of vitamin A, developed hypocalcemia and rickets. Supplementing chick and poult diets with extra vitamin D$_3$, can partially counter the deleterious effects of a high vitamin A diet, as measured by growth and skeletal deformities (Veltmann *et al.*, 1986). Work with rats suggests that excess dietary vitamin A decreases bioactive serum PTH and 1,25-(OH)$_2$ D$_3$. Aburto *et al.* (1998) show similar effects related to bone ash in birds fed high levels of vitamin A, while the toxicity can be corrected by supplements of 25 (OH) D$_3$ or 1,25 (OH)$_2$ D$_3$. It is unclear just how significant this interaction is at more normal levels of diet supplementation.

Chicks fed with an adequate vitamin D_3 diet and excess vitamin E develop hock deformities and rickets. With no added vitamin D_3, incidence of rickets is increased while with excess vitamin E almost all birds show rickets.

The recommended levels of vitamin D_3, presented in Table 4.4 are sufficiently high to produce normal growth, calcification, production and reproduction, in the absence of sunlight, provided that diets being fed contain adequate levels of calcium and phosphorus. As the ratio of calcium to phosphorus becomes wider or narrower, the requirement for vitamin D_3 increases. Also, the requirement for vitamin D_3 becomes higher if the source of phosphorus in the diet is of low availability. Mycotoxins may also significantly increase the requirement of vitamin D_3, possibly due to impaired absorption.

4.11.8 Signs of vitamin D_3 deficiency

Laying hens fed a vitamin D_3 deficient diet will exhibit loss of egg production within 2-3 weeks, and depending upon the degree of deficiency, shell quality will deteriorate almost instantaneously (Figure 4.12). Using a corn-soybean meal diet with no supplemental vitamin D_3, the shell quality, as assessed by deformation (Figure 4.12) decreases dramatically within 7d. Shell weight declines, due to D_3 deficiency, by about 150 mg daily. The less obvious decline in shell quality with suboptimal supplements (eg. 125 IU/kg, Figure 4.12) are more difficult to diagnose, especially since it is very difficult to assay vitamin D_3 in complete feeds.

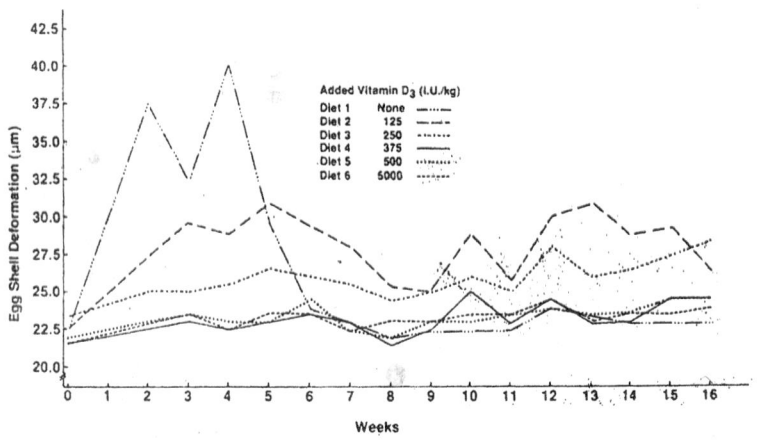

Figure 4.12 Eggshell quality of layers fed various dietary levels of vitamin D_3.

Soares and Ottinger (1988) showed a significant increase in plasma $1,25(OH)_2D_3$ of birds producing good vs poor eggshells. Feeding purified $1,25(OH)_2D_3$ improved the shell quality of these inferior layers, suggesting a potential inherent problem with metabolism of cholecalciferol. Monitoring $1,25(OH)_2D_3$ in immature birds, does not seem to be a good predictor of subsequent eggshell quality.

Retarded growth and severe leg weakness are the first signs noted when chicks receive a vitamin D_3 deficient diet. Also, beaks and claws will become soft and pliable. Chicks may have trouble walking and will take a few steps before squatting on their hocks. While resting, they often sway from side to side, suggesting some loss of equilibrium. Feathering is usually poor and an abnormal banding of feathers has been reported with colored breeds. With chronic vitamin D_3 deficiency, marked skeletal disorders are noted. The spinal column may bend downward and the sternum can also deviate to one side. These structural changes reduce the size of the thorax with subsequent crowding of the internal organs. Adding synthetic $1,25(OH)_2 D_3$ to the diet of TD susceptible chicks does reduce the incidence of this condition (Xu *et al.,* 1997). Although the response is not dramatic and is quite variable, results suggest that some leg abnormalities may be a consequence of inefficient metabolism of cholecalciferol. With chicks, a characteristic finding is a beading of the ribs at the junction of the spinal column along with a downward and posterior bending (Figure 4.13).Poor calcification can also be seen at the epiphysis of the tibia and femur. By dipping the split bone in a silver nitrate solution, and allowing it to stand under an incandescent light for a few minutes, the calcified areas are easily distinguished from the areas of uncalcified cartilage, (Figure 4.14). In the laying hen, signs of gross pathology are usually confined to the bones and parathyroid glands. Bones are soft and easily broken and the ribs may become

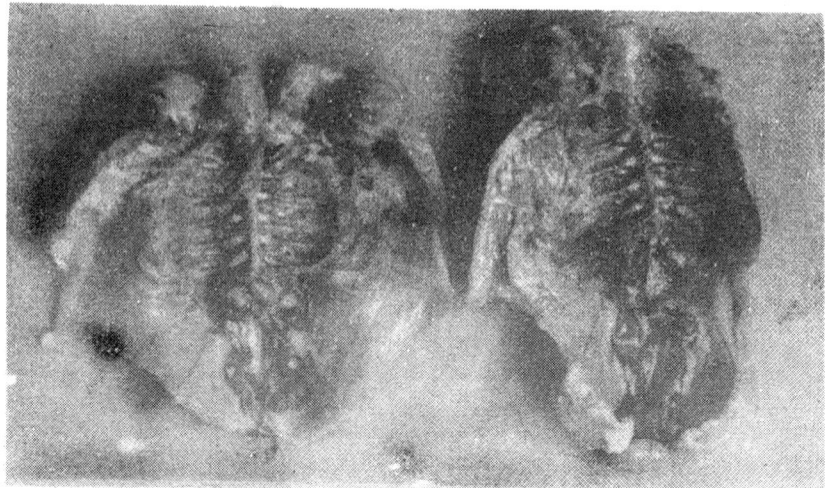

Figure 4.13 Beading of ribs in birds fed diets devoid of added vitamin D_3.

beaded. The ribs may also show spontaneous fractures in the sterno-vertebral region. Histological examination shows deficiency of calcification in the long bones, with excess of osteoid tissue, and the parathyroids are usually enlarged.

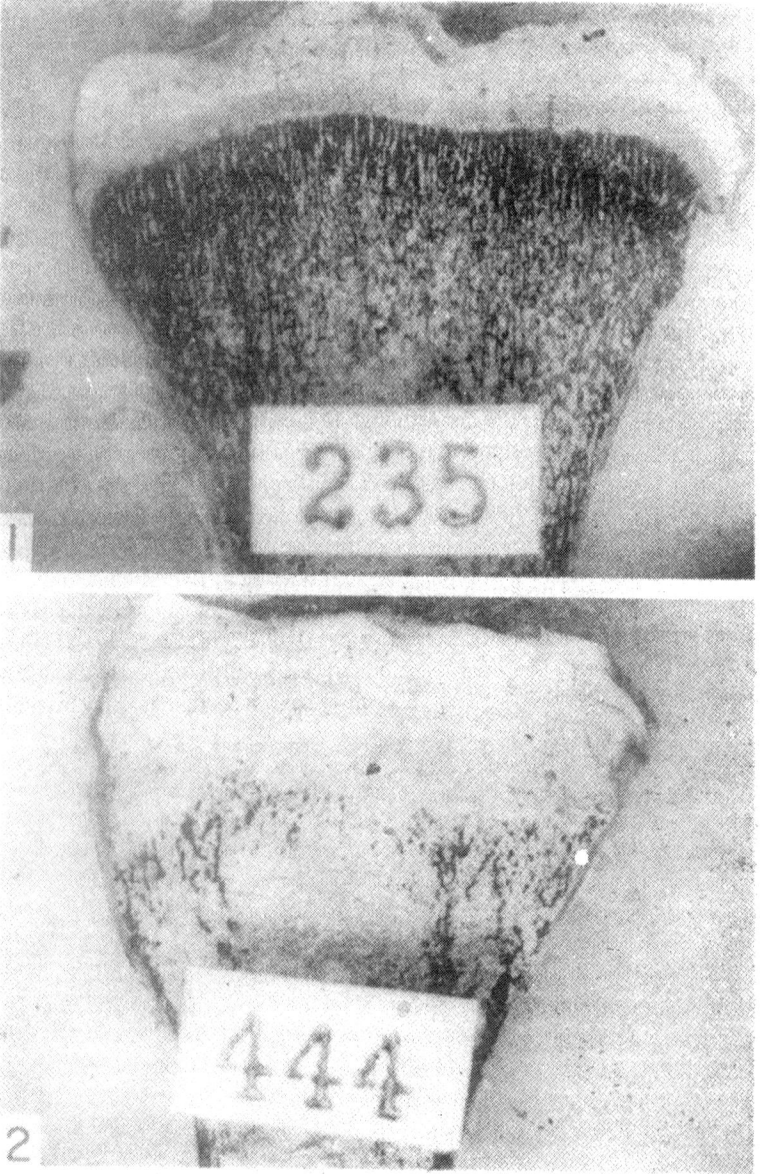

Figure 4.14 Normal bone calcification (1) in a tibia from a chick fed vitamin D₃ as compared with extremely poor calcification (2) in the tibia from a chick fed a vitamin D₃ deficient diet.

4.11.9 Hypervitaminosis D$_3$

Excessive intakes of vitamin D$_3$ produce a syndrome characterized by resorption of bone salts and abnormal deposition of calcium in the viscera and soft tissues. Doses of 300,000 to 600,000 IU in rats has produced resorption of calcium salts, rendering the bones brittle and ultimately leading to deformity and fracture. Smooth muscle is very susceptible to abnormal calcium deposition. The pathological sequences noted are, inflammation, cellular degeneration, and finally calcification. Calcium deposits are often found in the vascular system, and urinary and respiratory tract. Very high levels of cholecalciferol in chicks can lead to renal damage, due to calcification of the kidney tubules while the aorta and other arteries may also become calcified. Baker *et al.,* (1998) show no toxic effects of cholecalciferol fed at 250x requirement. However, 25(OH)D$_3$ is 5-10x more toxic than is vitamin D$_3$. Toxicity of vitamin D$_3$ and metabolites is always accentuated when diets are also high in calcium and phosphorus.

While adequate vitamin D$_3$ is essential for normal shell calcification, high doses can lead to an abnormality known as shell pimpling (Goodson-Williams *et al.,* 1987). Such eggs have extra deposits of calcium spread across the surface of the shell, some of which can break off and lead to physical breakage of the shell. The calcium content of the isthmus and uterus is increased when high levels of vitamin D$_3$ are fed, and so the hen appears to absorb and transport calcium to the shell gland faster than its uptake for normal calcification. While vitamin D$_3$ levels can be a factor in shell pimpling, it is not the sole cause.

4.12 VITAMIN E

Vitamin E is a group name that includes a number of closely related active compounds. Eight naturally occurring forms of the vitamin are known and they can be divide into two groups according to whether the side chain of the molecule is saturated or unsaturated. The four saturated forms are referred to as tocopherols (McDowell 1989) and are designated as α, β, and γ tocopherols. These are 6-hydroxychroman molecules, substituted at the 2-position by a 16-carbon isopranoid chain. Of these α is the most biologically active and most widely distributed. The β, γ and ε forms have around 25,10 and 1% of the activity, respectively, of the α form. The saturated forms, referred to as tocotrienols, have double bonds on the 16 carbon side chain at positions 3,7 and 11. These are of little interest nutritionally, as they have very low vitamin E activity.

Vitamin E was discovered by Evans and Bishop, (1922), as a fat soluble factor in vegetable oil, required for normal reproduction in rats. It was isolated by Evans, *et al.* in 1936. Early studies were made with a wide variety of experimental animals which led to the recognition of vitamin E deficiency as a cause of a number of different pathological conditions. It is now recognized that vitamin E is concerned in the normal functioning of most of the tissues in the body and preventing many deficiency diseases, in a number of animal species, as shown in Table 4.14.

Table 4.14 Pathology of vitamin E deficiency			
Condition	Tissue affected	Prevented by	
		Vitamin E	Selenium
1. Reproductive Failure Embryonic degeneration	Vascular system of embryo	Yes	No
Male Sterility		Yes	No
II. Liver, Blood, Brain, Capillaries, etc. Erythrocyte destruction	Blood (RBC hemolysis)	Yes	No
Blood protein loss	Serum albumin	Yes	Yes
Encephalomalacia	Cerebellum (Purkinje cells)	Yes	No
Exudative diathesis	Capillary walls	Yes	Yes
Steatitis	Depot fat	Yes	Yes
III. Nutritional Myopathies Nutritional muscular dystrophy	Skeletal muscle	Yes	No
Myopathy of gizzard	Gizzard, heart, skeletal muscles (mainly turkeys)	Yes	Yes

Vitamin E is required for normal fertility in the rooster and for normal reproductive performance of the hen. A deficiency with chicks can lead to lipid degeneration and hemolysis. With an acute deficiency, chicks may show one or more of the well defined deficiency diseases, such as encephalomalacia, exudative diathesis or muscular dystrophy. Although there are some similarities observed in the tissues of chicks suffering from all these diseases, it appears that there is no common metabolic defect responsible for all three conditions. Various specific dietary changes, unrelated to vitamin E content of the diet, appear to completely prevent one of the conditions while having no effect on the others. Of these the most important are the prevention of encephalomalacia with synthetic antioxidants, the effectiveness of inorganic selenium in prevention of exudative diathesis, and the role of cystine in preventing muscular dystrophy.

4.12.1 Chemistry of vitamin E

The chemical structure of vitamin E was elucidated by Fernholz (1938), and synthesized the same year by several groups of workers. The chemical structures of the tocopherols are shown in Figure 4.15 while Figure 4.16 shows some of the oxidation products. Figure 4.17 indicates the structure of some quinones that are also similar in structure to vitamin E, and that are known to exist in the body. The degradation of vitamin E in the body is similar to that shown in Figure 4.16 where tocopherol is converted to tocopherol quinone. This conversion product has no biological activity and cannot be directly converted to vitamin E. α-tocopheroxide is converted to tocopherol, to a limited extent, in the presence of vitamin C.

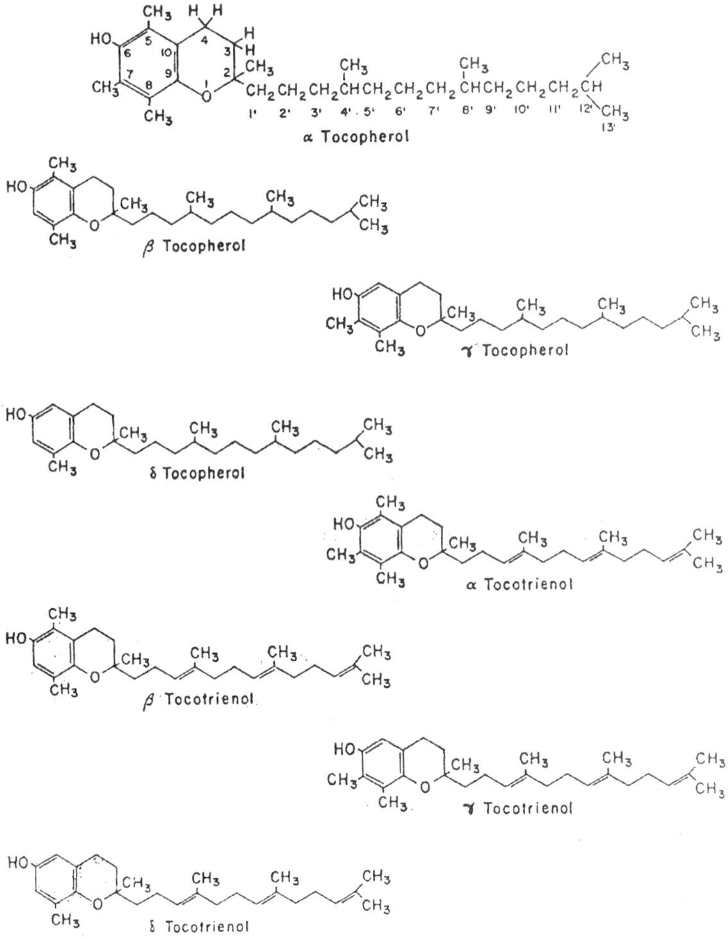

Figure 4.15 Chemical structures of naturally occurring tocopherols and tocotrienols.

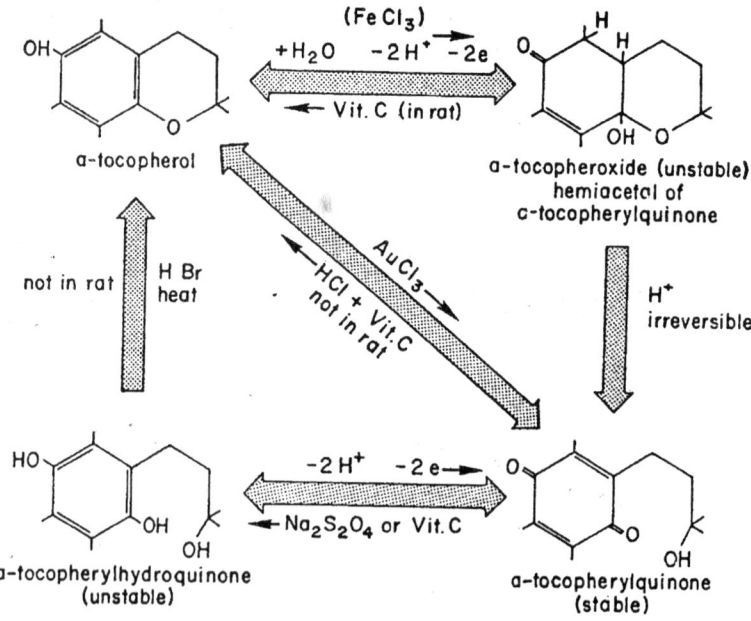

Figure 4.16 Oxidation products of α-tocopherol.

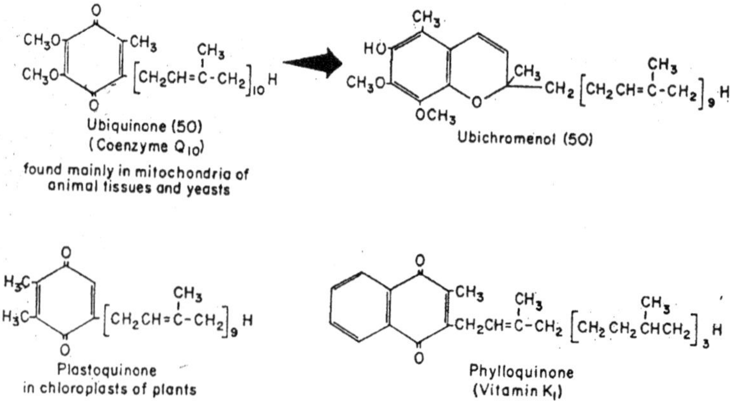

Ubiquinone (50)
(Coenzyme Q₁₀)
found mainly in mitochondria of
animal tissues and yeasts

Ubichromenol (50)

Plastoquinone
in chloroplasts of plants

Phylloquinone
(Vitamin K₁)

Figure 4.17 Structures of several metabolically active chemical compounds similar to vitamin E. Ubiquinone has from 6 to 10 isoprene units in the side chain (CoQ₆-CoQ₁₀).

The quinones, shown in Figure 4.16, demonstrate the similarities in chemical structure between vitamin K, and α-tocopherol. The action of quinone in hydrogen transport is depicted in Figure 4.18, and the relative biopotencies of the various forms of vitamin E are presented in Table 4.15.

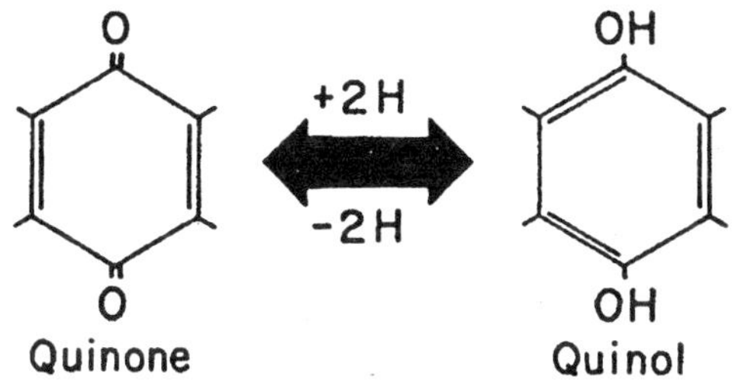

Figure 4.18 function of quinones in hydrogen transport.

Table 4.15 Relative biological activities of various forms and oxidation products of vitamin E	
Compound	Relative biopotency for resorption gestation prevention in female rats
d-α-tocopherol	100
β-tocopherol	30-35
γ-tocopherol	1-10
δ-tocopherol	0
ζ_1-tocopherol	30-40
ε-tocopherol	10
η-tocopherol	0
α-tocopheroxide	3-10
α-tocopheryl hydroquinone	0
α-tocopherylquinone	0
di-α-tocopherone	5

The d form of α-tocopherol is a slightly viscous, pale yellow oil, insoluble in water, but freely soluble in oils, fats and organic solvents. It has a melting point of 2.5-3.5° C and a boiling point of 200-220° C. It can be purified by molecular distillation and has a maximum absorption at 294 mμ and minimum absorption at 267 mμ. Since esterification usually improves its stability, commercial supplements are present as d-α-tocopherol acetate, or dl-α-tocopherol acetate. There are three centers of asymmetry in the molecule, and so there are 8 possible isomers. Vitamin E is synthesized from trimethylhydroquinone and isophytol, resulting in approximate equal proportions of the 8 isomers and the resultant mixture is known as all racemic--tocopherol or dl-α-tocopherol.

Vitamin E is very unstable, with oxidative destruction enhanced by minerals, and unsaturated fatty acids in a diet. When diets contain fish or other sources of polyunsaturated fatty acids in any appreciable amounts, an effective antioxidant should be added to prevent the oils from undergoing oxidative rancidity which destroys not only vitamin E, but is also detrimental to vitamins A and D_3. Today most commercial forms of vitamin E are prepared as acetates, by reacting the tocopherol with acetic anhydride. The α-tocopherol acetate, especially when encased in gelatin beadlets, is much more stable than the reactive natural alcohol. Natural sources of vitamin E are the vegetable oils, and for humans, the egg provides an excellent source of this vitamin. One International Unit of vitamin E is equivalent to 1 mg dl-α–tocohpherol acetate.

4.12.2 Absorption, transport and storage of vitamin E

Absorption appears to be mainly achieved through micellar formation in the intestine, similar to that described for vitamin A. While d and L-α–tocopherol are both well absorbed, a lower blood concentration is found with the L as compared to the d form. Both bile and pancreatic lipase are essential for maximum absorption, and when acetates are used, as is most common, then pancreatic esterase aids in initial cleavage. Any acetate absorbed is converted to the alcohol in the mucosal cells. The α-tocopherol is absorbed along with fatty acids as a lipid-bile-lipase micelle, and factors that influence micelle formation, (Chapter 1) influence vitamin E absorption. The efficiency of digestion and absorption of vitamin E varies with dietary inclusion level. At 10 IU/kg, there is about 98% uptake of vitamin E, while at 100 and 1,000 IU/kg, efficiency declines to 80 and 70% respectively. As with fats, absorbed tocopherol is transported to the liver via the portal vein. Such vitamin E in circulation has no known specific carrier protein, since it seems to bind to all classes of lipoprotein.

Vitamin E is stored in the liver and most fat depots. Adipose tissue accounts for 90% of body stores, although it is unlikely that this store is labile, since levels are little affected when birds are fed deficient diets and are showing signs of deficiency.

4.12.3 Metabolic functions of vitamin E

In view of the many tissues affected in the body by a vitamin E deficiency, it would appear that the vitamin has several different metabolic functions. However, it is believed that its main underlying function is its role as a natural antioxidant in the body. Major functions involving vitamin E are: (1) as a biological antioxidant; (2) in normal tissue respiration; (3) in normal phosphorylation reactions, especially of high energy phosphate compounds like creatine phosphate, and adenosine triphosphate; (4) in metabolism of nucleic acids; (5) in synthesis of ascorbic acid; (6) in synthesis of ubiquinone; (7) involved in sulfur amino acid metabolism; (8) in maintenance of low peroxide levels in the cells; (9) assist in maintaining an active immune system and (10) influence carcass lipid peroxidation. While many of the roles played by vitamin E in these various metabolic functions have been elucidated during the past several decades, there still appears to be a number of unanswered or unresolved questions concerning its many and varied functions in the body. Table 4.16 summarizes the major interrelations between vitamin E, selenium and antioxidants as they influence bird metabolism and function.

Table 4.16 Interrelation of vitamin E, selenium and synthetic antioxidants				
Syndrome	Signs	Prevented by		
		Vit E	Se	Synthetic antioxidants
Exudative diathesis	Subcutaneous edema, hemorrhage	+++	+++	
Muscular dystrophy	Muscle degeneration	+++	+	
Pancreatic atrophy	Small pancrease	+	+++	
Encephalomalacia	Cerebral lesions	++++	+	+

a. Vitamin E as an antioxidant:

While oxygen is vital for life of higher organisms, several toxic products result during the reduction of oxygen to water in the body. Presence of the super oxide anion (O_2), hydrogen peroxide ($H_2 O_2$) , and the hydroxyl radical (OH), as intermediates during this reaction, present serious problems to an animal as they are all potent oxidizing agents. The hydroxyl radical, the strongest oxidizing agent known, can also be formed from the breakdown of hydrogen peroxide. All the above oxidizing agents are a potential threat to living cells as they can cause damage to the protein and lipid fractions of the cells. Fortunately self-defence mechanisms exist in the body to scavenge these oxidizing agents, one of the most important being the enzyme glutathione peroxidase, present in mitochondrial matrix. Lipid membranes have an abundance of unsaturated fatty acids and are thus very susceptible to peroxide formation. The peroxidation of membrane lipids can in turn cause oxidation of the membrane proteins. These reactions are enhanced by the presence of metal ions, especially iron.

b. Immune system

Vitamin E enhances the immune system by stimulating glutathione peroxidase activity of the circulating neutrophyls and macrophages, and is also reported to stimulate the activity of T- lymphocytes. Increase in phagocytosis activity and antibody production against several antigens have also been reported. Erf *et al.* (1998) suggest that feeding 90 IU vitamin E/kg diet influences T-cell differentiation in the thymus and that there are altered proportions among T-cell subsets in both the thymus and spleen. These authors conclude that vitamin E added at levels beyond those needed to support optimal growth are beneficial to improving the immunocompetence of growing broilers. Likewise, Colnago *et al.* (1984) suggest that immunization against coccidiosis is enhanced by feeding moderately high levels (100 IU/kg) of vitamin E. There is also an indication of improved growth and liveability in birds fed higher levels of vitamin E, when the diet also contains mycotoxins such as T-2 and ochratoxin. In this situation, the beneficial effect of vitamin E is likely via its role as an antioxidant (Hoehler and Marquardt, 1996). Marsh *et al.* (1986) concluded that primary lymphoid organs are major targets for vitamin E (and selenium) deficiency and provide a possible mechanism by which immune function may be affected. Contrary to these results however, Fridman *et al.* (1998) show that a high intake of vitamin E (150 IU/kg) is detrimental to antibody production, since at these levels vitamin E becomes a prooxidant, rather than an antioxidant.

c. Cellular respiration

Vitamin E appears to be of particular importance in cellular respiration of heart and skeletal muscles. It is thought to act as a cofactor in the cytochrome-reductase portion of the NAD and succinate oxidase systems. The tocopherols also appear to be involved in the biosynthesis of DNA, probably by regulation of the incorporation of pyrimidine into nucleic acid structures.

d. Synthesis of coenzyme Q and vitamin C

Vitamin E is involved in the synthesis of vitamin C, possibly through its stimulation of coenzyme Q. Vitamin E is an antagonist to vitamin K coagulation functions as it can inhibit platelet aggregation by inhibiting peroxidation of arachidonic acid, which is required for the formation of prostaglandins involved in platelet aggregation. Excessive intake of vitamin A or carotene, increases the requirement for vitamin E, while excess vitamin E can deplete vitamin A reserves.

e. Meat quality

Post-mortem peroxidation invariably occurs in the muscle and fat depots of the carcass. The higher the polyunsaturated fat content of the carcass, the quicker, and the more severe, peroxidation will occur. There is an indication that high levels of vitamin E (100 IU/kg diet) fed for 3-4 weeks prior to slaughter, improves meat stability during storage. Vitamin E seems to slow down the rate of peroxidation, catalyzed by products such as iron derived from hemoglobin (Sheehy *et al.*, 1997). Even feeding high levels of vitamin E in only the 0-3 week period, is reported to improve the stability in meat harvested from 7 week old birds (Bartov and Frigg, 1992).

f. Antagonists

The requirement for vitamin E is increased with high dietary levels of polyunsaturated fatty acids (PUFA). Not only do PUFA oxidize vitamin E present in the diet and intestine, but also increase the metabolic requirement as PUFA are laid down in the body.

4.12.4 Vitamin E sparing factors

Some biological functions of vitamin E can be carried out in part, or full, by other chemically unrelated factors. Selenium, as a part of the enzyme glutathione peroxidase, spares vitamin E by destroying peroxides that are formed, before they can cause cell damage. Selenium is efficient in controlling exudative diathesis and muscular dystrophy but has little or no effect in relieving encephalomalacia. Sulfur amino acids are effective in controlling muscular dystrophy but are not effective against exudative diathesis and encephalomalacia.

Antioxidants also prevent the appearance of some of the symptoms of vitamin E deficiency. Vitamin C is also a powerful physiological antioxidant at the cellular level. Vitamin C is rapidly absorbed but also rapidly excreted. Thus, to maintain a good level in the body, vitamin C or its precursor glucose, must be constantly administered.

4.12.5 Mode of action of vitamin E and its relation to the biological action of selenium

Rotruck *et al.* (1973) and Noguchi *et al.* (1973) provided information which helped to show the separate activities of vitamin E and selenium in the protection of biological membranes. Selenium was shown to be an integral part of the enzyme, glutathione peroxidase, which destroys hydrogen peroxide and hydroperoxides in the plasma and in the aqueous medium of cells and organelles. Vitamin E appears to act within the lipid membrane of cells by preventing the formation of free radical and peroxides (Noguchi *et al.*, 1973). Phospholipids appear to have a special affinity for vitamin E, transporting and depositing d-α-tocopherol in that portion of the phospholipid which is most subject to initial attack by peroxides or hydroxyl free radicals, produced by the reactions of superoxide ions.

Thus, phospholipids may act as the first line of defense, in the prevention of exudative diathesis and the protection of vital mitochondria and microsomes, by preventing the formation of peroxides. Selenium in the aqueous portion of the cell represents the second line of defense, destroying peroxides that are formed before they can cause any further damage. Thus, for complete protection of mitochondria and microsomes from peroxidation, both vitamin E and selenium are required.

Although both selenium and other antioxidants spare the requirement for vitamin E for certain metabolic functions, it is still necessary that chicken diets contain adequate amounts of vitamin E.

4.12.6 Inhibitors, antagonists and factors which may destroy vitamin E

Following are some factors which influence vitamin E requirements

a. *Peroxidizing polyunsaturated oils:* Unsaturated vegetable oils will increase the requirement for dietary vitamin E. This is especially true if steps are not taken to prevent or reduce oxidative rancidity of the oil or if they are in the process of peroxidation when consumed by an animal. If they are completely rancid before being ingested, the only damage is a loss of vitamin E present in the diet. However, if they are undergoing oxidative rancidity when consumed, they can result in destruction of body stores of vitamin E, thereby leading to the onset of encephalomalacia in growing chickens, and low hatchability with breeders.

As the PUFA concentration of the diet is increased, it is advisable to increase the vitamin E level so as to prevent signs of encephalomalacia and other related disorders. The usual recommendation is to increase dietary vitamin E concentration by 30 IU/kg for each 1% increase in PUFA content of the diet. Table 4.17 indicates appropriate increments for dietary vitamin E for different fats, and these calculations are based on respective PUFA contributions of these fat sources

Table 4.17 Extra vitamin E need related to polyunsaturated fatty acids	
Fat	Vit E (IU/1% fat)
Tallow	2
Lard	4
Poultry	8
Canola oil	10
Coconut oil	0
Cottonseed oil	16
Fish oil	8
Flax oil	25
Corn oil	16
Palm oil	4
Soy oil	20
Sunflower oil	20

b. Pelleting: Since pelleting subjects feed to increased temperature and moisture, conditions which speed up most chemical reactions, both vitamin A and E can be destroyed unless the diets contains a sufficient level of an antioxidant.

c. Effects of iron salts: Ferric salts enhance oxidation reactions and thus can lead to reduced levels of dietary vitamin E, again unless the diet contains an antioxidant.

d. Flour bleaching agents: Nitrogen, chloride and chlorine oxide, at the concentrations used to bleach flour, can destroy much of the tocopherols in the flour. Also baking can further destroy a significant amount of the remaining vitamin E.

4.12.7   Signs of vitamin E deficiency

No clinical symptoms are noted in mature birds even if fed low vitamin E diets for a prolonged period. However, egg production may be slightly reduced, while hatchability will be markedly lowered, with embryos dying as early as the 4th day of incubation. Testicular degeneration may be noted in mature males fed a deficient diet for 6-8 weeks.

As mentioned previously, the three main deficiencies seen in chicks are encephalomalacia, exudative diathesis, and muscular dystrophy. The occurrence of these conditions, under practical conditions, depends on dietary and environmental factors that the birds are exposed to. Encephalomalacia is seen in commercial flocks if diets are low in vitamin E, or an antioxidant is either omitted or not present in sufficient quantities, or the diet contains a reasonably high level of an unstable, unsaturated fat.

For exudative diathesis to be present in a flock, the diet must be deficient in both vitamin E and selenium. In recent years, levels of selenium in soils have been depleted to the point that corn and soybeans are low in these nutrients, thus requiring that a dietary supplement be used to prevent the condition from appearing.

Symptoms of muscular dystrophy are rare in chicks as the diet has to be deficient in both sulfur amino acids as well as vitamin E. Since the sulfur amino acids are necessary for growth, a deficiency severe enough to induce muscular dystrophy is unlikely to occur under commercial conditions.

Signs of exudative diathesis and muscular dystrophy can be reversed in chicks by supplementation of the diet with liberal amounts of vitamin E assuming the deficiency is not too advanced. Encephalomalacia may or may not respond to vitamin E supplementation, depending on the extent of the damage to the cerebellum.

4.12.8 Encephalomalacia

The classical sign of encephalomalacia is ataxia as shown in Fig. 4.19. This condition results from hemorrhages and edema within the molecular and granular layers of the cerebellum (Figure 4.20), with pyknosis, and eventual disappearance of the Purkinje cells and separation of the molecular and granular layers of the cerebellar folia (Figure 4.21). Due to its inherently low level of vitamin E, the cerebellum is particularly susceptible to lipid peroxidation. Fuhrmann and Sallmann (1997) also suggest that altered aldehyde metabolism in the cerebellum, related to vitamin E and lipid unsaturates, is involved in the pathogenesis of encephalomalacia.

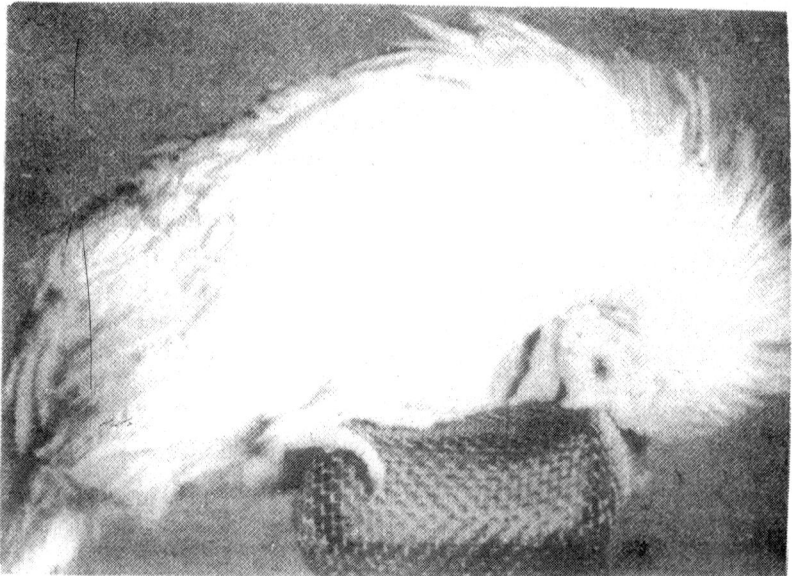

Figure 4.19 Encephalomalacia in a chick fed a vitamin E deficient diet.

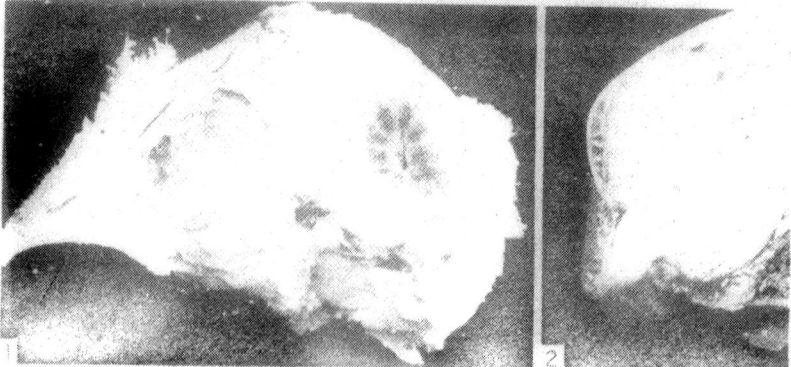

Figure 4.20 Longitudinal section through the brain of a chicken with encephalomalacia (1). Note the hemorrhages and edema of the cerebellum as compared with the cerebellum of a normal chick (2).

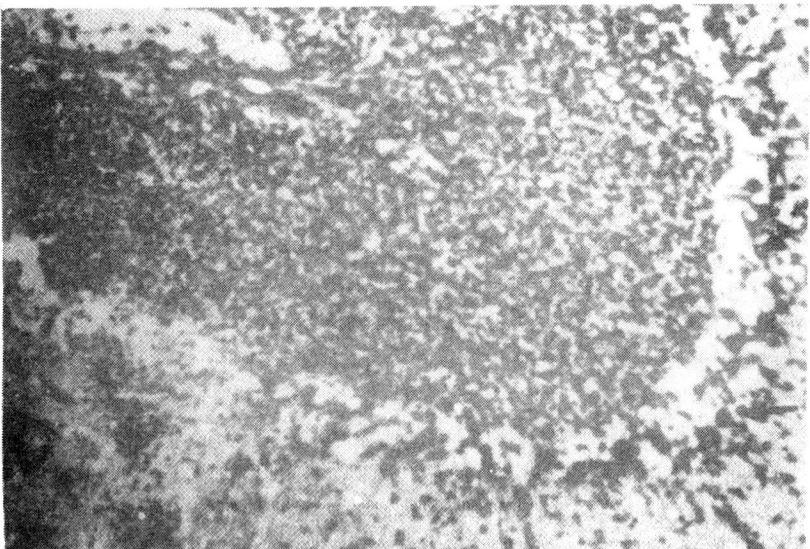

Figure 4.21 Photomicrograph of the cerebellar folia of a chick with encephalomalacia, H & E x 100. Note separation of molecular and granular layers with pyknosis (arrow) of the Purkinje cells and their complete disintegration from, and extensive hemorrhage of, the molecular layer (lower left).

In prevention of encephalomalacia, vitamin E functions as a biological antioxidant. The quantitative needs for vitamin E for this function depend on the amount of linoleic acid and PUFA's in the diet. Many workers have presented evidence showing that antioxidants, other than tocopherols, are capable of preventing signs of a vitamin E deficiency in animals. There is some controversy as to whether synthetic antioxidants prevent certain vitamin E deficient diseases, by completely replacing vitamin E in metabolic functions, or whether they are effective because they prevent destruction of limited vitamin E levels in the feed or reserves in the body. Over prolonged periods, it has been well demonstrated that antioxidants will prevent encephalomalacia in chicks when added to diets with very low levels of vitamin E, or when fed vitamin E depleted purified diets. Chicks hatched from breeders that are given additional dietary vitamin E are also less susceptible to lipid peroxidation in the brain. Surai *et al.* (1999) show a 2-10x increase in tissue concentration of day-old chicks hatched from breeders fed well fortified diets.

The fact that antioxidants can help prevent encephalomalacia, but fail to prevent exudative diathesis or muscular dystrophy in chicks, strongly suggests that in preventing encephalomalacia, vitamin E is acting as an antioxidant. Søndergaard *et al.* (1962), found that phytyl-ubichromenol, prevented encephalomalacia, and suggested that its presence in brewer's and torula yeast probably accounted for the yeast being effective in preventing this disease.

Antioxidants have been reported to prevent exudative diathesis and muscular dystrophy although the amounts required to do this were so high as to be almost toxic. Since vitamin E, in very low concentrations, effectively prevents exudative diathesis and muscular dystrophy, it has been hypothesized that this may be due to; (a) its participation in metabolic processes which are more specific than simple prevention of peroxidation within the body of the animal; or (b) a special affinity of phospholipids of capillary membranes, muscle cells and organelles for vitamin E, but not for synthetic antioxidants. The discovery that a low concentration of ethoxyquin prevents encephalomalacia has aided studies of exudative diathesis and muscular dystrophy in chicks. Complete prevention of encephalomalacia has been regularly achieved in experiments on exudative diathesis and muscular dystrophy by supplementing the basal diets with a 0.0125-0.025% ethoxyquin.

4.12.9 Exudative diathesis and interrelationship with selenium

Exudative diathesis (Figure 4.22), results in a severe edema caused by a marked increase in capillary permeability. Dam and Glavind, (1942), were the first to recognize it as a vitamin E deficiency while Goldstein and Scott (1956) reported that an alteration in blood proteins occurred as the disorder progressed. Electrophoretic patterns of the blood showed a decrease in albumin levels whereas exudative fluids contained a protein pattern similar to normal blood plasma.

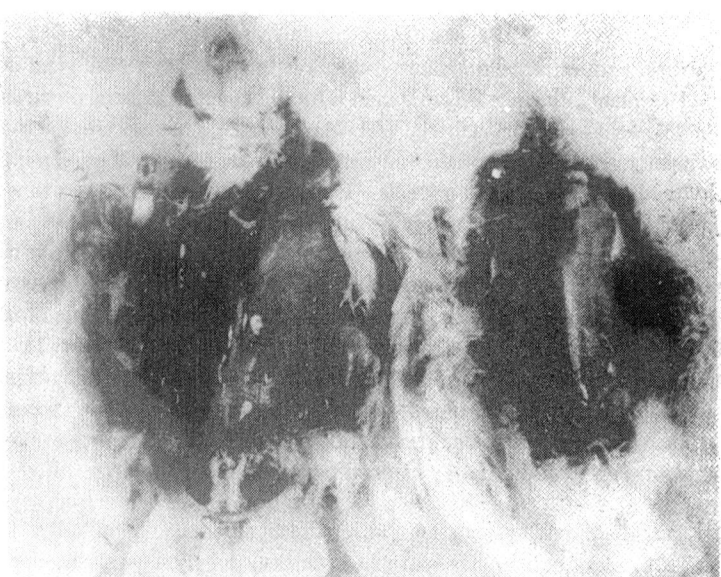

Figure 4.22 Exudative diathesis in chicks fed a vitamin E deficient diet, low in selenium but containing an antioxidant which prevents encephalomalacia. Note the severe edema.

For years it had been known that brewer's yeast, and several other natural food-stuffs, contained an unidentified factor which would prevent dietary necrosis of the liver in rats, when fed a vitamin E deficient diet. Following the discovery by Schwarz and Foltz (1957), that selenium, which was present in brewer's yeast, would prevent liver necrosis in rats, several groups of workers demonstrated that it would also prevent exudative diathesis in chicks (Scott *et al.,* 1957, and Stokstad *et al.,* 1957). Using a purified diet Nesheim and Scott (1958), showed that selenium, as sodium selenite (8 µg/100 g of diet) had a greater effect on promoting growth than did vitamin E alone. In the presence of adequate vitamin E, maximum growth was obtained with 4µg/100 g of diet of selenium, while without selenium growth was poor and chick mortality high between 5 and 8 weeks of age. Thus, it was demonstrated that selenium was an essential nutrient for the chick, and its metabolism was closely related to that of vitamin E.

Thompson and Scott (1970) provided evidence that selenium was a nutrient in its own right and always necessarily related to functions of vitamin E. These workers showed that a pancreatic exocrine dysfunction occurred in chicks, when fed a diet containing a low level of selenium but with a high level of vitamin E. Rotruck *et al.* (1973) discovered that selenium was an essential constituent of the enzyme glutathione peroxidase. Since glutathione peroxidase was known to function in the metabolic reduction of hydroperoxides, the nature of the interrelationship of selenium and vitamin E in preventing lipid peroxidation became apparent. The belief that selenium was exclusively involved in preventing pancreatic dysfunction has now been abandoned as it was shown that high dietary vitamin E levels, with very low levels of selenium, prevented pancreatic dysfunction in chicks. Thus, the disease actually results from loss in the tissues of total antioxidant protection. Further observations with other vitamin E - selenium related metabolic functions, supports the hypothesis that vitamin E and selenium serve to protect cells from oxidative stress.

4.12.10 Nutritional muscular dystrophy

A vitamin E deficiency, accompanied by a sulfur amino acid deficiency, results in a severe myopathy, especially of the breast muscle in chicks, by around 4 weeks of age. This condition is characterized by degeneration of the muscle fibers, usually in the breast, (Figure 4.23) but sometimes also in the leg muscles. Histological examination show Zenker's degeneration, with perivascular infiltration, and marked accumulation of infiltrated eosinophils, lymphocytes and histocytes. Accumulation of these cells in dystrophic tissue, results in a large increase in lysosomal enzymes, whose function appears to be the breakdown and removal of the products of dystrophic degeneration.

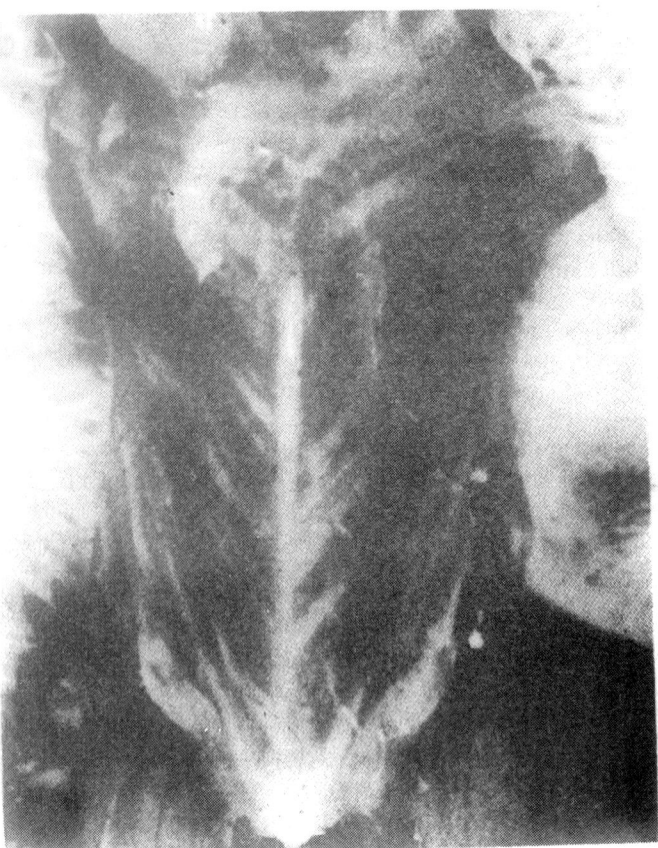

Figure 4.23 Nutritional muscular dystrophy in chicks fed a vitamin E deficient diet low in the sulfur amino acids. The diet contains an antioxidant and 0.1 ppm of selenium to prevent encephalomalacia and exudative diathesis. Note the white degenerated muscle fibers in both the breast and the thigh.

Initial studies involving the effects of dietary vitamin E on muscular dystrophy, (Dam *et al.*, 1952, and Nesheim and Scott, 1958) showed that the addition of 1 to 5 mg of selenium per kg of diet (much higher levels than necessary to prevent exudative diathesis), reduced the incidence of muscular dystrophy in chicks receiving a vitamin E deficient diet that was low in methionine and cystine, but did not completely prevent the disease. However, selenium was completely effective in preventing muscular dystrophy in chicks when the diet contained a low level of vitamin E, which by itself had been shown to have no effect on the disease.

Studies with chickens on the interrelationships between antioxidants, linoleic acid, selenium and sulfur amino acids have resulted in bringing some order to the confusion previously existing about the role of vitamin E in nutrition. It is now apparent that selenium and vitamin E play supportive roles in several processes, one of which is cystine metabolism and its role in the prevention of muscular dystrophy in the chicken. Glutathione peroxidase is soluble and is therefore located in the aqueous portions of the cell, while vitamin E is located mainly in the hydrophobic environments of membranes and in lipid storage cells. The overlapping manner in which vitamin E and selenium function in the cellular antioxidant system would suggest that they spare one another in the prevention of deficiency symptoms.

Dam *et al.* (1952), first reported the effectiveness of cystine in preventing muscular dystrophy in vitamin E deficient chicks. No other sulfur compound, including methionine, has been shown to possess dystrophy-preventing activity equal to that of cystine. Factors which block the conversion of methionine to cysteine interfere with the effectiveness of methionine in alleviating the condition, while compounds like guanidoacetic acid, which acts as a methyl donor and thus aid in the conversion of methionine to cystine, tend to alleviate the problem.

Factors which spare cystine in the body decrease the incidence or severity of dystrophy while the converse is true for compounds which enhance the metabolic requirement of cysteine. Dietary cholic acid, which in the chicken is converted to taurocholate, was shown to increase the rate of conversion of cysteine to taurine, and thus increased the severity of dystrophy. Lipoic acid, which prevents muscular dystrophy when added to a diet deficient in vitamin E and containing a marginal level of sulfur amino acids, has no effect on the condition when added to a diet deficient in sulfur amino acids. This suggests that lipoic acid, like taurocholic acid and taurine, acts by sparring cysteine for the role it plays in the prevention of dystrophy.

Thus, it was assumed that vitamin E and cystine act via two entirely different mechanisms, in their prevention of muscular dystrophy in chicks. However, more recent work has shown that the effect of cystine, in alleviating muscular dystrophy in the chick, is probably due to the role it plays in the glutathione peroxidase system. In the synthesis of glutathione peroxidase, cysteine is required. In vitamin E-selenium deficient animals, glutathione peroxidase demand increase, thus increasing the intracellular demand for cysteine. The protective effects of methionine and cystine are thus assumed to be related to satisfying the increased metabolic demand for cysteine.

Desai, *et al.* (1964) showed significant increases in peroxidation in muscle tissues of chickens with nutritional muscular dystrophy as evidenced by thiobarbituric acid (TBA) index of the unincubated muscle tissues. Activities of the lysosomal enzymes, acid phosphatase, β–glucurondiase, cathepsin, β–galactosidase, and ribonuclease also were increased. The increase in peroxidation and lysosomal enzymes were in direct proportion to the degree of muscular dystrophy measured in the chicks at 4 weeks of age. Studies showed no significant introduction of lysosomal enzymes before the visible symptoms of dystrophy appeared, indicating that the lysosomal enzymes are not the primary cause of the dystrophy. The high lysosomal enzyme activity occurring during the course of the disease apparently is involved mainly in the hydrolytic removal of the degradative products of the tissues. This process, in turn, appeared to facilitate a more rapid regeneration of the muscle tissues in dystrophic chicks during recovery, following addition to the diet of the sulfur amino acids.

The finding that sulfur amino acids are completely effective not only in prevention but also in treatment of nutritional muscular dystrophy under conditions of high peroxidizability of the muscle tissues indicates that the sulfur amino acids play a primary role in prevention of nutritional muscular dystrophy in the chick.

4.12.11 Toxicity of vitamin E

Vitamin E is one of the least toxic of the vitamins where signs are non-specific and most likely related to impairment of absorption or utilization of vitamins A and D_3. Consequently there have been reports of impaired bone calcification with toxic levels of vitamin E. Nockels *et al.* (1976) described a linear decrease in body weight of 5 week old birds as vitamin E content of the diet increased from 0 →64,000 IU/kg. At 4,000 IU/kg there was decreased pigmentation of the beak, shanks and feet, while at 8,000 IU/kg waxy feathers were noted. At the "high" concentrations of vitamin E used today in commercial diets (100-200 IU/kg) there does not seem to be any meaningful impairment to metabolism of other fat soluble vitamins, and even with mild vitamin D_3 deficiency "high" levels of vitamin E do not accentuate the problem (Bartov 1997).

4.13 VITAMIN K

In 1929, Dam, a student of the University of Copenhagen, observed that chicks fed a purified diet, low in lipids, developed subcutaneous and intramuscular hemorrhages, anemia and prolonged blood clotting time. In 1935 Dam, along with several other workers, recognized the existence of a new vitamin, naming it vitamin K, ("Koagulations" vitamin). Schonheyder, (1935), demonstrated that the prolonged blood clotting was not due to a lack of fibrinogen or thrombokinase, or from an accumulation of plasma anticoagulants, but rather a lack of blood thrombin, and in particular prothrombin. At the same time other workers demonstrated the existence of an anti-hemorrhagic factor in alfalfa and that such products were also synthesized by intestinal microbes.

Vitamin K has since been shown to be required for production of four blood proteins involved in blood clotting; these are prothrombin, plasma thromboplastin component, factor VII (proconvertin) and Stuart factor. Thus, a deficiency of vitamin K results in a markedly prolonged blood clotting time such that an affected chicken may bleed to death from a slight bruise or other injury. Even a borderline deficiency of vitamin K is of economic importance in broiler production because under these conditions hemorrhagic areas may occur in the legs or throughout the body which result in a high percentage of condemnations during inspection at the processing plant.

The general term vitamin K is now used to describe a group of quinone compounds that have characteristic anti-hemorrhagic effects. The basic molecule is a naphthoquinone and the various isomers differ in the nature and length of the side chain. Vitamin K extracted from plant material was named phylloquinone or vitamin K_1. Vitamin K from material that had undergone bacterial fermentation were named menaquinones, or vitamin K_2. The simplest form of the vitamin is the synthetic form, menadione or vitamin K_3, which has no side chain. Menaquinone is synthesized in the liver from ingested menadione or changed to a biologically active menaquinone by intestinal microorganisms.

Natural sources of vitamin K are fat soluble, stable to heat, and labile to oxidation, light and irradiation. In contrast to natural sources of vitamin K, some of the synthetic products, such as the salts of menadione, are water soluble. Like all fat soluble vitamins, vitamin K is absorbed in association with dietary fats, and requires the presence of bile salts and pancreatic juice for adequate uptake from the intestinal tract. The chemical structure of the most important natural vitamin K's are shown in Figure 4.24, while relative biological activity is shown in Table 4.18. Table 4.19 lists sources of vitamin K.

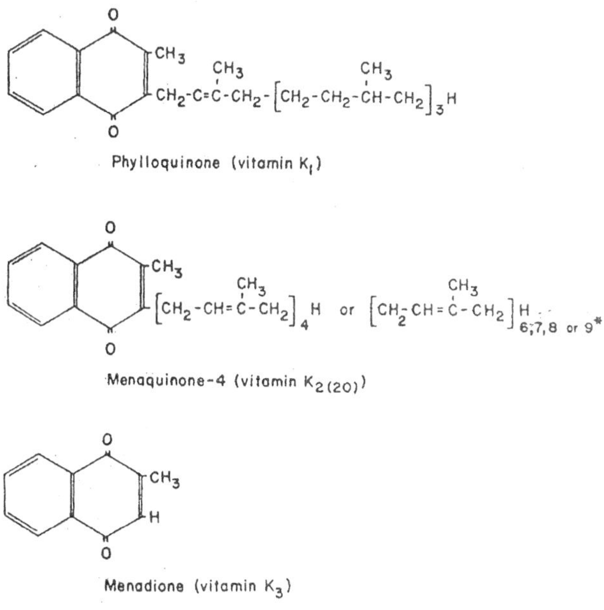

Phylloquinone (vitamin K_1)

Menaquinone-4 (vitamin $K_{2(20)}$)

Menadione (vitamin K_3)

Figure 4.24 Chemical structure of the vitamin K compounds.

Table 4.18 Relative biological activity of the vitamins K by chick bioassay*	
Form of vitamin K	Relative activity** (molar basis)
	%
Phylloquinone series:	
Phylloquinone-1 (vitamin $K_{1(5)}$)***	5
Phylloquinone-2 (vitamin $K_{10(10)}$)	10
Phylloquinone-3 (vitamin $K_{1(15)}$)	30
Phylloquinone-4 (natural vitamin $K_{1(20)}$)	100
Phylloquinone-5 (vitamin $K_{1(25)}$)	80
Phylloquinone-6 (vitamin $K_{1(30)}$)	50
Prenylmenaquinone series:	
Menaquinone-2 (vitamin $K_{2(10)}$)***	15
Menaquinone-3 (vitamin $K_{2(15)}$)	40
Menaquinone-4 (vitamin $K_{2(20)}$)	100
Menaquinone-5 (vitamin $K_{2(25)}$)	120
Menaquinone-6 (vitamin $K_{2(30)}$)	100
Menaquinone-7 (vitamin $K_{2(35)}$)	70
Menadione series:	
Menadione (vitamin K_3)	40-150****
Menadione sodium bisulfite (complex)	50-150****
Menadione dimethylpyrimidinol bisulfite	100-160****

*As reviewed by Griminger (Vitamins and Hormones 24: 605, 1966).
** Activity presented relative to that of pure phylloquinone.
***Number in parentheses after the K_1 or K_2 designates the number of carbons in the isoprene units; each unit has 5 carbon atoms.
****Activities of the synthetic vitamins K depend in part upon relative stabilities of the preparations used and on whether or not sulfaquinoxaline was present in the assay diet. Menadione and its derivatives has been shown to be less effective than phylloquinone in counteracting the antagonistic effects of sulfaquinoxaline.

Table 4.19 Sources of natural vitamins K	
Form of vitamin K	Sources
Phylloquinone (vitamin $K_{1(20)}$)	Green plants
Menaquinone-4 (vitamin $K_{2(20)}$)	Animal tissues, functional form
Menaquinone-6 (vitmain $K_{2(30)}$*)	Putrefying fish meal (small amount) - bacterial origin
Menaquinone-7 (vitamin $K_{2(35)}$*	Putrefying fish meal - Bacillus brevis, Mycobacterium tuberculosis, Bacillus subutilis, Lactobacillus casei
Menaquinone-8 (vitamin $K_{2(40)}$)	Sarcina lutea, Escherichia coli, Proteus vulgaris, Chromatium vinosum
Menaquinone-9 (vitamin $K_{2(45)}$)	Pseudomonas pyocyanea, Corynebacterium diphtheriae, Mycobacterium tuberculosis

*Isler et al (Helv. Chim. Acta 41:786, 1958) have shown that vitamin K_2 isolated by Doisy, instead of possessing 6-isoprenoid units, had 7.
The mother liquor from which K_2 was isolated contained a small amount of the vitamin with 6-isoprenoid units = $K_{2(30)}$*.

All biologically active vitamins K possess a 2-methyl-1,4-naphthoquinone nucleus. Phylloquinone has a phytyl side chain composed of four isoprene units, the first of which contains a double bond. This form is designated phylloquinone or vitamin K. Other natural forms of the vitamin contain side chains of varying numbers of isoprene units, with one double bond in each unit. Biologically active, synthetic vitamin K has been produced, usually containing no side chain. Synthesis of phylloquinone was achieved in 1939. However, synthetic phylloquinone and menaquinones are too expensive to be used commercially. The relative biological activities of vitamin K as determined by chick bioassay are presented in Table 4.18. Natural phylloquinone and menaquinones-4, -5 and -6 possess approximately equivalent biological activity.

Both phylloquinone and menadione are quite unstable during prolonged storage, and menadione is a lung irritant. Water soluble derivatives are menadione sodium bisulfate (MSB) and menadione sodium bisulfite complex(MSBC) which has an excess of sulfite, and further improves stability. Another common menadione salt is menadione dimethyl pyrimidinol bisulfite (MPB). The sodium bisulfite salt contains 52% menadione, while the complex contains 33% menadione. The activity of menadione salts and other compounds cannot be calculated simply from their menadione content, since the size and structure of side chains seems to influence biological activity. MSBC seems to have the same activity as does menadione, even though the former is only 33% menadione. Likewise MPB is claimed to have twice the activity of menadione, on a weight basis. MSBC is highly soluble in water, while MPB is much less soluble.

4.13.1 Sources of vitamin K

There are two major natural sources of vitamin K. Phylloquinone (vitamin K_1) is present in plant food sources, particularly green leafy vegetables. The menaquinones (vitamins K_2) are produced by the bacterial flora in animals, and are especially important in providing the vitamin K requirements of man and most other mammals. However, the chick does not receive sufficient vitamin K from intestinal microbial synthesis. Biologically active synthetic vitamin K is produced commercially on a large scale. These represent the major forms of supplementary vitamin K used in poultry feeds. Sources of natural vitamins K are listed in Table 4.19. Most forms of vitamin K apparently are converted in the liver to menaquinone.

4.13.2 Absorption of vitamin K

Phylloquinone, the menaquinones and menadione require the presence of some dietary fat and bile salts for optimum absorption from the intestinal tract. Feeding a bile acid sequestrant, reduces the absorption of vitamin K in chicks, suggesting that the formation of lipid bile salt micelles is needed for optimum absorption. Menadione bisulfites and phosphates are relatively water-soluble and therefore presumably are absorbed satisfactorily from low fat diets.

Wostman and Knight (1965) found no antagonism of vitamin A on absorption of vitamin K in germ-free rats at the usual "requirement" levels of the vitamins. But when dietary vitamin A was increased to ten times the requirement, an antagonism was apparent.

The vitamin K of animal tissues is menaquinone-4 and when either a menaquinone or a phylloquinone are given to animals the side chain is removed, probably by the microrganisms in the gut, and a new side chain attached to the nucleus by the animal, thus forming menaquinone-4, the form found in the liver. However, Griminger and Brubacher (1966) showed that a major portion of the phylloquinone which they fed to chicks was absorbed and deposited in the liver intact, and that as such it had equally as good biological activity upon prothrombin synthesis as the menaquinone-4 which they found in the chick's liver following feeding of menadione. It appears likely, therefore, that menaquinone-4 is produced only if menadione is fed, or if the intestinal microorganisms degrade the dietary K_1 or K_2 to menadione. The formation of menaquinone-4 is not obligatory for metabolic activity, since phylloquinone is equally active in bringing about synthesis of the K-dependent blood clotting proteins.

The efficiency of vitamin K absorption is variable depending on the form in which the vitamin is administered. There are reports indicating that menadione is completely absorbed while phylloquinone absorption is only 50%. Further work has indicated that while menadione is well absorbed it is poorly retained while the opposite is true of phylloquinone.

4.13.3 Metabolic functions of vitamin K

A vitamin K deficiency results in increased blood coagulation time, because the vitamin is required for the synthesis of (factor II) prothrombin. Prothrombin is subsequently converted to thrombin, which in turn, activates conversion of fibrinogen to fibrin to form the actual blood clot. Other important plasma clotting factors (VII, proconvertin; IX, Christmas; and X, Stuart-Power also depend on vitamin K for their synthesis. These blood clotting proteins are synthesized in the liver in inactive precursor forms, and then converted to biologically active proteins by action with vitamin K (Suttie,1980). With a deficiency, vitamin K administration brings about a return to normal levels of the above coagulation factors in 5 to 7 hours. During the active conversion of the above inactive precursor proteins, carboxylation of glutamic acid residues takes place, involving the vitamin K dependent carboxylase enzyme systems, resulting in γ-carboxyglutamic acid being formed in the protein molecules. The presence of γ-carboxyglutamic acid confers calcium binding properties to blood clotting proteins, which allows them to function in protein-Ca^{++}—phospholipid interactions, necessary for the activation of certain enzymes.

There are a number of other body functions involving vitamin K other than blood coagulation, such as bone mineralization, skin metabolism, etc. While it is appar ent these functions involve a number of proteins, many of the metabolic pathways have not been identified.

The blood clotting mechanism can apparently be stimulated by intrinsic as well as extrinsic systems. All the factors necessary for coagulation are present in the plasma for the intrinsic system. In the extrinsic system, injury to the skin or other body tissues frees thromboplastin which in the presence of various factors and calcium changes prothrombin to thrombin in the blood. Thrombin facilitates the conversion of soluble fibrinogen into insoluble fibrin, which in turn polymerizes into strands and eventually the blood clot is formed, (Griminger, 1984a). The final active component in both the intrinsic and extrinsic systems appears to activate the Stuart factor, leading to activation of prothrombin. The various steps involved in blood clotting are shown in Figure 4.25. The action of vitamin K is indicated at four different sites in the above reactions, however, the most critical need for vitamin K is in the synthesis of prothrombin in the liver. Determination of the rate of conversion of prothrombin to thrombin in the presence of added thromboplastin is the best assay of the vitamin K status of an animal. It is now recognized that vitamin K deficient animals synthesize vitamin K dependent proteins but in an inactive form. Vitamin K is needed to convert these inactive protein precursors to biologically active compounds.

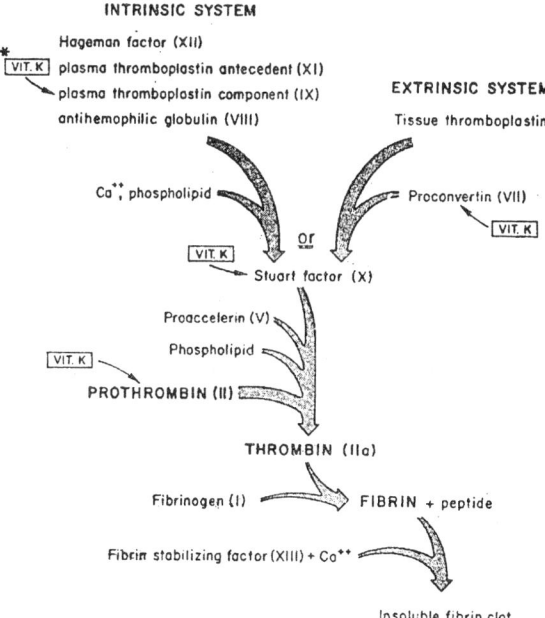

Figure 4.25 Reactions involved in blood clotting.

4.13.4 Signs of vitamin K deficiency

Impairment of blood coagulation is the major clinical sign of vitamin K deficiency in all animals. With a severe deficiency, subcutaneous and internal hemorrhages may be noted which can prove fatal. A vitamin K deficiency results in a reduction in prothrombin content of the blood, and in the young chick, plasma levels may be as low as 2% of what is considered a normal level. Since the prothrombin content of newly hatched chicks is only about 40% that of adult birds, the young chick is readily affected by a vitamin K deficient diet. A carryover of vitamin K from the dam to eggs, and subsequent hatched chick has been demonstrated, and so breeder diets should be well fortified with the vitamin.

Griminger and Brubacher (1966) found four times as much vitamin K in eggs of hens fed phylloquinone as in eggs of hens fed an equivalent level of menadione. The maximum amount of phylloquinone found was 25 µg per yolk. When menadione was fed, menaquinone-4 was found in the egg; when phylloquinone was fed, phylloquinone was the only form present in the egg. Vitamin K carryover, which is notably poor, may be of great importance, since Kohane, *et al.* (1960) reported a hemorrhagic syndrome in day-old chicks which they attributed to a deficiency of vitamin K in the diet of the parents.

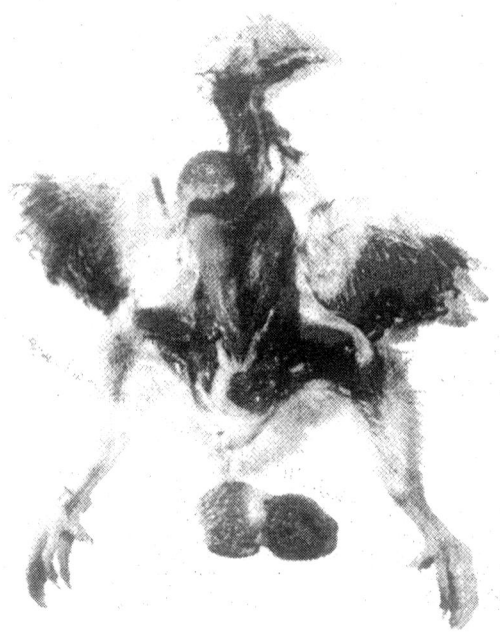

Figure 4.26 Generalized hemorrhage due to severe vitamin K deficiency in a young chick.

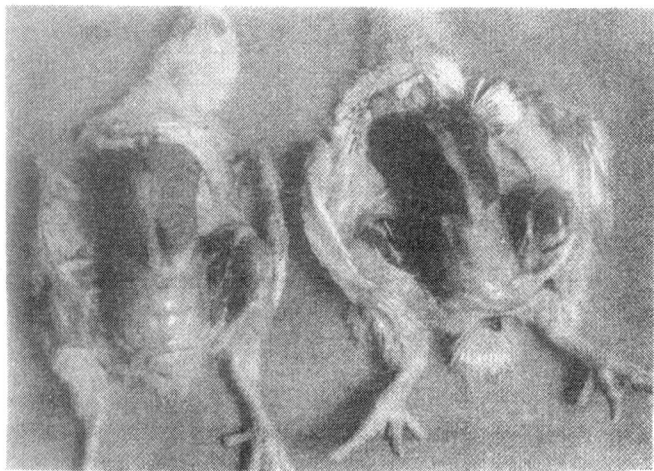

Figure 4.27 Bird on left shows muscle hemmorhage as a result of feeding a diet devoid of supplemental vitamin K.

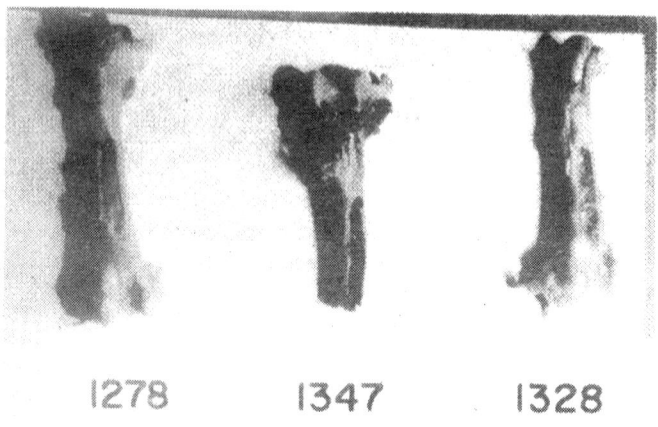

1278   1347   1328

Figure 4.28 Hypoplastic bone marrow (1278, 1328) from vitamin K deficient chicks as compared with the normal bone marrow from a vitamin K-fed chick (1347).

Gross deficiency of vitamin K results in such a prolonged blood clotting time that severely deficient chicks may bleed to death from a slight bruise or other injury (Figure 4.26). Borderline deficiencies often cause small hemorrhagic blemishes. Hemorrhages may appear on the breast, legs, wings, in the abdominal cavity and on the surface of the intestine (Figure 4.27). Chicks show an anemia which in part may be due to loss of blood but also to the development of a hypoplastic bone marrow (Figure 4.28). Although blood clotting time is a fairly good measure of vitamin K deficiency, a more accurate measure is obtained by determining the "prothrombin time". Prothrombin times in severely deficient chicks may be extended from a normal of 17-20 seconds to 5-6 minutes or longer. There are no major heart lesions seen in vitamin K deficient chicks, as occurs more commonly in pigs.

A number of conditions can influence the possibility of a vitamin K deficiency appearing in poultry. These include, low dietary levels of the vitamin, low levels in the maternal diet, degree of intestinal synthesis, extent of coprophagy, presence of sulfur drugs and other feed additives in the diet, and the presence of disease. Chicks suffering from coccidiosis can have severe damage to their intestinal wall, and besides absorption being depressed, the chicks could bleed excessively. Antimicrobial agents can suppress intestinal synthesis of vitamin K and thus the bird may be completely dependent on the diet for its total supply of the vitamin.

In poultry, there is little intestinal synthesis due to the short digestive tract of the bird. For the young chick, the large intestine or colon, which is the major site of bacterial synthesis, makes up only around 6% of the total intestinal tract and for the adult only 7%, (Griminger, 1984b). Similar comparisons would be 13% for the dog and 28% for the rabbit. Also for poultry, the synthesis takes place at the distal end of the intestinal tract, thus allowing for very little absorption. Rate of food passage through the digestive tract may also be a factor. After a meal, it takes about 3 hours for food passage through the tract of a bird while for the pig a similar figure would be 18 hours, (Griminger 1984b). Synthesis of vitamin K does, however, occur in bacteria resident in the bird's digestive tract. Such vitamin K remains inside the bacterial cell, rather than being an excretory product, and so the only benefit to the bird arises from bacterial cell digestion or coprophagy. Berdanier and Griminger (1968) showed quite inefficient uptake of MSBC given anally to vitamin K deficient chicks.

4.13.5   Antivitamins, inhibitors and metabolic interrelationships

The antivitamin effects of sulfa drugs is well established, as is the effect of dicumarol. Dicumarol is used as an anticoagulant in human medicine, for those people with cardiovascular problems in order to avoid intravascular blood clots. It has been reported that vitamin K_1 is competitive with dicoumarol, while menadione, even at high dosages, was not. Vitamin K_1 has been shown to be effective in overcoming the inhibitory effect of warfarin, a common anticoagulant rodenticide, on blood clotting. The structures of several antivitamins are shown in Fig. 4.29.

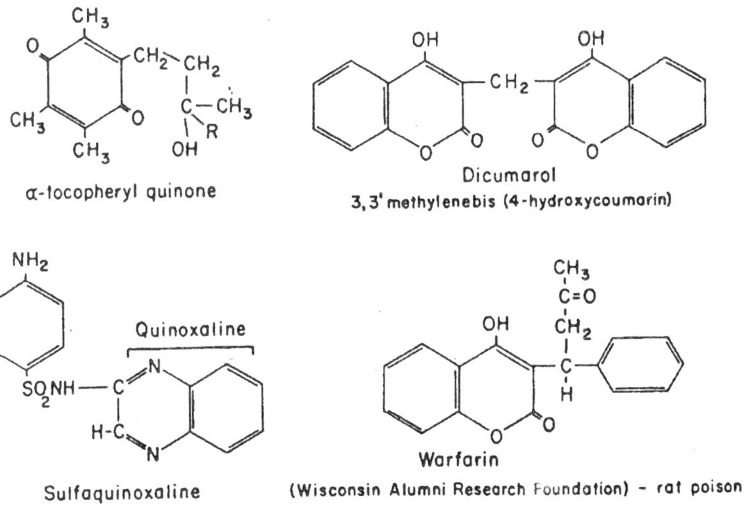

Figure 4.29 Antivitamin K compounds.

4.13.6 Vitamin K requirements

When birds are fed a practical diet without any stress agents, the minimum requirement can be met with as little as 0.6 mg of vitamin K/kg of diet. However, if coccidiosis is a problem or other factors are present that can result in reduced intestinal synthesis, or absorption, much higher levels are recommended. With simplified diets, containing solvent extracted soybean meal, and little vegetable oil, and usually just a single cereal grain, vitamin K supplementation is necessary in order to achieve optimum performance and reduced flock mortality. Most diets contain supplements of 2-4 mg vitamin K/kg diet.

4.13.7 Vitamin K toxicity

Vitamin K toxicity is quite rare, because it takes some 1,000 x normal diet levels (Table 4.9) to cause problems. Signs of toxicity are hemolytic anemia and liver toxicity, likely due to the quinone moiety.

4.14 THIAMIN (VITAMIN B₁)

T hiamin is considered to be the oldest known vitamin with the deficiency disease
beriberi having been recognized in China in 2600 B.C. Eijkman (1897) working in a hospital in Java, noted that chickens suffering from polyneuritis showed
symptoms similar to beriberi in humans, when fed a diet of polished rice. He noted
the condition did not occur if brown rice or rice polishings were fed. Jansen and
Donath, (1926) who were successors to Eijkman and coworkers in the Indonesian
laboratory, succeeded in crystallizing the vitamin in pure form. The structure of
thiamin was established by Williams and Cline (1936) and it's synthesis achieved
by the same laboratory (Cline *et al*, 1937). Lohmann and Schuster discovered
the diphosphate ester of vitamin B₁, cocarboxylase, which decarboxylates pyruvic acid, forming acetaldehyde and carbon dioxide. The structure of thiamin, its
cleavage products and its oxidation product (thiochrome), as well as the structure
of thiamin pyrophosphate (cocarboxylase) are shown in Figure 4.30. The structures of three anti-thiamin compounds (pyrithiamin, oxythiamin and amprolium)
are presented in Figure 4.31.

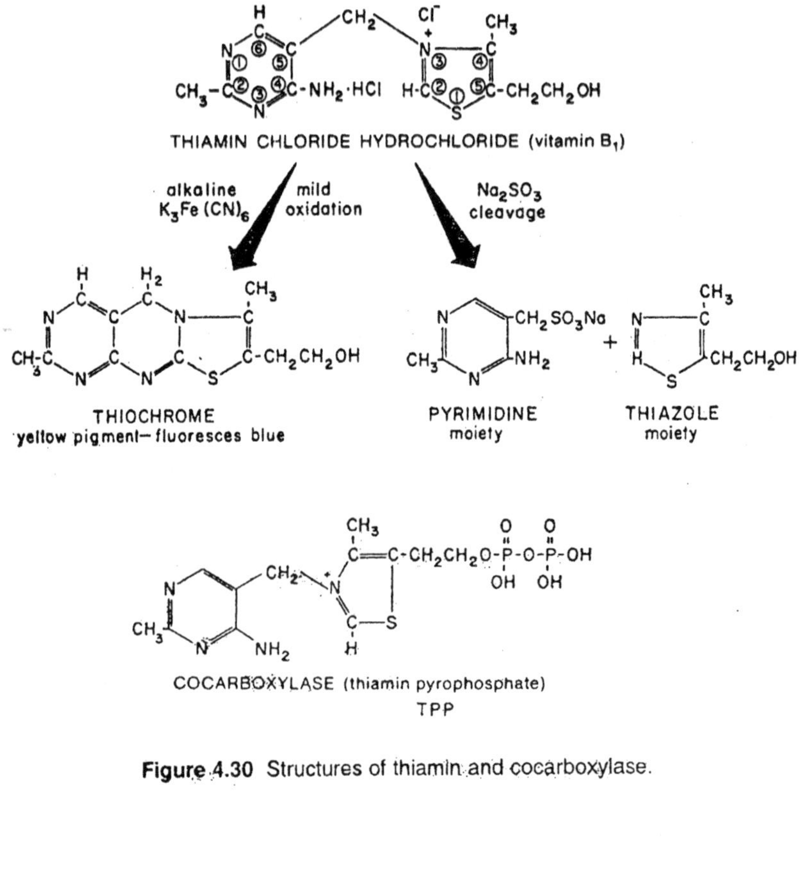

Figure 4.30 Structures of thiamin and cocarboxylase.

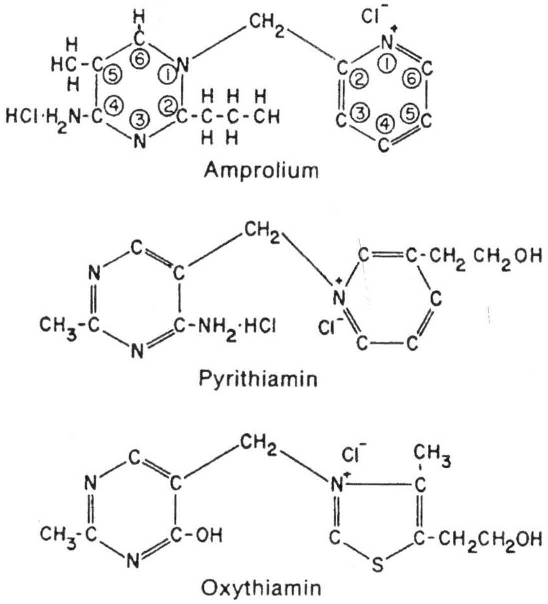

Amprolium

Pyrithiamin

Oxythiamin

Figure 4.31 Structures of some antithiamin compounds.

4.14.1 Properties of thiamin

As indicated in Figure 4.30, vitamin B_1 is isolated in pure form as thiamin hydrochloride. It crystallizes as white, monoclinic plates in rosette-like clusters. It has a characteristic odor and taste. It is very soluble in water, fairly soluble in glycerol, and 95% ethanol. It is insoluble in fats or fat solvents. In ordinary atmosphere, thiamin hydrochloride takes up moisture, forming a hydrate. The pure material, therefore, should be kept sealed or it will gain weight. When pure thiamin hydrochloride is needed for standard solutions is should be dried. It is stable to 100° C for 24 hours. It can be sterilized at 120° C in aqueous solution unless the pH is above 5.5, whereupon it is destroyed rapidly. Analytical analysis for thiamin is conducted by oxidation to thiochrome, which shows a characteristic blue fluorescence in ultraviolet light. One International Unit of vitamin B_1 activity is equivalent to about 3 µg of crystalline thiamin hydrochloride (one gram of thiamin hydrochloride=333,000 I.U.)

The cereal grains and their byproducts, soybean meal, cottonseed meal, peanut meal, and alfalfa meal are all relatively rich sources of thiamin. Thus, under ideal conditions, practical poultry rations contain adequate thiamin without the addition of special high thiamin feed supplements. The thiamin content of feedstuffs is shown in Table 4.20. Thiamin appears to be readily digested and released from natural sources. Although readily absorbed and transported to the cells through-out the body, it is not stored to any great extent. Excessive doses appear quickly in the urine.

Table 4.20 Thiamin content of feedstuffs (ppm)	
Feedstuff	Thiamin content
Alfalfa meal, dehydrated	3.9
Barley	3.4
Beans	5.0
Corn	3.0
Corn germ meal	10.9
Cottonseed meal, solvent extracted	6.4
Distillers dried solubles	6.8
Eggs, whole	3.4
Fish meal	2.0
Hominy feed	7.2
Meat and bone meal	0.1
Milk, cow's	0.4
Milo	3.9
Oats	5.2
Peanut meal	12.0
Peas	9.0
Rice bran	22.5
Rice, brown	3.2
Sesame meal	10.0
Soybean meal	4.0
Soybeans	11.0
Sunflower seed meal	20.0
Wheat bran	8.0
Wheat	5.5
Wheat middlings	12.0
Whey, dried	8.0
Yeast, dried brewers	95.0

Under certain conditions a thiamin deficiency in a poultry feed may be created. Thiamin is very unstable to heat under neutral and alkaline pH conditions. Tests show that while no destruction occurs in 1% HCl during 7 hours at 100° C, over 90% destruction occurs under the same conditions at pH 7, and 100% destruc-tion in 15 minutes at pH 9. Poultry diets, and especially pelleted diets, should not contain alkaline salts in sufficient quantities to produce an alkaline reaction in the feed. Processing of feedstuffs also may destroy thiamin. Most of the thiamin in meat meal is lost during processing. Since the thiamin of fish is in the water-soluble fractions, fish meal contains little unless the fish solubles fraction is included with the meal. Bisulfite ions are very destructive of thiamin, cleaving the mole-cule into the pyrimidine and thiazole parts. The enzyme thiaminase, capable of destroying thiamin, exists in fish and in other materials, including the heart and spleen of warm-blooded animals. Certain microorganisms have been shown to produce thiaminases and although these may be produced in the intestinal tract, highest concentrations have been found in feces. Thiamin deficiency occurs only when these organisms are present and significant levels of microbial thiaminas-es are recycled via coprophagy.

Oxythiamin is a potent antagonist of thiamin. When this compound is present in the diet, much more thiamin is required to prevent a deficiency. Many natural feedstuffs such as beans and mustard seed contain antithiamin compounds. The coccidiostat, amprolium, acts by interfering with the thiamin metabolism of the oocysts, while at recommended levels it does not interfere with the thiamin metabolism of the chicken. Excess amprolium in the feed and drinking water, however, could cause a thiamin deficiency.

4.14.2 Functions of thiamin

The tricarboxylic acid cycle (TCA) governs the metabolic energy supply in the body. The vitamins niacin, riboflavin, and thiamin play major roles in the function of this cycle and thiamin is the coenzyme for all enzymatic carboxylations of keto acids. Hence, one of its main functions is in the oxidative decarboxylation of pyruvate to acetate, which in turn is combined with coenzyme A to enter the TCA cycle.

Thiamin pyrophosphate is a coenzyme in the transketolase reaction that is part of the oxidative pathway (pentose phosphate cycle) of glucose metabolism, that occurs in the cell cytoplasm of liver, brain, adrenal cortex and kidney. Thiamin also plays a role in the synthesis of ribose, which in turn is needed for nicotinamide adenine dinucleotide phosphate (NADPH) formation, which is essential in the breakdown of carbohydrates to form fatty acids. Some of the metabolic activities involving thiamin are shown in Fig. 4.32.

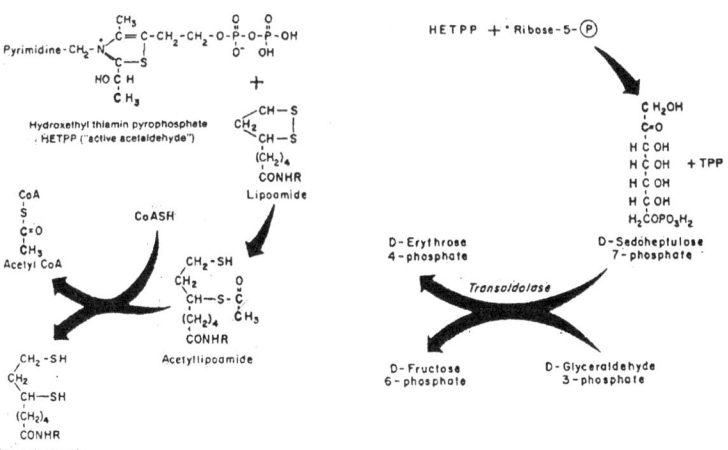

Figure 4.32 Examples of reactions in which α-hydroxyethyl thiamin pyrophosphate ("active aldehyde") participate. Formation of acetyl CoA and of D-sedoheptulose 7-phosphate.

While little is known about the exact function of thiamin in nervous tissues, some of its possible functions have been suggested as follows: (a) involved in the synthesis of acetylcholine which transmits nerve impulses; (b) participates in the passive transport of sodium in certain membranes which is important for transmission of nerve impulses at the membrane of the ganglionic cells, and (c) preventing a reduction in the activity of transketolase in the pentose phosphate pathway (that follows a thiamin deficiency) thus reducing the synthesis of fatty acids and the metabolism of energy in the nervous system.

4.14.3 Requirements of thiamin

Diet composition can have a marked influence on thiamin requirements. Since the vitamin is closely involved in carbohydrate metabolism, high dietary carbohydrate levels, in relation to other energy sources can influence requirement. When a high carbohydrate diet is fed, body reserves can become depleted more rapidly than when a diet contains liberal quantities of protein and fat. Indeed, the thiamin sparing action of fats and proteins have been known for some time.

Thornton and Schutze, (1960), showed that Leghorn birds have a higher thiamin requirement and deposit more thiamin in their eggs, than do heavier breeds. Thiamin requirements are obviously higher if a diet contains anti-thiamin additives. Chicks fed *Fusarium moniliforme*, have been shown to develop polyneuritis, which could be reversed with thiamin injections (Fritz *et al.*, 1973). Feed contaminated with Fusarium has been reported to be quite low in thiamin as compared to non-contaminated feed. Endoparasites which compete with the host for thiamin, also increase the bird's requirement.

While many practical type diets appear to have sufficiently high levels of thiamin to meet requirements, thiamin supplementation is recommended for all practical diets. There is some microbial intestinal synthesis of thiamin. The amount of synthesis depends somewhat on the type of carbohydrate present in the diet, being favored by cooked (dextrinized) starches as compared with glucose or sucrose. This does not provide a dependable thiamin source for the chicken, however, since most of the synthesis apparently occurs too far down the intestinal tract for efficient absorption to occur.

Olkowski and Classen (1996) suggest that even with supplements of 2-4 mg/kg diet, blood thiamin content of young birds declines over time. These workers cite evidence for an involvement of thiamin in heart physiology, and question the chick's thiamin status as it relates to the common occurrence of heart disorders in growing meat birds. In a subsequent study, Olkowski and Classen (1999) showed that thiamin nutrition of the breeder hen has a measurable effect on status of the young chick. Feeding 8 vs 0 mg supplemental thiamin/kg of breeder diet almost doubled the day-old chick's thiamin reserve.

4.14.4 Deficiency symptoms

Polyneuritis in birds represents the later stages of a deficiency of thiamin, probably caused by a build up of the intermediates of carbohydrate metabolism. Since the brain's immediate source of energy results from the degradation of glucose, it is dependent on biochemical reactions involving thiamin. In the initial stages of a deficiency, lethargy and head tremors may be noted. A marked effect on appetite is also noted in birds fed a thiamin deficient diet. Poultry are also susceptible to neuromuscular problems, resulting in impaired digestion, a general weakness, stargazing and frequent convulsions.

In mature birds polyneuritis may be noted approximately 3 weeks after they are fed a thiamin deficient diet. As the deficiency progresses muscle paralysis is noted, beginning with the toes, and progressing to the legs, wings and neck. The bird may sit on its flexed legs, and draw back its head in a star-gazing position. Retraction of the head is due to paralysis of the anterior neck muscles. Soon after this stage, the chicken loses the ability to stand or sit upright and topples to the floor, where it may lie with the head still retracted (Fig 4.33). It has also been reported that the body temperature of a bird will drop with a thiamin deficiency, while respiration rate decreases. Testicular degeneration in males may be noted and the heart may show a slight degree of atrophy.

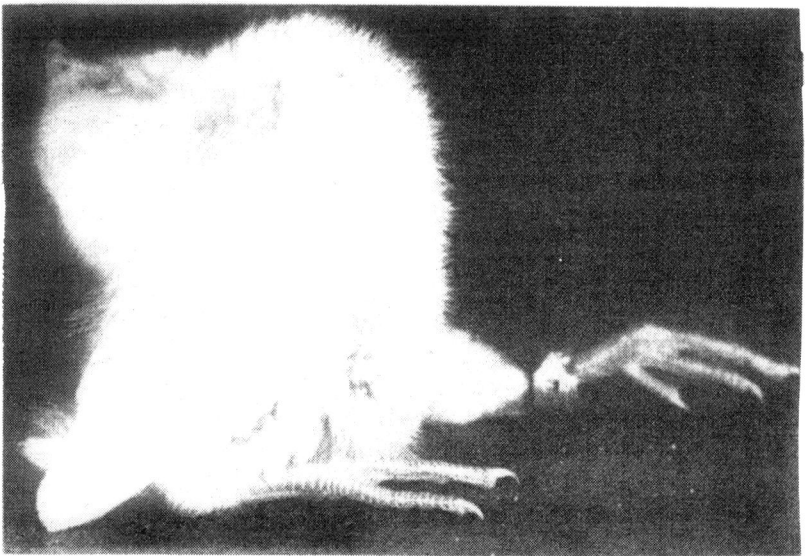

Figure 4.33 Polyneuritis in a thiamin deficient chick. Muscle paralysis causes extended legs and retraction of the head.

Gries and Scott (1972) studied the comparative pathologies of thiamin, riboflavin, pantothenic acid and niacin deficiencies. All four deficiencies caused degeneration of the cells lining the crypts of Lieberkuhn and vacuolations (hyaline bodies) in the pancreatic acinar cells. These four vitamins act as coenzymes required for energy transfer metabolism. Their absence in the highly metabolically active cells of the duodenum and pancreas causes changes which are similar to those of cellular anoxia. Of all nutrients, a deficiency of thiamin has the most marked effect upon appetite. Animals consuming a thiamin deficient diet soon show severe anorexia. They lose all interest in feed and will not resume eating unless given thiamin. If a severe deficiency has developed, the thiamin must be force-fed or injected to induce the chickens to resume eating, even though fresh feed containing thiamin has been placed before them.

4.14.5 Thiamin toxicity

Very high levels of thiamin have been administered without toxicity. Some evidence in humans indicates that doses of 5-10 mg thiamin per kg body weight may have analgesic effects upon the peripheral nervous system. In chickens, it takes some 700 x requirement level in order to induce toxicity (Table 4.9). Signs of toxicity are blockage of nerve transmissions and laboured breathing, with death usually occurring due to respiratory failure.

4.15 RIBOFLAVIN (VITAMIN B$_2$)

With the water-soluble vitamin B complex, the heat stable fraction became known as vitamin B$_2$, differentiating it from the heat-labile anti-beriberi fraction called B$_1$. It soon become apparent that the B$_2$ fraction contained a number of other growth factors, which were eventually recognized as nicotinic acid, pantothenic acid, vitamin B$_{12}$, biotin and folic acid.

In the 1930's researchers isolated what they called the Old Yellow Enzyme, a respiratory enzyme composed of a protein and a pigment, later shown to be flavin mononucleotide (FMN). Thus, riboflavin was found to be a cofactor before it was discovered in free form. The synthesis of riboflavin was accomplished by European workers. Although commonly referred to as vitamin B$_2$, it was also know as vitamin G for some time, as well as names such as ovoflavin, uroflavin, lactoflavin and heptoflavin.

4.15.1 Structure and properties of riboflavin

Riboflavin consists of a substituted isoalloxazine ring with a D-ribityl-side chain attached to the nitrogen in position 9. Its structural formula and some closely related derivatives are shown in Figure 4.34. Structures of the two most important riboflavin-containing coenzymes, FMN and FAD, are shown in Figure 4.35.

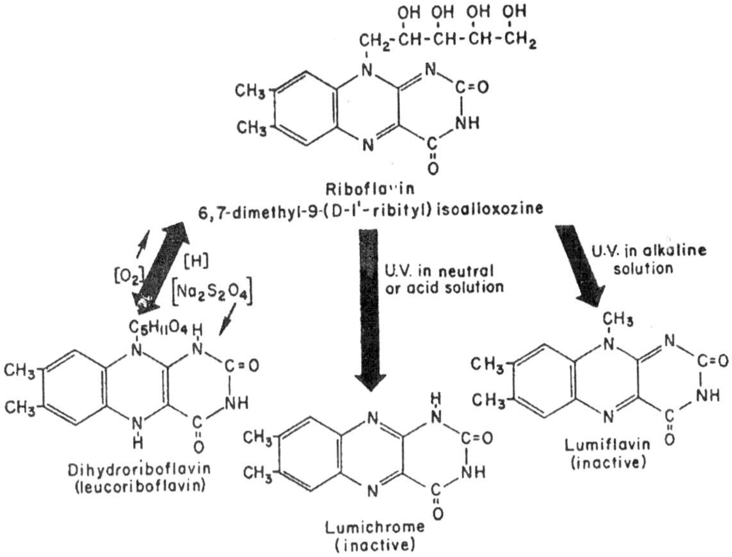

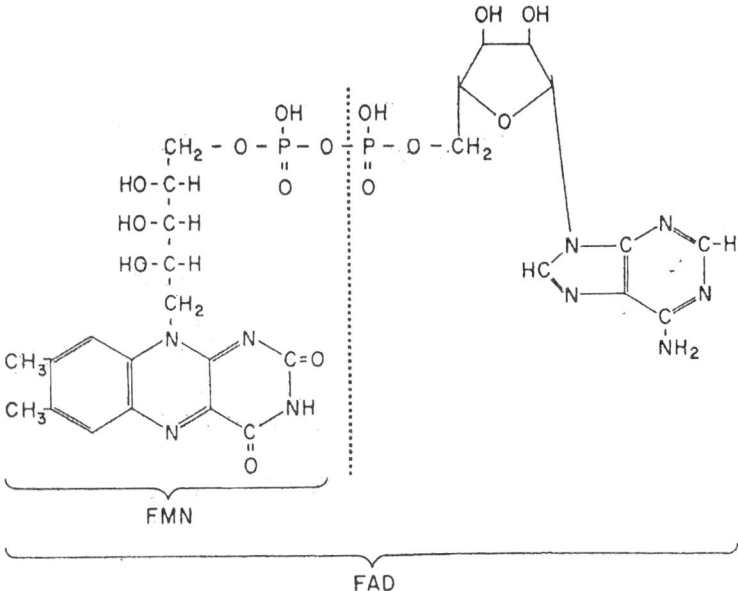

Figure 4.34 Structural formula of riboflavin and some compounds produced by either reduction or the action of ultraviolet light.

Figure 4.35 Flavin mononucleotide, riboflavin, 5'-phosphate (FMN) and flavin adenine dinucleotide (FAD).

Riboflavin is found in three forms, the free dinucleotide, and as flavin mononucleotide (FMN) and flavin adenine dinucleotide (FAD), the two coenzyme derivatives (Figure 4.34). Riboflavin is only slightly soluble in water, but readily soluble in dilute basic or strong acidic solution. It is quite stable to heat in neutral or acid conditions but not alkaline solutions and is quite susceptible to destruction by light, especially under moist conditions.

Riboflavin forms orange-yellow crystals of three types, depending upon solvents and methods of crystallization; it is sparingly soluble in water, less soluble in ethanol and cyclohexane, and insoluble in fat and fat solvents. If heated slowly from 250°C, it decomposes at 280°C. Riboflavin shows absorption maxima at 220-225, 266, 371 and 447μm. It is destroyed by alkalies and by light, but is quite stable in mineral acids in the dark. When dry, it is not affected appreciably by light, but in solution it is quickly destroyed. Riboflavin produces a strong green fluorescence when irradiated with blue or ultraviolet light. Fluorescence maximum is at pH 6 or 7. Visible or ultraviolet irradiation of alkaline solutions converts riboflavin to lumiflavin; irradiation of acid or neutral solutions produces lumichrome with small amounts of lumiflavin (Figure 4.34). Riboflavin is reversibly reduced by sodium hydrosulfite and other reducing agents to the colorless, non-fluorescing form dihydroriboflavin (leucoriboflavin). It may be reoxidized to riboflavin by shaking in air or by addition of a suitable oxidizing agent.

Riboflavin, covalently bound to protein, is degraded in the intestine to its phosphorylated forms (FAD and FMN) which are hydrolyzed by phosphatases to release the vitamin for absorption. It enters the mucosal cells of the small intestine where it is absorbed by an active as well as a passive process, proportional to its concentration. Free riboflavin is phosphorylated in the mucosal cells to FMN, by the enzyme flavokinase (Cooperman and Lopez, 1984). It then enters the portal system where it binds to plasma albumin, and is transported to the liver, where it is converted to FAD.

There is an autosomal recessive disorder in chickens called renal riboflavinuria, in which the riboflavin binding protein is absent. Eggs from such hens become riboflavin deficient resulting in dead embryos around the 14th day of incubation. Riboflavin is not stored to any extent in the body, with intakes in excess of immediate needs rapidly excreted in the urine. Thus, a continuous dietary intake is essential for optimum well being of the bird.

4.15.2 Sources of riboflavin

Riboflavin is synthesized by green plants, yeast, fungi, and autotrophic bacteria. Riboflavin is not synthesized by any animal, but the symbiotic organisms inhabiting the gastrointestinal tract can make an important contribution to the animal's needs. This is especially true in ruminants where the entire requirement is supplied by the rumen microflora as soon as the rumen becomes functional. Many microorganisms synthesize more riboflavin than they need. The production of riboflavin by industrial fermentation with *Clostridium acetobutylicum* from whey, molasses or other fermentable substrates represents an important commercial source of the vitamin, especially for animal needs. It is also produced in large quantities by chemical synthesis.

Since riboflavin is needed for cellular respiration, it is probably present in all plant and animal cells, although few foods contain large quantities. In plants, the site of synthesis of riboflavin is not known, although the greatest concentration is in the leaves. Yeast is the most potent natural source of riboflavin (up to 125 μg/gm); other good sources are liver, milk and eggs. A considerable loss of riboflavin may occur in certain feedstuffs due to exposure to light. The riboflavin of the various feedstuffs is not equally available upon ingestion. For example, drying of yeast and heat-treatment of certain feedstuffs may increase the riboflavin availability.

Gamma irradiation of foods has been found to destroy up to 10% of riboflavin, whereas thiamin under similar conditions may suffer 70-95% decomposition to its thiazole and pyrimidine moieties.

4.15.3 Functions of riboflavin

Riboflavin forms the prosthetic part of over a dozen enzymes in the animal body. Among these are cytochrome reductase, lipoamide dehydrogenase, xanthine oxidase, L- and d-amino acid oxidases, histaminase, and others, all of which are vitally associated with oxidation-reduction reactions involved in cell respiration. Riboflavin is essential for growth and tissue repair in all animals.

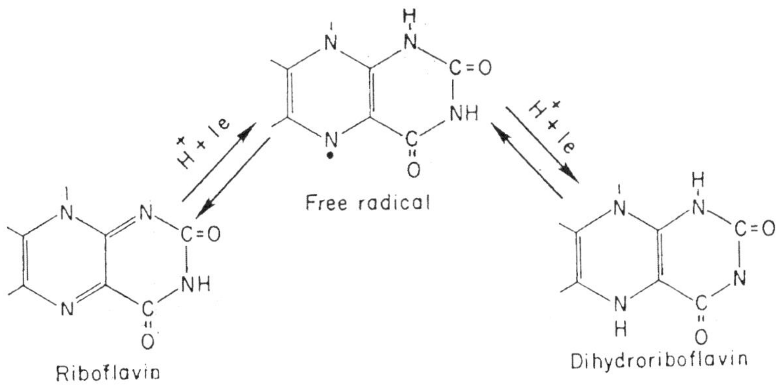

Figure 4.36 Free radical intermediate involved in hydrogen and electron transport.

When FMN and FAD and the flavin protein enzymes are exposed to ordinary intensities of visible light, they readily form free radicals. These light-induced free radicals appear to be identical to those formed during oxidation-reduction processes in the enzyme-catalyzed reactions of metabolism. In hydrogen transfer by flavin coenzymes, the reaction appears to occur by acceptance of one hydrogen atom at a time and in so doing the coenzyme changes as follows: flavin ↔ semiquinone ↔ dihydroflavin. The structural changes in the coenzyme are shown in Figure 4.36.

The main function of FMN and FAD is to transfer hydrogen between the nicotinic acid-containing coenzymes, NAD and NADP, and the iron porphyrin cytochromes. Thus, these enzymes are a part of the chain which carries hydrogen from substrates (carbohydrates, amino acids, lipids, etc.) to molecular oxygen, forming water. These flavoprotein pathways are the most important means of electron transport in both mitochrondria and microsomes.

4.15.4 Specific reactions involving riboflavin-containing enzymes

The riboflavin-containing enzymes may be arbitrarily classified as follows: (1) reduced pyridine nucleotide dehydrogenases; (2) mitochondrial metabolite dehydrogenases – coupled to respiratory chain; and (3) oxidases. Some specific reduced pyridine nucleotide dehydrogenases are shown in Figure 4.37 while mitochondrial dehydrogenases are shown in Figure 4.38. The sequence of electron acceptors in the early stages of the respiratory chain indicates that coenzyme Q (ubiquinone) acts between flavoprotein and cytochrome b. Some common oxidases requiring FAD or FMN are shown in Figure 4.39.

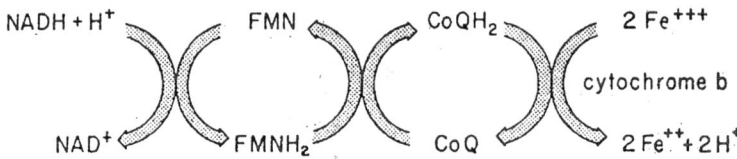

(a) NADH dehydrogenase of mitochondria

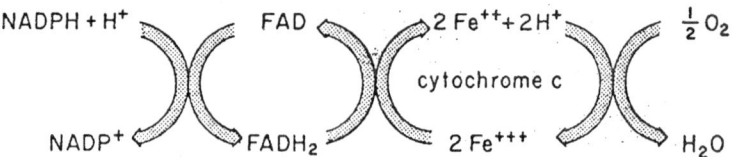

(b) NADPH-cytochrome c reductase of microsomes

Figure 4.37 Specific reduced pyridine nucleotide dehydrogenases requiring FMN or FAD.

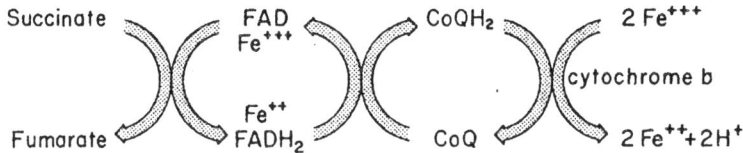

(a) Succinate dehydrogenase

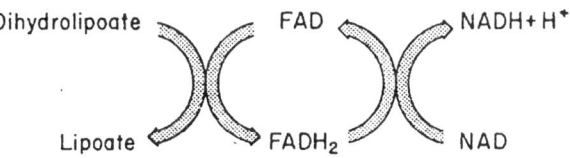

(b) Lipoyl dehydrogenase (Straub's diaphorase)

Figure 4.38 Some mitochondrial dehydrogenases requiring FAD.

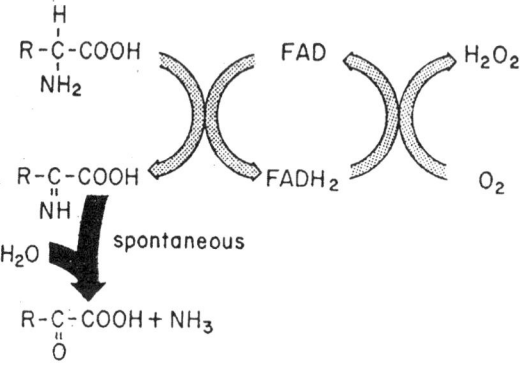

(a) Amino acid oxidase of liver and kidney

(b) Xanthine oxidase of liver
   (also may use other purines as substrates)

Figure 4.39 Important oxidases requiring FMN or FAD.

Seven metalloflavoproteins containing copper, iron or molybdenum have been characterized. Among these are cuproflavoprotein in butyryl-CoA-dehydrogenase; xanthine oxidase – an iron and molybdenum-containing flavoprotein; aldehyde oxidase, a molybdoflavoprotein; and DPNH-cytochrome reductase, containing iron. Anti-riboflavin compounds may result from chemical changes in either the isoalloxazine nucleus or in the ribityl side chain. Some anti-riboflavin compounds are shown in Figure 4.40.

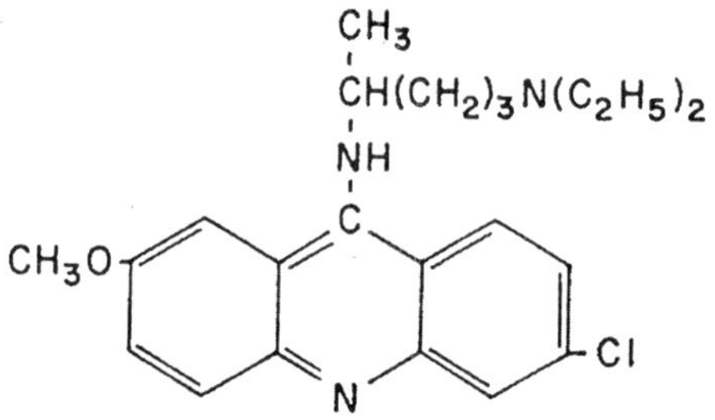

Atabrine (Quinacrine)

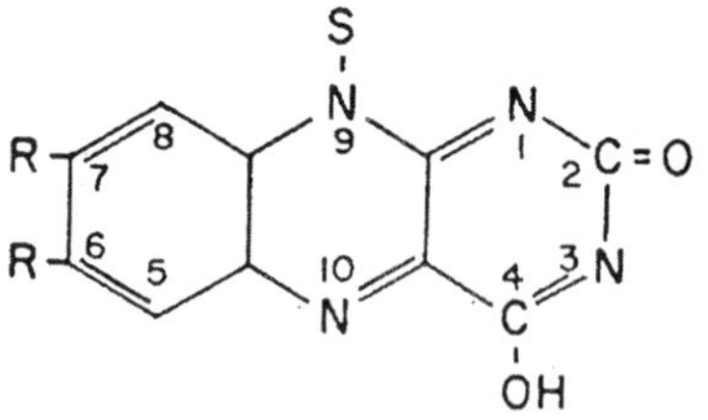

Riboflavin	R = CH$_3$	S = D-ribityl
Diethyl	R = C$_2$H$_5$	S = D-ribityl
Dichloro	R = Cl	S = D-ribityl
Isoriboflavin	CH$_3$ in 5 & 6	S = D-ribityl
D-araboflavin	R = CH$_3$	S = D-arabityl
D-galactoflavin	R = CH$_3$	S = D-dulcityl

Figure 4.40 Anti-riboflavin compounds resulting from changes in either the isoalloxazine nucleus, as in Atabrine, or in the side chains.

4.15.5 Riboflavin requirements and toxicity

Riboflavin requirements are detailed in Table 4.4. NRC (1994) estimates are 3.6 mg/kg for broilers and 2.5 mg/kg for laying hens. Ruiz and Harms (1988) indicate a need for 2.8 mg riboflavin supplement/kg diet in order to promote growth and prevent leg paralysis in broilers. In this study, the corn-soy diet itself contained 2.6 mg riboflavin/kg. Chung and Baker (1990) suggest that around 60% of the riboflavin naturally found in corn and soybean meal is available to the bird. Olkowski and Classen (1998) also indicate a need for around 2 mg/kg diet as supplemental riboflavin for young birds. For laying hens, Squires and Naber (1993) suggest a need for around 4.4 mg/kg diet for optimum egg production and hatchability and that the egg albumin should containing around 2.5µg riboflavin/g. Because of increased urine loss of riboflavin in situations of excess intake, toxic effects are very rare, and it probably requires intakes of around 200x requirement to cause metabolic problems.

4.15.6 Riboflavin deficiency

Many tissues may be affected by riboflavin deficiency. It appears, however, that the two most severely affected tissues are the epithelium and the myelin sheaths

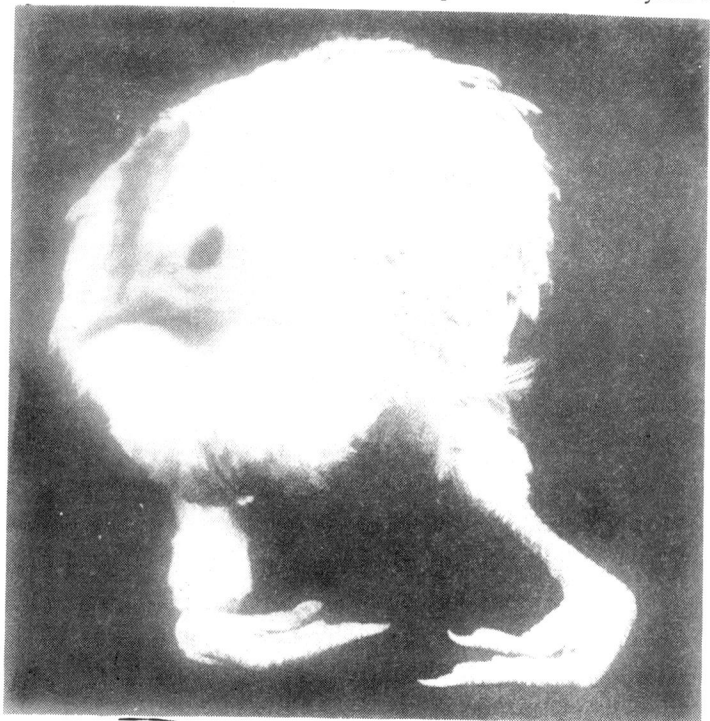

Figure 4.41 Curled toe paralysis in a riboflavin-deficient chick.

of some of the main nerves. Changes in the sciatic nerves produce curled-toe paralysis in growing chickens. Bootwalla and Harms (1990) showed a 10% incidence of curled-toe paralysis for broilers within 21d of receiving a corn-soy diet devoid of supplemental riboflavin. When chicks are fed a diet deficient in riboflavin, their appetite is fairly good but they grow very slowly, become weak and emaciated, and diarrhea occurs between the first and second weeks. Deficient chicks do not move about, except when forced to do so and then frequently walk on their hocks with the aid of their wings. The toes are curled inward (Figure 4.41), both when walking and when resting on their hocks. The leg muscles are atrophied and flabby and the skin is dry and harsh. In advanced stages of deficiency, the chicks lie prostrated with their legs extended, sometimes in opposite directions.

Postmortem examination shows no marked abnormalities of the internal organs. The characteristic sign of riboflavin deficiency is a marked enlargement of the sciatic and brachial nerve sheaths with the sciatic nerves usually showing the most pronounced effects (Figure 4.42). Histological examination of the affected nerves show definite degenerative changes in the myelin sheaths which when severe, pinch the nerve, producing a permanent stimulus which causes the curled-toe paralysis. Dilations of the duodenal crypts of Lieberkühn and vacuolation of the pancreatic acinar cells, though severe, are not specific for riboflavin deficiency, since these pathologic changes occur also in deficiencies of thiamin, niacin or pantothenic acid.

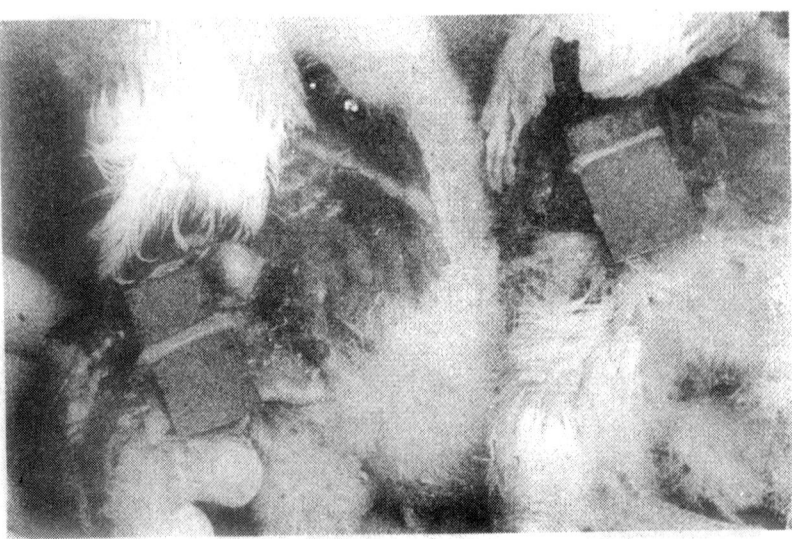

Figure 4.42 Enlarged sciatic nerve in bird fed a diet devoid of supplemental riboflavin.

The signs of riboflavin deficiency in the hen are decreased egg production, increased embryonic mortality and an increase in size and fat content of the liver. Hatchability declines quickly after hens are fed a riboflavin-deficient diet, and can be returned to near normal within 7 days after addition to the diet of adequate amounts of riboflavin. The embryos which fail to hatch from the eggs of hens receiving riboflavin-low diets are dwarfed and show a high incidence of edema, degeneration of the Wolffian bodies, and may show a characteristically defective down, referred to as clubbed down. The nervous system of these embryos shows degenerative changes much like those described in deficient chicks. White (1998) showed that the effects of riboflavin deficiency first appear at 10d of incubation, when embryos become hypoglycemic and accumulate intermediates of fatty acid oxidation. Although flavin-dependent enzymes are depressed with a riboflavin deficiency, the main effect seems to be an impaired fatty acid oxidation, which is obviously a critical function in the developing embryo. There is an autosomal recessive trait which blocks the formation of riboflavin binding protein needed for transport of riboflavin to the egg. While the adults appear normal, their eggs fail to hatch regardless of diet riboflavin content. As eggs become deficient in riboflavin, the egg albumen loses its characteristic yellow tinge, and in fact albumen color score has been used to assess riboflavin status of birds.

Chicks receiving diets only partially deficient in riboflavin may recover spontaneously, indicating that the requirement rapidly decreases with age. A 100 µg injection should be sufficient for treatment of riboflavin deficient chicks, followed by incorporation of an adequate level in the diet. However, when the curled-toe deformity is long standing, irreparable damage has occurred in the sciatic nerve, and the administration of riboflavin no longer cures the curled-toe condition.

4.16 NIACIN (NICOTINIC ACID)

In the early 1900's researchers reported that pellagra in humans was similar in most respects to black tongue in dogs, and suggested that the two diseases were of the same causative origin. Using a diet that consistently produced black tongue in dogs, scientists assayed many foods for their pellagra-preventing properties and discovered that brewer's yeast was a source of a factor that prevented the condition. Daily doses of 15-30 gms of brewer's dried yeast or a water extract of 15 gms of yeast prevented pellagra in humans.

The isolation of nicotinamide from NADP and NAD gave the original clue of the importance of nicotinic acid in metabolism, and quickly thereafter led to the discovery of its role in preventing pellagra. It was subsequently shown that black tongue in dogs could be cured with a single dose of 30 mg of nicotinic acid or nicotinamide.

Niacin had been known to chemists since the mid 1880s, long before it was recognized as an essential nutrient between 1911 and 1913. Funk had isolated it from yeast and rice polishings in the course of trying to identify the water soluble anti-beriberi factor. However, interest was lost in niacin when it was found ineffective in curing beriberi. Funk found that beriberi was cured more rapidly when niacin was administered along with the antiberiberi factor. Warburg and coworkers in 1935 showed that niacin functioned as part of a hydrogen transport system.

Pellagra, meaning rough skin, appeared in Europe in the early 1700s when corn was introduced from America, and became an important foodstuff in southern Europe. Pellagra was first reported in the USA in 1864 and in the early 1900s it was estimated that 20,000 deaths occurred annually. Indeed, even as late as 1941, five years after the cause of pellagra was known, 2,000 people were reported to have died from the disease. Clinical signs were often referred to as the four D's: dermatitis of skin exposed to the sun, dementia, diarrhea and death.

In 1914, Goldberger, a U.S. public health bacteriologist, was assigned the task of identifying the cause of pellagra. While their studies appeared to confirm that the condition was dietary related, the medical profession did not want to believe that the condition was a nutritional problem rather than the popular "germ theory" of disease. Goldberger and his associates injected themselves with biological materials from people suffering from pellagra and demonstrated that the condition was of a non-infectious nature. At about this time an important step was the discovery that dogs, as laboratory animals, would come down with a pellagra-like disease (black tongue). Thus, the dog became important in studies leading to the discovery of a cure for pellagra.

Following the discovery that an extract of liver would cure pellagra, Elvehjam and co-workers (1937) isolated nicotinamide from liver as the factor that would cure black tongue in dogs and pellagra in humans. In 1945, Krehl and co-workers showed that the amino acid tryptophan was effective in the treatment of pellagra. The conversion of tryptophan to niacin explained why diets rich in animal proteins prevented and cured pellagra.

4.16.1 Structure and properties of niacin

Chemically, niacin is the simplest of the vitamins having the chemical formula, CH_5O_2N. The chemical structures of nicotinic acid and nicotinamide, and the coenzymes NAD and NADP are shown in Figure 4.43. Both nicotinic acid and nicotinamide (niacinamide) possess the same vitamin activity, as the free acid is converted to the amide in the body. Nicotinamide functions as a component of the two coenzymes, nicotinamide adenine dinucleotide (NAD) and nicotinamide adenine dinucleotide phosphate (NADP). Both are white, odorless crystalline solids, soluble in water and alcohol, are resistant to heat, air, and alkali and are thus quite stable in feeds.

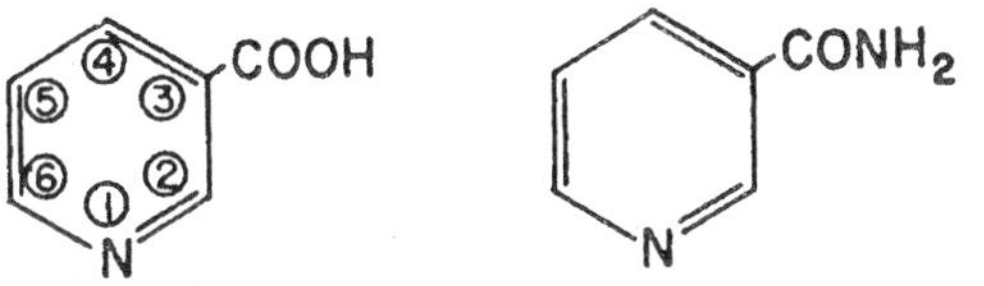

Nicotinic acid (pyridine-3-carboxylic acid) Nicotinamide (3-pyridinecarboxylic acid amide)

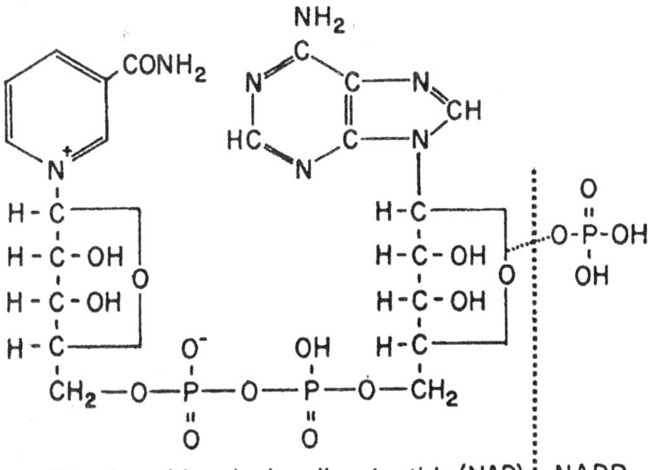

Nicotinamide adenine dinucleotide (NAD) : NADP

Figure 4.43 Structures of nicotinic acid, nicotinamide, nicotinamide adenine dinucleotide (NAD) and nicotinamide adenine dinucleotide phosphate (NADP).

Niacinamide, one of the most common forms of synthetic niacin used in poultry diets, is produced by ammoniation of β-picoline. The resultant β-cyano-pyridine is then hydrolysed to yield niacinamide. Nicotinamide is soluble in ether, but nicotinic acid is not; thus the amide can be separated from nicotinic acid in aqueous solutions by repeated shakings with ether. Nicotinic acid sublimes without decomposition at 236.6°C; nicotinamide melts at 128-131°C. The absorption maximum for nicotinic acid is 236 mμ. Nicotinic acid is stable in boiling acid or base while nicotinamide is converted to nicotinic acid under these conditions.

For biological activity, the pyridine molecule must have a change in the 3-position. Any change at positions 2, 4, 5 or 6 yields an inactive compound with the exception of quinolinic acid which readily decarboxylates to form nicotinic acid (Figure 4.44).

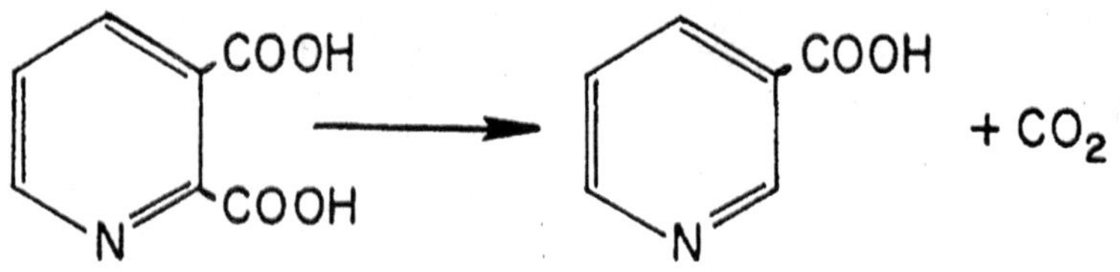

Figure 4.44 Decarboxylation of quinolinic acid to form nicotinic acid.

Nicotinic acid is widely distributed in grains and their byproducts and in protein supplements, although levels are low and much of it is unavailable (Manoukas *et al.*, 1968). Nicotinic acid is the form of the vitamin present in plants while nicotinamide is the metabolic form in animals. Ruiz and Harms (1988) suggest equal biopotency of niacin and niacinamide for young broilers, although Oduho and Baker (1993) conclude that nicotinamide has higher potency (124%) compared to nicotinic acid.

4.16.2 Metabolic functions

Nicotinic acid is the vitamin component in two important enzymes. Prior to the elucidation of their chemical structures, they were referred to as coenzyme I and coenzyme II. For a time they were termed DPN and TPN. They are now known as nicotinamide adenine dinucleotide (NAD) and nicotinamide adenine dinucleotide phosphate (NADP), respectively.

Since nicotinic acid is the form present in plants, and thus the most common form in feed, the body has an efficient mechanism for converting nicotinic acid to NAD, as follows:

a. nicotinic acid + 5-phosphoribosyl-P-P → nicotinic acid mono nucleotide + P-P$_I$

b. nicotinic acid mononucleotide + ATP→ deamido-NAD + P-P$_I$

c. deamido-NAD + glutamine + ATP → NAD + glutamate + P-P$_I$

Nicotinamide goes through the nicotinic acid mononucleotide intermediate. There appears to be no direct conversion of nicotinic acid to nicotinamide in the animal body.

The coenzymes NAD and NADP are involved in carbohydrate, fat and protein metabolism and are especially important in the metabolic reactions which furnish energy to the animal. The general reaction of NAD and NADP in hydrogen and electron transport is shown in Figure 4.45.

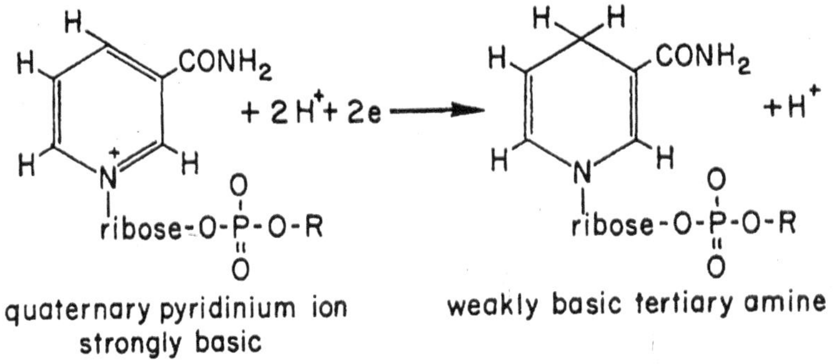

$$NAD^+ + 2\ H^+ + 2e \longrightarrow NADH + H^+$$

Figure 4.45 The function of NAD and NADP in the stereospecific transfer of hydrogen and electrons.

Some of the most important metabolic roles are:

1. Carbohydrate metabolism

 - anaerobic and aerobic oxidation of glucose

 - Krebs cycle

2. Lipid metabolism

 - glycerol synthesis and breakdown

 - fatty acid oxidation and synthesis

 - steroid synthesis

 - oxidation of C_2 units via the Krebs cycle

3. Protein metabolism

 - degradation and synthesis of amino acids

 - oxidation of carbon chains via the Krebs cycle

4. Rhodopsin synthesis (Figure 4.4).

Examples of enzyme reactions of NAD and NADP in dehydrogenases are shown in Figure 4.46. Some of these enzymes show a strict specificity for NAD or for NADP, while others utilize these coenzymes equally well. Some catalytic activities of NAD and NADP which are coupled with oxidation-reduction reactions were shown in Figure 4.37.

I. Dehydration of primary and secondary alcohols

$$R-CH_2OH + NAD^+ \text{ or } NADP^+ \longleftrightarrow R-CHO + NADH + H^+$$

Example: Alcohol dehydrogenase (NAD)

$$\underset{R_1}{\overset{R}{>}}CHOH + NAD^+ \text{ or } NADP^+ \longleftrightarrow \underset{R_1}{\overset{R}{>}}C = O + NADH + H^+$$

Example:
(a) lactate dehydrogenase (NAD) – liver, heart, NAD $>$ NADP
(b) malate dehydrogenase (NAD $>$ NADP)
(c) β-glycerophosphate dehydrogenase (NAD)
(d) isocitrate dehydrogenase (NAD; NADP)
(e) β-hydroxy acyl CoA dehydrogenase (NAD)

II. Oxidative decarboxylation

$$R-\overset{O}{\overset{\|}{C}}-COOH + NAD^+ + CoASH \xrightarrow[\text{TPP}]{\text{lipoic acid}} R-\overset{O}{\overset{\|}{C}}\sim SCoA + NADH + H^+ + CO_2$$

Example: Pyruvic dehydrogenase
α-ketoglutaric dehydrogenase

Figure 4.46 Specific enzyme reactions of NAD and NADP in various types of dehydrogenases.
(The general reactions are indicated as requiring either NAD or NADP; specificities for either NAD or NADP are shown in the specific examples.)

In mammals nicotinic acid is excreted largely as N-methyl nicotinamide, or as the two oxidation products of this compound, the 4-pyridone or 6-pyridone of N-methyl nicotinamide. In the chicken, however, nicotinic acid is conjugated with ornithine as either α- or δ-nicotinyl ornithine or dinicotinyl ornithine as shown in Figure 4.47.

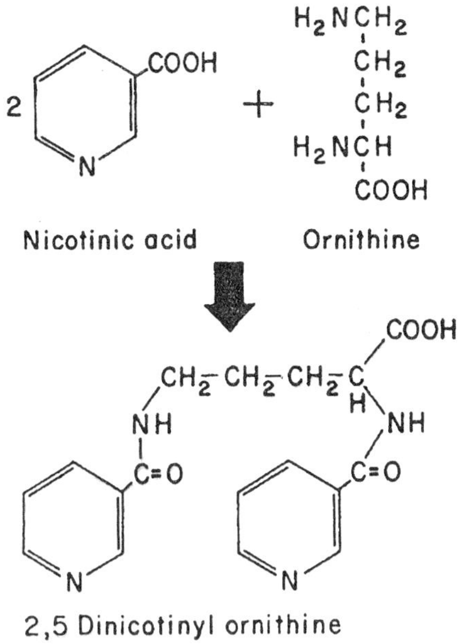

Figure 4.47 Urinary excretion products of nicotinic acid (niacin) metabolism in the chicken. (The 2- and 5-mononicotinyl ornithines are also known to exist.)

4.16.3 Niacin requirements

Two phenomena may cause wide variations in niacin requirements under certain conditions. These are: (1) nicotinic acid is synthesized in the animal body from tryptophan; thus the niacin requirement depends upon the tryptophan content of the diet; (2) much of the nicotinic acid present in many foods and feedstuffs is in a bound form that is not available to birds. It is released by treating the food materials with alkaline solutions, but this rarely happens to poultry diets. Other conditions also may increase or decrease niacin requirements. Some anti-nicotinic acid compounds are shown in Figure 4.48. Other phenomena which may alter niacin requirements are the effects that various diets may have on the nicotinic acid synthesis by the gastrointestinal microflora.

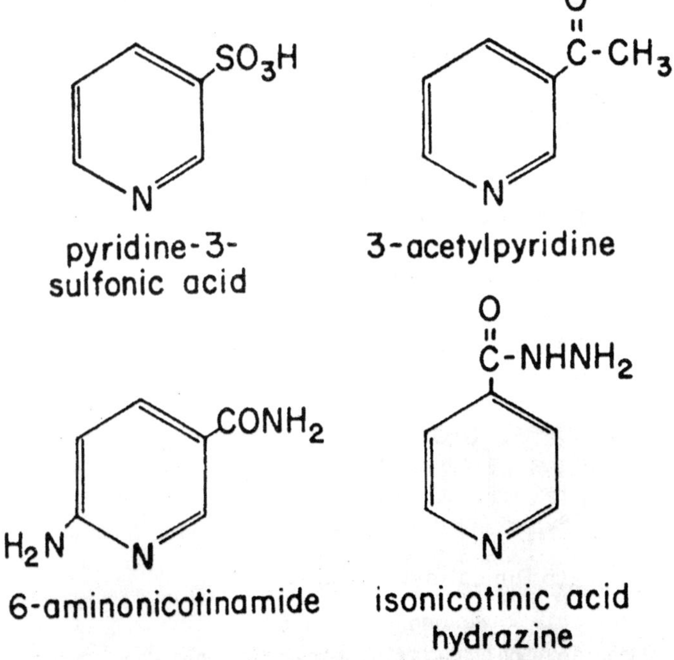

Figure 4.48 Antivitamins of nicotinic acid.

In view of these findings, it is difficult to establish the niacin requirement of the chick unless the tryptophan level is specified and it is known that the diet is adequate in pyridoxine, since this vitamin is needed in the synthesis of nicotinic acid from tryptophan. Because the pyridoxine level is adequate in most practical diets, the niacin requirement is most influenced by the tryptophan content of these diets. Modern poultry diets containing considerable quantities of corn do not contain marked excesses of tryptophan. It is usually necessary, therefore, to supplement these diets with niacin in order to meet the chicken's requirement. Waldroup *et al.* (1985) suggest that broiler chickens may benefit from adding as much as 99 mg/kg niacin to a corn-soy diet already containing 22 mg/kg. Contrary to these results, Ruiz and Harms (1990) suggest no need to add supplemental niacin to corn-soy diets for 3-7 week old birds.

4.16.4 Conversion of tryptophan to nicotinic acid

Because most diets for chickens do not contain large excesses of tryptophan above the level needed for tissue growth, a better understanding is needed of the control mechanisms involved in channeling more or less tryptophan into the synthesis of nicotinic acid. The chemical reactions involved in conversion of tryptophan to nicotinic acid mononucleotide in the animal body are shown in Figure 4.49. The intermediate compounds, some side reactions, and the reactions which require either pyridoxine or riboflavin are shown.

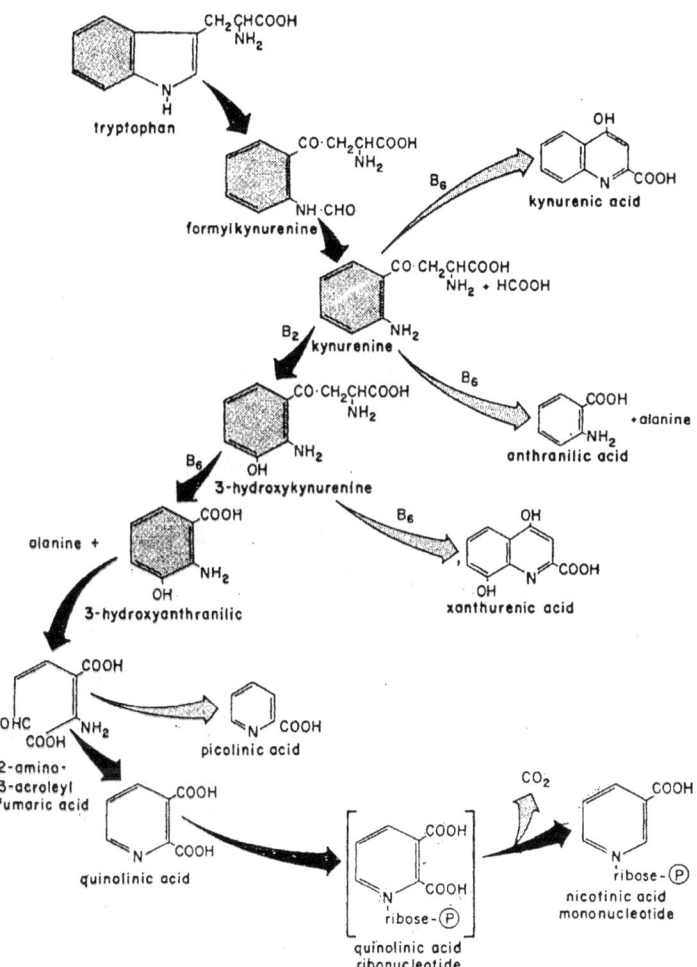

Figure 4.49 Conversion of tryptophan to nicotinic acid plus some known side reactions. Note the reactions which require pyridoxine (vitamin B_6) or riboflavin (vitamin B_2).

It is apparent that pyridoxine is of primary importance in many of the reactions. In animals receiving little or no dietary nicotinic acid, therefore, prevention of niacin deficiency via biosynthesis of the vitamin depends not only on adequate dietary tryptophan but also upon an adequate level of pyridoxine.

Animals differ widely in their ability to synthesize niacin from tryptophan. Studies by DiLorenzo (1972) indicate that this is probably due to inherent differences in liver levels of picolinic carboxylase, the enzyme which diverts one of the intermediates (2-amino, 3-acroleylfumaric acid) toward the glutaryl-CoA pathway instead of allowing this compound to condense to quinolinic acid which is the immediate precursor of nicotinic acid.

The relative distribution of picolinic acid carboxylase in livers of various animal species is shown in Table 4.21. The levels shown bear a very close inverse relationship to experimentally determined niacin requirements: i.e. the cat has so much of this enzyme that it cannot convert any of its dietary tryptophan to niacin. Thus the cat has an absolute requirement for niacin *per se*. Conversely, the rat diverts very little of its dietary tryptophan to carbon dioxide and water, and thus is very efficient in converting tryptophan to niacin. The duck has a very high niacin requirement (approximately twice as high as chickens). DiLorenzo was able to make genetic selection of two strains of chickens, one having a high niacin requirement (40 mg/kg on a low tryptophan diet), the other having a low niacin requirement (20 mg/kg of diet). When the tryptophan content of the diet provided a slight excess of this amino acid over the basic tryptophan requirement, the niacin requirements of the two strains were 15 mg/kg and 5 mg/kg of diet respectively.

Table 4.21 Picolinic acid carboxylase activity	
Species	*Units/g liver (wet basis)*
Cat	30,500
Lizard	29,640
Duck	17,330
Frog	13,720
Turkey	9,230
Cow	8,300
Pig	7,120
Pigeon	6,950
Chicken (high niacin-requiring strain)	5,380
Rabbit	4,270
Mouse	4,260
Guinea pig	3,940
Chicken (low niacin req. strain)	3,200
Man	3,180
Hamster	3,140
Rat	1,570

Data on chickens, turkeys and ducks are from DiLorenzo (1972); all others summarized by Ikeda et al (1965).

In practical nutrition, the sparing effect of tryptophan on niacin requirements is perhaps of limited importance, since tryptophan is rarely provided much in excess of requirements for protein synthesis. Even when tryptophan is available, efficiency of conversion is limited. Oduho and Baker (1993) suggest conversion of tryphophan:niacin to be about 50:1. In waterfowl, the ratio is even greater at around 170:1 (Chen, 1996).

4.16.5 Niacin deficiency and toxicity

A niacin deficiency is characterized by severe metabolic disorders of the skin and digestive organs. The first signs noted are usually loss of appetite, retarded growth, general weakness and diarrhea. While there is good evidence to indicate that poultry, even embryos, are able to synthesize niacin, the rate of synthesis is too slow, especially with modern fast-growing birds.

While there have been reports (Ruiz and Harms, 1990), that broilers do not respond, in terms of growth and feed utilization to niacin supplementation, other reports, (Waldroup *et al.,* 1985), have shown responses under similar conditions. It has been clearly established that the chick does have a requirement for niacin, where a deficiency produces an enlargement of the tibiotarsal joint, a bowing of the legs, poor feathering and dermatitis on the head and feet (Figure 4.50).

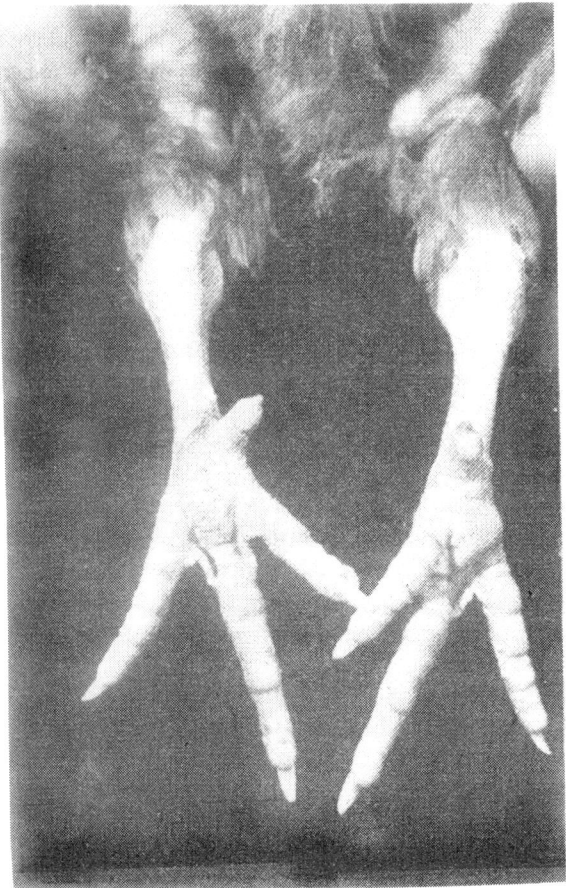

Figure 4.50 Enlarged tibiotarsal joint of a chick fed a niacin deficient diet.

A niacin deficiency in the chick can also result in black tongue. In this condition, at around two weeks of age, the tongue and mouth cavity, as well as the esophagus, can become distinctly inflamed. In the hen, a loss of weight and a reduction in egg production, as well as a marked decrease in hatchability, results from feeding a niacin deficient diet. Turkeys, ducks, pheasants and goslings are much more severely affected with a niacin deficiency than are chickens. It is suggested that their apparent higher requirement is related to their less efficient conversion of tryptophan to niacin. Ducks and turkeys show a severe bowing of the legs and an enlargement of the hock joint with a niacin deficiency. The main difference between the leg condition noted with a niacin deficiency and the perosis condition seen with a manganese and choline deficiency, is that with a niacin deficiency, the Achilles tendon seldom slips from its condyles.

Supplementation of a deficient diet usually brings about a rapid return to normal conditions for most birds, unless the deficiency has progressed to a relatively severe state. While niacin toxicity is quite rare, niacin is used as a vasodilator in humans suffering from conditions of vasoconstriction. Signs of toxicity in humans are a marked flushing of the skin and "tingling" of the extremities. Toxic levels of niacin (100x requirement) cause vasodilation, skin lesions, elevated serum transminases and alkaline phosphatase. Johnson *et al.* (1995) noted a decrease in tibia thickness and bone strength in birds fed 7,500 ppm niacin although growth rate and feed intake were unaffected.

4.17 PYRIDOXINE (B_6)

Vitamin B_6 refers to three compounds, pyridoxol, (pyridoxine), pyridoxal, and pyridoxamine, whose activity is equivalent in animals but not in microorganisms. The vitamin acts as a component of a number of enzyme systems involved in the metabolism of carbohydrates, fats, and especially protein.

Symptoms of pyridoxine deficiency were first described for rats in the 1920's. In studies to produce pellagra in experimental animals, rats fed a vitamin B_2-deficient diet exhibited severe dermatitis (acrodynia) analogous, to human pellagra. The rat pellagra preventative factor was not vitamin B_2 and the term vitamin B_6 was proposed as the name of the new rat acrodynia-preventing factor.

Isolation of the vitamin in crystalline form was reported by several laboratories in 1938, and its chemical synthesis was accomplished in 1939. The structure of the vitamin was first explained by Kuhn and co-workers who named it adermin as it was believed that the only clinical sign of a deficiency was skin dermatitis. However, this name was later discarded when evidence arose indicating that nondermal symptoms were noted with a deficiency of the vitamin. In view of its pyridine structure, the name pyridoxine was proposed, which was widely adopted. However, when later studies with bacteria identified the pyridoxal and pyridoxamine active compounds, official action was taken to use vitamin B_6, as the approved name for the vitamin.

The term vitamin B_6 refers to a complete class of three compounds. Pyridoxine (pyridoxol) refers specifically to the primary alcohol form, pyridoxal to the alde-hyde, and pyridoxamine to the 4-aminomethyl compound.

By 1945, research in numerous laboratories had established that pyridoxine was involved not only in preventing dermatitis, but also in prevention of symptoms of the central nervous system and certain types of anemia. This vitamin was found to be of primary importance in numerous enzyme systems involved in metabolism of animals and microorganisms. Elucidation of the existence of the three forms of vitamin B_6 (pyridoxol, pyridoxal and pyridoxamine) as well as the enzyme forms (pyridoxal phosphate and pyridoxamine phosphate) of the vitamin, resulted from studies with microorganisms.

4.17.1 Discovery of pyridoxal and pyridoxamine

Snell and associates reported the presence in animal tissues of a compound termed pseudopyridoxine which was more potent than pyridoxol in the nutrition of certain lactic acid bacteria. In studying the tyrosine decarboxylation mechanism of bacteria, it was found that more pyridoxine and nicotinic acid were required for decarboxylase production than were needed for maximum growth of these lactic acid bacteria. These workers later showed that pseudopyridoxine, present in acid autoclaved yeast extract or produced from pyridoxine by heating with cystine or with dilute hydrogen peroxide, was very active in providing the necessary cofactor for decarboxylation of tyrosine. Unaltered pyridoxol was found to be inactive for this function. Pyridoxal and pyridoxamine seemed equally effective for the growth of *Streptococcus-lactis R* (approximately 8000-9000 times as potent as pyridoxol); that pyridoxal was 1000-1500 times more potent for the growth of *Lactobacillus casei* than either pyridoxol or pyridoxamine; and that all three pyridoxine derivatives promoted equal growth of the yeast, *Saccharomyces carlsbergensis*. These results demonstrated not only the two important metabolic forms of pyridoxine, but also provided an excellent assay for measuring each of the three forms in natural materials. Soon after the discovery of pyridoxal, pyridoxal phosphate was synthesized and shown to be the coenzyme form.

4.17.2 Structure and properties of B_6

The structures of the three vitamin B_6 forms, as well as the coenzyme pyridoxal phosphate, and several anti-vitamins and excretory products, are shown in Figure 4.51, while the functions of pyridoxal phosphate and pyridoxamine phosphate are shown in Figure 4.52.

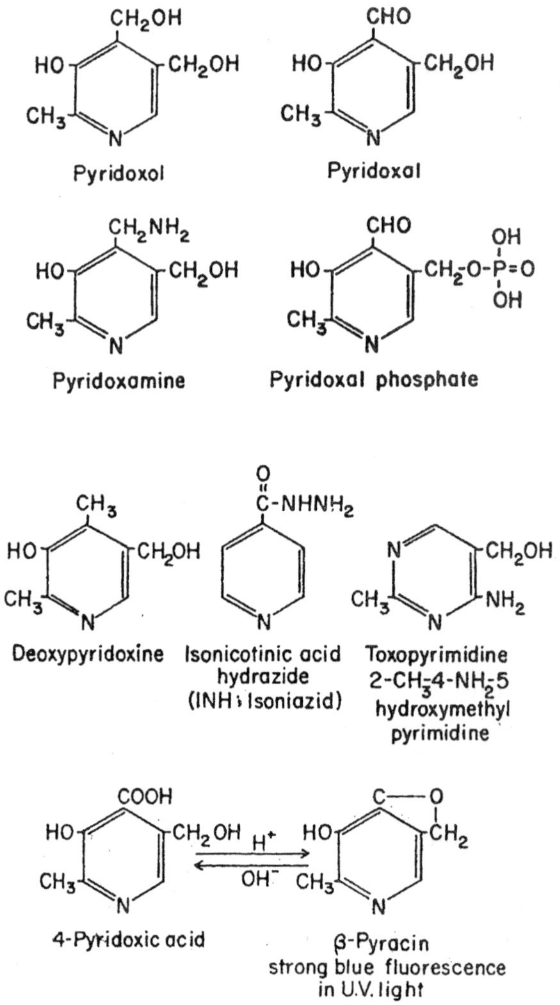

Figure 4.51 Structural formulas of pyridoxol, pyridoxal and pyridoxamine, the coenzyme form pyridoxal phosphate, the excretory product 4-pyridoxic acid and three anti-pyridoxine compounds.

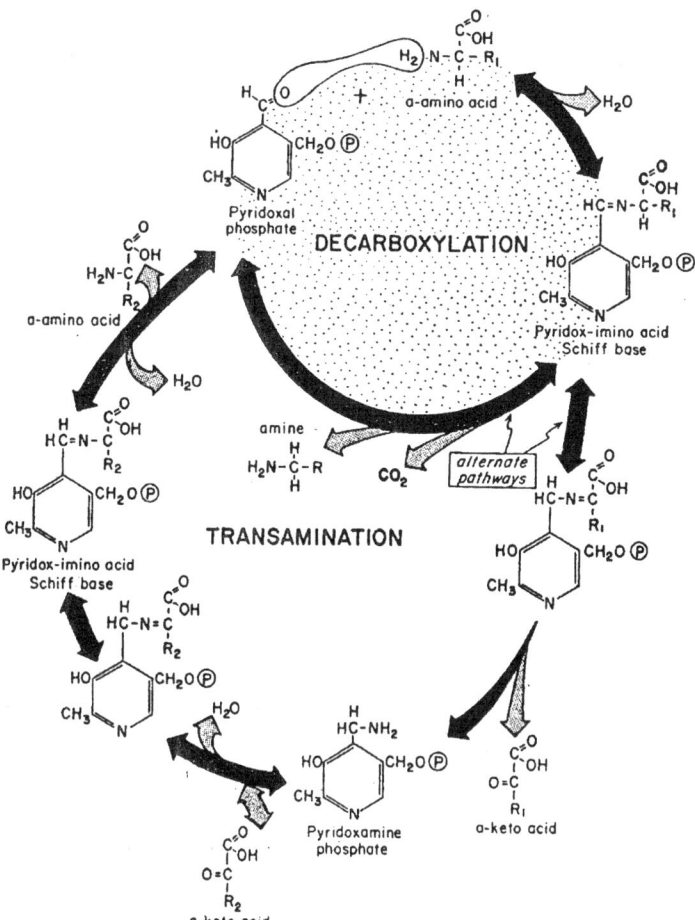

Figure 4.52 The function of pyridoxal phosphate and pyridoxamine phosphate in decarboxylation and transamination of amino acids.

Pyridoxine exists in pure synthetic form as the hydrochloride, which appears as white platelets or birefringent rods from alcohol-acetone solution. It is stable to heat, acids and alkalis but is readily oxidized to pyridoxal in the presence of mild oxidizing conditions. Strong oxidizing agents will readily convert pyridoxal to the biologically inactive compound, 4-pyridoxic acid. Pyridoxol is very soluble in water, ethanol and propylene glycol, sparingly soluble in acetone and insoluble in fats or fat solvents. It shows absorption maxima of 291 mμ at pH 2.1. Pyridoxol melts at 160°C, while the hydrochloride sublimes with decomposition at 205-212°C.

Several vitamin B_6 antagonists exist (Figure 4.51) which either compete for reactive sites of apoenzymes or react with pyridoxal phosphate to form inactive compounds. Presence of B_6 antagonists in flaxseed has been demonstrated.

Digestion of vitamin B_6, first involves splitting off of the vitamin as it is bound to the protein of most foods. Pyridoxine has been shown to be absorbed from all sections of the small intestine, with minimum amounts absorbed in the cecum and crop. All vitamin B_6 compounds are absorbed in the dephosphorylated form, and they are rapidly transported to the liver where they are converted into pyridoxal phosphate, which is the most active form of the vitamin. Both riboflavin and niacin function in the phosphorylation of vitamin B_6. Pyridoxal and pyridoxal phosphate are associated mainly with plasma albumin and red blood cell hemoglobin. Only small amounts of B_6 are stored in the body, and thus a constant supply of the vitamin is required in the diet.

The basic action of pyridoxal phosphate in decarboxylation and transamination is brought about by the reaction of the α-amino group of the amino acid with the aldehyde group in position 4 of pyridoxal phosphate. This reaction takes place because pyridoxal phosphate is capable of forming an imine or a Shiff base whereby the oxygen of the aldehyde group is replaced and the α-amino nitrogen of the amino acid is attached to the aldehyde carbon by a double bond, as shown in Figure 4.52. This reaction is involved in the amination of dl-methionine hydroxyanalogue in the process of its conversion to the essential amino acid, l-methionine. Reactions of amino acids, which are catalyzed by pyridoxal phosphate enzymes, are transamination, decarboxylation, desulfhydrations. However Saroka and Combs (1986) suggest that while pyridoxine deficiency can limit methionine metabolism, the levels found in even unsupplemented corn-soy diets, are adequate for utilization of methionine hydroxy analogue.

Pyridoxine enzymes are also involved in a number of other reactions, which are not necessarily involved with α-amino or α-keto acids. Among these are (a) oxidation of amines such as the conversion of histamine to imidazole acetaldehyde plus ammonia; (b) phosphorylase activity of muscle; (c) amino acid transport. All three known amino acid transport systems, (1) neutral amino acids and histidine, (2) basic amino acids, and (3) proline and hydroxyproline, appear to require pyridoxal phosphate.

4.17.3 Sources of vitamin B_6

Vitamin B_6 occurs in most foods as phosphate protein complexes of the three basic vitamin compounds. The vitamin is widely distributed in muscle, liver, green vegetables and whole grains. Pyridoxine is the predominant form found in plants while pyridoxal and pyridoxamine are found in animal products. The vitamin B_6 in all feedstuffs is influenced by processing and subsequent storage, with losses as high as 70% being reported (Shideler, 1983) although more normally the range is less than 40%.

4.17.4 Requirements for B_6

A minimum of research has been done on investigating the requirements for poultry. Part of the reason for this is that practical diets have usually been considered to have sufficiently high levels of the vitamin. However, there are a number of factors that should be considered when formulating diets for modern strains of poultry. One factor is that today's birds are consuming less feed per unit of product produced and thus, vitamin intake levels are less than a decade or so ago, unless the diet is supplemented. Also some birds, especially turkeys and broilers, are fed higher protein diets, which will increase the need for pyridoxine. There have been reports that there is decreased deposition of vitamins in eggs as birds age (Robel, 1983). It is well known that hatchability also decreases with age of breeder. Thus, with less vitamins being deposited in the egg, and with higher rates of production, serious consideration should be given to vitamin B_6 supplementation of breeder diets. The bioavailability of vitamin B_6 in feedstuffs may not be as high as earlier work has suggested. A range of from 45 to 65% for the availability of the vitamin in corn and soybean meal has been reported. Several reports have indicated that in a premix containing minerals, a significant amount of vitamin B_6 activity can be lost (Verbeeck, 1975; Adams, 1982), while similar losses may be encountered with pelleted and extruded feed (Gadient, 1986). Today, most poultry diets will be supplemented with 3-4 mg pyridoxine/kg.

4.17.5 Deficiency and toxicity of B_6

The diseases common to a vitamin B_6 deficiency are retarded growth, dermatitis, convulsions and anemia. Since a predominate role of the vitamin is in protein metabolism, a deficiency can result in reduced nitrogen retention. Dietary protein is not well utilized and thus nitrogen excretion increases. A deficiency can result in a marked rise in iron and a fall in copper levels in the serum, and iron utilization appears to be markedly decreased. The resulting anemia is believed to be the result of a disturbance in the synthesis of the protoporphyrins. Anemia is often noted with ducks but seldom seen with chickens and turkeys. Blalock and Thaxton (1984) indicated a microcytic, normochromic polycythemia in B_6 deficient chicks. There was an increased number of smaller red blood cells. Classical anemia does not occur, although over time this may develop because of reduced erythrocyte membrane integrity. The young chick may show nervous movements of the legs when walking, and often undergo spasmodic convulsions leading to death. During these convulsions, the chicks may run about aimlessly, flapping their wings and falling with jerking motions. These symptoms can be distinguished from those of encephalomalacia by the greater intensity of activity during the seizure, resulting from the pyridine deficiency, which results in complete exhaustion and death. A marked gizzard erosion has been noted in vitamin B_6 chicks (Daghir and Haddad, 1981). Such gizzard erosion is prevented by inclusion of 1% taurocholic acid to the diet, leading to the speculation that pyridoxine is involved in taurine synthesis, and that this is important for gizzard integrity. With pyridoxine deficiency, Masse *et al.* (1994) showed that collagen maturation was incomplete and so this vitamin is essential for integrity of the connective tissue matrix. A chronic, or borderline deficiency can result in perosis, with one leg usually being crippled and one or both middle toes bent inward at the first joint (Gries and Scott, 1972).

In adult birds, a pyridoxine deficiency results in reduced appetite leading to reduced egg production and a decline in hatchability. A severe deficiency can cause a rapid involution of the ovary, oviduct, comb and wattles, as well as the testes in cockerels. Feed consumption in B_6-deficient hens and cockerels declines sharply but inanition is not responsible for the marked effects of vitamin B_6 deficiency upon sexual development. Although a partial molt is observed in some hens, the molt is not serious and hens returned to normal egg production within two weeks following repletion with a normal dietary level of pyridoxine (Weiss, 1976).

Pyridoxine toxicity causes ataxia, muscle weakness and uncoordination at levels approaching 1000 times requirement. However, more moderate levels of pyridoxine (20-50x requirement) have been shown to adversely affect the metabolism of xenobiotics such as chloramphenicols (Atef *et al.*, 1993). At these same levels, pyridoxine has been shown to reduce the adverse effect of some biogenic amines, such as spermidine.

4.18 PANTOTHENIC ACID

Pantothenic acid deficiency was first described in the chick by Norris and Ringrose (1930). In the course of studying the growth factor then referred to as vitamin B_2, these workers noted the occurrence of a pellagra-like syndrome in chicks which later was shown to be due to a deficiency of pantothenic acid. Studies of pantothenic acid during the 1930s were closely associated with studies of pyridoxine. Both were fractions of the vitamin B_2 complex found together in yeast and liver and both were extracted from these materials with water. Pyridoxine was adsorbed on Fuller's earth from which it could be eluted, and was referred to as the eluate factor, whereas pantothenic acid was not adsorbed on Fuller's earth and was therefore called the filtrate factor. Concentrates of the filtrate factor free of other known vitamins were shown to cure dermatitis in chicks but not in rats. Thus, one of the early names for pantothenic acid was the chick anti-dermatitis factor.

In completely independent studies concerned with the "bios factors" required for growth of yeasts, particularly *Saccharomyces cerevisiae*, scientists concentrated the vitamin in relatively pure solution and determined many of its properties. These workers noted that the compound could be obtained from a variety of plants and tissues and therefore gave it the name pantothenic acid meaning an acid found everywhere. It was soon recognized that the filtrate factor, the anti-dermatitis factor and the unknown factor required by yeast and lactic acid bacteria were identical and were in fact pantothenic acid. At this time it was also discovered that β-alanine could replace pantothenic acid for the growth of some microorganisms. Another cleavage product was an α-hydroxy-γ–lactose. When this lactone was coupled with β-alanine, racemic pantothenic acid was formed. The lactone became known as pantoic lactone and its free acid as pantoic acid.

The metabolically active form of pantothenic acid was discovered and the biochemical function of the vitamin was worked out in 1946-1947 by Lippman and associates, who found that the coenzymes required for the acetylation of sulfon-amide contained 10% pantothenic acid in a bound form. The name coenzyme A was given to this compound to designate that it is a coenzyme of acetylation.

4.18.1 Structure and properties of pantothenic acid

The chemical structure of pantothenic acid is presented in Figure 4.53. The structure of coenzyme A has been discussed previously in Chapter 2 and is shown in Figure 2.21.

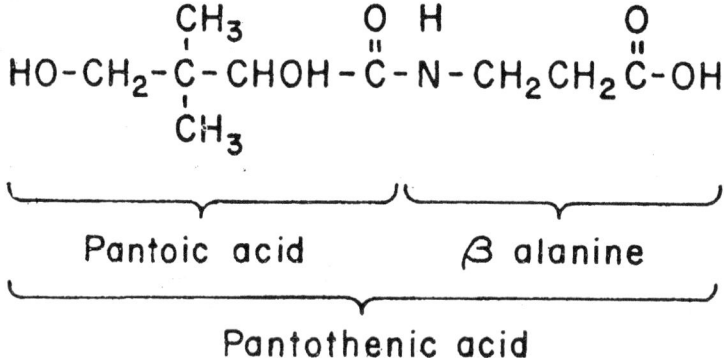

Figure 4.53 Structure of pantothenic acid.

Cleavage of the pantothenic acid or coenzyme A molecules into various moieties is carried out by specific enzymes. Attack by intestinal phosphatase yields panteth-eine (LBF) plus adenosine and phosphoric acid (cleavage by liver enzyme) yields pantothenic acid if pantetheine is the substrate, or 3-phospho-ADP pantothenic acid if coenzyme A is the substrate. Determination of pantothenic acid requires that it be freed from the coenzyme prior to analysis.

Free pantothenic acid is an unstable, highly hygroscopic, viscous oil easily destroyed by acids, bases and heat. It is soluble in water and ethyl acetate, moderately soluble in ether, but insoluble in benzene and chloroform. Calcium pantothenate is the dry form of the vitamin used commercially. It is prepared both as the pure d-form or the racemic dl mixture. Only the d- form is effective as a vitamin, thus the racemic mixture has only half the potency of d- calcium pantothenate.

Pantothenic acid is found in feedstuffs in bound forms, largely as coenzyme A, but the free form can also be present. Pantothenic acid must be freed from the bound forms, in the digestive process, before it can be absorbed. The vitamin is probably absorbed from the digestive tract by diffusion and is converted in the epithelial tissues to coenzyme A and other compounds where the vitamin is a functional group (Sauberlich, 1985). While poultry store little pantothenic acid in the body, most of it is found in red blood cells as coenzyme A.

4.18.2 Sources of pantothenic acid

Values for the pantothenic acid content of feedstuffs which were obtained by microbiological procedures performed before modern methods were devised for liberating the vitamin from its bound form (Coenzyme A), are now known to be much too low. Pantothenic acid is universally distributed in all living cells. The richest known source of pantothenic acid is royal jelly (510 µg/gm dry weight) of bees. Liver, yeast, eggs and green leafy plants are good sources, while seeds contain little pantothenate.

Pantothenate is fairly stable in feedstuffs during long periods of storage. There may be some loss due to heating during processing, especially if held at high temperatures (100-150°C) for long periods of time. Prolonged heat treatment of dietary ingredients was the original procedure for obtaining pantothenate-deficient chick diets. In the usual pelleting process, however, only small amounts are lost.

4.18.3 Metabolic role of pantothenic acid

Pantothenic acid is the prosthetic group of coenzyme A (Figure 2.13) an important coenzyme involved in many reversible acetylation reactions in carbohydrate, fat and amino acid metabolism. The complete enzyme system consists of a specific protein (apoenzyme) combined with the coenzyme moiety. Coenzyme A may act as an acyl acceptor and the acyl group may be passed to other acceptors. It facilitates condensation reactions such as the formation of citrate from oxaloacetate and acetate in the Kreb's Cycle and also acts as a receiver of acetyl radicals formed in the β-oxidation of fatty acids. Acetyl CoA is involved in synthesis of acetylcholine, acetylglucosamine, and in the biosynthesis of steroids. Malonyl CoA is of primary importance in the biosynthesis of fatty acids. Coenzyme A derivatives of fatty acids are involved in synthesis of triglycerides and phospholipids. Pantothenate is intimately involved in fatty acid synthesis and metabolism. Acetyl CoA is converted to Malonyl CoA which reacts with another activated fatty acid, yielding a product that is lengthened by two carbon chains. Consequently fatty acids that contain an even number of carbon atoms predominate in *de novo* synthesized fat. Thus, pantothenic acid through coenzyme A is of fundamental importance in the metabolism of all cells.

Maragondakis *et al.* (1972) found that genetically obese mice fed normal diets had liver acetyl CoA carboxylase activities at least six-fold higher than those of their lean siblings. On fasting and refeeding with a fat-free diet, the lean siblings showed marked increases in liver acetyl CoA carboxylase, which increased to levels equal to those of the obese mice. Using an inhibitor of acetyl CoA carboxylase, it was possible to depress fat synthesis by about 50% in the obese mice, accompanied by a striking reduction in body weight. Goodridge (1972) has shown that the acetyl CoA carboxylase of chicken liver is markedly inhibited by palmitoyl CoA. These data suggest that long chain acyl CoA's may produce a specific feedback which regulates fatty acid synthesis via their effects upon acetyl CoA carboxylase.

4.18.4 Requirements of pantothenic acid and interrelation with other vitamins

Most poultry diets will contain supplements of around 12-14 mg pantothenate/kg. There has been very little work published on requirements for pantothenate in the last 20 years. Bootwalla and Harms (1991) and Harms and Nelson (1992) suggest that SCWL pullets to 6 weeks and broiler chicks to 21d do not require supplementation. In their studies the corn and soybean meal provided about 4.8 mg pantothenate /kg diet, and this seemed adequate to support growth and development.

There seems to be an interrelation between metabolism of panthothenate and vitamin B_{12}. The pantothenate requirement of chicks obtained from B_{12} depleted hens appears greater than that of chicks hatched from normal hens. Liver pantothenate of chicks supplied an adequate amount of vitamin B_{12} is markedly decreased compared with the free pantothenic acid found in the livers of chicks receiving no dietary vitamin B_{12}. The vitamin B_{12} concentration in the livers of chicks receiving no dietary B_{12} was reduced as the pantothenic acid content of the diet was increased. Dietary pantothenate, however, has no effect on the vitamin B_{12} content of livers obtained from chicks receiving adequate amounts of vitamin B_{12}.

4.18.5 Deficiency and toxicity of pantothenic acid

The major lesions seen with a pantothenic acid deficiency in experimental animals involves the nervous system, the adrenal cortex and the skin. A deficiency may result in reduced egg production; however, a marked drop in hatchability is usually noted prior to this event. Embryos from pantothenate deficient hens have been observed to have subcutaneous hemorrhages and severe edema, with most of the mortality showing up during the later part of the incubation period.

In chicks, the first signs are reduced growth and feed consumption, poor feather growth, with feathers becoming ruffled and brittle, followed by a rapidly developing dermatitis. Corners of the beak and the area below the beak are usually the worst affected but the condition is also noted on the feet. In severe cases the skin of the feet may cornify and wart-like lumps occur on the balls of the feet. The foot problem often leads to bacterial infection (Figure 4.54).

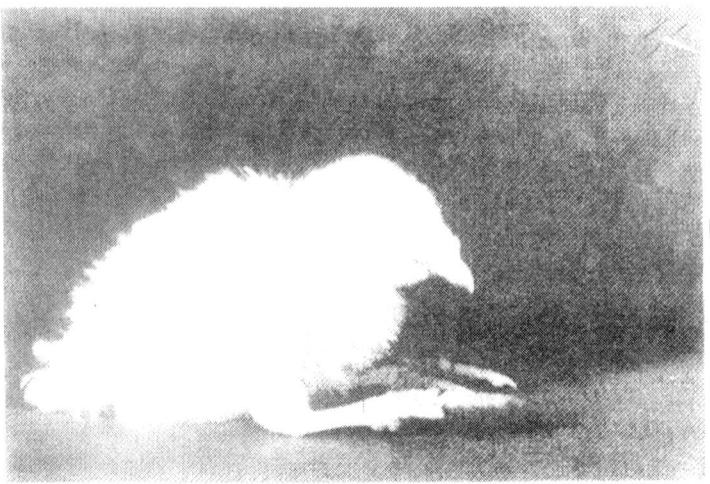

Figure 4.54 Pantothenic acid deficient chick showing the typical deficiency syndromes of stunted growth, poor feathering, encrustations around beak and eyes, and dermatitis of the feet.

Liver concentration of pantothenic acid is reduced during a deficiency, with the liver becoming atrophied and a faint to dirty yellow color noted. Nerve fibers of the spinal cord can show myelin degeneration. Pantothenic acid deficient chicks show lymphoid cell necrosis in the bursa of Fabricius and thymus, together with lymphocytic paucity in the spleen.

The foot condition noted in chicks, as well as the poor feathering, is difficult to differentiate from a biotin deficiency. With a pantothenic acid deficiency, dermatitis of the feet is usually noted first on the toes in contrast to a biotin deficiency where it primarily affects the foot pads, and is usually more severe than that noted with a pantothenic acid deficiency. Ducks do not show the usual signs noted for chickens and turkeys, except for retarded growth. However, mortality can be quite high with ducks. Pantothenate can become toxic at around 2,000 mg/kg where reduced growth rate associated with liver damage is seen.

4.19 BIOTIN

The discovery of biotin and its importance in nutrition stems from two lines of research, one by microbiologists, and the other by animal nutritionists. In the early 1930s, a new factor was discovered called coenzyme-R which was required for respiration in legume nodule bacteria, *Rhizobia*. Subsequently, a substance in crystalline form was extracted from boiled yolks of duck eggs and was extremely potent as a source of bios II necessary for the growth of yeast. This substance was termed biotin.

Concurrently, others were studying a toxic condition discovered to occur in animals fed raw egg white. Researchers described in detail the histological changes that occur in the skin due to animals eating raw egg white and called the protective factor vitamin H from the German word Haut, meaning skin. In 1940, these same workers found that vitamin H, biotin and co-enzyme R were the same substance. It therefore became evident that the feeding of raw egg white to chickens and to mammals created a deficiency of a nutrient which was essential for the nutrition of animals, yeasts and certain bacteria. The structure and properties of biotin were described in 1942 and the product finally synthesised in 1943.

4.19.1 Structure and properties of biotin

The structures of d-biotin and some of its derivatives and associated compounds, are shown in Figure 4.55. The structure of biotin includes a sulfur atom in its ring (as does thiamin) with a transverse bond across the ring. Biotin with its unique structure contains three asymmetric carbon atoms, and thus can have eight different isomers. Of these, only d-biotin contains vitamin activity. Free biotin crystallizes from water as long white needles, has a melting point of 233°C, is soluble in dilute alkali and hot water, and almost completely insoluble in fats and organic solvents. While biotin is relatively stable, under normal storage conditions it is gradually destroyed by ultraviolet light.

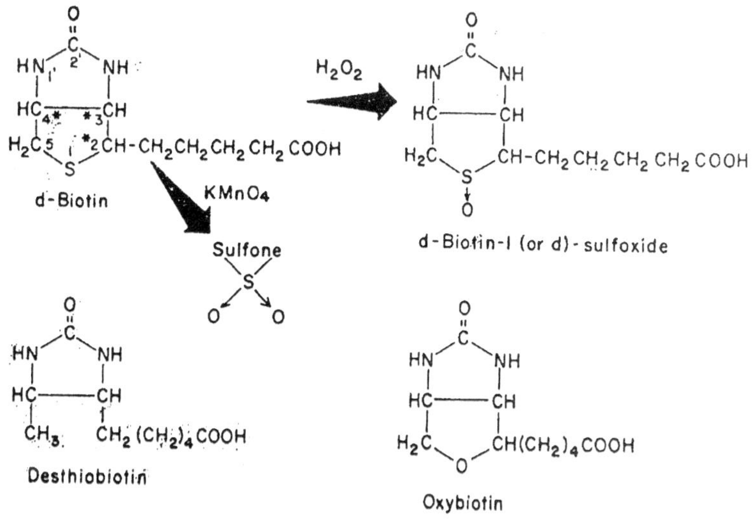

Figure 4.55 Structures of biotin and some derivatives.

Biotin exists in natural feedstuffs in both bound and free forms, with much of this biotin apparently not available to the chicken. There are estimates of only around one half of the biotin in feedstuffs being available (Frigg, 1984, 1987), while some estimates report zero availability in wheat. Fruit, vegetables and milk, contain appreciable quantities of free biotin while the biotin in animal tissues and plant seeds is often bound to lysine or protein. Biotin appears to be absorbed as the intact molecule in the first half of the small intestine (Bonjour, 1984). McCormick and Olson (1984), reported that biotin is transported as a free water-soluble component of plasma, and is taken up by the cells through active transport and attached to its apoenzymes. All cells contain biotin but larger quantities are found in liver and kidney. Biotin metabolism in animals is difficult to interpret as biotin-producing microbes in the intestinal tract and cecum can result in biotin excretion in urine and feces, which together exceed total dietary intake.

4.19.2 Metabolic functions of biotin

Biotin is an essential coenzyme in carbohydrate, fat and protein metabolism and is involved in the conversion of carbohydrate and protein to fat. It also plays an important role in maintaining blood glucose levels from the metabolism of fat and protein when carbohydrate intake is low. As a component of several carboxylating enzymes, it can transport carboxyl units and fix carbon dioxide in tissues. Biotin acts in combination with adenosine triphosphate as a coenzyme specializing in the transfer of CO_2 radicals.

Specific biotin dependent reactions in carbohydrate metabolism are as follows:

- Carboxylation of pyruvic acid to oxaloacetic acid

- Conversion of malic acid to pyruvic acid

- Interconversion of succinic acid and propionic acid

- Conversion of oxalosuccinic acid to α-ketoglutaric acid

Biotin enzymes are important in protein synthesis, amino acid deamination, purine synthesis and nucleic acid metabolism. Biotin is very important for optimum hatchability of eggs, and so is an essential nutrient of the developing embryo, and biotin status of the young chick is greatly affected by nutrition of the dam. The uptake of biotin by the yolk follicle is facilitated by specific receptors and the transport of biotin bound to protein carriers in the plasma. Two biotin binding proteins have been isolated from yolk and plasma (Whitehead, 1995). One is a high-affinity and the other a low affinity binding protein. The high affinity protein is found in almost constant levels regardless of biotin nutrition, while the low affinity binding protein increases in response to increased biotin intake. Yolk biotin level seems to plateau with dietary levels of around 250 µg/kg, assuming the bird eats about 100 g feed/day. Albumen biotin levels are about half that found in the yolk, for any given dietary situation. Albumen contains a potent binding protein, avidin, and it is unlikely that any biotin in the albumen is available to the developing embryo.

4.19.3 Deficiency and toxicity of biotin

During biotin deficiency, dermatitis of the feet and the skin around the beak and eyes (Figure 4.56) is similar to that described under the section on pantothenic acid. Thus, in making a differential diagnosis between biotin and pantothenic acid deficiency, it is usually necessary to examine the composition of the diet fed and decide which vitamin is more likely to be deficient in the ration. This can be checked by feeding the diet to two groups of chicks, supplementing the feed from one group with biotin, the other with pantothenic acid. Perosis is also a characteristic deficiency symptom of biotin avitaminosis. In 1942, Jukes and Bird, using a purified diet containing all known nutrients except biotin, demonstrated that the injection of crystalline biotin at a level which supplied approximately 2 µg of biotin daily was sufficient to completely prevent perosis but did not completely prevent the dermatitis.

Bain *et al.* (1988) also describes footpad dermatitis as well as enlargement and deviation of the distal tibiotarsus in biotin deficient birds. With marginal biotin deficiency, status of birds is improved by feeding antibiotics and impaired by feeding lactobacilli (Buenrostro and Kratzer, 1983). It appears that the intestinal microflora compete with the bird for available biotin, and in this respect dietary carbohydrate type can influence the bird's status. Bauer and Griminger (1980) conclude that dextrin reduces intestinal biotin levels, especially in the ceca, while feeding sorbitol enhances cecal biotin production.

While signs of classical biotin deficiency as shown in Figure 4.56 are quite rare, occurrence of Fatty Liver Kidney Syndrome (FLKS) is more important to commercial poultry producers. FLKS was first described in Denmark in 1958, but it was not until the late 1960s that it became a major concern, especially in Europe and Australia. Chicks around 3 weeks of age would become lethargic, unable to stand and die within hours of first showing such signs. Mortality was usually quite low at 1-2%, but periodically would reach 20-30%. Post-mortem examination revealed pale liver and kidney with accumulation of fat (Figure 4.57).

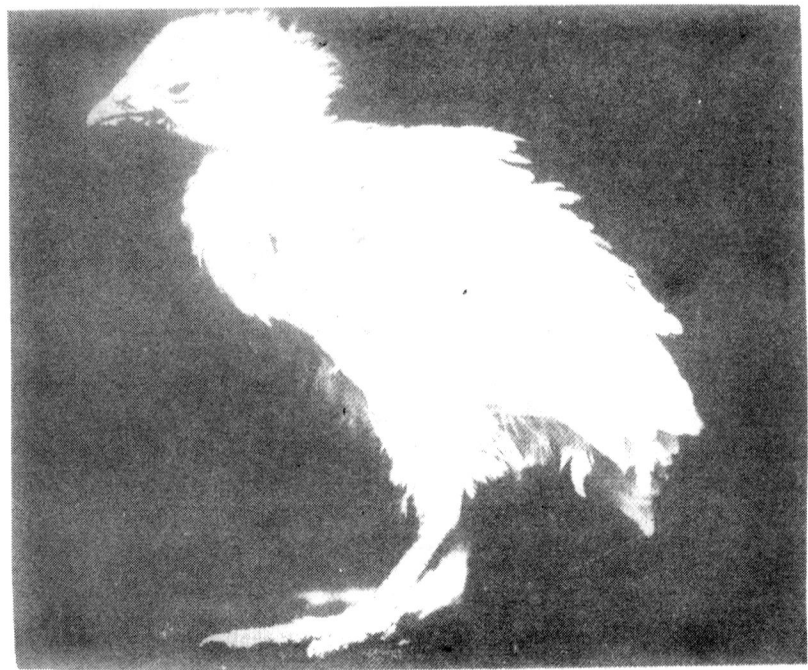

Figure 4.56 Biotin deficient chick.

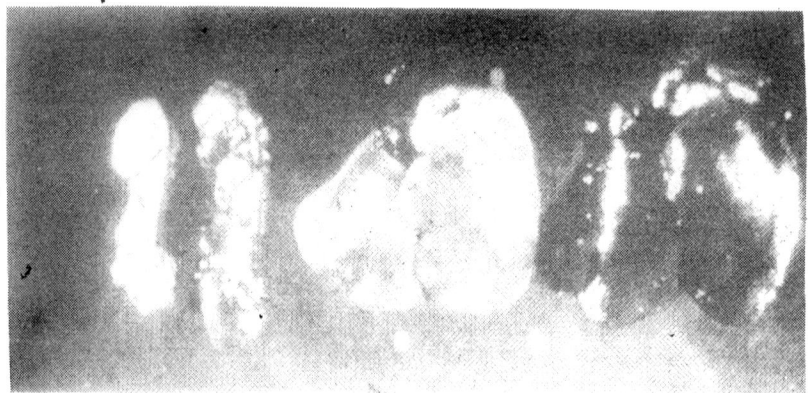

Figure 4.57 Pale liver and kidney of bird with fatty liver and kidney syndrome induced by inadequate dietary biotin (Courtesy Dr. C. Whitehead).

The condition was usually confined to wheat-fed birds, and was most problematic in low fat, high energy diets. High vitamin supplementation corrected the problem, and biotin was isolated as the causative agent. At that time, little synthetic biotin was available to the feed industry, and it is now known that biotin in wheat

has exceptionally low availability. The trigger of high-energy diets led to investigation of biotin in carbohydrate metabolism. Chicks suffering from FLKS are
invariably hypoglycemic. Whitehead *et al.* (1976) showed that biotin's involvement in two key enzymes, namely pyruvate carboxylase and acetyl Co-A
carboxylase was crucial in etiology of FLKS. Acetyl Co-A carboxylase appears
to preferentially sequester biotin, such that with low biotin availability and need
for high *de novo* fat synthesis (high energy, low fat diet), pyruvate carboxylase
activity is severely compromised. Even with this imbalance, birds are able to grow.
However, with a concurrent deprivation in feed intake or increased demand for
glucose, hypoglycemia develops leading to adipose catabolism and the characteristic accumulation of fat in both liver and kidney. Birds with FLKS rarely show
signs of classical biotin deficiency (Figure 4.56). Whitehead *et al.* (1976) conclude
that such signs are only seen in high fat diets, while FLKS is more common in
low fat, high carbohydrate diets.

Plasma biotin levels less than 100 ng/100 ml have been reported as indicative of
a deficiency. However more recent evidence suggests that plasma biotin levels
are quite insensitive to the bird's biotin status, and that biotin levels in the liver
or kidney are more useful indicators. Plasma pyruvic carboxylase is positively
correlated to dietary biotin concentration, and levels plateau much later than does
the growth response to biotin.

Embryos are also quite sensitive to biotin status. There are reports of congenital
perosis, ataxia and characteristic skeletal deformities in embryos and newly hatched
chicks when the dams are fed a low biotin diet. The deformities were prevented
by adding biotin to the diet. These embryonic deformities consisted of a shortened tibiotarsus which was bent posteriorly, a much shortened tarsometatarsus,
shortening of the bones of the wing and of the skull, and shortening and bending
of the anterior end of the scapula. Hatchability increased as the biotin content of
the eggs increased from 2 to approximately 10μg per egg. Others have reported
syndactylin, an extensive webbing between the 3rd and 4th toes of biotin deficient embryos. Such embryos are chondrodystrophic and characterized by
reduced size, parrot beak, crooked tibia and shortened or twisted tarsometatarsus.

Birds are very tolerant of high levels of biotin, and because the vitamin is excreted intact, toxicity is very rare.

4.19.4 Biotin antagonists

Avidin is a glycoprotein secreted by the mucosa of the oviduct of the hen into the
albumen of the egg. It combines stoichiometrically with biotin (ratio of one molecule avidin to one molecule biotin); therefore, if fed in the diet, it renders biotin
unavailable to the animal. Since the avidin-biotin complex is not degraded by
proteolytic digestion, when biotin is combined in this way, it is nonabsorbable and

nutritionally unavailable. Dosing animals with biotin in excess of the binding capacity of avidin for the vitamin prevents or cures lesions of biotin deficiency. Avidin is denatured by moist heat, thereby preventing its binding with biotin. Thus, biotin deficiency does not occur when heated egg white is consumed. The amount of biotin present in the yolk of the egg is approximately equivalent to the biotin-binding capacity of the white of an egg. Therefore consumption of raw whole eggs by animals usually does not create a biotin deficiency. White and Hughes (1981) have reported the existence of a biotin-binding protein in egg yolk that is quite different from avidin. They found a relationship between the level of this yolk biotin-binding·protein and the biotin requirement for hatchability.

Streptavidin, first isolated from *Streptomyces* cultures is a more potent biotin-binding protein than egg avidin. Streptavidin has been shown to be present in some poultry litters and has been isolated from *Streptomyces avidini* and *Streptomyces lavendula* taken from soil samples. It is quite possible that these biotin antagonists may have been responsible for biotin deficiencies which have been reported to occur from time to time in commercial broilers.

Biotin is inactivated in diets undergoing oxidative rancidity. Ninety-six per cent inactivation of pure biotin has been reported within 12 hours by addition of partially rancid ethyl linoleate. In the presence of α-tocopherol, this inactivation amounted to only 40% after 48 hours *in vitro* incubation at 37°C. Imidazolidone caproic acid is also an anti-biotin compound.

4.20 FOLACIN (FOLIC ACID)

Folacin is a general term used to describe folic acid and related compounds that exhibit biological activity of the vitamin. A condition referred to as tropical macrocytic anemia, observed in pregnant women in Bombay, was first reported in 1931, where an extract from autolyzed yeast would prevent or relieve the condition. It was found that the factor, also present in liver, differed from the pernicious anemia factor, and that it was different from thiamin, riboflavin and nicotinic acid. Similar results were obtained by other workers using an extract from brewer's yeast that they called vitamin M.

In 1938, workers at California, and Cornell reported the existence of an unidentified factor required for growth and the prevention of anemia in chicks. The California workers referred to it as the U and the Cornell workers, the R factors. Subsequent researchers extracted a compound from spinach that was required for growth of several strains of bacteria and named this factor folic acid. Confusion existed in the 1940's concerning these various factors because folic acid appeared to be active for both microorganisms and animals whereas concentrates of vitamin M and factor R were active for animals but not microbes. It was subsequently shown that incubation of vitamin M and factor R concentrates with rat liver enzymes caused a marked increase in folic acid activity for several microorganisms. Thus, the various studies had shown that folic acid existed in nature in both free and bound forms. Crystalline folic acid was isolated in 1943 and the structure and synthesis demonstrated in 1946.

4.20.1 Structure and properties of folacin

Much of the folacin in foodstuffs is found conjugated with varying numbers of glutamic acid molecules. The structures of folic acid and a number of its compounds are shown in Figure 4.58. Its chemical structure contains three distinct parts, namely: 1) a pteridine nucleus, 2) amino benzoic acid and (3) glutamic acid. The chemical name for folic acid is pteroylglutamic acid. Much of the folic acid in natural feedstuffs is conjugated with varying numbers of extra glutamic acid molecules. In these bound forms, it is inactive for the assay with microorganisms and as a metabolite in the animal body. However, chicken pancreas, liver and kidney contain enzymes capable of releasing free folic acid from the respective conjugates. The activities of these conjugases are influenced by cysteine, ascorbic acid and a number of other factors. The active forms of folic acid may contain a formyl group or a methyl group attached to the number 5 or number 10 nitrogen of the compound, or the methylene group between nitrogens 5 and 10 (Figure 4.58).

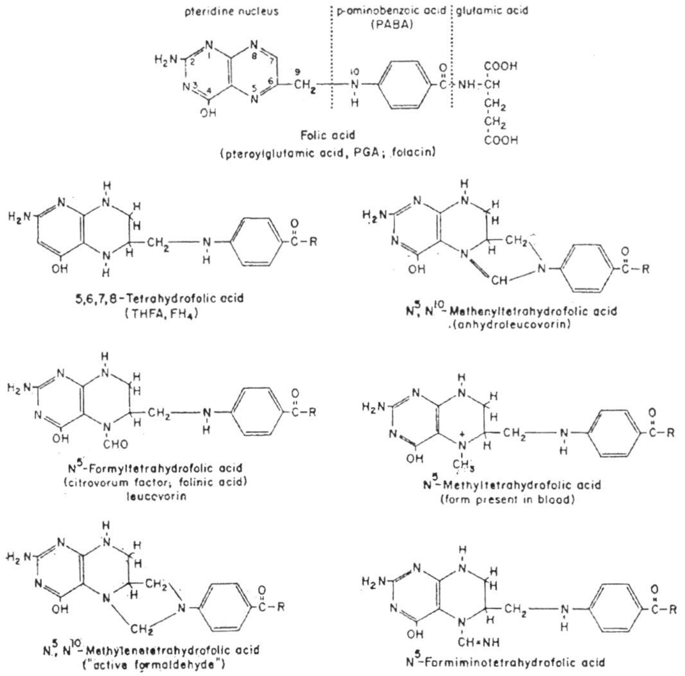

Figure 4.58 Structures of folic acid compounds. -R is one or more glutamic acid molecules.

Folacin is a yellowish-orange crystalline powder, which is tasteless, odorless, and insoluble in alcohol, ether and other organic solvents. The salt form is readily soluble in hot water while the acid form is only slightly soluble. It is fairly stable to air and heat, in neutral and alkaline solutions, but unstable in acid solutions. Polyglutamate forms of folacin are degraded to pteroylmonoglutamate prior to being transported across the intestinal wall. Several conjugase enzymes are responsible for the hydrolysis of the long chain polyglutamates to the monoglutamates before being taken up by the mucosal cells (Rosenberg and Newmann, 1974). After hydrolysis and absorption, dietary folates are transported via the plasma as monoglutamate derivatives, mainly as 5-methyl-tetrahydrofolate (THF), which is the active form of a group of enzymes called pteroproteins. The derivatives are taken up by the cell, where the major form of folacin in the cell, pteroylpolyglutamate, is built up in a stepwise manner by the enzyme polyglutamate synthetase. Specific binding proteins, that bind folacin and polyglutamates are known to exist in many tissues and body fluids.

4.20.2 Sources of folic acid

Folic acid is distributed widely in nature mainly as the THF acid derivatives, generally possessing three or more glutamic acid residues. While leafy green materials, organ meats, various nuts, soybeans, and animal products are relatively good sources of the vitamin, cereals, milk and eggs are usually poor sources. Only limited amounts of free folacin are found in natural products.

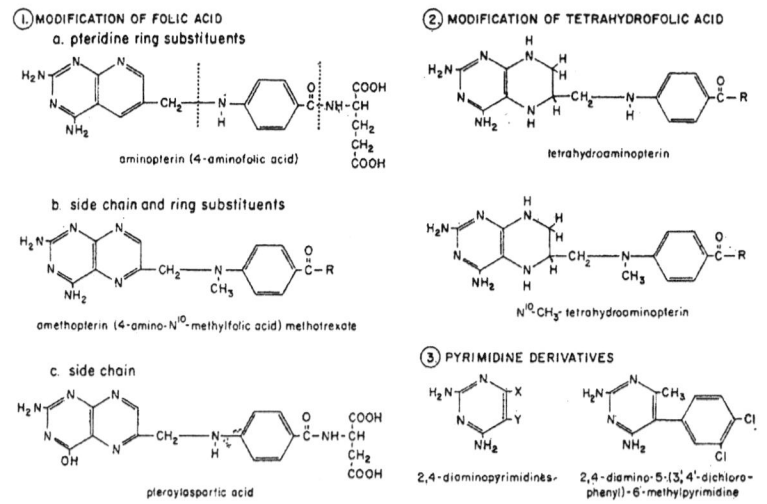

Figure 4.59 Structures of folic acid antagonists

There are folacin antagonists that block the conversion of pteroylmonoglutamic acid to THF, by binding dihydrofolic acid reductase, or blocking the transfer of single carbon units from THF to acceptors such as in the synthesis of methionine or purines. Structures of some of the folacin antagonists are shown in Figure 4.59. Folacin is sensitive to light and heat, especially in acid solution. Crystalline folacin, produced by chemical synthesis, is available to the feed industry in various dilutions.

4.20.3 Functions of folacin

Folic acid is indispensable in its role of transferring single carbon units, a role similar to that of pantothenic acid in transferring two carbon units. Some biochemical relationships of one-carbon units are shown in Figure 4.60. These one carbon units are usually produced during amino acid metabolism and are used in metabolic interconversions of amino acids and in the biosynthesis of purine and pyrimidine components of nucleic acids.

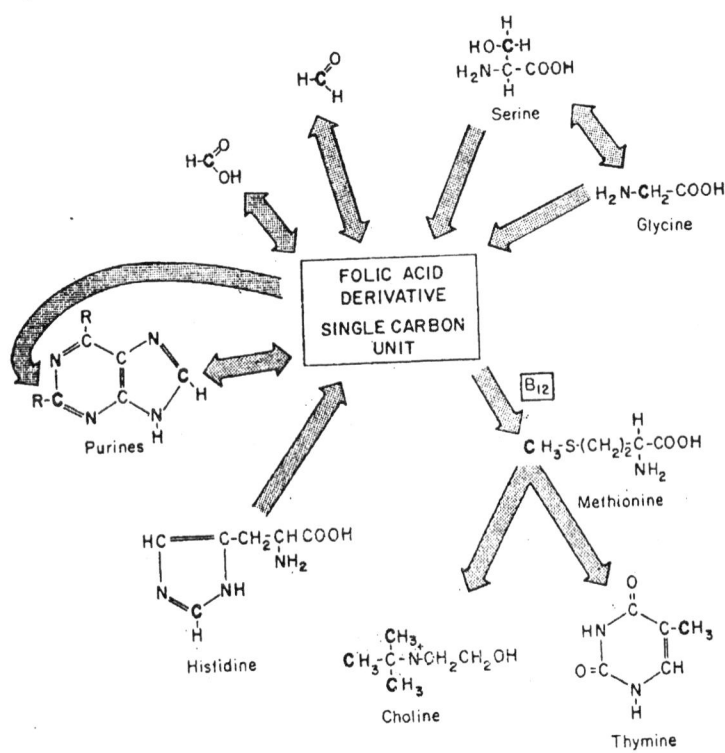

Figure 4.60 Compounds requiring single carbon units in their synthesis.

The important function of folic acid is in binding single carbon units to the vitamin molecule and thus transforming them to active forms so these can, by specific reduction or oxidation reactions, be transferred to appropriate acceptors. Pteroylpolyglutamates are considered to be the acceptors and donors of one carbon units in amino acid and nucleotide metabolism, while the monoglutamate is merely the transport form.

Since adenine and guanine (purine bases), as well as thymine (a pyrimidine base), are nucleic acid constituents, a deficiency of folic acid results in reduced cell formation and metabolism. In the absence of adequate nucleoproteins, synthesis and maturation of primordial red blood cells does not take place and hematopoiesis is inhibited at the megaloblast stage. As a result of this megaloblastic arrest, a typical macrocytic anemia is noted. Vitamin B_{12} is also necessary for reduction of one- carbon compounds and together with folacin, participates in the biosynthesis of labile methyl groups. Folacin has been reported to be necessary for maintenance of the immune system, which is probably mediated through its role in DNA synthesis.

4.20.4 Deficiencies and toxicities of folacin

A folacin deficiency in experimental animals, results in a macrocytic (megaloblastic) anemia and leukopenia (reduced white blood cells). Tissues with a rapid turnover, like epithelial lining, gastrointestinal tract, epidermis and bone marrow, as well as cell growth and tissue regeneration, are principally affected.

Poultry seem more susceptible to a folacin deficiency than do other farm animals. A deficiency results in poor feathering, slow growth, an anemic appearance and also perosis. As anemia develops, the comb becomes waxy white and pale mucous membranes in the mouth are noted (Siddons, 1978). Rennie *et al.* (1993) suggests that erythrocyte phosphoribosylpyrophosphate concentration is elevated in folate deficient chicks, and that this can be used as a diagnostic tool. Maxwell *et al.* (1988) described macrocytic anemia as the major sign in birds fed semi-purified folate deficient diets. These same authors also describe damage to liver parenchymal cells that also had depleted glycogen reserves. While turkey poults show some of the same symptoms as chickens, mortality is usually higher, and the birds develop a spastic type of cervical paralysis that results in the neck becoming stiff and extended. Poults will die within two days of exhibiting such signs unless folacin is administered.

The abnormal feather condition in chickens leads to weak and brittle shafts. Because folacin, along with lysine and iron, is required in feather pigmentation, a depigmentation occurs in colored feathers due to a deficiency of the vitamin. The appearance of Barred Plymouth Rock chicks fed graded levels of folic acid is shown in Figure 4.61. While a deficiency of folacin can result in reduced egg production, the main sign noted with breeders is a marked decrease in hatchability associated with an increase in embryonic mortality, usually during the last few days of incubation.

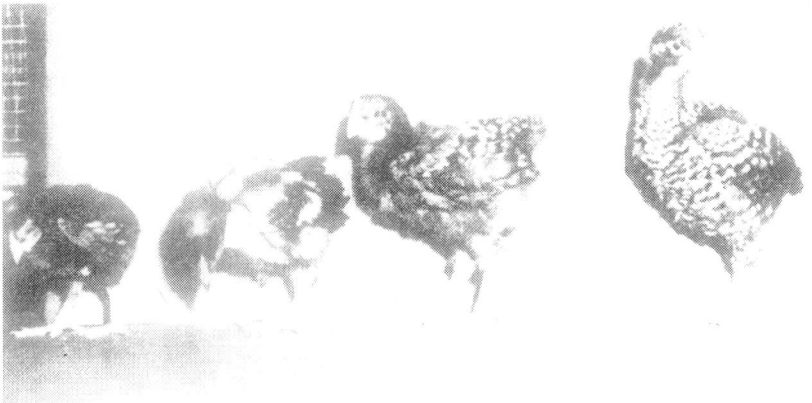

Figure 4.61 Chick (1) fed a folic acid deficient diet shows stunted growth, extremely poor feathering and perosis. Chick (2) received a small amount of folic acid which permitted some feather growth but feathers show typical depigmentation. Chick (4) positive control was fed adequate folic acid, and (3) was fed diet marginal in folic acid.

Such embryos have deformed beaks and a bending of the tibiotarsus is often noted (Froehli, 1987).

While birds can also exhibit perosis, histologically the lesions seen are different from those occurring as a consequence of choline or manganese deficiency. Abnormal structure of the hyaline cartilage, and retardation of ossification are noted with folacin deficiency.

It has been reported that choline is more effective in controlling perosis when the diet contains adequate levels of folacin. Others workers have suggested that there is a sparing effect of folic acid on choline requirement and also that the converse applies (Young *et al.,* 1955). Increasing the protein content of a diet has been shown to increase the severity of perosis in chicks receiving diets low in folic acid. With high protein diets there is an increased folacin demand for uric acid synthesis.

Birds are very tolerant of high levels of folacin, with up to 5,000x normal intake being needed to induce toxicity. Renal hypertrophy has been described under such conditions.

4.20.5 Requirements for folacin

While intestinal microbial synthesis can be a factor in helping to meet the requirements of a number of animals, this is not the case with poultry, due to their short gastro-intestinal tract and with much of the synthesis being too far along the tract for any meaningful absorption to take place. Folacin requirements increase as diet protein level increases. Also, it has been demonstrated that in birds subjected to disease such as reovirus infection, lesion scores are much higher with diets low in folacin (Cook *et al.*, 1983). The type of medication administered to a flock can also affect the folic acid requirement of the birds. It has been shown that sulfur drugs significantly enhance the need for supplemental folic acid as will feed containing mycotoxins.

Gradient (1986) reported that folic acid was very sensitive to heat, light and moisture, and so it is necessary to keep feed fresh and dry. Adams, (1982) has reported a marked increase in the destruction of the vitamin if minerals are present in a premix. Most commercial poultry diets will contain folacin supplements of around 1-1.5 mg/kg. Rennie *et al.* (1993) indicated that all folate dependent pathways are normalized with dietary folate supplements of 1 mg/kg. In a latter publication, this same group concluded that pelleted diets needed supplements of 2.5-3.0 mg folic acid/kg (Whitehead *et al.*, 1995). Ryu *et al.* (1995) showed that 1.2–1.3 mg folic acid/kg diet was adequate for normal broiler growth.

4.21 VITAMIN B_{12}

Vitamin B_{12} was discovered in 1948. It was the last of the vitamins to be identified and the most potent, as very low concentrations are needed to meet animal requirements. It is also unique in that it is only synthesized in nature by microorganisms, and so there is none in plant products. It is also a unique nutrient in that cobalt is an integral part of its molecule.

In 1824, Combe described a fatal anemia, called pernicious anemia, (apparently only seen in humans) and suggested that it was related to a digestive tract disorder. Some 100 years later it was shown that eating raw liver, would alleviate this fatal disease. Castle (1929) suggested that pernicious anemia was due to an interaction of a dietary (extrinsic) factor, and an intrinsic factor produced by the stomach. Mixing beef muscle with gastric juice prevented the anemia, and thus the gastric juice contained the intrinsic factor while the beef contained the extrinsic factor. During World War II, efforts were made to eliminate expensive and scarce animal proteins from the diets of farm animals. The use of all-vegetable protein diets reduced the rate of growth in chickens and pigs and decreased the hatchability of eggs. Increasing the protein level of the diet made matters worse. The deficiency was corrected by an unknown factor present in liver, fish meal or cow manure. Cornell workers called the unknown substance the animal protein factor. Cary *et at.* (1946) demonstrated the presence in purified liver extracts of a "factor X" necessary for rat growth which others named Zoopherin. As research progressed, it became apparent that these factors might be identical. Since the factor was present in cow manure, it was postulated that it was synthesized by the microorganisms of the rumen. It was also shown that an organism isolated from hen's feces could synthesize a factor effective in promoting chick growth and in treating pernicious anemia.

At about this time, two groups of workers in the U.S.A. and in England, reported the isolation of vitamin B_{12}. The American team was aided by a microbiological assay for the "animal protein factor while the British group tested all of their fractions on pernicious anemia patients in relapse. The key to the isolation of vitamin B_{12} was the use of chromatography in which, finally, the red color of the vitamin was followed in the chromatographs.

4.21.1 Properties and metabolism of B_{12}

Vitamin B_{12} is the generic name for a group of compounds having B_{12} activity. These compounds have very complex structures and among their unusual features is the content of 4.5% cobalt. Adenosylcobalamin and methylcobalamin are natural occurring forms while cyanocobalamin is a synthetic product. However, it is the most common form used in clinical and commercial practice because of its availability and stability.

Vitamin B_{12} is a red crystalline hygroscopic substance, soluble in water and alcohol, but insoluble in acetone, chloroform and ether. Oxidizing and reducing agents, and exposure to sunlight destroys its activity. Losses due to feed processing are low as the vitamin is quite heat stable. The structure of the co-enzyme form of vitamin B_{12} is shown in Figure 4.62. Cyanocobalamin is the usual form in which the vitamin is isolated. In the presence of anions like cyanide, and light, the 5'-deoxyadenosine

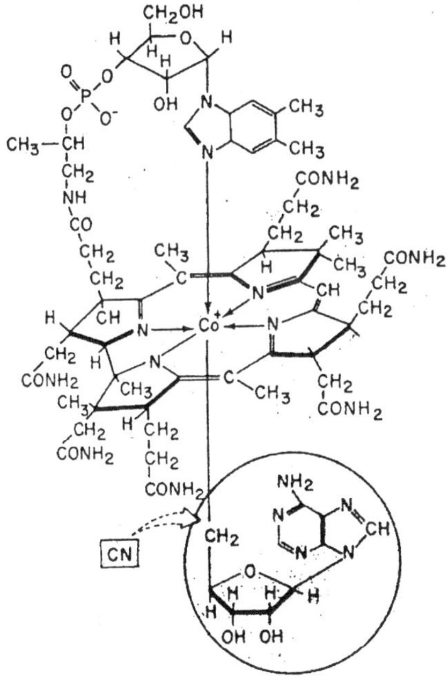

Figure 4.62 Cobamide coenzyme, the structure of the coenzyme form of vitamin B_{12}. The usual form in which vitamin B_{12} is isolated has the cyanide group replacing the 5' deoxyadenosine shown in the shaded area.

is replaced by cyanide and the cobalt is oxidized to the trivalent state. Several other biologically active forms are known which differ in having other anions, such as hydroxy, chloro, bromo, sulfato or nitro groups in place of the cyano group attached to the cobalt atom of the vitamin. Vitamin B_{12} is a chelate. While it is theoretically possible for other polyvalent cations to replace cobalt in the vitamin B_{12} structure, no such analogous compounds have been described.

4.21.2 Absorption of B_{12}

Pernicious anemia in humans is due to failure of absorption of vitamin B_{12}. A heat-labile protein known as the intrinsic factor is required to carry vitamin B_{12} across the intestinal mucosa and into the blood stream. The B_{12}-intrinsic factor complex is resistant to proteolysis and taken up by specific receptor sites in the ileum. The basic defect in patients with pernicious anemia is a degenerative change in the gastric mucosa, which ceases to elaborate and secrete the glycoprotein intrinsic factor. When this occurs, dietary vitamin B_{12} is no longer absorbed, thus producing a deficiency that leads to pernicious anemia. Addisonian pernicious anemia is characterized by megaloblastic arrest of erythrocyte maturation in the bone marrow, macrocytic anemia, leukopenia, and progressive neurologic degeneration.

4.21.3 Studies on intrinsic factor, B_{12}-binding proteins and B_{12}- releasing factors

Sonneborn and Hansen (1970) discovered in chickens two substances that bind vitamin B_{12} one in the serum and the other in the proventriculus. Although these proteins differ in molecular weight it appears that the serum binder may be the same as the proventricular binder with a secretory piece added to it, since an antibody elicited in rats against the proventriculus binder reacts against both binders. Earlier studies with rats and mice also indicated the existence of two immunologically different substances that bind vitamin B_{12}. These were called intrinsic factor (a glycoprotein) and transcobalamin II, found in the gastric mucosa and the serum, respectively. Transcobalamin has been shown to be synthesized in the liver and is the transport carrier for the vitamin. Some cases of macrocytic anemia have been reported in which failure to absorb B_{12} in the presence of intrinsic factor was corrected by intestinal secretions, suggesting that these individuals lacked an intestinal releasing factor for the vitamin B_{12}-intrinsic factor complex.

4.21.4 Sources of vitamin B_{12}

The primary origin of vitamin B_{12} in nature is microbial synthesis. There is no convincing evidence that the vitamin is produced in the tissues of higher plants or animals. It is synthesized by many bacteria and actinomycetes but apparently not by yeasts or by most fungi. Chemical synthesis was achieved in 1973 as a result of an extensive 11 year study in the U.S.A. and Europe. Vitamin B_{12} is widely distributed in foods of animal origin such as meat, milk, eggs and fish.

Its presence in the tissues of animals is due to the ingestion of vitamin B_{12} in animal foods or from intestinal or rumen synthesis. The organs of ruminants are richer in vitamin B_{12} than are those of most non-ruminant animals.

Plant products are practically devoid of vitamin B_{12}. The vitamin B_{12} reported in higher plants in small amounts, may result from synthesis by soil microorganisms, and/or contamination with insect excreta. Certain species of algae have been reported to contain appreciable quantities of vitamin B_{12} (up to 1 µg/gm of solids), although again such B_{12} may be of bacterial origin.

4.21.5 Functions of B_{12}

Vitamin B_{12} is stored mainly in the liver, however, kidney, heart, spleen, and brain also contain appreciable quantities. While a significant quantity of B_{12} is excreted via the bile, at least 65 to 70% of this is reabsorbed in the ileum through sequestering by glycoproteins.

Vitamin B_{12} is an essential part of several enzyme systems with most reactions involving the transfer or synthesis of one-carbon units (e.g. methyl groups). A close relationship exists between vitamin B_{12} and methionine, choline and folacin, in a number of metabolic functions. While the most important function of vitamin B_{12} is in the metabolism of nucleic acids and proteins, it also functions in carbohydrate and fat metabolism. A summary of the functions of vitamin B_{12} are as follows:

a) purine and pyrimidine synthesis

b) methyl group transfer

c) protein synthesis

d) carbohydrate and fat metabolism

Vitamin B_{12} also plays a role in promoting red blood cell synthesis and maintaining the integrity of the nervous system. A deficiency of B_{12} will precipitate a folacin deficiency due to blocking the utilization of folacin derivatives, since a vitamin B_{12} containing enzyme removes the methyl group from methylfolate, which is a step in the regeneration of tetrahydrofolate, necessary in the synthesis of thymidylate. Because vitamin B_{12} is important in protein synthesis it is believed that the growth depression seen with a B_{12} deficiency is due to impaired protein synthesis. Methylmalonyl CoA carboxylmutase is the vitamin B_{12} coenzyme responsible for conversion of propionyl CoA to succinyl CoA. Morrow et al. (1969) have shown that this reaction is important in gluconeogenesis. Detection of methylmalonic acid in urine is a much used test of vitamin B_{12} deficiency.

4.21.6   Requirements for B_{12}

The vitamin B_{12} requirements of the chicken depend upon the levels of several other nutrients in the diet. The relationship between vitamin B_{12} and pantothenic acid has been discussed earlier. Excess protein in the diet increases the need for vitamin B_{12}. The vitamin B_{12} requirement also appears to depend upon the levels of choline, methionine and folic acid in the diet and is interrelated with ascorbic acid metabolism in the body. Patel and McGinnis (1980) found that growth and efficiency of feed utilization were depressed upon addition of 10 and 20% fat unless the chick's diet contained adequate vitamin B_{12}. Isoenergetic substitution of glucose for the fat also depressed growth unless B_{12} was added. This indicates that vitamin B_{12} is important in the metabolism of excess energy. Squires and Naber (1992) suggest that laying hens require 8 µg B_{12}/kg diet in order to maintain an optimal concentration of vitamin B_{12} in the yolk, which is around 2 µg/100 g yolk. Yolk vitamin B_{12} content is very responsive to diet concentration of this vitamin. There has been a suggestion that increased levels of vitamin B_{12} aid in the utilization of under-processed soybeans. However studies by Ward et al. (1986) failed to confirm this assertion.

4.21.7   Deficiency and toxicity of B_{12}

In growing chickens a deficiency of B_{12} results in reduced weight gain and feed intake, along with poor feathering and nervous disorders. While a deficiency may lead to perosis, this is probably a secondary effect due to a dietary deficiency of methionine, choline or betaine as sources of methyl groups. Vitamin B_{12} may alleviate the perosis condition due to its effect on the synthesis of methyl groups. Further clinical signs reported in poultry are anemia, gizzard erosion, and fatty infiltration of heart, liver and kidneys. Laying hens appear to be able to maintain body weight and egg production in spite of a dietary deficiency of vitamin B_{12}, however, egg size has been reported to be reduced. With breeders, hatchability can be markedly reduced, however, several months may be needed for the symptoms to appear. Olcese et al. (1950) summarized changes noted in embryos from B_{12} deficient breeders as follows:

- a general hemorrhagic condition

- varying degrees of fatty liver

- heart may be enlarged and irregular in shape

- kidneys pale and sometimes showing hemorrhages

- myopathy of the legs and sometimes perosis

- fewer myelinated fibers in the spinal cord

- high incidence of malpositioned embryos with many embryos dying around the 17th day of incubation.

Vitamin B_{12} is reported to be toxic with dietary inclusion of around 5 mg/kg. Signs of toxicity are unclear, especially with many older reports, since results are likely confounded with toxic effects of fermentation residues, inadvertently included with B_{12} during manufacture.

4.22 CHOLINE

Choline is considered an essential nutrient and produces classical signs of deficiency when absent from a diet. While choline is classified as one of the B-complex vitamins it does not entirely satisfy the classical definition of a vitamin. Unlike all other B-vitamins, choline can be synthesized in the liver, is required in relatively high amounts and functions as a structural constituent, rather than as a coenzyme. Choline was recognized as an essential nutrient long before most other vitamins were discovered.

Choline was named by Strecker (1862), being isolated from hog bile, while the structure was established by Bayer (1867) as the quaternary ammonium compound, β-hydroxyethyl- trimethylammonium hydroxide. Best and Huntsman (1932) showed that choline was the active constituent of purified lecithin, which they had previously shown to prevent excess liver deposition in rats, whereas the other components of lecithin, such as glyceride and fatty acids, were ineffective in this regard.

In studies with chicks and turkeys, Jukes (1940) showed that choline was required for both growth and prevention of perosis, where the amount of choline necessary for prevention of perosis was greater than that required for normal growth. Arsenocholine also prevented perosis but betaine was completely ineffective. Methionine or a mixture of methionine and ethanolamine was ineffective for prevention of perosis in chicks. Such studies led to the realization of the interdependence of choline, methionine and betaine in poultry nutrition studies. Contrary to these findings, McGinnis et al. (1944) reported that under certain conditions, betaine and methionine were effective in preventing perosis and in enhancing growth of choline deficient chicks. They postulated that in preventing perosis, betaine and methionine were acting by furnishing methyl groups for the conversion of choline precursors in the natural feedstuffs, into choline. This hypothesis was based upon the fact that methionine and betaine prevented perosis when fed in natural diets but not in purified diets.

Almquist and Grau (1944) differentiated between the growth-promoting and the perosis-preventing effects of choline in young chicks. Using a purified diet containing known amounts of methionine, cystine and other nutrients required by chicks (with the exception of choline or choline precursors), these investigators showed that betaine caused a growth response but failed to prevent perosis whereas arsenocholine prevented perosis but did not promote growth. Addition of both arsenocholine and betaine produced maximum growth. It was also shown that a combination of arsenocholine and additional methionine could produce maximum growth in the absence of added betaine.

These early studies showed, therefore, that choline performs at least three functions in animals: It is required (1) *per se* for acetylcholine and (2) *per se* for prevention of perosis, and (3) via betaine as a source of methyl groups for the formation of creatine and other compounds requiring methyl groups. It was shown that choline itself cannot act as a methyl donor but must first be oxidized to betaine. Other work has indicated that in the prevention of perosis, choline is required for the phospholipids needed for normal maturation of the cartilage matrix of the bone. Most body choline is found in the phospholipid form with only a relatively small amount as free or phosphorylated choline derivatives.

4.22.1 Structure and properties of choline

The chemical structures of choline, and some other related compounds are shown in Figure 4.63.

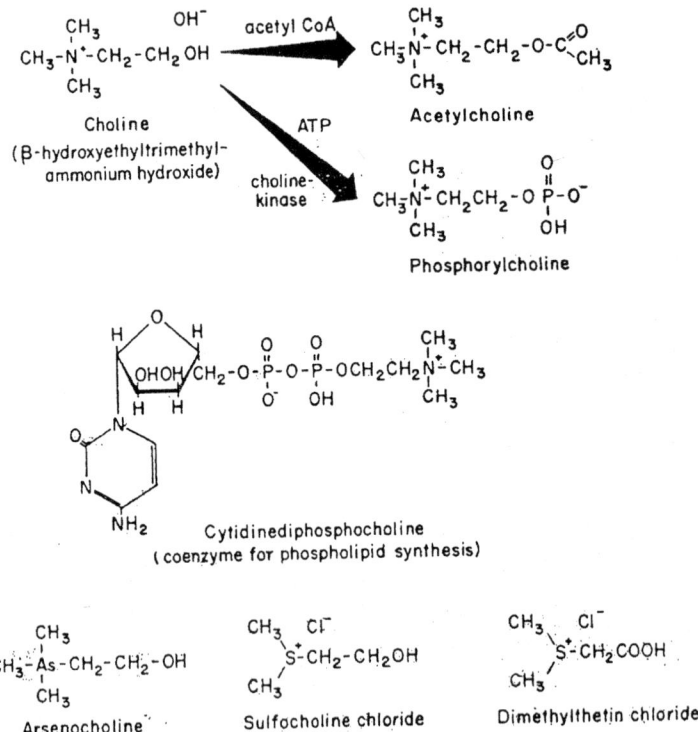

Figure 4.63 Structures of choline and related compounds.

Choline is a colorless, viscous, alkaline, hygroscopic liquid. It is soluble in water, formaldehyde and alcohol and has no definite melting or boiling point. Choline chloride, a deliquescent white crystal, is produced by chemical synthesis for use in the feed industry.

Choline is widely distributed in nature either as free choline, acetylcholine, or as more complex phospholipids and their metabolic intermediates. It is a structural part of the lecithins which accounts for its presence in all plant and animal cells. Choline is present in natural feedstuffs as lecithin, with less than 10% present as the free base or sphingomyelin. Choline is released from lecithin and sphingomyelin, by digestive enzymes, however, around 50% of ingested lecithin enters the thoracic duct intact (Chan, 1984). Absorption of choline takes place in the jejunum and ileum, by an energy and sodium dependent carrier mechanism. Only one third of ingested choline seems to be absorbed with the remainder being metabolized by microorganisms in the intestine to trimethylamine, which is either deposited in meat or eggs or excreted via the urine approximately 6 to 12 hours after consumption. With consumption of an equivalent amount of choline as lecithin, less trimethylamine is excreted and it takes longer to appear in the urine.

4.22.2 Functions of choline

Choline has four main functions in the animal body:

a) It is essential for building and maintaining cell structure. As a phospholipid, it is structurally part of lecithin phosphatidylcholine and also sphingomyelins. Choline is incorporated into phospholipid by being converted first to phosphoryl choline to cytidine-diphosphate choline and then by reaction with phosphatidic acid to lecithin. The intact choline molecule appears to be required in prevention of fatty liver and hemorrhagic kidney in rats and mice, and perosis in chickens.

b) It plays an essential role in liver fat metabolism, preventing abnormal fat accumulation and promoting its transport from the liver as lecithin or by increasing fatty acid catabolism in the liver. In view of the above, choline has been referred to as a lipotropic factor.

c) It is necessary for the synthesis of acetylcholine, which is required for the transmission of nerve impulses. Acetylcholine is released at the termination of the parasympathetic nerves and functions in transmitting nerve impulses from presynaptic to postsynaptic fibers of the sympathetic and parasympathetic nervous system.

d) Choline is also a source of labile methyl groups, which function in the formation of methionine from homocystine and of creatine from guanidoacetic acid. It is necessary for choline to be converted to betaine in order to be a source of methyl groups. While betaine has been reported to perform some methylation functions similar to those of choline, it cannot prevent perosis, fatty liver or hemorrhagic kidney syndromes.

Various metabolic functions and synthesis of choline are shown in Figure 4.64.

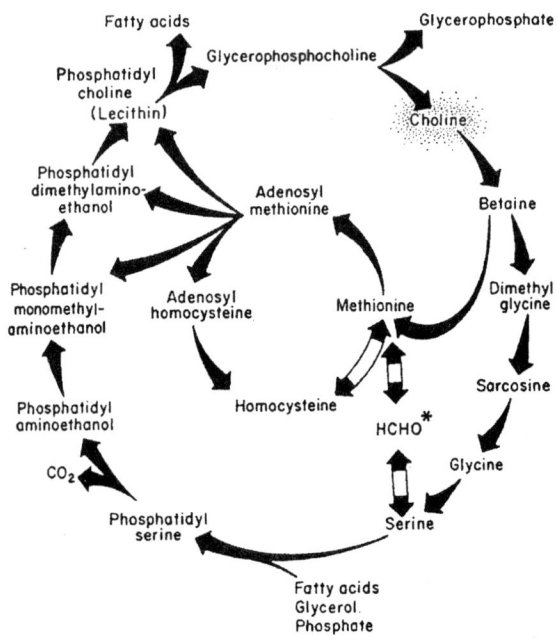

Figure 4.64 Metabolic pathway for the synthesis of choline, methyl groups and phospholipids.
*Folic acid is required as the carrier of single carbon units and vitamin B_{12} functions in the synthesis of methyl groups from these single carbon units.

4.22.3 Sources of choline

All naturally occurring fats contain some choline, with glandular meal, egg yolk and brain being the richest animal sources, while germs of cereals, legumes and oil seed meals are the best plant sources. Since betaine can spare choline, ingredients like wheat and its by-products, which are relatively high in betaine can meet part of the choline requirement for poultry. The availability of choline in natural feedstuffs has not been well established, however, Molitoris and Baker (1976), reported that availability of choline in several soybean products ranged from 60 to 75%.

Choline is available to the feed industry as the chloride salt, in liquid dilutions of 50, 60 or 70%. These products can be very corrosive and special handling and storage equipment is necessary. Since the commercially available products need to be added in large quantities and are very hygroscopic they are not suitable for incorporation into vitamin premixes and so are added directly to poultry feeds as separate inclusions.

4.22.4 Biosynthesis of choline

Unlike the other vitamins, choline can be synthesized by various animals, although in many cases not in sufficient amounts or rapidly enough to satisfy all the needs for this vitamin. Choline is synthesized in rat liver apparently by the methylation of a microsomal-bound phosphatidyl ethanolamine substrate. The methyl groups for choline synthesis apparently are all transferred from S-adenosyl methionine where probably two methyl transferase enzymes are involved. One enzyme system is needed for the initial methylation of the phosphatidyl ethanolamine and one for the other two methyl groups required to complete the synthesis. The ethanolamine portion of the choline molecule arises from serine. Apparently, all choline synthesis, at least in rats, occurs in liver since the microsomal system for incorporation of methyl groups into phosphatidyl ethanolamine is not found in other tissues (Figure 4.65).

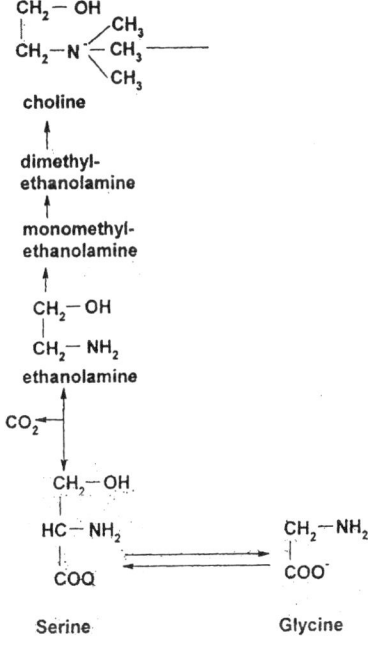

Figure 4.65 Synthesis of choline from glycine.

Monomethylethanolamine or dimethylethanolamine can serve as a source of choline in a choline deficient chick diet if sufficient methyl groups are supplied. The young chick is unable to synthesize monomethylethanolamine, but if the first methyl group is already on the ethanolamine molecule the remainder of the synthesis can be performed. Chick liver can synthesize microsomal monomethylethanoamine and choline from S-adenosyl methionine much in the same way as can rat liver microsomes. Therefore it appears that choline deficiency in young chicks is perhaps not due to lack of ability to synthesize choline but more likely to lack of ability to synthesize it at a rate sufficient for the needs of the bird. This also has been suggested as the reason for the high choline requirement of the guinea pig. The possibility also exists that a system may be present for methylating free monomethyl- and dimethylethanolamine, which could explain their effectiveness as choline precursors.

The rate of choline synthesis in chickens apparently increases with age since it is difficult to produce a choline deficiency in growing chicks over 8 weeks of age and since, as indicated above, laying hens seem to have considerable ability to synthesize choline. March (1981) found no effect upon egg production, egg size, relative yolk and albumen weights or mortality following addition of choline (1000 mg/kg) to laying diets containing either soybean meal or rapeseed meal even though liver fat was reduced about 25% by the choline supplementation.

4.22.5 Choline requirement

While choline in the strictest sense is not a vitamin, as many animals including the laying hen can apparently synthesize sufficient to meet their requirements, it does fulfill the definition of a vitamin for the young chick. Without a dietary supplement, the young chick does not perform optimally and can develop perosis. Because of the importance of folic acid and vitamin B_{12} in the synthesis and metabolism of choline, dietary levels of these vitamins together with methionine can have a significant influence on the choline requirement of the young bird.

While eggs contain a relatively high level of choline, and thus the laying hen must have a high metabolic requirement, it is difficult to demonstrate a need for added choline in the hen's diet. Thus, the hen can apparently synthesize sufficient choline to meet her requirement. Despite a lack of evidence that the hen has a dietary choline requirement, the addition of choline to a practical laying ration markedly reduces fat in the liver of the hen. The NRC (1994) indicates choline requirement for young birds at around 1300 mg/kg diet and 1050 mg/kg for layers consuming 100 g feed daily. Choline requirement will be affected by methionine level of the diet, and these previous values assume methionine requirements are met.

Arsenocholine, triethylcholine, and sulfocholine have all been found to spare choline for phospholipid synthesis and lipotropic effects. Studies with radioactive compounds have shown that to a limited extent these compounds can be incorporated into phospholipids in place of choline. Leach and associates have shown that the immature cells of the cartilage matrix of the bones of perotic chicks are very low in lecithin but contain increased amounts of cephalin. This apparently represents an attempt on the part of the bird to substitute ethanolamine for choline for the necessary phospholipids for cartilage cell growth. Cell immaturity appears to be the main cause of perosis.

Hormones also appear to affect the choline requirement. Female rats are much less susceptible to choline deficiency than are male rats. High doses of diethylstilbestrol given to young male chicks will markedly increase their growth rate when they are fed a choline deficient diet and will also reduce the incidence and severity of perosis in chicks. The exact mechanism whereby this hormone appears to spare the choline requirement is not known.

4.22.6 Deficiency and toxicity of choline

In addition to poor growth, the outstanding sign of choline deficiency in chicks is perosis. Perosis is first characterized by pinpoint hemorrhages and a slight puffiness about the hock joint. This is followed by an apparent flattening of the tibiometatarsal joint that is caused by a rotation of the metatarsus. The metatarsus continues to twist and may become bent or bowed so that it is out of alignment with the tibia. When this condition exists, the leg cannot adequately support the weight of the bird. The articular cartilage is displaced, and the Achilles tendon slips from its condyles. Perosis is not a specific deficiency sign since it appears with several nutrient deficiencies. Derilo and Balnave (1980) describe perosis as well as kidney lesions in choline deficient broilers. Kidneys were either swollen with petichial hemorrhages, or of normal size with more general large size hemorrhages.

Eggs contain approximately 12-13 mg of choline per gm of dried whole egg and a large egg contains about 170 mg of choline, found almost entirely in the phospholipids. Thus, there appears to be a considerable need for choline to produce an egg. In spite of this situation, several investigators have been unable to produce a marked choline deficiency in laying hens even when highly purified diets, essentially devoid of choline, were fed to laying hens for a prolonged period of time. The choline content of eggs was not lowered by prolonged feeding of a choline deficient diet, and so the laying hen must be able to synthes considerable amounts of choline. The choline requirement of laying hens can be influenced by the choline level in the diet of the growing pullet. Pullets which received choline-free diets after 8 weeks of age were apparently able to synthesize of the choline required for optimum egg production. Those that had received choline supplements in the growing diet required supplemental choline in the laying diet for maximum egg production and for maintaining liver fat at a relatively low level. The deficiency signs noted in these hens were a reduction in egg production and an increase in the fat content of the liver. Even under these circumstances, however the choline content of the egg was not affected by the low choline diet. Choline deficiency is usually more difficult to produce in other species than in chickens and turkeys Rats do not require a source of choline in the diet if sufficient methionine is provid-ed to supply the methyl groups necessary for choline synthesis. Similarly, young pigs do not require a source of choline if the methionine level of the diet is suffi-ciently high. Guinea pigs, however seem to behave much like chicks in that even with high protein diets adequate in methionine, choline deficiency is easily produced. To produce a choline deficiency in rats, it is generally necessary to feed a diet low in protein and in methionine. Under these circumstances choline deficiency in the rat results in an increase in liver fat and the appearance of kidney lesions. Compounds such as choline, methionine and betaine, which prevent the fatty liver syndrome in rats, are termed lipotropic compounds. Factors, which influence either synthesis or transfer of methyl groups, will also have considerable influence on choline deficiency. Thus, in rats, vitamin B_{12} is often omitted from the diet by investigators wishing to produce a choline deficiency, to reduce the *de novo* synthe-sis of methyl groups and thus further reduce the methyl groups available for choline synthesis. Folic acid deficiency exaggerates a choline deficiency because methyl transfer is affected.

The bird tolerates high levels of choline because it needs some 20-30,000 mg/kg diet in order to induce toxicity, the signs of which are reduced erythrocyte number. There are reports of high levels of pyridoxine alleviating such toxicity.

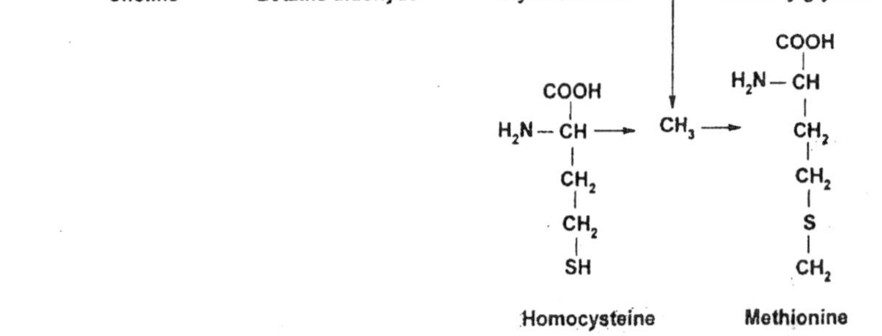

Figure 4.66 Role of choline in synthesis of methionine.

4.22.7 Choline:Methionine interrelation

Choline and methionine are usually the two major methyl donors in metabolism. In many feeding scenarios however, there should be limited transmethylation from methionine, because this implies an excess of this nutrient above its requirement for protein synthesis. Choline can spare methionine as a source of transmethylation, but obviously it cannot spare methionine in its role for protein synthesis. Methyl groups from choline can also aid in the synthesis of methionine from transmethylation of homocysteine (Figure 4.66). Homocysteine can therefore replace methionine as long as there is adequate choline available for methylation. Demethylation of methionine to yield homocysteine likewise can provide methyl groups for choline synthesis. This reaction occurs as a prelude to cysteine synthesis from methionine. While the demethylation of methionine to form homocysteine is reversible, the transulfuration of homocysteine is not a reversable reaction, meaning that methionine cannot be synthesised via transulfuration and methylation of cysteine. Methionine becomes the essential amino acid. Virtually all homocysteine in the body will be derived from methionine, since it is virtually absent in most feed ingredients. Transmethylation seems to be independent of requirements for folic acid and vitamin B_{12} the co-factors required in *de novo* methyl synthesis.

4.22.8 Trimethylamine and fishy taint

Trimethylamine (TMA) has a characteristic fishy taint and can be produced from choline by action of intestinal microbes. As long ago as the 1930s it was recognized that some laying hens would produce eggs with a fish taint, even though there was no fish meal or fish oil in the diet. In the 1970s the problem received particular attention in Europe, where brown egg birds fed rapeseed had a high incidence of this problem. Rapeseed meal was found to contain sinapine, the choline ester of sinapinic acid, which is a precursor of TMA. Choline *per se* can also be converted into TMA, and in humans at least, this is the fate of up to 50% of dietary choline. Most TMA is oxidised and excreted as trimethylamine oxide which has no fishy taint. Numerous strains of brown egg bird lack the ability to produce TMA oxidase enzyme. In chickens, much of the TMA synthesis seems to occur in the ceca. Emmanuel *et al.* (1984) showed extensive fishy taint in eggs of birds fed 0.5% choline in a wheat-based diet. When these same birds were cecectomized, the taint problem was virtually eliminated.

4.23 VITAMIN C

Vitamin C, or ascorbic acid, is only known to be required by man, most primates and guinea pigs. A deficiency results in scurvy, which is characterized by edema, emaciation and diarrhea. These conditions have been known and feared since ancient times. Over many years it was shown that scurvy could be cured or prevented by the consumption of fresh meat or fruit, with citrus being the most potent source of the scurvy-preventing factor. In 1928, Szent-Gyorgyi isolated a substance from orange, cabbage juice, and ox adrenal glands, that he called hexuronic acid, that cured scurvy, and which is now called vitamin C. In 1933 Richstein, synthesized hexuronic acid, which was shown to have the same activity as the natural product and thus was recognized as the vitamin.

4.23.1 Structure and properties of vitamin C

Vitamin C occurs in two forms, either the reduced ascorbic acid (ascorbate is the ionized form) or the oxidized dehydroascorbic acid (Figure 4.67). Both ascorbic acid and dehydroascorbic acid have biological activity, although further oxidation leads to irreversible production of inactive diketogutonic acid. This change occurs under moderate conditions of temperature and pressure, and so ascorbic acid is very prone to oxidation under conditions of commercial feed manufacture. Because of the ease of oxidation of ascorbic acid, one of its roles is as a metabolic antioxidant.

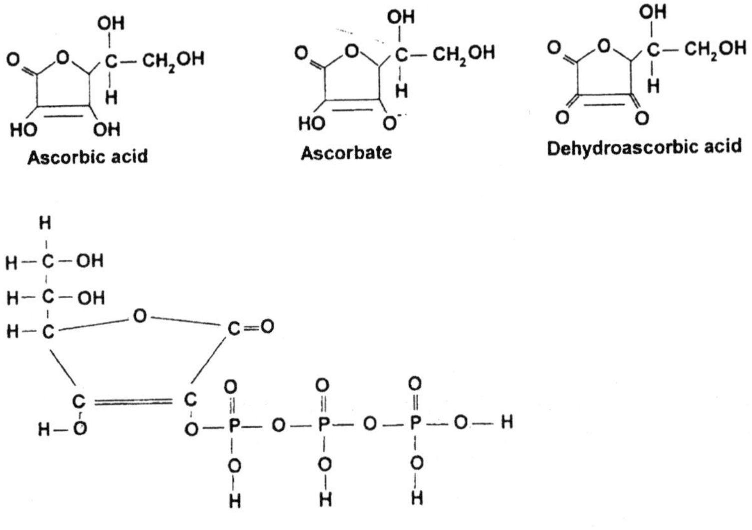

Ascorbic acid   Ascorbate   Dehydroascorbic acid

L-Ascorbyl- 2-Triphosphate

Figure 4.67 Forms of vitamin C

Ascorbic acid is a white-yellow powder, soluble in water giving a strong acid solution. Stability is improved under acid conditions. Ascorbic acid is classically produced from glucose, through intermediates of sorbitol→ L-sorbose → diacetone sorbose → diacetone 2 ketogulonic acid → L ascorbic acid. Modern techniques now allow production of the immediate precursor directly from D-glucose. Because ascorbic acid is so unstable, feed forms are usually polyphosphates such as the form shown in Figure 4.67. With high temperature pelleting, there is often loss of 85-95% of pure ascorbic acid, while most stable products such as Stay-C® retain around 80% of their potency under similar conditions.

4.23.2 Metabolic functions of vitamin C

Vitamin C is required for hydroxylation of proline residues necessary for the synthesis of procollagen, where it serves as a specific antioxidant. The hydroxylation process is assisted by Fe^{2+} to which it is tightly bound and needed for activation of oxygen. The ferric ion is then reduced in the inactivated enzyme, by the action of ascorbic acid which itself is converted to dehydroascorbic acid. The classical signs of scurvy in humans are in fact due to failure of collagen synthesis.

Because the bird synthesises its own vitamin C, then the role of exogenous ascorbate in collagen synthesis is not entirely clear. Vitamin C has been reported to improve leg bone condition in stressed birds. Under these conditions it is not known if vitamin C is beneficial in terms of precollagen synthesis, which is a precursor to bone formation, or more directly in its role of activation of 25(OH) D_3 – 1 – hydroxylase enzyme. Thus the conversion of 25(OH) D_3 to both 1 25(OH)$_2$ D_3 and 24, 25(OH)$_2$ D_3 is dependent on supply of vitamin C. Farquharson *et al.* (1993) reported a reduced incidence of TD in broilers (40→11%) when the diet was supplemented with vitamin C. Supplements of 1, 25(OH) $_2D_3$ completely eliminated TD. In these studies supplements of both ascorbic acid and 1, 25(OH)$_2D_3$ had the same effect on some key bone resorption marker enzymes.

In most animals the highest concentration of vitamin C is found in the adrenals. Birds contain much less adrenal vitamin C than do mammals (180 vs. 400 mg/100g) but this is still much more than found in other tissues such as muscle (4 mg/100g). The high adrenal content of vitamin C leads to the speculation of its role in adrenal hormone synthesis, and associated stressor reactions. In mammals, but not in young birds, injection of ACTH results in sudden depletion of ascorbic acid in the adrenals. In fact adrenal depletion of ascorbic has been used as an indicator of ACTH release in mammals. There seems to be a similar, but less defined response in older laying hens, suggesting in birds at least an age dependent maturation in this process. Vitamin C therefore plays a role in hydroxylation of amino acids such as phenylalanine that can be converted into adrenalin (Figure 4.68).

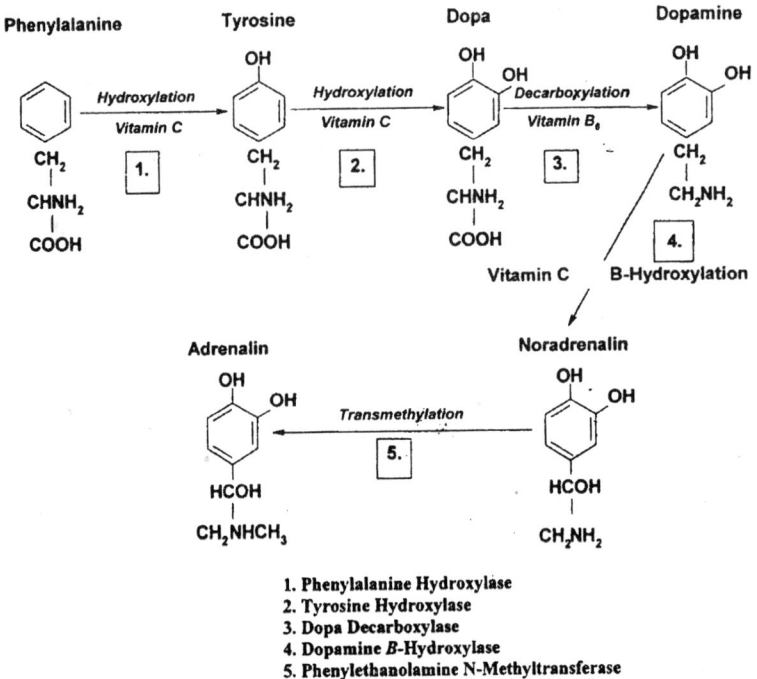

1. Phenylalanine Hydroxylase
2. Tyrosine Hydroxylase
3. Dopa Decarboxylase
4. Dopamine *B*-Hydroxylase
5. Phenylethanolamine N-Methyltransferase

Figure 4.68 Hydroxylation of phenylalanine in synthesis of adrenalin.

There are numerous reports of the benefit to supplemental vitamin C during periods of stress, and especially heat stress. McKee and Harrison (1995) show elevated feed intake, and growth of birds fed 300 ppm ascorbic acid when subjected to multiple stresses of beak trimming, heat and coccidial infection. Ascorbic acid also resulted in reduced plasma corticosterone and heterophil:lymphocyte ratio. Whether such effects are mediated via the adrenal cortex is unclear at this time. For example Kutulu and Forbes (1994) show that young birds voluntarily select a diet high in ascorbic acid (selection also aided by color difference of diets) when environmental temperature is suddenly changed from 26°C to 37°C. Within 3 days, birds voluntarily doubled their ascorbate intake. Vitamin C seems to ameliorate the increase in corticosteroid production common to heat stress situations. Pardue and Thaxton (1986) cite evidence of bursal involvement in adrenal ascorbate metabolism. Following bursectomy, there is depletion of adrenal ascorbic acid concentration, unless birds are concurrently treated with ACTH. Freeman (1967) suggests that failure of researchers to detect changes in adrenal ascorbic acid levels of stressed birds is due to the rapidity of change. During handling stress for example, adrenal ascorbic acid levels decline within 10 minutes, but are normal again (assuming the stress is removed) within 30 minutes. Adrenal ascorbic acid depletion is considered a classical stress response in chickens (Siegel, 1971).

Kratzer *et al.* (1996) indicate that for reasons unknown, soybean meal and other plant proteins such as cottonseed meal cause a marked elevation in plasma ascorbic acid of birds, compared to birds fed animal proteins. Balnave *et al.* (1991) suggest that water supplements of 1 g/L of ascorbic acid can prevent the occurrence of loss in shell quality due to saline (2g/L) drinking water. Interestingly this treatment could not correct an already established inferior shell quality.

4.23.3 Requirements, synthesis and toxicity of vitamin C

As previously discussed, all galliform birds synthesise vitamin C in the kidney, where d-glucose is converted to d-glucuronolactone and then 2-keto-gulonolactone which spontaneously converts to ascorbic acid. Some songbirds that require exogeneous vitamin C lack the enzyme L-gulonolactone oxidase in the kidney microsomes. There are no reported mutant galliform strains that lack this enzyme, a situation that would be of interest to researchers. The biosynthesis of vitamin C is however limited in very young birds, and increases with age up to about 60d of age (Figure 4.69). It is unclear whether this is a normal progression for ascorbate synthesis or whether the young chick would benefit from dietary supplements.

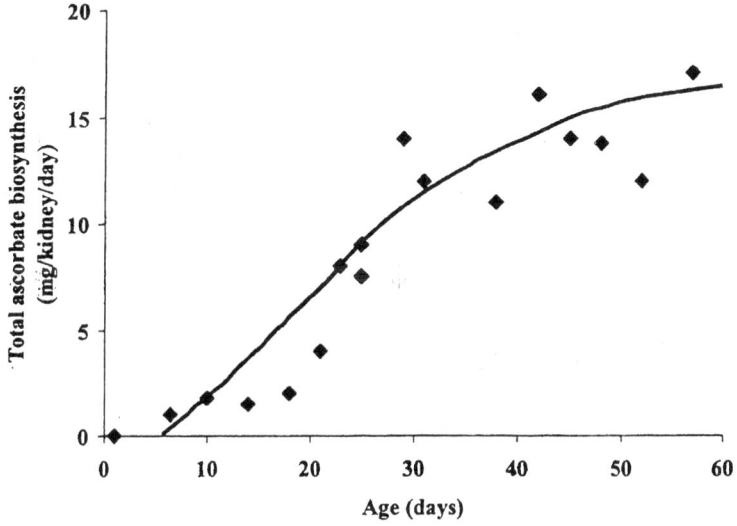

Figure 4.69 Influence of aging on ascorbate biosynthesis.
(adapted from Hornig and Frigg, 1979).

As previously described, it is essential to provide stable forms of vitamin C, such as polyphosphates, especially if diets are pelleted. There is some indication that moderate supplements (100 ppm) of ascorbic acid have only marginal effects on plasma levels, and that at least 250 ppm are needed for meaningful changes to occur. Response to dietary supplements are quite rapid, with plasma levels plateauing some 12 hr after administration and then returning to normal 24 hr after the supplement is withdrawn. Under stress situations, there is good evidence for dietary supplements of 250-300 ppm vitamin C for most classes of bird.

Vitamin C toxicity occurs at 20-30 times normal intake where there is interference with mixed function oxidase systems in the liver. One sign is excess accumulation of iron in the liver.

4.24 ESSENTIAL FATTY ACIDS

Although the essential fatty acids (EFA) are not vitamins by definition, dietary deficiency can result in a disease, or condition, similar to that noted with some vitamin deficiencies. Since it was known that dietary carbohydrate can be converted into fat in the body, and that essential fat constituents like phospholipids and cholesterol can be synthesized in the body, led to the early established view that a source of dietary lipids was not essential for growth or normal well-being of an animal. The finding that components of fat, other than the fat soluble vitamins, were dietary essentials was first reported by Evans and Burr (1926) in their work with rats. They noted a foot pad dermatitis, cessation of growth, necrosis of the tail, and eventually death, when a fat free diet was fed. They showed that this condition could be cured by certain polyunsaturated fatty acids, but not with any of the fat soluble vitamins. The name essential fatty acids was used to describe these compounds. Reiser (1950) showed that chicks could not survive beyond the fourth week if fed a fat free ration. Machlin and Gordon (1960) found that adding safflower oil or linoleic acid, but not linolenic acid, to a purified diet, resulted in an almost immediate growth response in chicks.

Linoleic, arachidonic, and linolenic acids were originally designated as EFAs. However, subsequent studies showed that arachidonic acid can be synthesized from linoleic acid. Since linolenic acid appears to only be required by fish, linoleic remains as the only EFA required by animals.

4.24.1 Structures and properties of essential fatty acids

The chemical structures of linoleic and arachidonic acid as well as other fatty acids with essential fatty acid activity are shown in Figure 4.70. Linoleic acid is a colorless oil that melts at −12°C, is soluble in ether, absolute alcohol and other fat solvents and has an iodine value of 181. Arachidonic acid is an oil that melts at −49.5°C, and has an iodine value of 33.5 (Scott et al., 1982).

Linoleic and arachidonic acid are readily oxidized in air and can be easily destroyed in feeds unless stabilized by natural or synthetic antioxidants. Because linolenic acid is readily oxidised it is a very important component of drying oils which are used in oil paints. Arachidonic acid is 5, 8, 11, 14 eicosatetraenoic acid (Figure 4.70), a fatty acid containing 20 carbons and 4 double bonds. Linolenic acid, sometimes considered an essential fatty acid for some functions in rats and trout, is 9, 12, 15 octadecatrienoic acid and it is normally found in nature in the cis form.

Linoleic acid   (9,12 octadecadienoic acid)
$$CH_3-CH_2-CH_2-CH_2-CH_2-CH = CH-CH_2-CH =$$
$$CH-CH_2-CH_2-CH_2-CH_2-CH_2-CH_2-CH_2-COOH$$
γ-Linolenic acid   (6,9,12 octadecatrienoic acid)
$$CH_3-CH_2-CH_2-CH_2-CH_2-CH = CH-CH_2-CH =$$
$$CH-CH_2-CH = CH-CH_2-CH_2-CH_2-CH_2-COOH$$
8,11,14-Eicosatrienoic acid
$$CH_3-CH_2-CH_2-CH_2-CH_2-CH = CH-CH_2-CH =$$
$$CH-CH_2-CH = CH-CH_2-CH_2-CH_2-CH_2-CH_2-COOH$$
Arachidonic acid   (5,8,11,14 eicosatetraenoic acid)
$$CH_3-CH_2-CH_2-CH_2-CH_2-CH = CH-CH_2-CH =$$
$$CH-CH_2-CH = CH-CH_2-CH = CH-CH_2-CH_2-CH_2-COOH$$
Linolenic acid   (9,12,15 octadecatrienoic acid)
$$CH_3-CH_2-CH = CH-CH_2-CH = CH-CH_2-CH =$$
$$CH-CH_2-CH_2-CH_2-CH_2-CH_2-CH_2-CH_2-COOH$$

Figure 4.70 Structural relationships among unsaturated fatty acids.

All of the fatty acids that have essential fatty acid activity contain double bonds in the 6,7 and 9,10 position, counting from the terminal methyl group instead of the customary carboxyl group. Thus, it appears that certain fatty acids are essential because of the inability of animals to synthesize a double bond between carbons 6 and 7 counting from the terminal methyl group. The nomenclature often used in describing these fatty acids gives an indication of the location of the double bond in relation to the terminal methyl group. Thus linoleic acid is C18:2ω6 and arachidonic acid is C20:4ω6 in this nomenclature. Linolenic acid, C18:3ω3 belongs to the ω3 series of fatty acids and oleic acid, C18:1ω9, to the ω9 series. The relationship between these families of fatty acids is shown in Figure 4.71. Arachidonic acid can be synthesized only from linoleic acid but not from oleic or linolenic acid. Linolenic acid is not an essential acid for chickens. Linoleic and linolenic acid come only from the diet, whereas oleic acid is synthesized readily by animals. During severe linoleic acid deficiency 5,8,11 eicosatrienoic acid, which arises form oleic acid (Figure 4.71) accumulates in body lipids and has been used as an indicator of EFA deficiency.

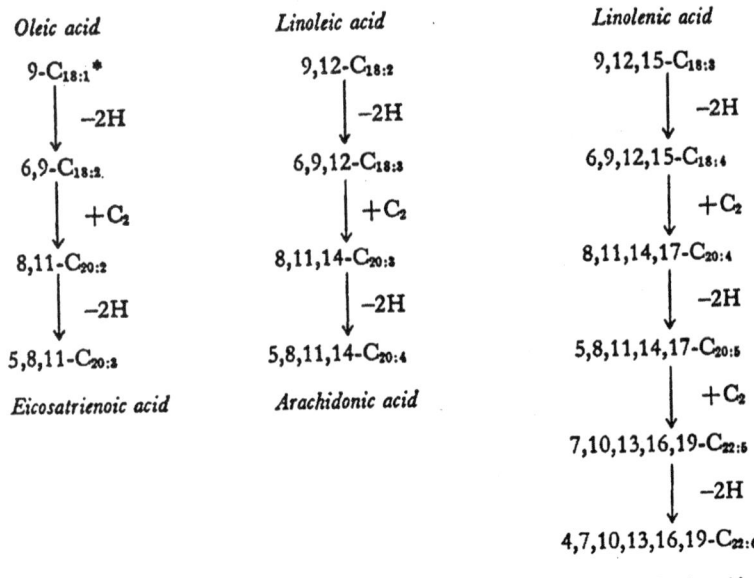

Figure 4.71 Metabolic transformations of some unsaturated fatty acids.

*The fatty acids are identified by the position of the double bond and number of carbon atoms and number of double bonds. Thus oleic acid is $9\text{-}C_{18:1}$; where 9 = carbon numbered from the carboxyl end which contains the double bonds; C_{18} = number of carbon atoms; and :1 = number of double bonds.

The most important metabolic function of linoleic acid may be as a precursor for a wide group of compounds called prostaglandins. These are formed by elongation and destruction of linoleic acid to di-homo-α-linolenic acid ($C20:3\omega6$) and arachidonic acid ($C20:4\omega6$) and from long chain fatty acids, unsaturated in the $\omega3$ position ($C20:5\omega3$, eicosapentaenoic acids). Production of prostaglandins requires the action of prostaglandin synthetase, which functions in forming the cyclopentane ring. Changes in saturation and oxidation made to the fatty acid chain, both inside and outside the cyclopentane ring, give rise to the three series of prostaglandins.

Almost all cells are capable of either producing or of being influenced by prostaglandins. There are many known prostaglandins in the body, most having a very short half-life, and their main function appears to be to raise or lower cellular cyclic nucleotide levels. Functions in which prostaglandins are known to play a role are; blood clotting, renal free water excretion, renal blood flow, reproduction, bronchoconstriction, gastro-intestinal motility and water loss, endocrine function, neurotransmitter release and perhaps immune function.

While linoleic (18:2, ω-6) and linolenic acid (18:3, ω-3) are recognized as metabolically essential fatty acids for the chicken, only linoleic has been found to have a dietary requirement. Alpha-linolenic acid appears to be important in the development of specialized membranes found in the retina and the nervous system. These membranes contain relatively high concentration of ω-3 PUFA that can originate from 18:3(ω-3). Certain PUFA, derived from linolenic and α-linolenic acid are used in the synthesis of a number of eicosanoids, which are important in embryonic development, reproduction, immunological responses and bone development in poultry. Of interest in the past few years has been the concentration of ω-3 linolenic derivatives in eggs. There appears to be an increasing body of evidence that these compounds are important in human health.

4.24.2 Sources of essential fatty acids

The major sources of linoleic acid in feedstuffs are the vegetable oils. Safflower oil contains 75% linoleic acid, whereas corn oil, soybean oil and cottonseed oil all contain approximately 50% linoleic acid. Yellow corn is the major source of linoleic acid in most feed formulas. Diets composed of corn and soybean meal with no further supplementation are likely to be just adequate in linoleic acid for chick growth and marginal for maximum egg size. Chickens that are fed diets containing milo, barley or wheat instead of corn as the major grain may receive suboptimal quantities of linoleic acid. Supplementation in the form of fats containing appreciable quantities of this fatty acid may improve performance in some cases. Corn distiller's dried solubles contain nearly 10% corn oil and is a good source of linoleic acid for chicks and hens.

4.24.3 Symptoms of an essential EFA deficiency in poultry

In the young chick a linoleic acid deficiency results in reduced growth rate and as the condition progresses a build up of fat occurs in the liver. Several investigators have reported that linoleic acid deficient chicks are more susceptible to a respiratory infection. In the laying hen it is difficult to demonstrate a linoleic acid requirement. However, a linoleic acid deficiency has been shown to result in smaller egg size and reduced hatchability for breeders, with a marked increase in early embryonic mortality. A deficiency in the male can lead to impaired spermatogenesis resulting in lower fertility.

4.24.4 Essential fatty acid requirements for poultry

The linoleic acid requirements of the newly hatched chick can be significantly affected by the carryover in the egg. However, most studies indicate that chicks hatched from normal eggs require around 1% linoleic acid in their diet to grow and function normally. For the laying hen, the level has been reported to vary from 0.25 to 1.5% of the diet. There seems to be an effect of linoleic acid on egg size. Layers may not respond to linoleic acid in a corn-based diet because these often provide 1-1.5% linoleic acid. However in wheat-based diets, that may contain as little as 0.5% linoleic acid, résponse to linoleic acid is often seen. For example, March and McMillan (1990) show increased egg size in birds fed supplements of safflower oil, rather than tallow, using a wheat-based diet.

4.25 UNIDENTIFIED GROWTH FACTORS (UGF'S)

Nutritionists in the 1910's and 1920's schooled in the concepts of Kellner and Voit, were primarily students of energy metabolism. To believe that accessory food factors such as vitamins were essential for metabolism in animals was a difficult doctrine to accept. Writing on the nutrition of man in different climates, Voit stated that 'unquestionably it would be best if one could feed only pure chemical compounds, for example, pure protein, fat, sugar, starch and ash constituents, or mixtures of these. However, inasmuch as man and animals rarely tolerate tasteless mixtures, it is necessary in most cases to choose foods as they are provided by nature. It probably would be possible to repeat tests with the natural food products by using the pure substances, although the results yielded thereby might not be essentially different.' This statement shows that Voit had no appreciation of the possible existence of accessory food factors such as vitamins and essential trace minerals.

With the discoveries of Eijkman and of McCollum showing the existence of a water soluble vitamin B and a fat soluble vitamin A, thereby supplying proof that animals cannot live without these accessory factors, nutritionists were forced to accept the importance of vitamins. Vitamin C was quickly included in the group. When Evans reported the existence of a fat soluble factor necessary for reproduction, it required only about two years for acceptance of vitamin E. Following this, 4-6 years were needed to bring about a realization that vitamin B was composed of at least two factors, vitamin B_1 required for prevention of polyneuritis, and vitamin B_2 required for growth. Then, the 1930s became the era of discovery of B vitamins. The vitamin B_2 complex was shown to be made up of riboflavin, pantothenic acid, pyridoxine, biotin, nicotinic acid and folic acid. Choline, although water soluble, is not ordinarily included in the vitamin B_2 complex.

With the isolation and synthesis of folic acid in the early 1940's many believed that all of the unidentified factors (usually referred to as unidentified growth factors or UGF) had been discovered and that there were no more factors needed for optimum nutrition. One reason for this supposition was the fact that completely synthetic diets of known nutrient composition, containing all of the recognized vitamins and minerals and adequate in essential amino acids, would support growth and development in young weanling rats.

Conclusions drawn from this work failed to consider the alterations in nutritional requirements produced by three important phenomena: (1) carryover of nutrients from the dam to her offspring; (2) intestinal microbial synthesis of nutrients; and (3) nutrient interrelationships where one nutrient may spare the amount of another. Thus, since the discovery of folic acid, numerous UGFs have been reported from time to time. Some have been shown to be associated with trace mineral nutrition, others to imbalances in the dietary levels of two or more essential nutrients, particularly in amino acid nutrition.

The discovery of vitamin B_{12} as the unknown activity termed the 'animal protein factor' responsible for special growth promoting effects and for improvements in reproduction of poultry, is an excellent example of the fallacy of assuming that no more factors exist simply because animals can survive on synthetic diets. The discovery of vitamin B_{12} was delayed because this vitamin is stored in the liver and is transferred by the hen to the egg. The progeny of hens that have received high levels of vitamin B_{12} in the breeding diet contain enough vitamin B_{12} to survive and grow normally for several weeks on diets deficient in the vitamin. Several groups of workers have reported the existence of unidentified growth factors for chicks or of factors required for egg production and hatchability. Some of these factors have already been shown to represent phenomena resulting from alterations in the balance or availability of some of the known nutrients.

Since the discovery of vitamin B_{12} many cases have been reported of growth stimulation resulting from the addition of natural materials to purified diets. Many of the growth responses obtained have been traced to relationships between known nutrients, such as natural chelates in corn distiller's dried solubles which improved the utilization of zinc in a purified diet containing soybean. Discovery of the essentiality of selenium probably represents the most spectacular recent discovery coming from UGF research. However, demonstrable responses in growth or other criteria are still being reported from studies on the addition of complex ingredients to highly purified diets. Fish solubles, dried whey, brewer's yeast, and corn distiller's dried soluble and other fermentation residues are the major special ingredients often added to poultry rations as potential sources of unrecognized nutritional factors.

Identification of the active principles in these materials has proved to be very difficult. At best, growth responses are small, often non-reproducible, making significant assays of isolated fractions impossible. Response often is affected by environment. In one series of experiments, chicks were shown to respond to corn distiller's solubles under normal laboratory conditions but not in a germ-free environment. Field reports have suggested that practical rations containing sources of UGF are superior to unsupplemented feeds under conditions of disease or other environmental stresses.

Many nutritionists consider it unlikely that there are still nutrients waiting to be identified. Likewise it is unlikely that we will ever show a requirement for such obscure nutrients as tin, boron or other minor trace elements. However, many commercial nutritionists still recognize the fact that more complex diets, although perhaps not economical, at times provide an improved performance beyond that expected from calculated nutrient supply. Inclusion of ingredients such as fish meal, brewers grains and yeasts and fermentation solubles may well be acting as antibiotics or probiotics in some manner, and so advantageously affecting the bird's intestinal microflora. In the future, as classical antibiotics come under closer scrutiny from regulatory agencies, we may see a renewed interest in UGF's.

SELECTED REFERENCES

Aburto, A., H.M. Edwards and W.M. Britton, 1998. The influence of vitamin A on utilization and amelioration of toxicity of D_3 25 (OH) and I, 25 $(OH)_2$ in young broiler chickens. Poultry Sci. 77:585-593.

Adams, C.R., 1982. In Vitamins - The Life Essentials. Nutr. Int. NFIA, Des Moines, Iowa.

Almquist, H.J. and C.R. Grau, 1944. Interrelationship of methionine, choline, betaine and arsenocholine in the chick. J. Nutr. 27:263.

Ameenuddin, S., M.L. Sunde and M.E. Cook, 1985. Essentiality of vitamin D_3 and its metabolites in poultry nutrition: A review. Wld. Poultry Sci. J. 41:52-63.

Aslam, S.M., J.D. Garlich and M.A. Qureshi, 1998. Vitamin D deficiency alters the immune response of broiler chicks. Poultry Sci. 77:842-849.

Atef, M., M.S.M. Hafy and M.I.A. El-Azia, 1993. Effect of pyridoxine on the distribution of chloramphenicol and its residues in the chicken. Br. Poultry Sci. 34:161-166.

Bain, S.D., J.W. Newbrey and B.A. Watkins, 1988. Biotin deficiency may alter tibiotarsal bone growth and modeling in broiler chicks. Poultry Sci. 67:590-595.

Baker, D.H., R.R. Biehl and J.L. Emmert, 1998. Vitamin D_3 requirement of young chicks receiving diets varying in calcium and available phosphorus. Br. Poultry Sci. 39:413-417.

Balnave, D., D. Zhang and R.E. Moreng, 1991. The use of ascorbic acid to prevent the decline in eggshell quality observed with saline drinking water. Poultry Sci 70:848-852.

Bar, A., S. Edelstein, V. Eisner, I. Ben-Gal and S. Hurwitz, 1982. Cholecalciferol requirements of young turkeys under normal conditions and during recovery from rickets. J. Nutr. 112:1779-1786.

Bartov, I., 1997. Moderate excess of dietary vitamin E does not exacerbate cholecalciferol deficiency in young broiler chicks. Br. Poultry Sci. 38:442-444.

Bartov, I., and M. Frigg, 1992. Effect of high concentrations of dietary vitamin E during various age periods on performance, plasma vitamin E and meat stability of broiler chicks at 7 weeks of age. Br. Poultry Sci. 33:393-399.

Bauer, K.D. and P. Griminger, 1980. Effect of dietary carbohydrates and biotin level on cecal size and biotin concentration of growing chickens. Poultry Sci. 59:1493-1498.

Berdanier, C.D. and P. Griminger, 1968. In vitro and in vivo absorption of three vitamin K analogues by chicken intestine. Int. J. Vit. Res. 38:376-382.

Best, C.H. and M.E. Huntsman, 1932. The effects of components of lecithin upon deposition of fat in the liver. J. Physiol. 75:405.

Blalock, T.L. and J.P. Thaxton, 1984. Hematology of chicks experiencing marginal vitamin B_6 deficiency. Poultry Sci. 63:1243-1249.

Bonjour, J.P., 1984. In Handbook of Vitamins. Publ. Dekker, N.Y.

Bootwalla, S.M. and R.H. Harms, 1990. Reassessment of riboflavin requirement for SCWL pullets 0-6 weeks of age. Br. Poultry Sci. 31:779-784.

Bootwalla, S.M. and R.H. Harms, 1991. Reassessment of pantothenic acid requirement for SCWL pullets from 0-6 weeks. Poultry Sci. 70.80-84.

Bryden, W., 1991. Tissue depletion of biotin in chickens and the development of deficiency lesions and the fatty liver kidney syndrome. Avian Path. 20:259-269.

Buenrostro, J.L. and F.H. Kratzer, 1983. Effect of lactobacillus inoculation and antibiotic feeding of chickens on availability of dietary biotin. Poultry Sci. 62:2022-2029.

Chan, M.M., 1984. *In* Handbook of Vitamins. Publ. Dekker, N.Y.

Chen, B.J., 1996. Efficiency of tryptophan-niacin conversion in chickens and ducks. Nutr. Res. 16(1) 91-104.

Chung, T.K. and D.H. Baker, 1990. Riboflavin requirement of chicks fed purified amino acid and conventional corn-soybean meal diets. Poultry Sci. 69:1357-1363.

Cline, J.K., R.R. Williams and J. Finkelstein, 1937. Crystalline vitamin B_1. XVII. Synthesis of vitamin B_1. J. Am. Chem. Soc. 59:1052.

Coelho, M.B., 1994. Vitamin stability in expanders. Feed Management 45(8) p 10-15.

Colnago, G.L., L.S. Jensen and P.L. Long, 1984. Effect of selenium and vitamin E on the development of immunity to coccidiosis in chicks. Poultry Sci. 63:1136-1143.

Cooperman, J.M. and R. Lopez, 1984. *In* Handbook of Vitamins. Publ. Dekker, N.Y.

Daghir, N.J. and K.S. Haddad, 1981. Vitamin B_6 in the etiology of gizzard erosion in growing chickens. Poultry Sci. 60:988.

Dam, H. and J. Glavind, 1942. Factors influencing capillary permeability in the vitamin E- deficient chick. Science 96:235.

Dam, H., I. Prange and E. Søndergaard, 1952. Muscular degeneration (white striations of muscles) in chicks reared on vitamin E deficient, low fat diets. Acta Pathol. Microbiol. Scand. 31:172.

DeLuca, H.F., 1988. The vitamin D story: a collaborative effort of basic science and clinical medicine. FASEB J. Mar 1; 2(3):224-236.

DeLuca, H.F., 1980. Some concepts emanating from a study of the metabolism and function of vitamin D. Nutr. Reviews 38:169.

Derilo, Y.L. and D. Balnave, 1980. The choline and sulphur amino acid requirements of broiler chickens fed on semi-purified diets. Br. Poult. Sci. 21:479-487.

Desai, I.D., C.C. Calvert, M.L. Scott and A..L. Tappel, 1964. Peroxidation of lysosomes in nutritional muscular dystrophy of chicks. Proc. Soc. Exp. Biol. Med. 115:462.

DiLorenzo, R.N., 1972. Studies on the genetic variation in tryptophan-nicotinic acid conversion in chicks. Ph.D. Thesis, Cornell Univ.

Emmanuel, B., Y.K. Goh, R. Berzins, A.R. Robblee and D.R. Clandinin, 1984. The entry rate of trimethylamine and its deposition in eggs of intact and cecectomized chickens fed rations containing rapeseed meal or supplementary choline. Poultry Sci. 63:139-143.

Erf, G.F., W.G. Bottje, T.K. Bersi, M.D. Headrick and C.A. Fritts, 1998. Effects of dietary vitamin E on the immune system in broilers: altered proportions of CD4T cells in the thymus and spleen. Poultry Sci. 77:529-537.

Evans, H.M. and K.S. Bishop, 1922. On the relation between fertility and nutrition. Am. J. Physiol. 63:396.

Evans, H.M. and G.O. I   r, 1926. A new dietary deficiency with highly purified diets. Proc. Soc. Exp. Biol. Mec. 24:740.

Evans, H.M., I.H. Emerson and G.A. Emerson, 1936. The isolation from wheat germ oil of an alcohol,α-tocopherol, having the properties of vitamin E. J. Biol. Chem. 113:319.

Farquhsarson, C., J.S. Rennie, N. Loveridge and C.C. Whitehead, 1993. Effect of ascorbic acid and I,25(OH)$_2$D$_3$ on bone cell metabolism in relation to the development of TD. Proc. WPSA Spring Mtg. Paper #23.

Fernholz, E., 1938. Constitution of alpha tocopherol. J. Am. Chem. Soc. 60:700

Freeman, B.M., 1967. Effect of stress on the ascorbic acid content of the adrenal gland of *gallus domesticus*. Comparative Biochem. Physiol. 23:303-309

Fridman, A., I. Bartov and D. Sklan, 1998. Humoral immune response impairment following excess vitamin E nutrition in the chick. Poultry Sci. 77:956-962.

Frigg, M., 1984. Studies of biotin deposition in hens' eggs. Proc. XVII WPSA. Helsinki. p 420- 421.

Fritz, J.C. et al. 1973. Toxicogenicity of moldy feed for young chicks. Poultry Sci. 52:1523-1530.

Froehli, D.M., 1987. Importance of folic acid in turkey diets explored. Feedstuffs. April 27 p 26.

Fuhrmann, H. and H.P. Sallmann, 1997. Unsaturated aldehydes in plasma, liver and brain of chickens in response to dietary vitamin E and fat type. Nutrition Res. 17:363-378.

Gadient, M., 1986. The effect of pelleting on the nutritional quality of feed. Proc. Maryland Nutr. Conf. p 73-78.

Garabedian, M., Tanaka, Y., Holick, M.F. and H.F. DeLuca, 1974. Response of intestinal calcium transport and bone calcium mobilization to dihydroxyvitamin D$_3$ in thyroparathyroidectomized rats. Endocrinology 94:1022-1027.

Goldstein, J. and M.L. Scott, 1956. An electrophoretic study of exudative diathesis in chicks. J. Nutr. 60:349.

Gonnerman, W.A., S.V. Toverud, W.K. Ramp and G.L. Mechanic, 1976. Effects of dietary vitamin D and calcium on lysyl oxidase activity in chick bone. Proc. Soc. Exp. Biol. Med. 151:453-456.

Goodridge, A.G., 1972. Regulation of acetyl CoA carboxylase by palmitoyl CoA. Federation Proc. 31:459.

Goodson-Williams, G., D.A. Roland and J.A. McQuire, 1987. Eggshell pimpling in young hens as influenced by dietary vitamin D$_3$. Poultry Sci. 66:1980-1986.

Gries, C.L. and M.L. Scott, 1972. The pathology of pyridoxine deficiency in chicks. J. Nutr. 102:1259.

Gries, C.L. and M.L. Scott, 1972. The pathologies of thiamin, riboflavin, pantothenic acid and niacin deficiencies in the chick. J. Nutr. 102:1269.

Griminger, P., 1984ab. Vitamin K in nutrition: deficiency can be fatal. Feedstuffs. Sept. 10 p 24:Sept 17 p 24.

Griminger, P. and G. Brubacher, 1966. The transfer of vitamin K$_1$ and menadione from the hen to the egg. Poultry Sci. 45:512.

Harms, R.H. and D.S. Nelson, 1992. A lack of response to pantothenic acid supplementation to a corn-soy broiler diet. Poultry Sci. 71:1952-1955.

Hoehler, D. and R.R. Marquardt, 1996. Influence of vitamins E and C on the toxic effects of ochratoxin and T-2 toxin in chicks. Poultry Sci. 75:1508-1515.

Holick, M.F., H.K. Schnoes and H.F. DeLuca, 1971. Identification of 1,25- dihydroxy-cholecalciferol, a form of vitamin D_3 metabolically active in the intestine. Proc. Nat. Acad. Sci. 68:803.

Hornig, M.P. and M. Frigg, 1979. Effects of age on biosynthesis of ascorbate in chicks. Archiv. Fur. Gefluegel. 43:108-112.

Jansen, B.C.P. and W.F. Donath, 1926. The isolation of the anti-berberi vitamin. Mededeel. Dienst. Volksgezondheid Nederl.-Indie, Part 1:186

Johnson, N.E., X.L. Qui, L.D. Gantz and E. Ross, 1995. Changes in dimensions and mechanical properties of bone in chicks fed high levels of niacin. Food and Chem. Toxicol. 33:265-271.

Jukes, T.H., 1940. Effect of choline and other supplements on perosis. J. Nutr. 20:445.

Jukes, T.H. and F.H. Bird, 1942. Prevention of perosis by biotin. Proc. Soc. Exp. Biol. Med. 49:231.

Karrer, P., R. Morf and K. Schöpp, 1931. Vitamin A from fish oils. Helv. Chim. Acta 14:1036; 1431.

Keane, K.W., R.A. Collins and M.B. Gillis, 1956. Isotopic tracer studies on the effect of vitamin D on calcium metabolism in the chick. Poultry Sci. 35:1216.

Koch, E.M. and F.C. Koch, 1941. The provitamin D of the covering tissues of chickens. Poultry Sci. 20:33.

Kohane, J., Z. Okonowski and E. Cuperstein, 1960. Field cases of vitamin K deficiency in day- old chicks. Refuah Vet. 17:216.

Kratzer, F.H., H.J. Almquist and P. Vohra, 1996. Effect of diet on growth and plasma ascorbic acid in chicks. Poultry Sci. 75:82-89.

Kutulu, H.R. and J.M. Forbes, 1994. Self-selection for ascorbic acid by broiler chicks in response to changing environmental temperature. Br. Poultry Sci 35:820-821.

Leeson. S. and J.D. Summers, 1997. Commercial Poultry Nutrition - 2nd Ed Publ. University Books, Guelph, Ontario.

Lessard, M., D. Hutchings and N. Cave, 1997. Cell mediated and humoral immune responses in broiler chickens maintained on diets containing different levels of vitamin A. Poultry Sci. 76:1368-1378.

Loosli, J.K., 1988. *In* Animal Science Handbook, CRC Press, Boca Raton, FL.

Machlin, L.J. and R.S. Gordon, 1960. The requirement of the chicken for certain unsaturated fatty acids. Poultry Sci. 39:1271.

Manoukas, A.G., R.C. Ringrose and A.E. Teera, 1968. The availability of niacin in corn, soybean meal and wheat middlings for the hen. Poultry Sci. 47: 1836-1842.

Maragondakis, M.E., H. Hankin and J.M. Wasvary, 1972. Acetyl coenzyme A carboxylase inhibition in genetically obese mice. Federation Proc. 31:475 Abs.

March, B.E., 1981. Choline supplementation of layer diets containing soybean meal or rapeseed meal as protein supplement. Poultry Sci. 60:818.

March, B.E. and C. MacMillan, 1990. Linoleic acid as a modulator of egg size. Poultry Sci. 69:634-639.

Marsh, J.A., G.F. Combs, M.E. Whitacre and R.R. Dietert, 1986. Effect of selenium and vitamin E dietary deficiencies on chick lymphoid organ development. Proc. Soc. Exp. Biol. Med. 182:425-436.

Masse, P.G. et al., 1994. Vitamin B_6 deficiency:experimentally induced bone and joint disorder. Br. J. Nutr. 71:919-932.

Maxwell, M.H., C.C. Whitehead and J. Armstrong, 1988. Haematological and tissue abnormalities in chicks caused by acute and subclinical folate deficiency. Br. J. Nutr. 59:73-80.

McCormick, D.B. and R.E. Olson, 1984. *In* Nutrition Reviews, Present Knowledge in Nutrition. Publ. Nutr. Foundation Washington, D.C.

McDowell, L.R., 1989. Vitamins in Animal Nutrition. Publ. Academic Press, N.Y.

McGinnis, J., L.C. Norris and G.F. Heuser, 1944. Influence of diet on chick growth-promoting and antiperotic properties of betaine, methionine and choline. Proc. Soc. Exp. Biol. Med. 56:197.

Mckee, J.S. and .P.C. Harrison, 1995. Effects of supplemental ascorbic acid on the performance of broiler chickens exposed to multiple concurrent stressors. Poultry Sci. 74:1772-1785.

Mehansho, H., and L.M. Henderson, 1980. Transport and accumulation of pyridoxine and pyridoxal by erythrocytes. J. Biol. Chem. 255:119001-11907.

Molitoris, B.A. and D.H. Baker, 1976. Assessment of the quantity and biologically available choline in soybean meal. J. Anim. Sci. 42: 481-489.

Morrow, G., L.A. Barnes, V.H. Auerback, A.M. DiGeorge, T. Ando and W.L. Nyhan, 1969. Observations on the coexistence of methylamalonic acidemia and glycinemia. J. Pediatr. 74:680.

Nesheim, M.C. and M.L. Scott, 1958. Studies on the nutritive effects of selenium for chicks. J. Nutr. 65:601.

Nockels, C.F., D.L. Menge and E.W. Kienholz, 1976. Effect of excessive dietary vitamin E on the chick. Poultry Sci. 55:649-652.

Noguchi, T., A.H. Cantor and M.L. Scott, 1973. Mode of action of selenium and vitamin E in prevention of exudative diathesis in chicks. J. Nutr. 103:1502.

Norris, L.C. and A.T. Ringrose, 1930. The occurrence of a pellagrous-like syndrome in chicks. Science 71:643.

O'Rowski, A.A. and H.L. Classen, 1998. The study of riboflavin requirement in broiler chickens. Int. J. Vit. Nutr. Res. 68:316-327.

Oduho, G.W. and D.H. Baker, 1993. Quantitative efficacy of niacin sources for chicks: Nicotinic acid, nicotinamide, and tryptophan. J. Nutr. 1323:2201-2206.

Olcese, O., J.R. Couch, J.H. Quisenberry and P.B. Pearson, 1950. Congenital anomalies in the chick due to vitamin B_{12} deficiency. J. Nutr. 41:423.

Olkowski, A.A. and H.L. Classen, 1996. The study of thiamine requirement in broiler chickens. Int. J. Vit. Nutr. Res. 66:332-341.

Olkowski, A.A. and H.L. Classen, 1998. The study of riboflavin requirement of broiler chickens. Int. J. Vit. Nutr. 68: 316-327.

Olkowski, A.A. and H.L. Classen, 1999. The effects of maternal thiamine nutrition on thiamine status of the offspring in broiler chickens. Int. J. Vit. Nutr. Res. 69:32-40.

Pardue, S.L. and J.P. Thaxton, 1986. Ascorbic acid in poultry: A review. Wld. Poultry Sci. J. 42:107-123.

Patel, M.B. and J. McGinnis, 1980. The effect of vitamin B_{12} on the tolerance of chicks for high levels of dietary fat and carbohydrate. Poultry Sci. 59:2279.

Reinhardt, T.A. and F.G. Hustmyer, 1987. Role of vitamin D on the immune system. J. Dairy Sci. 70:952-962.

Reiser, R., 1950. The essential role of fatty acids in rations for growing chicks. J. Nutr. 42:319.

Robel, E.J., 1983. The effect of age of breeder hen on the levels of vitamins and minerals in turkey eggs. Poultry Sci. 62: 1751-1756.

Rotruck, J.T., et al., 1973. Selenium: biochemical role as a component of glutathione perioxidase. Science 179:588.

Rennie, J.S., C.C. Whitehead and J. Armstrong, 1993. Biochemical response of broiler chicks to folate deficiency. Br. J. Nutr. 69:801-808.

Ruiz N. and R.H. Harms, 1988. Riboflavin requirement of broiler chicks fed a corn-soybean diet. Poultry Sci. 67:794-799.

Ruiz, N. and R.H. Harms, 1988. Comparison of the biopotencies of nicotinic acid and nicotinamide for broiler chicks. Br. Poultry Sci. 29:491-498.

Ruiz, N. and R.H. Harms, 1990. The lack of response of broiler chickens to supplemental niacin when fed a corn-soybean meal diet from 3-7 weeks of age. Poultry Sci. 69:2231-2234.

Ruiz, N, R.D. Miles and R.H. Harms, 1983. Choline, methione and sulfate interrelationships in poultry nutrition. Wld. Poultry Sci. J. 39:185-198.

Ryu, K.S., K.D. Roberson, G.M. Pesti and R.R. Eitenmiller, 1995. The folic acid requirement of starting broiler chicks fed diets based on practical ingredients. Poultry Sci. 74:1447-1455.

Saroka, J.M. and G.F. Combs, 1986. The lack of effect of a pyridoxine deficiency on the utilization of the hydroxyl analogue of methionine by the chick. Poultry Sci. 65:764-768.

Schønheyder, F., 1935. The anti-hemorrhagic vitamin of the chick. Nature 135:653.

Schwarz, K. and C.M. Foltz, 1957. Selenium as an integral part of factor 3 against dietary liver degeneration. J. Am. Chem. Soc. 79:3292.

Scott, M.L., J.G. Bieri, G.M. Briggs and K. Schwarz, 1957. Prevention of exudative diathesis by Factor 3 in chicks on vitamin E-deficient Torula yeast diets. Poultry Sci. 36:1155 (abstract).

Sheehy, P.J.A., P.A. Morrissey and D. J. Buckley, 1997. Advances in research and application of vitamin E as an antioxidant for poultry meat. Proc. XII European Symposium on Quality of Poultry Meat. P 425-436.

Shen, H., J.D. Summers and S. Leeson, 1981. Egg production and shell quality of layers fed various levels of vitamin D_3. Poultry Sci. 60:1485-1490.

Siegel, H.S., 1971. Adrenals, stress and the environment. Wld. Poultry Sci. J. 27:327-335.

Sklan, D., D. Melamed and A. Friedman, 1994. The effect of varying levels of dietary vitamin A on immune response in the chick. Poultry Sci. 73:843-847.

Soares, J.H. and M.A. Ottinger, 1988. Potential role of $1, 25 (OH)_2$ in eggshell calcification. Poultry Sci. 67:1322-1328.

Soares, J.H., Jr., M.R. Swerdel and E.H. Bossard, 1978. Phosphorus availability. 1. The effect of chick age and vitamin D metabolites on the availability of phosphorus in defluorinated phosphate. Poultry Sci. 57:1305.

Søndergaard, E., M.L. Scott and H. Dam, 1962. Effects of ubiquinones and phytylubichromenol upon encephalomalacia and muscular dystrophy in the chick. J. Nutr. 78:15.

Sonneborn, D.W. and H.J. Hansen, 1970. Vitamin B_{12} binders of chicken serum and chicken proventriculus are immunologically similar. Science 168:591.

Squires, M.W. and E.C. Naber, 1992. Vitamin profiles of eggs as indicators of nutritional status in the laying hen: Vitamin B_{12} study. Poultry Sci. 71:2075-2082.

Squires, M.W. and E.C. Naber, 1993. Vitamin profiles of eggs as indicators of nutritional status in the laying hen: Vitamin A study. Poultry Sci. 72:154-164.

Squires, M.W. and E.C. Naber, 1993. Vitamin profiles of eggs as indicators of nutritional status in the laying hen. Riboflavin study. Poultry Sci. 72:483-494.

Stoewsand, G.S. and M.L. Scott, 1964. Influence of high protein diets on vitamin A metabolism and adrenal hypertrophy in the chick. J. Nutr. 82:139.

Stokstad, E.L.R., E.L. Patterson and R. Milstrey, 1957. Factors which prevent exudative diathesis in chicks on Torula Yeast diets. Poultry Sci. 36:1160.

Surai, P.F., R.C. Noble and B.K. Speake, 1999. Relationship between vitamin E content and susceptibility to lipid peroxidation in tissues of the newly hatched chick. Br. Poultry Sci. 40:406-410.

Suttie, J.W., 1980. The metabolic role of vitamin K. Fed. Proc. 39:2730.

Thornton, P.A. and J.V. Shutze, 1960. The influence of dietary energy level, energy source and breed on the thiamine requirement of chicks. Poultry Sci. 39:192.

Veltmann, J.R., L.S. Jensen and G.N. Rowland, 1986. Excess dietary vitamin A in the growing chick. Effect of fat source and vitamin D. Poultry Sci. 65:153-163.

Waldroup, P.W. et al., 1985. The effects of increased levels of niacin supplementation on growth rate and carcass composition of broiler chickens. Poultry Sci. 64:1777-1784.

Ward, N.E., J.E. Jones and D.V. Maurice, 1986. Vitamin B_{12} nutrition of chickens fed raw soybean meal. Poultry Sci. 65:106-113.

Wasserman, R.H., A.N. Taylor and F.A. Kallefelz, 1966. Vitamin D and transfer of plasma calcium to intestinal lumen in chicks and rats. Am. J. Physiol. 211:419.

Weis, F.G., 1976. An investigation of the role of fiber, kilocalories and vitamin B_6 on serum and egg cholesterol, body parameters and reproduction in the laying hen. M.Sc. Thesis, Cornell Univ.

White, H.B., 1998. Sudden Death of chickens embryos with hereditary riboflavin deficiency. J. Nutr. 126:13035-13075.

White, H.B. and A.R. Hughes, 1981. Biotin-binding proteins in chicken eggs and biotin requirements of chicken embryos. Poultry Sci. 60:1454.

Whitehead, C.C., 1995. Biotin in Adult Poultry. Publ. Roche Animal Nutr. #2036.

Whitehead, C.C., R. Blair, D.W. Bannister, A.J. Evans, W.G. Siller and R. Morley-Jones, 1976. The involvement of biotin in preventing the FLKS in chicks. Res. Vet. Sci. 20:180-184.

Whitehead, C.C., J.S. Rennie and M. Frigg, 1995. Folic acid requirements of broilers. Br. Poult. Sci. 36:113-121.

Williams, R.R. and J.K. Cline, 1936. Synthesis of vitamin B_1. J. Am. Chem. Soc. 58:1504.

Windaus, A., H. Lettré and F. Schenck, 1935. 7-Dehydrocholesterol. Ann. 520:98

Wolbach, S.B. and D.M. Hegsted. 1952. Vitamin A deficiency in the duck. Skeletal growth and central nervous system. Arch. Pathol. 54:548.

Woollam, D.H.M. and J.W. Millen, 1955. Effect of vitamin A deficiency on the cerebrospinal fluid pressure of the chick. Nature 175:41.

Wostman, B.S. and P.L. Knight, 1965. Antagonism between vitamins A and K in the germfree rat. J. Nutr. 87:155.

Xu, T., R.M. Leach, B. Hollis and J.H. Soares. 1997. Evidence of increased cholecalciferal requirement in chicks with TD. Poultry Sci. 76:47-53.

Young, R.J., L.C. Norris and G.F. Heuser, 1955. The chick's requirement for folic acid in the utilization of choline and its precursors betaine and methylaminoethanol. J. Nutr. 55:353.

Minerals

Most of our knowledge about the metabolism and essentiality of minerals has occurred over the last 100 years. In the early 1900's it was realized that there was a constant ash component of most tissues and that fasting animals quickly went into negative sodium balance. Subsequent studies outlined daily needs for calcium and iron in humans.

Up to the early 1950's 13 minerals had been identified as essential; these being the major elements calcium, phosphorus, potassium, sodium, chlorine, sulfur and magnesium, and the trace micro elements; iron, iodine, copper, manganese, zinc and cobalt. By 1959, molybdenum, selenium and chromium had been added to this list. Since that time, additional trace elements such as nickel, fluorine, silicon, vanadium, tin, and arsenic, have also been added to the list of essential minerals. Classification of minerals as major or trace elements depends upon their concentration in the body. Those minerals which are of particular nutritional importance along with their approximate concentrations in the body of the chick, are shown in Table 5.1.

TABLE 5.1 Comparison of body minerals with diet levels commonly fed to chicks.		
	Body content per kg fat free mass	Diet inclusion per kg
Na (g)	1.2	1.8
K (g)	2.0	7.0
Cl (g)	0.7	2.2
Ca (g)	4.0	10
P (g)	3.4	5
Mg (g)	0.2	-
Mn (g)	0.1	.07
Fe (mg)	40	80
Cu (mg)	1.5	10
Zn (mg)	30	60
I (mg)	0.3	0.4
Se (mg)	0.2	0.3

5.1 GENERAL MINERAL METABOLISM AND INTERACTION

All of the essential minerals are known to have at least one or more catalytic function in cells. Some minerals are bound to the protein of enzymes, while others are present in prosthetic groups as chelates, which are compounds formed between an organic molecule and a metallic ion held within the organic molecule as if by a claw.

Elements such as Na^+, K^+ and Cl^-, have primarily an electrochemical function to maintain acid-base balance as well as osmotic control of water distribution in the body (Mongin, 1968; Hurwitz et al., 1973; Sauveur and Mongin, 1978). Other elements such as the cations Ca^{++}, Mg^{++}, and anions, SO_4^-, PO_4^-, also play a significant role in the acid-base status of an animal. The appropriate dietary balance of these electrolytes is usually assessed by the level of the cations versus the anions, where an imbalance can have an acidic or alkaline type effect. One of the problems in trying to calculate a cation: anion balance, is the marked difference in absorption between the various naturally occurring minerals and dietary mineral supplements. Thus, calculating a dietary balance may not be close to what the body receives as a supply of cations and anions.

Calcium and phosphorus have structural roles as essential components of the skeleton, while sulfur plays a role in the structural synthesis of proteins. Magnesium functions structurally, electrochemically, and catalytically. Other elements have unique functions such as iron, which is an essential part of the heme molecule, necessary for the haemochromagens, which are important in respiration. Cobalt is a component of vitamin B_{12}, while iodine forms part of the hormone thyroxin.

Some elements such as calcium and molybdenum can interfere with the absorption and activity of other minerals. The interaction of minerals with each other is an important factor in animal nutrition, because an imbalance of minerals, as distinct from a simply deficiency, is important in diagnosing certain nutritional disorders. Also a number of minerals can be toxic if intake is excessive. This is particularly true of copper, selenium, fluorine, vanadium and arsenic. Copper and fluorine are cumulative poisons, the bird not being able to effectively excrete them and so over time a build up in the tissues results in toxicity. The interaction between minerals at sites of absorption, transport and metabolism creates an added complexity to their study as essential nutrients. Some, but not all, of the important potential interactions between minerals are shown in Figure 5.1. Many minerals are therefore influenced by interaction with 2-6 other major minerals.

A number of elements, including fluoride, nickel, silicon, tin, vanadium and chromium, have been shown to produce important beneficial effects in the animal body, but have not yet been classified, as nutritionally essential. Cadmium and vanadium belong to a special category because of their detrimental effects, yet they do not quite belong to the group of obviously toxic elements such as lead, arsenic, beryllium and tungsten. Many important interrelationships exist among the various inorganic elements and also among these elements with vitamins, amino acids, and other nutrients.

Of the thirteen essential inorganic elements, eight are cations. These are calcium (Ca^{++}), sodium (Na^+), potassium (K^+), magnesium (Mg^{++}), manganese (Mn^{++}), zinc (Zn^{++}), iron (Fe^{++}) and copper (Cu^{++}). Five minerals are either anions

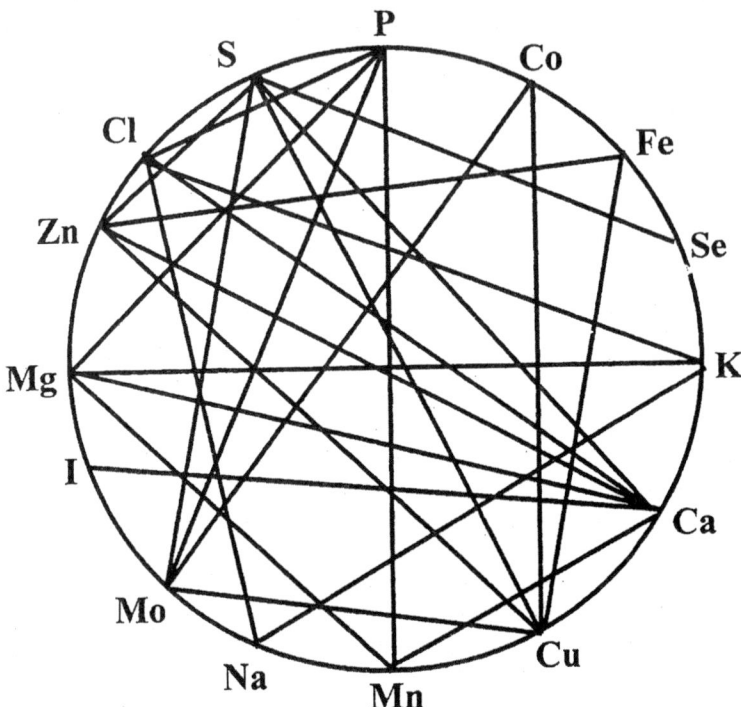

Figure 5.1 Mineral interrelationships

or are usually found in anionic groupings. Theses are chloride (Cl⁻), iodide (I⁻), phosphate (PO_4^-), molybdate ($MoO_4^=$) and selenite ($SeO_3^=$). It appears quite likely that under natural conditions selenium is supplied mainly in its organic form as seleno-methionine.

Numerous factors may alter the availability of the essential anions and cations. The most soluble and therefore most absorbable form of any of the essential elements should be the simple ionic state of the atom or ionic group of atoms (for example, as Ca^{++}, Mg^{++}, Mn^{++}) However, many electronegative compounds in nature are looking for a cation with which it can share its electrons, thereby forming a stable compound. Often the resultant compound is highly insoluble in water but nevertheless dissociates to a sufficient extent in the intestinal tract to allow absorption of the essential cation. This is usually brought about by the influence of the gastric acidity of hydrochloric acid in the stomach, which converts the cations temporarily into chloride salts, which for all essential cations have a considerable degree of ionic dissociation and therefore good absorption from the intestinal tract. Thus even copper sulfide, manganese oxide or zinc oxide, which are highly insoluble chemical compounds, are converted to copper chloride, manganese chloride or zinc chloride by the action of the hydrochloric acid in the proventriculus. This allows absorption of much of the copper, manganese and zinc even when consumed in the form of highly insoluble compounds. Absorbability of such anionic groups as phosphate depend upon the crystal structure, total amount in the diet and the ratio of calcium to phosphate.

Soon after the discovery that manganese was required for prevention of perosis in chicks, studies were undertaken to determine the effects of various manganese compounds and modes of administration of the element upon the requirements for prevention of perosis. It was found that the amount of dietary manganese required by the chick is approximately 25-50 times that needed if the element is administered in soluble form by injection. Studies were conducted to determine the reason why a very high level of manganese is needed in the diet to provide the relatively small needs for metabolism. These studies showed that one thing which interferes with manganese absorption, is the presence in the diet of excess calcium and phosphorus. After becoming solubilized by the gastric acidity and then entering the alkaline environments of the duodenum, excess calcium and phosphorus reforms in a flocculent precipitate of calcium phosphate. This adsorbs manganese and carries it through the intestinal tract, thereby creating a manganese deficiency unless the dietary level of manganese is in excess of that removed by the calcium-phosphate precipitate. Other recent studies using high levels of calcium in the diet show markedly increased zinc requirement. It is likely that zinc is also adsorbed on insoluble calcium-phosphate precipitates in the intestinal tract.

Colloids such as particles of clay, insoluble salts of aluminum, magnesium, iron and other elements, are strongly adsorptive of cations, and this adsorption occurs both through chemical union with highly electro-negative areas of the colloid surface and through attraction of the cation by physical forces (such as occurs in adsorption of elements by charcoal).

In most common feed ingredients such as corn and soybean meal, availability of most nutritionally important minerals, is around 50-70%. The main site of mineral absorption is the lower duodenum through to the upper jejunum. Some sodium will be absorbed in the ileum and even the rectum.

5.2 ORGANIC CHELATES

It is now recognized that organic chelates of minerals are important factors influencing absorption of these elements. The ideal chelating compound is one that will release the mineral in the ionic form at the intestinal wall, or that can be absorbed as the intact chelate. Such a chelate may markedly enhance the absorption of a mineral by preventing its conversion to an insoluble chemical compound in the intestine, or by preventing its strong adsorption on an insoluble colloid.

Unlike the high energy covalent bonding, which normally binds atoms together, a metal chelate is formed as a ring structure, resulting from the attraction between positive charges of certain polyvalent cations, at any two or more sites of high electronegativity in a chemical compound. The bonds are referred to as coordinate bonds.

The word chelate comes from the Greek word chele meaning claw, which is an appropriate term for the manner in which the polyvalent cations are held by the metal binding agents. The organic substances which bind to the metal are called ligands. Some chelates hold the metal so firmly that the metal can become almost completely unavailable to either plants or animals (e.g. phosphorus in phytic acid). However, many chelates are highly absorptive and protect the mineral from forming an insoluble complex. This type of chelate is referred to as a sequestering agent.

Three types of chelates are recognized in biological systems:

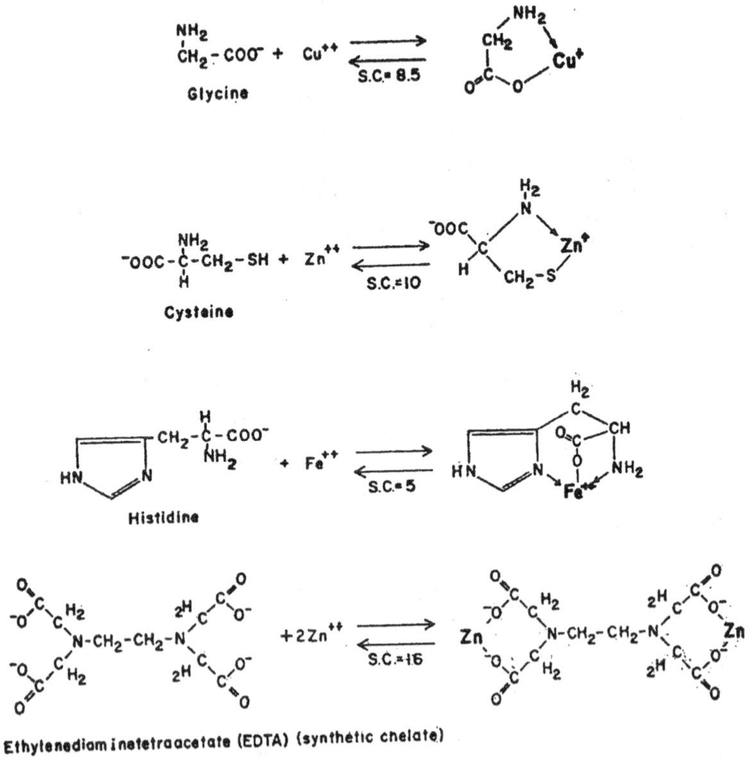

Figure 5.2 Group I. chelates. Chelates which serve to transport and to store metal ions. S.C.–Stability constant.

Group I   Chelates that serve to transport and to store metal ions. With this type of chelate the metal requires a ligand with such chemical and physical properties that the chelate is able to be absorbed, transported in the blood stream, and pass across cell membranes, where the metal ion is deposited at the site where needed:

eg: Amino acids, especially cysteine and histidine, are effective metal binding agents and may be of primary importance in the transport and storage of minerals throughout the body;

eg: Ethylenediaminetetraacetic acid (EDTA) and similar synthetic ligands, are known to improve the availability of zinc as well as other minerals. These chelates are used in medicine to hasten excretion of heavy metals, like lead, from patients poisoned with such compounds.

Examples of the above type of chelates are shown in Figure 5.2.

Group II   These chelates are essential in metabolism. A number of chelates exist in the body in a structure in which the metal ion is present in a chelate form, which is required for it to perform its metabolic function. Hemoglobin, the cytochrome enzymes and vitamin B_{12} are examples. Structure of the heme portion of hemoglobin and cytochrome-c is shown in Figure 5.3

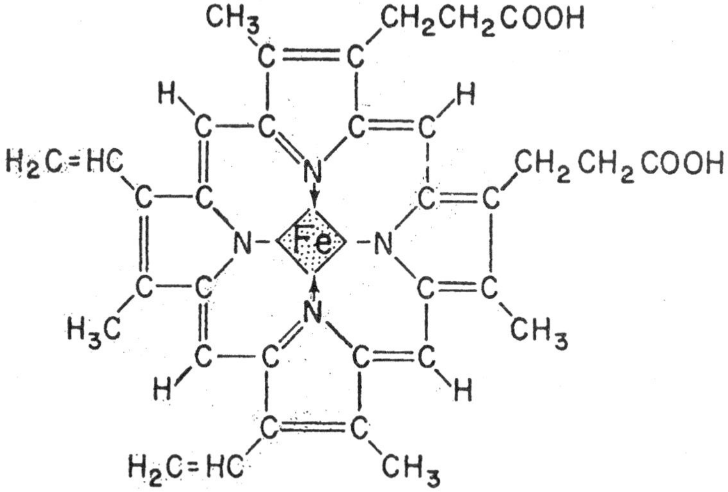

Figure 5.3 Group II chelates. Heme, the chelate portion of hemoglobin, and the cytochromes.

Group III   Chelates, which interfere with utilization of essential cations. Some metal chelates are probably formed by accident and have no biological purpose or value. Chelates such as the phytic acid-zinc chelate, may interfere with normal metabolism by rendering an essential mineral unavailable for its needed metabolic function. Examples of such chelates are shown in Figure 5.4

The affinity of a chelate for a metal ion may be expressed quantitatively as a stability constant. The general (1:1) interaction between a chelating agent or ligand (L) and a cation (M^{++}) may be expressed as $L + M^{++} \leftrightarrow MC$ where C is the constant.

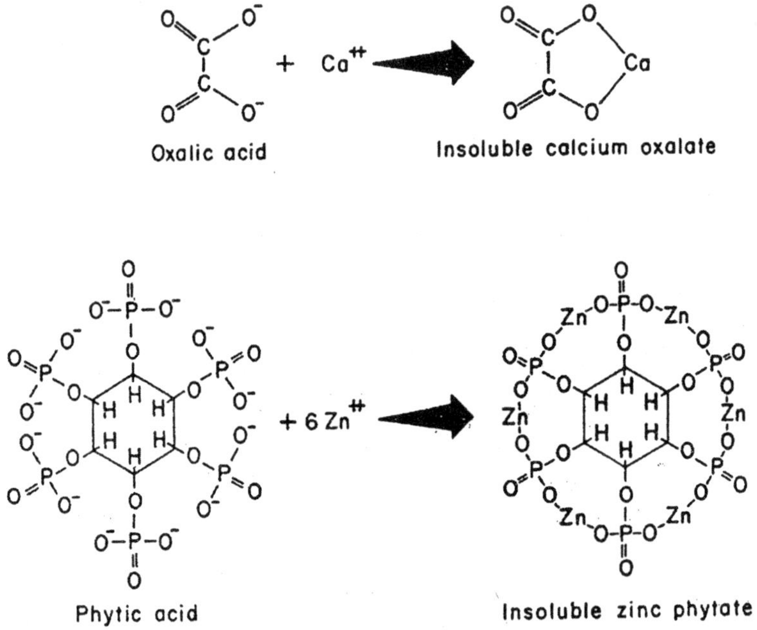

Oxalic acid   Insoluble calcium oxalate

Phytic acid   Insoluble zinc phytate

Figure 5.4 Group III chelates. Chelates which interfere with absorption of certain cations.

The equilibrium constant K, for the formation of these chelates, may be expressed mathematically as follows:

$$K_f = \frac{[MC]}{[M^{++}][L]}$$

K_f thus represents the number of moles of chelated metal ion in relation to the product of the number of moles of metal ion and of ligand remaining in free state in the system. The log K_f is the stability constant.

The stability constants presented in Table 5.2 show that with a wide variety of ligands, the stability of the chelates formed with copper are greatest and that with each ligand, the stability of the chelate ranges in decreasing order for copper, nickel, zinc, cobalt, iron, manganese and magnesium respectively.

TABLE 5.2 Stability constants (log K_t) of some common chelates (1:1 ratios of ligand: metal ion in H_2O at 20°C)							
Ligand	Cu++	Ni++	Zn++	Co++	Fe++	Mn++	Mg++
Glycine	8.5	6	5	5	4	3	2
Cysteine	*	10	10	**	6	4	4
Histidine	10.5	9	7	7	5	4	4
Histamine	10	7	5	5	4	?	?
Ethylenediamine	11	8	6	6	4	3	?
Ethylenediaminetetraacetate (EDTA)	19	18	16	16	14	13.5	9
Guanosine	6	4	4.5	3	4	3	?
Oxalic acid	6	5.5	5	4.5	4.5	4	3
Salicylic acid	11	7	7	7	6	6	?
Tetracycline	8	6	5	5	5	4	4

*Cysteine is decomposed by copper
** Cobalt-cysteine chelate is formed but only with 3:1 ratio of cobalt:cysteine, whereupon Stability constant is 16 [Albert, A., 1962. Federation Proc. 20(3):137]

The metal ion having a higher stability constant theoretically can replace a metal ion of lower stability constant in a chelate or at least the chelate with the higher stability constant will be formed before that of a lower constant. With a higher level of copper in the diet this element may replace the ions having lower stability constants, such as zinc, iron or manganese, in chelates of these metal ions. The very high stability constants for EDTA with all of the mineral elements shown above clearly demonstrate the reason that EDTA can so successfully act as a metal scavenger and, when present in a system in adequate concentration, pick up all of the polyvalent transition cations even in competition with most other chelating agents.

Kratzer et al. (1959), found that the availability of zinc in soybean meal for the chick, was markedly improved by adding EDTA to the diet. Other workers confirmed Kratzer's finding and also showed that there were a number of natural chelates which improved zinc utilization for the chick. Zinc chelates with stability constants of 15 to 16 are optimum for maximum utilization of zinc. In comparing the effects upon zinc utilization in chicks of EDTA, and a variety of other chelating agents having higher and lower stability constants, Kratzer and associates obtained the results presented in Figure 5.5. Chelating agents with zinc stability constants below 11 produced very little improvement in zinc utilization, probably because they did not compete with phytic acid and other substances in the intestinal tract. Kratzer, in studying how EDTA functioned, demonstrated that its chelate is absorbed from the intestine and metabolized by the bird. Thus, like Group 1 chelates, it acts as a carrier for the polyvalent transition trace minerals. It was shown in *in vitro* studies that maturing reticulocytes produced hemoglobin much more rapidly if the medium contained EDTA or other metal binding agents, thus indicating that the chelating agents were functioning in passing the metal ions across cell walls.

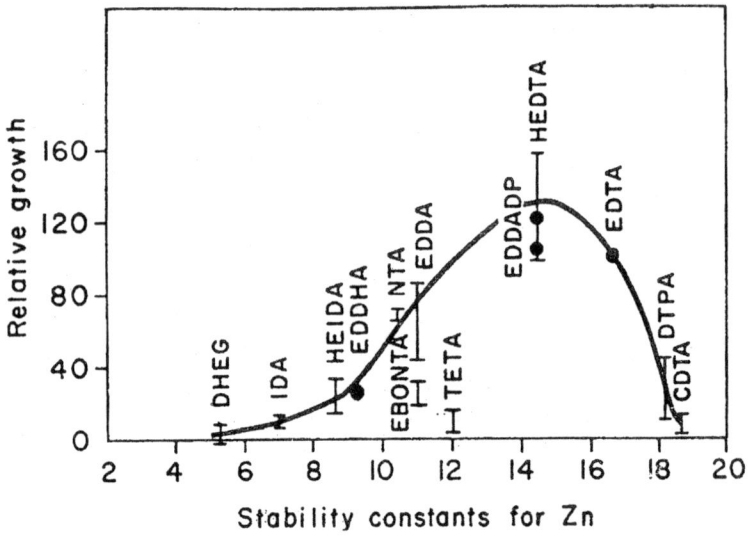

Figure 5.5 The relative growth of chicks fed chelating compounds with a range of zinc stability constants. (From Vohra and Kratzer, 1964).

It is obvious that chelates are important in regulation of many reactions that we now take for granted. An example would be the function of calcium and phosphorus needed by the osteoblasts for bone deposition. These minerals must be presented at the site of deposition in a ratio of two parts calcium to one part phosphorus. If these minerals were transported to the deposition site in this ratio as inorganic elements, at the blood pH of 7.3, calcium phosphate would precipitate. It is known that the parathyroid hormone regulates the amount of soluble calcium in the blood, which is influenced to some extent by the phosphorus content of the blood.

It is also known that some antibiotics form chelates with calcium and other polyvalent cations. Diets high in calcium are known to interfere with the antimicrobial activity of antibiotics. Simple amino acids, peptides, and perhaps whole proteins may have important chelating functions in the body. The reaction compounds formed between sugars and lysine, which render the lysine unavailable for incorporation into tissue proteins, may serve a useful purpose since this type of sugar-amino acid compound is an excellent chelating agent.

5.3 CALCIUM

5.3.1 Calcium, phosphorus and vitamin D₃.

Calcium and phosphorus are often discussed together as they are closely related in metabolism, especially in bone formation. In the growing chicken the major portion of calcium in the diet is used for bone formation while for the laying hen, the major portion is used for eggshell synthesis. Calcium is also important for blood clotting and is required along with potassium and sodium for normal heart rhythm, as well as playing a role in acid-base balance in the body. Phosphorus also plays an important role in bone formation, but has other very important functions in the metabolism of carbohydrates and fats. It enters into the composition of important constituents of all living cells, and the salts formed from it play an important role in acid-base balance.

The nutritional requirements and interrelationships of calcium, phosphorus and vitamin D_3 were shown to be closely interrelated in the formation of bone. Not only were particular dietary levels of calcium and phosphorus required but also the proper ratio of one to the other was considered extremely important. Wilgus, (1931) reported that the available phosphorus requirement was 0.5%, while the ratio of calcium to phosphorus for the growing chick, was between 1.0:1 and 2.2:1. A ratio of 2.5:1 appeared borderline, while a ratio of 3.3:1 was found to produce a high incidence of rickets and leg abnormalities.

As previously described in Chapter 4, vitamin D_3 is essential for intestinal uptake and subsequent metabolism of calcium. Unless otherwise stated, the following discussion assumes an adequate vitamin D_3 status in the bird.

5.3.2 Calcium metabolism

Calcium is the most abundant mineral in the body with 97% of it found in bone. It is also an essential constituent of all living cells and extracellular fluids. It is required for activity of a number of enzyme systems including those necessary for the transmission of nerve impulses and the contractile properties of muscle.

A dietary deficiency of calcium can result in:

a) growth retardation

b) decreased feed intake

c) increased basal metabolic rate

d) reduced activity and sensitivity

e) rickets or osteoporosis

f) abnormal posture and gait

g) susceptibility to internal hemorrhages

h) increased urine volume

i) reduced life span

j) reduced egg production and thin shells

k) tetany

Chemical changes noted are a rapid reduction in serum calcium level with losses of calcium and magnesium from the body. Bones of deficient animals are markedly demineralized with ash and calcium contents reduced to about half normal levels.

Calcium levels in the body are regulated by parathyroid hormone and calcitonin. With low levels of plasma calcium, parathyroid hormone stimulates mobilization of bone calcium and an increase in kidney resorption. Parathyroid hormone also stimulates the production of $1, 25 (OH)_2 D_3$ in the kidney, which further enhances kidney resorption of calcium, as well as increased calcium uptake from the intestine. Low plasma phosphorus also induces $1, 25 (OH)_2 D_3$ production with greater bone mobilization. However, in this situation, there is increased calcium loss by the kidneys and so calcium deficiency can be induced.

Calcitonin has the opposite effect to that of parathyroid hormone, although results are not always as clearly defined compared to its effect in mammals. Calcitonin inhibits bone resorption, the target cells being osteoclasts. Within minutes of administering calcitonin osteoclastic activity ceases. Calcitonin is produced in significant amounts in mammalian thyroid glands (Bussolati and Pearse, 1967). In most other vertebrates, including birds, the secretory cells are found in small glands in the neck called ultimobranchial bodies, which are separate from the thyroid glands. In mammals, calcitonin causes a reduction in blood calcium by arresting the calcium absorption from bone. Bélanger and Copp (1972) found that the inhibition of bone resorption is due to decreased osteocytic activity. However, the precise role of the ultimobranchial bodies and of calcitonin on calcium metabolism in birds is a matter of controversy (Copp, 1970; Brown et al., 1970).

Calcium exists in plasma as both bound and ionized forms. The level of serum proteins is a major determinant to the quantity of bound calcium, although parathyroid hormone and vitamin D_3 tend to also influence this balance. Some plasma calcium is chelated, mainly with citrate and phosphate. Table 5.3 shows levels of total and ionized plasma calcium in immature and mature birds. There is a characteristic increase in total calcium level at onset of maturity, associated with shell calcification.

TABLE 5.3 Plasma calcium and phosphorus levels of pullets at various ages			
Age	Total plasma calcium	Ionized plasma calcium	Plasma inorganic phosphorus
Weeks	(mg %)		
2	8.62	4.00	5.44
18	9.72	4.87	4.51
25	27.45[1]	6.60	1.91

[1]A White Leghorn strain with significantly lower eggshell breaking strength also had a significantly lower total plasma calcium at the onset of egg production (Combs, *et al.*, 1979).

Calcium is also important for muscular contractions brought about by interaction between myosin and actin components of muscle. Actin and myosin are restrained from interaction by maintenance of a low cytosol calcium level. In a non-active muscle the calcium is stored in the sarcoplasmic reticulum. The Ca^{++} cystol concentration is maintained at less than 1 μm. Nerve impulse causes release of Ca^{++} leading to levels of 10 μm, which initiates muscle contraction. The intermediate messengers responsible for Ca^{++} transport are tropin and tropomyosin. However, the most important nutritional roles of calcium are bone modeling and eggshell formation.

5.3.3 Bone modeling - structure of bone

Calcium constitutes almost one third of the weight of fat-free dried bone. While bone is composed largely of calcium phosphate, it also contains approximately 13% calcium carbonate, 2% magnesium phosphate, and 5% of other substances with 0.5 - 3% present as citrates. Fluoride deposition is most rapid in bones where metabolic activity is greatest. At low levels fluoride may be an important if not essential component of bone. Excess fluoride produces osteosclerosis, the first signs of which appear in the vertebrae.

The crystal lattice of the phosphate of bone is comparable to that of apatitic calcium phosphate, of which hydroxyapatite is the best known mineralogical example. Studies on synthetic and biological hydroxyapatites have indicated that the apatite portion of bone mineral does not contain the ideal stoichiometry, $Ca_{10}(PO_4)_6(OH)_2$, but instead is approximately 10% deficient in calcium. Infrared studies indicate that the missing electronic charge in the calcium deficient apatites is made up by hydrogen bonding between orthophosphate ions in sufficient quantity to achieve neutrality. When bone apatites are heated to temperatures between 300° to 600°C there is a condensation of some orthophosphate ions to pyrophosphate. Since the pyrophosphate produced by heat is a result of dehydration and condensation of hydrogen connected phosphate groups, this change can be taken as a measure of the non-stoichiometry of the mineral. Immature bone yields more heat producible pyrophosphate than does mature bone.

New bone is formed by initial deposition of an organic matrix, which is predominantly collagen fibrils. In some nutritional deficiency situations, such as tibial dyschondroplasia, the collagen fibrils fail to become mineralized, and so bones are soft and/or grow in unusual directions. Both calcium and phosphorus are transported to the active growth plate, and need to be in such a concentration as to precipitate crystals of hydroxyapatite. Osteoblasts participate in bone formation (ossification) and are seen at the surface of the organic matrix or already deposited bone surface. The deposition of mineral into the collagen and mucopolysaccharide organic precursor, is directly controlled by the osteoblastic activity. Osteoclasts on the other hand are responsible for the removal of inorganic bone material. Unlike osteoblasts, osteoclasts are multinucleated, leading to the supposition that they are derived from aggregations of osteoblasts. Osteoblastic and osteoclastic activity can occur concurrently, although it is more common to see the dominance of one cell type at any one time. Parathyroid hormone stimulates osteoclastic activity, while calcitonin has the opposite effect. The important interrelations between the developing inorganic matrix and the active living phase is via fine lacunae, or channels, that are well endowed with capillary blood vessels. Derangement of these lacunae and/or their capillary invagination seems to be a common factor in many leg abnormalities. This probably accounts for the fact that numerous metabolic derangements may induce remarkably similar types of leg disorders. Under ideal conditions, the cortical, or compact bone is deposited by osteoblasts on the inner edge of the subperiosteal boundary and in order to prevent excessive thickening, osteoclasts reabsorb material at the boundary with the marrow cavity. Normal development therefore, relies on the continual deposition and reabsorption of bone. It is interesting to note that the majority of skeletal abnormalities relate to problems with deposition, rather than the reabsorption of bone at the growth plate. In the young bird, the marrow cavity is composed almost exclusively of myeloid tissue, while in the adult, this is replaced by adipose tissue. In older birds, long bones represent a major store of adipose tissue.

Medullary bone is unique to adult females, where a spongy-type bone replaces the marrow in the cavity of the long bones. It is assumed that this labile calcium reserve is the major skeletal contributor of calcium during shell formation. Presumably the role of medullary bones in shell formation is to augment calcium supplies during the dark period, when the hen consumes little feed. This bone is then replaced in the interim between successive shell formations. The interlacing bone spicules are similar in gross appearance to cortical bone in the epiphysis of the long bone. In medullary bone, the spicules are surrounded by red marrow and blood sinuses.

Both the longitudinal growth and thickness of bone are controlled by the activity at the growth plate in the metaphysis region. The zone of active hypertrophy is recognized by its hardness and especially its opaqueness. In normal bone, the proliferating zone is a relatively narrow band, although certain nutrient deficiencies lead to the thickening and widening of this zone and associated non-ossified cartilage. Bone growth is accomplished through two basic processes. First, there is the formation of the bone matrix (collagen fibers and mucopolysaccharides) followed by calcification, mainly as $Ca_3(PO_4)_2$. Osteoblasts are responsible for the synthesis of basic collagen units, which tend to increase in size with distance from the site of synthesis. Calcification occurs on the matrix parts that are more mature, and once ossification has occurred the osteoblast reverts to a quiescent osteocyte. There is still some controversy as to the mechanisms with which unmineralized collagen matrices become impregnated with calcium. Either nucleation sites exist on the collagen molecules, or so-called matrix residues actively accumulate calcium and phosphorus ions to levels required for precipitation. Berthet-Colominas et al. (1979) suggests that when collagen is calcified, minerals penetrate throughout the fibrils, becoming crystalline in the so-called hole region and amorphous between the collagen molecules. These two mineral forms probably account for differences in the labile nature of various minerals within certain bone, and the rate with which they are affected during nutritional inadequacy.

Osteoclasts bring about resorption of bone during growth and/or repair situations. Such osteoclasts invaginate medullary bone during shell calcification, and are responsible for the gradual internal erosion of bone surface as normally occurs with elongation and growth in width of the bone. There are marked differences in the rates at which different bones are ossified. There has been a suggestion of there being some set biological time limit to normal ossification, and so this may have implications to the industry situation of marketing broilers at ever decreasing ages. Bone formation in the zone of ossification therefore results in gradual replacement of hypertrophic cartilage. The multiplying chondrocytes at the growth plate are arranged in parallel columns aligned with the bone shaft, and this is the basis of the calcifiable matrix. Calcium, phosphorus and other nutrients are supplied by invading blood vessels, originating from the base of the growth plate, such that calcified hypertrophic cartilage is eventually replaced by inorganic bone material. In birds, the chondrocytes at the top end (epiphysis) of the growth plate are supplied with separate blood vessels that enter the articular cartilage in the joint region. There is no joining of these two separate blood supply systems. Growth of bone is therefore dependent upon regular blood supply of nutrients to the active growth plate.

Two very important functions take place as the pullet matures. There is an increase in blood calcium levels brought about by estrogens and an increase in carbonic anhydrase, which is involved in supplying the carbonate portion of the calcium carbonate in the shell. Just prior to the pullet reaching sexual maturity, estrogen, released from the maturing ovary and acting in parallel with the androgens, induces the formation of medullary bone in the narrow bone cavities, especially in the long bones. This bone formation occupies virtually the complete marrow cavity of the femur by the time the first egg is due to be calcified. During this time, the total skeletal weight of the pullet increases by 15 to 20 grams, representing the storage of around 4 to 5 grams of additional calcium. Medullary bone formation can be influenced by dietary levels of calcium and vitamin D_3 and can be called upon, at any time during eggshell formation, to ensure optimum shell deposition (Candlish, 1971).

Pelanger and Taylor (1967), reported that reabsorption of medullary bone (osteolysis) is under the influence of enlarged osteocytes during eggshell calcification. In the case of the hen being in negative calcium balance, when she is not receiving enough dietary calcium to meet her requirements for shell formation, secretion of parathyroid hormone is markedly increased. This results in calcium being mobilized from cortical bone, to help meet requirements. However, with an acute calcium deficiency, egg production ceases, and medullary bone is gradually resorbed.

In the immature pullet, medullary bone deposition is initiated some 5-6 weeks prior to maturity, depending upon photoschedule. Calcium level of the diet is sometimes increased at this time, so as to accommodate this bone remodelling. However excess calcium can be detrimental leading to kidney dysfunction as a result of a more alkaline urine. Such high calcium diets (3-4%) are most problematic if administered to birds exposed to viruses (eg: infectious bronchitis) which, themselves, target kidney tissue.

5.3.4 Eggshell formation

In adult birds, most of our interest in calcium metabolism relates to eggshell formation. Although the eggshell is composed essentially of calcium carbonate, metabolism of both calcium and phosphorus are important for the 20-23 hr process of egg calcification. Although we have gained considerable knowledge about shell calcification over the last 30 years, we are still unable to prevent the age dependent decline in shell quality that naturally occurs throughout a one-year production cycle.

Following ovulation, the ovum receives an envelope of albumen, and is then coated with a netting of keratin fibers that form the inner shell membrane. As the egg moves down the isthmus, it acquires a second or outer membrane, composed of coarser protein fibers, which serve as the base for shell formation. As the egg passes through the isthmo-uterine junction, the cores of the mammillary knobs of the eggshell, which appear to be chemically bound to the outer shell membrane fibers, are laid down, (Figure 5.6). Thus, by the time the egg reaches the shell gland the mammillary cores and the nucleation of the calcite crystals, have already taken place. Shell formation in the shell gland consists mainly of crystal growth with concommitant matrix deposition. The palisade, or spongy layer gives the

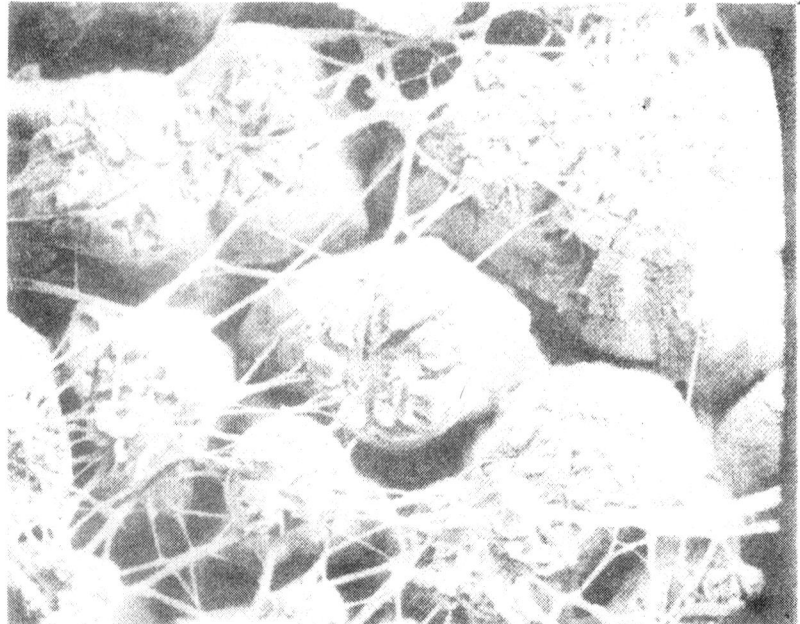

Figure 5.6 Mammillary cores showing attachment to fibers of outer shell membrane.

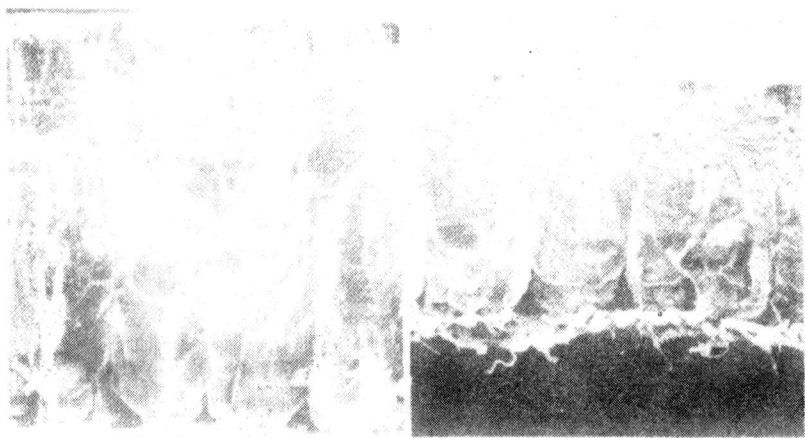

Figure 5.7 Ultrastructure of the eggshell showing (left) thick palisade layer of a strong shell and (right) thin palisade layer of a weak shell.

shell its main strength and thickness. The palisade layer is of uniform consistency and appears to act as the cement between the mammillary crystals. There is an indication that shell strength is correlated with integrity and thickness of the palisade layer (Figure 5.7). The final construction of the egg is the formation of the cuticle, the porous outer covering of the shell. Besides being the first line of defense in combating invading microorganisms, the cuticle also functions in helping to maintain the strength of the shell.

The egg remains in the shell gland for about 20 hours. During the first 5 hours calcium carbonate deposition increases rapidly to a maximum rate of approximately 300 mg/hr. The first 5 hours of slow calcification coincide with the formation of the mammillary knobs, and also during this period water and electrolytes move across the shell membrane into the albumen. Figure 5.8 shows the deposition of total minerals in an eggshell over a 24 h ovulation cycle.

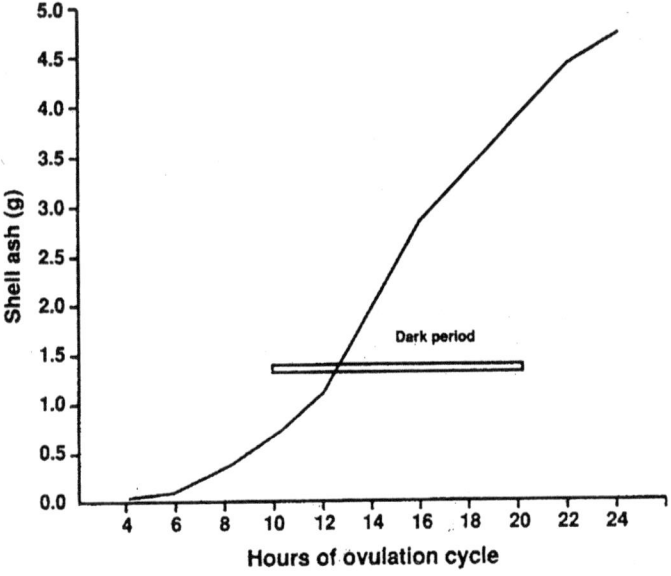

Figure 5.8 Shell mineral deposition over a 24h ovulation cycle (Source M. Clunies PhD Thesis, University of Guelph, 1987)

In the first 6 hours of the 24 h laying cycle, there is virtually no shell deposition. This is the time of albumen and shell membrane secretion, and the time of redeposition of medullary bone. From 6-12 hr about 400 mg of calcium are deposited, while the most active period is the 12-18 hr period when around 800 mg of shell calcium accumulates. This is followed by a slower deposition of about 500 mg in the last 6 hr, for a total of around 1.7 g shell calcium, depending upon egg size. Most shell calcification therefore takes place when birds are not feeding in the dark period. Consequently, a portion of the calcium for shell calcification is derived from resorbed medullary bone. Clunies *et al.* (1992) indicate the active laying hen to have around 740 mg total medullary calcium reserve, of which most is in the femur (290 mg) and tibia (230 mg) with the remainder in the humerus and other bones. On a calcium deficient diet, this reserve will decline to about 50 mg calcium, at which time, either the ovary will shut down or the bird will start to, destroy cortical bone in an attempt to sustain shell calcification.

Because bone is composed of calcium phosphate, there is concommitant release of phosphorus during mobilization of calcium from medullary bone. Declining cyclic (24 h) levels of estrogen are probably the key to initiation of osteoclastic medullary activity, mediated by the action of parathyroid hormone (Etches, 1987). This hemeral effect of estrogen is probably responsible for daily cyclic changes seen in plasma calcium of non-layers, or layers during a non-shell forming day.

Calcium balance in the laying hen is thus regulated by estrogen, parathyroid hormone, $1, 25 (OH)_2 D_3$ and perhaps calcitonin. A schematic representation of daily calcium and phosphorus balance is given in Figure 5.9.

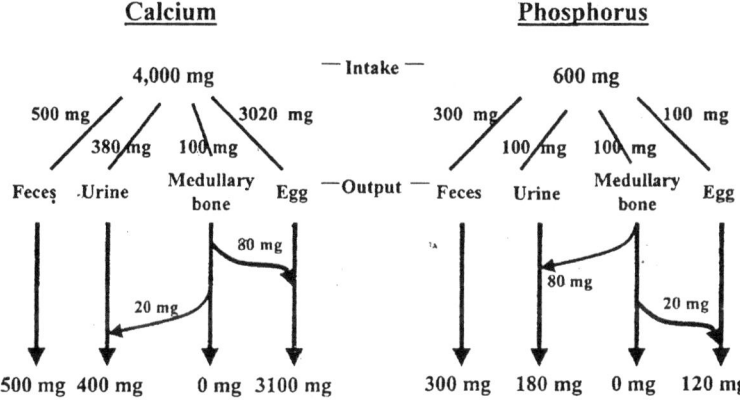

Figure 5.9 Schematic of daily calcium balance in a laying hen.

In this schematic, the overall balance of medullary mineral reserves is given as zero. In reality, it can be slightly positive or negative. Over time there is an indication of greater occurrence of daily negative balance, and this has been related to a decline in shell quality over time. Al-Batshan *et al.* (1994) indicated that decline in shell quality with age is also correlated with reduced rate of uptake of calcium from the duodenum. For a given age of bird, there is an indication that shell quality is correlated with plasma levels of calcium binding vitellogenin levels (Grunder *et al.*, 1980).

While most nutritional studies on eggshell quality centre on metabolism of calcium and phosphorus it must be remembered that carbonate is an integral part of the shell. Carbonate metabolism and acid:base balance in general can therefore influence the process of shell formation. Deposition of calcium carbonate on the forming shell is probably maintained through the continuous secretion of bicarbonate by the shell gland. Bicarbonate formation, within the shell gland mucosa, is brought about by the catalyzed hydration of metabolic carbon dioxide to bicarbonate by carbonic anhydrase. The formation of HCO_3 in the mucosa of the shell gland, and its precipitation as calcium carbonate in the shell, are accompanied by the release of hydrogen ions, which in turn must be buffered in the shell gland fluid. The sequence of events leading up to shell deposition is dependent, in large part, on maintaining normal acid-base in both the blood and shell gland fluid.

In cold weather the hen may have a respiration rate as low as 29 cycles per minute, which can increase to several hundred as the hen hyperventilates in very hot weather. Hyperventilation can decrease blood CO_2 to such an extent that shell thickness is reduced by up to 12% (Mueller, 1966). Mongin (1968), reported that eggshell thickness was improved with hens kept in an atmosphere rich in carbon dioxide. An increase in CO_2 in a poultry house, will eventually lead to an acidosis condition, which will be compensated for by reabsorption of bicarbonate from the kidney, thus increasing blood bicarbonate level.

A number of workers have attempted to increase the bicarbonate level of the blood by feeding sodium bicarbonate to the hen. If the diet is high in chloride, the chloride ions will be the main anion in the blood and bicarbonate will increase very little. By reducing dietary chloride, an improvement in shell quality may be noted, brought about by increased bicarbonate reabsorption from the kidney. This scenario again demonstrates the importance of maintaining proper acid-base balance in order for the hen to optimize metabolic functions in her body. Cipera (1980), found that C_{14} entered into the carbonate portion of the shell, for hens injected with C_{14} labelled bicarbonate, glucose or acetate suggesting that the hen is capable of producing adequate bicarbonate ions from glucose or acetate and so does not need a dietary supply.

5.3.5 Calcium nutrition for eggshell calcification

There is still considerable variation in calcium nutrition of layers, aimed at optimizing shell calcification. In some instances calcium is kept constant, while other nutritionists favor a gradual increase over time, usually accompanied by a concommitant decrease in diet phosphorus concentration. As calcium concentration of the diet is increased there is an increase in eggshell specific gravity (thicker shell) associated with elevated plasma calcium and decreased plasma phosphorus (Table 5.4, Roland and Gordon, 1997).

TABLE 5.4 Effect of diet calcium on layer physiology				
Diet calcium (%)	Egg specific gravity	Bone density (g/cm^2)	Serum	
			Ca mmol/L	P mg/L
2.5	1.082	0.199	1.42	6.77
3.0	1.084	0.218	1.46	5.70
3.5	1.086	0.229	1.51	5.45
4.0	1.087	0.240	1.51	5.06
4.5	1.088	0.243	1.51	4.93
5.0	1.089	0.239	1.53	4.83
Adapted from Roland and Gordon (1997)				

In practice the proportion of calcium in the diet will be adjusted according to feed intake so as to ensure 4-4.5 g calcium intake daily. For White Leghorns consuming 90-100 g feed daily, this equates to calcium concentrations of from 4.4-5.0%. In general, the higher the calcium concentration of the diet, the better the shell thickness and shell quality. Unfortunately with diet concentrations much above 5%, a proportion of eggs will contain extra pimples of calcite on the shell, which can break-off and puncture the shell. Also because calcium is usually supplied as some form of carbonate with only 38% calcium, 5% diet calcium necessitates a 13% inclusion of calcium carbonate which limits the space available in the diet for ensuring an adequate supply of other nutrients. Roush *et al.* (1986) indicate the importance of maintaining an optimum ratio of calcium:phosphorus for maximizing shell yield (Figure 5.10)

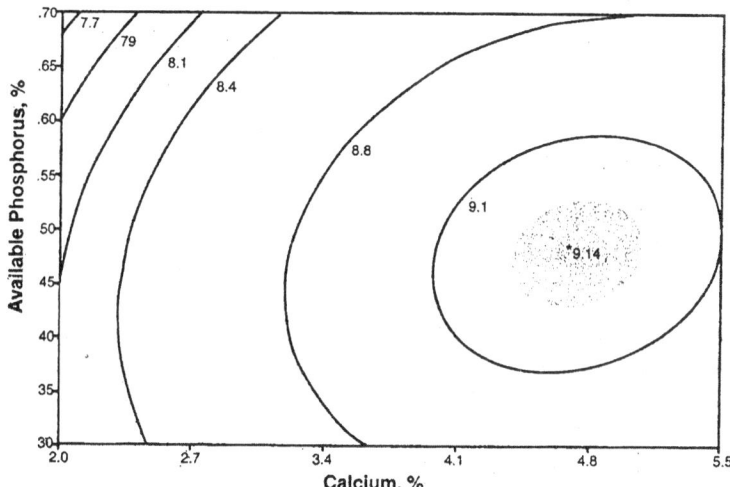

Figure 5.10 Response surface of eggshell percentage with varying % diet of calcium and phosphorus (adpted from Roush et al 1986).

There has been considerable discussion and research conducted about the form of calcium carbonate used in layer diets. Limestone and oystershell are the usual options and both contain around 38% calcium. Oystershell is regarded as an 'insoluble' slow-release form of calcium, and so residues remain in the digestive tract for some time. Limestone, depending on particle size and physical structure, is more soluble, and there is little retention in the gut.

The period of maximum shell accretion usually occurs in the dark period, when birds are not eating. Calcium supply at this time is therefore from feed remaining in digesta or from medullary bone. Oystershell and larger particles of limestone are retained in the gizzard and so provide some calcium for shell accretion at this time. Fine particle limestone leaves the digestive tract much more quickly, and so birds fed this source of calcium have to rely more heavily on medullary bone reserves. For example Rao *et al.* (1992) show very little residence time in the gizzard for particles < 0.84 mm. Particles >1.8 mm have much longer residence time. Particle size relates to 'solubility', an *in vitro* measure of dissociation in dilute hydrochloric acid over time. Zhang and Coon (1997) suggest that larger particles of limestone and/or those of lower solubility are retained longer in the gizzard. *In vivo* studies however, show much less difference in disappearance of calcium from various sources and this fact may be the basis of the considerable variation reported in results for limestone vs. oystershell.

Supplying some calcium as large particle limestone or oystershell within a mash diet does allow the bird some degree of ingredient self-selection. It has been proposed that this innate action by the bird is the reason behind any improvement related to oystershell feeding, rather than there being an issue of calcium solubility over time. Mongin and Sauveur (1974) were one of the first to show a specific appetite for calcium in the bird. When offered a choice feeding situation involving calcium, layers voluntarily consume about the normal amount of calcium, but only at specific times of the day. As shown by Chah (1972) there is a distinct peak in voluntary demand for calcium in the last 5-6 hours of the light period (Figure 5.11). This time coincides with the period of active shell calcification, and presumably leaves a residue of calcium in the digesta when the dark period occurs. Layers cannot exercise this cyclic demand for calcium when fed a compound mash diet that contains small particle limestone. Calcium self-selection is possible with oystershell, since it has different physical characteristics than the remainder of the feed.

Mongin and Sauveur (1979) indicate that this late day peak in voluntary calcium intake occurs even when shell calcification is suppressed, suggesting that the action is governed to some degree by estrogen, the light/dark cycle and/or the process of ovulation or oviposition. These same authors conclude that voluntary calcium intake of the immature pullet is around 1.15 g/d, and that of the rooster 0.74g/d. One week prior to first ovulation intake of calcium increases to 2.6 g/d, and then to 3.8 g/d when shell calcification commences.

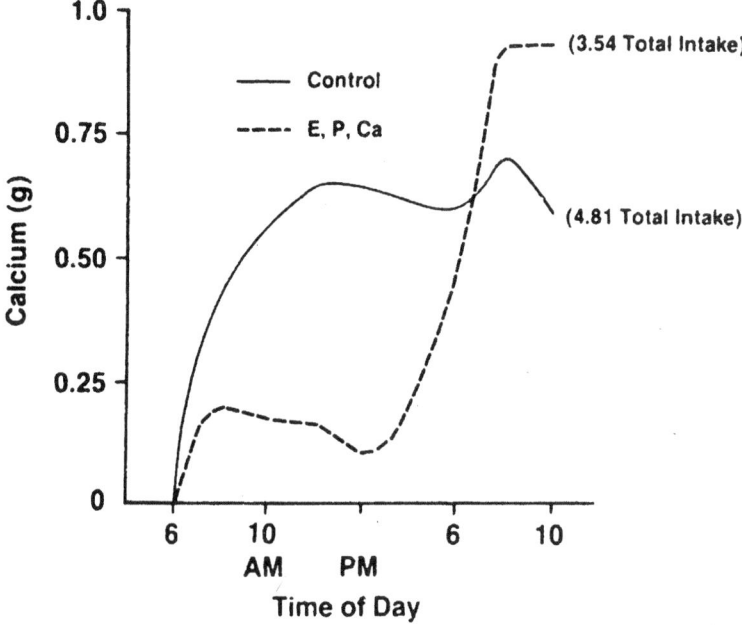

Figure 5.11 Calcium intake on egg forming days (Chah, 1972).

With a deficiency of calcium, the layer will first show loss of eggshell integrity and in some cases, subsequent loss in bone structure. If the deficit is large, ovulation often ceases and so there is no excessive bone resorption. With marginal deficiencies of calcium, ovulation often continues, and so the bird relies more heavily on bone resorption. Total medullary bone calcium reserves are limited and so after production of 3-4 eggs on a marginally calcium deficient diet, cortical bone may be eroded with associated loss in locomotion. As calcium content of the diet decreases, there is a transient (1-2 d) increase in feed intake, followed by a decline associated with reduced protein and energy needs for egg synthesis. Calcium deficiency is exacerbated by high levels of dietary chloride (0.4 – 0.5%). In such dietary situations, there is greater benefit to feeding sodium bicarbonate. In normal hens, which have been depleted of calcium by feeding a calcium deficient diet, egg production and eggshell calcium return to normal in 6 to 8 days after the hens are returned to a diet adequate in calcium. After three weeks the leg bones will be completely recalcified. The finding that the adrenal gland is enlarged in calcium deficiency indicates that this is a stress in the classical sense. Suggested levels of calcium for layers are given in Table 5.5. These data assume adequate daily intakes of available phosphorus (400 mg) and vitamin D_3 (300 IU).

TABLE 5.5 Calcium levels in layer diets (% diet)			
Feed intake (g/d)	Weeks of age		
	18-28	28-48	48+
80	4.70	-	-
85	4.40	4.65	-
90	4.20	4.40	4.60
95	3.95	4.15	4.38
100	3.75	3.95	4.15
105	-	3.76	3.95
110	-	3.60	3.80
115	-	-	3.60

5.3.6 Cage layer fatigue and bone breakage in layers

Young birds up to 30 weeks of age sometimes suffer from Cage Layer Fatigue (CLF) while older layers suffer from brittle bones. Both conditions relate to impaired calcium metabolism (in some way), although neither can always be corrected or prevented by supplying adequate or extra calcium.

As its name implies CLF is a syndrome most commonly associated with laying hens held in cages, and so its first description by Couch (1955) coincides with commercial acceptance of this housing system. Apart from the cage environment, CLF also seems to need a high egg output to trigger the condition, and for this reason, it has been most obvious in White Leghorn strain birds. At around the time of peak egg output, birds become lame and are reluctant to stand in the cage. Because of the competitive nature of the cage environment, affected birds usually move to the back area of the cage, and death can occur due to dehydration/starvation because of their reluctance to drink or eat. The condition is rarely seen in floor-managed birds and this leads to the assumption that exercise may be a factor. In fact, removing CLF birds from the cage during the early stage of lameness and placing them on the floor usually results in a complete recovery. However, this practice is usually not possible in large commercial operations. In the 1960-70s up to 10% mortality was common, although now the incidence is considered problematic if 0.5% of the flock is affected. There is no good evidence to suggest an association of CLF to general bone breakage in layers, although the two conditions are often described as part of the same general syndrome. Today, general bone breakage of older birds, especially during handling at the end of the laying cycle, is now more problematic than CLF.

Birds suffering from CLF are usually found on their sides, with their legs outstretched if they are in a non-competitive environment. In a cage, birds often crouch in the back corner away from general activity. If birds are identified early, they seem alert and are still producing eggs. The bones seem fragile, and there may be broken bones. Dead birds may be dehydrated or emaciated, simply due to the failure of these birds being able to eat or drink. The ribs may show some beading (Riddel, 1975) although the most obvious abnormality is a reduction in the density of the medullary bone trabeculae. There is also significant evidence of osteoblast activity, although little osteoid is present. Riddel *et al.* (1968) suggest that paralysis *per se* is often due to fractures of the fourth and fifth thoracic vertebrae causing compression and degeneration of the spinal cord. If birds are examined immediately after the paralysis is first observed, there is invariably a partly shelled egg in the oviduct, and the ovary contains a rich hierarchy of follicles. If birds are examined some time after the onset of paralysis, then the ovary is often regressed, due to reduced nutrient intake. Rowland and Foutz (1990) describe CLF as either osteoporosis of the cortical bone or osteomalacia of the medullary bone. If this is correct, then it is assumed that hens will respond rapidly to the treatment of osteomalacia but slowly to that for osteoporosis. Likewise, Rowland and Foutz (1990) suggest that an osteoporotic lesion strongly implies that optimizing the skeletal mass prior to maturity is critical in preventative nutrition. Bone composition is consistent with birds being deficient in calcium, and so mineralization is abnormal. Depending upon the stage of any eggshell formation, there may be considerable osteoclastic activity in the medullary bone. In extreme cases, there may be an erosion of the cortical bone since it is assumed that this acts as a reservoir to help supplement the mobile medullary reserves when extreme calcium deficiency occurs.

CLF is obviously due to an inadequate supply of calcium available for shell calcification, and the bird's plundering of unconventional areas of its skeleton for such calcium. Because the availability of other nutrients, and the status of phosphorus and vitamin D_3 in the diet and their availability, affect calcium metabolism, diet composition in general must be reviewed. Birds fed diets deficient in calcium, phosphorus, or vitamin D_3 will show cage layer fatigue assuming there is a high egg output. Scott *et al.* (1977) fed diets containing 1 or 3.5% Ca for 4 wks prior to expected maturity, and found that 1% Ca was inadequate for maximum bone mineralization and normal bone ash content. In this later context, birds fed only 1% pre-lay calcium had 35% bone ash, while those birds fed 3.5% Ca had 40% bone ash. Feeding a more extensive series of diets Leeson *et al.* (1986) showed only a small increase in Ca retention of pre-lay birds when fed diets containing 0.9 up to 3.5% Ca from 19 wk of age up to the time of the 4th egg. Low calcium diets resulted in reduced early eggshell quality, although there were no apparent changes in the bone histology of birds examined after producing their 15th egg. Keshavarz (1989) however suggests that the reappearance of CLF in some commercial flocks may be a result of too early sexual maturity due to the genetic selection for this trait coupled with early light stimulation. Feeding a layer diet containing 3.5% Ca vs. a grower diet at 1% Ca, as early as 14 wk of age, was beneficial in terms of an increase in the ash and calcium content of the tibiotarsus (Table 5.6). Feeding a high calcium diet as early as 14 wk of age seems unnecessary, and in fact, may be detrimental in terms of kidney urolithiasis. As suggested by Keshavarz (1989) changing from a low to a high calcium diet should coincide with the observation of secondary sexual characteristics, and especially comb development, which usually precedes first oviposition by 14-16 d.

TABLE 5.6 Diet calcium and bone characteristics of young layers in response to pre-lay diet calcium		
Time of change to 3.5% Ca	**Tibiotarsus**	
	Ash (%)	Ca (mg/g)
20 wks	53.5c	182b
18 wks	55.7b	187b
17 wks	59.3b	202b
16 wks	58.9b	199b
15 wks	58.4b	197b
14 wks	57.9b	196b
Adapted from Keshavarz (1989)		

There have been surprisingly few reports on the effect of vitamin D_3 on CLF in young birds. It is assumed that D_3 deficiency will impair calcium utilization, although there are no reports of testing graded levels of this nutrient as a possible preventative treatment. The other major nutrient concerned with skeletal integrity is phosphorus and as expected phosphorus deficiency can accentuate effects of CLF. While P is not directly required for shell formation, it is essential for the replenishment of Ca, as $CaPO_4$, in medullary bone during successive periods of active bone calcification. Without adequate phosphorus in the diet, there is a failure to replenish the medullary Ca reserves, and this situation can accelerate or precipitate the onset of CLF and other skeletal problems. Garlich et al. (1982) found the femur of P-deficient birds to have a reduced mineral content, although the organic matrix was little affected. For this reason, they suggested that the measurement of bone ash expressed per unit of external bone volume could be used as an indicator of osteoporosis in layers. Depending upon the level of feed intake, CLF will be minimized if layers are fed a diet providing > 3.5% Ca, 0.4% available phosphorus, and 1500 IU vitamin D_3/kg for at least 14 d prior to first oviposition. Once CLF is observed, there is little advantage to diet manipulation of the whole flock, because the immediate nutrient needs of affected birds are different from the remainder (majority) of the flock. Birds will likely recover if they can gain access to feed and water.

CLF may relate to bone breakage in older hens, although a definitive relationship has never been quantitated. It is suspected that as for CLF in young birds, bone breakage in older birds results as a consequence of impaired calcification of the skeleton over time. This is again related to a high egg output coupled with restricted activity within the cage environment. Few live birds have broken bones in the cage, the major problem occurring when these birds are removed from their cages and transported to processing units. Apart from the obvious welfare implications, broken bones prove problematic during the mechanical deboning of the muscles. Wilson (1991) recently studied preconditioning with various levels of calcium and phosphorus as it influences bone strength in older hens. Birds that did not lay for more than 3 wks prior to examination, had an increased radius bone strength. Bone shear strength increased with the increased bone ash content, but unfortunately diet manipulation had no effect on bone ash. Ruff and Hughes (1985) indicated that humerus strength could be increased by increasing levels of both Ca and P provided that the ratio of Ca:P was maintained at 1.3:1 (immature birds). Merkley (1991) concludes that there is no evidence to suggest that any diet nutrients fed in excess of those required for optimum shell quality are in any way beneficial to the skeletal integrity of older hens. There is an indication however that fluorine given at 300 ppm in the water of growing pullets can significantly improve bone breaking strength and increase the bone ash of younger birds, although this treatment has not been followed through for older birds. As with CLF, bone breakage in older hens is much worse for caged rather than floor managed birds. Harms and Arafa (1986) found bone-breaking strength to gradually decrease throughout early egg production and that this was most evident for cage rather than floor housed birds.

At this time, we do not know how to improve the bone integrity of older laying hens, without adversely affecting other traits of economic significance. For example, Roland (1987) clearly shows that the bone breaking strength in older birds can be increased by feeding high levels of vitamin D_3. Unfortunately this treatment also results in an excessive pimpling of the eggshells, and these extra calcium deposits on the shell surface readily break off causing leakage of the egg contents. It may be possible to improve the skeletal integrity of older birds by causing cessation of ovulation for some time prior to slaughter. Presumably the associated reduction in the drain on body calcium reserves would allow re-establishment of the integrity of the susceptible medullary bones. Currently such a feeding strategy is uneconomical, although consideration of bird welfare may provide the impetus for research in this area.

5.3.7 Calcium requirements for young birds

For young birds up to time of sexual maturity, calcium requirements are met with diet levels of 0.8-1.0%. At day of age, the requirement is close to 1.0% of the diet, assuming available phosphorus levels are 0.45-0.50%. There needs to be a calcium:phosphorus ratio of 2:1 in the diet, and so, if for some reason higher levels of available phosphorus are fed, then calcium levels must be increased accordingly.

5.3.8 Calcium toxicity

Birds are quite tolerant of dietary calcium levels, since there is a negative correlation between diet calcium concentration and percentage absorption. However, even with reduced absorption there can be higher levels of plasma calcium that either influence phosphorus balance and/or structure of the kidney. Most signs of calcium toxicity are those of phosphorus deficiency, many of which are often indistinguishable from a calcium deficiency. For example, offering layers a continuous supply of free-choice oystershell, as a separate feed, often causes production of soft-shelled eggs. The reason for failure in shell calcification is increased kidney excretion of calcium phosphate, and so medullary bone reserves are not replenished between successive cycles of calcification. Toxicity of calcium is often explainable on the basis of changes to digesta pH where high levels affect the solubility of other minerals (Shafey, 1993).

In growing pullets from 10-18 weeks of age, abnormally high levels of calcium can lead to kidney urolithiasis. Excess calcium causes urolith formation in the kidney, which can damage it's structure. Such uroliths are commonly composed of calcium sodium urate. Urates are rarely found in other regions of the body, and death usually occurs as a result of toxin accumulation. Urolithiasis is most common in pullets fed high calcium layer diets starting 4-5 weeks prior to maturity. The condition is made worse by concomitant infectious bronchitis. Lent and Wideman (1994) suggest that urolithiasis can be prevented or treated by using urine acidifiers such as ammonium sulphate or methionine hydroxy analogue.

5.4 PHOSPHORUS

Although the major role of phosphorus is as a component of bone, phosphorus is also an essential component of organic compounds involved in almost every aspect of metabolism. Phosphorus plays an important part in muscle coordination, energy, carbohydrate, amino acid and fat metabolism, nervous tissue metabolism, normal blood chemistry, skeletal growth and transport of fatty acids and other lipids. Phosphate is an important part of the nucleic acids, DNA and RNA. It is a component of many coenzymes and is involved in the storage and transfer of energy in phosphorylated compounds of glucose and its derivatives of other sugars, and such high energy compounds as adenosine di- and triphosphate, and creatine phosphate.

Blood contains approximately 35 – 45 mg of phosphorus per 100 ml, of which about 10% is in the form of inorganic phosphate. Normally there is an inverse relationship between serum diffusible calcium and serum inorganic phosphate.

A deficiency of phosphorus or a wide imbalance in the Ca:P ratio of the diet can cause rickets, because either element in excess precipitates the other in the intestine. Blood levels of Ca and P under these conditions are reduced. Administration of vitamin D_3 will prevent, lessen or cure either low P or low Ca rickets if the deficiency is not too severe. Beryllium in the diet also may cause severe rickets, believed to be due largely to the formation of insoluble beryllium phosphate which prevents the absorption of phosphate from the intestine.

Vitamin D_3 also influences the absorption of phosphorus as well as that of calcium from the digesta. Phosphorus levels also seem to influence regulation of vitamin D_3 metabolites while stimulation of $1,25\ (OH)_2D_3$ by the kidney in response to low calcium is dependent on parathyroid hormone. The situation with phosphorus seems independent of hormone action. Phosphate depletion may simply induce renal synthesis of $1,\ 25\ (OH)_2\ D_3$ directly.

5.4.1. Availability of dietary phosphorus

Most phosphorus is derived from animal protein ingredients such as meat meal or concentrated mineral supplements such as calcium phosphate. The phosphorus present in cereals and vegetable proteins is of variable digestibility, and this situation is now of great interest to nutritionists.

Inorganic phosphate sources that are mined in various regions of the world are relatively unavailable to birds unless these phosphates are heat-treated in such a way as to convert the native rock phosphates into available forms such as α- or β-tricalcium phosphates. Hydrated forms of phosphates are also less available, probably because of reduced solubility. The most common forms of phosphate used today are mono- or di-calcium phosphate or deflorinated rock phosphate (Table 5.7).

TABLE 5.7 Common sources of phosphorus (%)				
	Ca	P	Na	P availability
Monocalcium PO_4	17	23	0.10	98
Dicalcium PO_4	25	18	0.02	97
Deflorinated PO_4	32	18	5.50	95
Monosodium PO_4	-	20.0	15.0	95
Disodium PO_4	-	22.0	29.0	98
Meat and bone meal	11.0	6.0	0.60	90
Fish meal (60%)	6.5	3.5	0.50	92

Keshavarz (1994) indicates that monobasic calcium phosphate $Ca(H_2PO_4)_2$ $2H_2O$ is very acidogenic and causes shell quality problems at 150 mEq/kg. Dibasic calcium phosphate ($CaHPO_4$) on the other hand is less problematic, since birds can tolerate up to 1,000 mEq/kg without undue problems. Most inorganic phosphate supplements are 95-98% available to the bird, assuming there are no contaminants, and heat treatment has been adequate. Table 5.7 indicates availability of phosphorus in meat, bone meal and fish meal to be around 90% available although Waldroup and Adams (1994) conclude that in terms of growth and bone ash accretion in young birds, phosphorus in meat meals and poultry by-product meals is of comparable availability to that of monocalcium phosphate.

Accounting for availability of phosphorus in plant material is much more complicated. A proportion of plant phosphorus will be present as phytic acid, which is poorly digested by the bird. At neutral pH, the phosphate groups in phytic acid have one or two negatively charged ions, and so these can chelate with metal ions (Figure 5.12). If bonding is across two phosphate groups, as shown for calcium in Figure 5.12 the association is strong. If bonding is within a phosphate group the association is much weaker, but minerals are still unavailable to the bird. Because of its prevalence in the digesta, calcium is a common component of phytic acid. In many cereals, 60-70% of phosphorus will be as phytic acid. Digestibility of this phytate molecule varies from 0-50%, depending upon the ingredient and the age of the bird. Young birds are much less able to 'digest' phytate, while up to 50% availability is often claimed for mature birds. Phytate will also chelate with copper, zinc, manganese and iron, making these minerals unavailable. The 'digestion' of phytate occurs as a result of action from natural plant phytases or phytase synthesis by intestinal microbes. There are controversial reports of endogenous phytase production in the intestinal brush border (Sebastian *et al.*, 1998). Heat treatment of a diet, as occurs with pelleting and/or extrusion does not seem to improve the digestibility of phytate phosphorus (Edwards *et al.*, 1999).

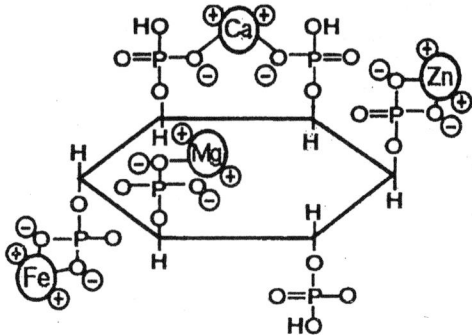

myo inositol hexakis phosphate

Figure 5.12 Phytate structure

Of more recent interest is the application of exogenous phytase enzymes. Fungal and bacterial phytases can be added to poultry diets, and there is a dramatic increase in digestibility of phosphorus, calcium, and other trace minerals (Sebastian *et al.*, 1996). This situation is of commercial significance because phosphorus is an expensive nutrient, and excretion of undigestible phosphorus is becoming an environmental concern. A typical inclusion rate will be 600 phytase units/kg of diet which is claimed to be equivalent to around 0.1% available phosphorus and up to 0.2% calcium in the diet.

Because phytic acid also complexes with proteins, there are reports of improved amino acid and energy availability in diets containing phytase. Namkung and Leeson (1999) recorded a 1-2% improvement in digestibility of amino acids, and 1-1.5% improvement in AMEn of a diet containing 600 IU phytase/kg. Rojas and Scott (1969) showed some time ago that the metabolizable energy values of several different types of cottonseed meal were improved by treatment with phytase. The almost complete hydrolysis of the phytin in the meals not only released the phosphorus for utilization by chicks but also appeared to free some protein from a protein-phytate complex, and apparently reduced the gossypol toxicity of the glanded cottonseed meals. Phytase hydrolysis of the phytin also produced a marked reduction in the zinc requirement of the chicks, providing further evidence of the detrimental effects of the chelation of zinc by phytate upon the availability of dietary zinc.

5.4.2 Phosphorus requirements for growth and egg production

As previously discussed, the bird is adaptable to a wide range of diet phosphorus concentration, as long as a balance with calcium is maintained at around 1:2, P:Ca. Roberson *et al.* (1993) suggest however, that the dietary Ca:AvP ratio required for optimum bone integrity in young chicks may be greater than 2.2:1. Because phosphorus is a relatively expensive nutrient, excess is usually avoided in a diet. Most diets for birds up to 6 weeks of age will contain around 0.4 – 0.45% available phosphorus. As the bird gets older, diet concentration is reduced, such that for 16 week old immature pullets, 0.35-0.38% available phosphorus is usually adequate. For mature males, or non-laying hens, phosphorus requirement is met with diet levels of from 0.25-0.30% available phosphorus.

Phosphorus needs of the layer are closely associated with needs for calcium, and the dynamics of medullary bone. When there is osteoclastic activity in medullary bone, plasma phosphorus levels will increase, because of release of both calcium and phosphorus from the bone. Mongin and Sauveur (1979) show the classic peak in plasma phosphorus that occurs at night time when medullary activity is greatest. Most of this phosphorus will be excreted in the urine, since there is no immediate metabolic need for this increased pool (Figure 5.13).

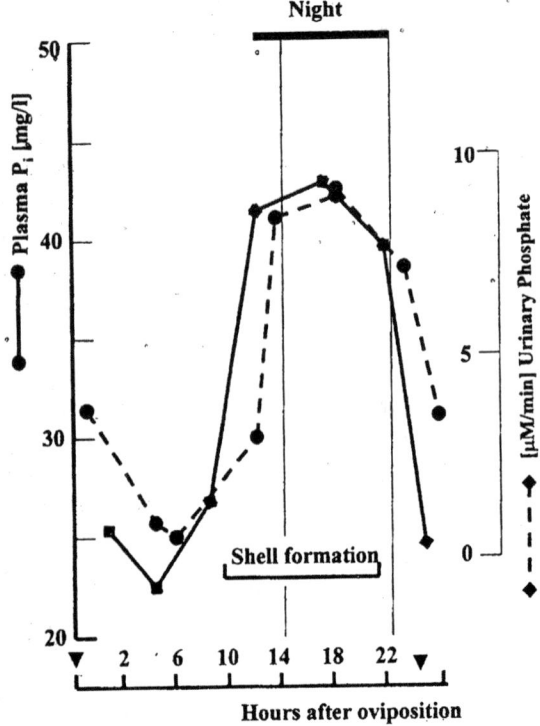

Figure 5.13 Plasma and urinary phosphorus levels in relation to the ovulatory cycle (adapted from Mongin and Sauveur, 1979).

Section 5.3.5 detailed the calcium flux of layers in relation to particle size of calcium carbonate. It was concluded that finer particle size limestone would necessitate greater medullary bone resorption, and by association, this means a greater need for phosphorus. Because most of the released bone phosphorus is excreted in the urine, the bird needs extra phosphorus to replenish medullary bone even at times when there is no shell calcification.

The phosphorus requirement of the young laying hen is around 400 mg/day declining to as low as 300 mg/day towards the end of the production cycle. Keshavarz (2000) provides evidence for decreasing the available phosphorus content of the layer diet from 0.35 → 0.30 → 0.25% in the 30-42, 42-54 and 54-55 week periods respectively. Under commercial conditions, phosphorus levels some 10-15% higher than this are often required for optimum performance. The reasons for this higher than theoretical phosphorus need are not readily understood.

Too high a level of phosphorus will lead to a decline in eggshell quality, likely due to an associated induced deficiency of calcium. Consistently high plasma levels of phosphorus are correlated with reduced shell quality. A deficiency of phosphorus will likewise result in impaired calcium metabolism. Harms *et al.* (1999) in feeding older laying hens just 0.3% total phosphorus for 56 d, describe signs of sporadic ovulation in individual birds, associated with random regression of oocytes. Severe deficiency or lack of availability of phosphorus in the diet results in early loss of appetite, weakness and death within a period of 10 to 12 days. A less severe deficiency causes rickets and poor growth, but apparently does not reduce the phosphorus level of the blood to an extent that it interferes with the availability of phosphorus for the formation of high energy phosphates, DNA, RNA and enzymes. Even during starvation, catabolism of bone releases sufficient phosphorus for the organic phosphates needed by the body and also results in a continuous loss of phosphorus into the urine.

5.5 SODIUM, POTASSIUM AND CHLORIDE

These three elements play a major and integrated role in osmotic regulation of body fluids and maintaining acid-base balance in the body. Hence, it is difficult to discuss the function of one without reference to the others.

It is interesting to compare aquatic and terrestrial life systems and the role played by these three elements in maintaining body functions. It has been postulated that life began in the sea, and that when animals became terrestrial their external environment changed, but their cells did not. In order to function normally animals had to maintain the level of electrolytes in their external environment within rather narrow limits. Thus, the living systems external environment became its internal environment, which today is known as the extracellular fluid. In feeding animals today, nutrients essential to the living cells, must be presented in a form they can use while concommitantly not appreciably changing the level or balance of electrolytes in their internal environment (extracellular fluid). The sea is rich in sodium but almost devoid of potassium, and both plants and animals have a high requirement for potassium. The separation in the cell and extracellular fluids of sodium and potassium and their close interaction with each other is one of the fundamentals of life. Hence, the need for a thorough knowledge of the function of sodium, potassium and chloride is necessary for an understanding of cell physiology and animal metabolism.

5.5.1 Electrolyte balance

While requirements for the three individual elements have been clearly defined, there is currently an understanding of the need to achieve a balance between cation and anion supply. Most commonly, electrolyte balance is described by the simple formula of Na+K-Cl expressed as mEq/kg of diet. In most situations it seems as though an overall diet balance of 250 mEq/kg is optimum for normal physiological functions. In reality, electrolyte imbalance does not occur, because the buffering systems in the body ensure the maintenance of near normal physiological pH. In extreme situations the need for buffering capacity seems to adversely affect other physiological conditions, thereby producing or accentuating potentially debilitating situations. While the primary role of electrolytes is in maintenance of body water and ionic balance, the requirements for elements such as sodium, potassium and chlorine cannot be considered individually because it is the overall balance that is important. Electrolyte balance, also referred to as acid-base balance, is affected by three major factors, namely the balance and proportion of these electrolytes in the diet, endogenous acid production and the rate of renal clearance.

In most situations, birds will attempt to maintain the balance between cations and anions in the body such that physiological pH is maintained. If conditions in the body result in a shift towards acid or base conditions, the normal physiological defense mechanism is to alter metabolic processes such that normal conditions prevail. In reality, electrolyte imbalance *per se* rarely occurs because these regulatory mechanisms must ensure optimum cellular pH and osmolarity. Electrolyte imbalance can therefore more correctly be described as the mechanisms that must occur in the body so as to achieve normal physiological pH. In extreme situations, such modifications in regulatory mechanisms seem to adversely affect other physiological systems, and so produce or accentuate potentially debilitating conditions. Tibial dyschondroplasia and respiratory alkalosis are examples of electrolyte imbalance. It is the cation:anion balance of the diet that provides the major mechanism for influencing electrolyte balance in the body when feeding poultry. Mongin (1980) describes cellular cation:anion balance as:

$$mEq \ (Na^+ + K^+ + Ca^{++} + Mg^{++}) - mEq \ (Cl^- + SO_4^= + H_2PO_4^- + HPO_4^=)$$

Mongin (1980) rationalizes that, in fact, only Na, K and Cl are likely to be involved in homeostasis, and this certainly makes diet formulation more easy. Ion balance is usually expressed in terms of mEq of the various electrolytes, and for an individual electrolyte this is calculated as Mwt ÷1,000. This unit is used on the basis that most minerals are present at a relatively low level in feeds. As an example calculation, the mEq for a diet containing 0.17% Na, 0.8% K and 0.22% Cl can be developed as follows:

a) Sodium

Mwt = 23.0 ∴ Eq = 23 g/kg, ∴ mEq = 23 mg/kg

Diet contains 0.17% Na = 1700 mg/kg = $\dfrac{1700 \ mEq}{23}$ = 73.9 mEq

b) Potassium

Mwt = 39.1 ∴ Eq = 39.1 g/kg, ∴ mEq = 39.1 mg/kg

Diet contains 0.80% K = 8000 mg/kg = $\frac{8,000}{39.1}$ mEq = 204.6 mEq

c) Chloride

Mwt = 35.5 ∴ Eq = 35.5 g/kg, ∴ mEq = 35.5 mg/kg

Diet contains 0.22% Cl = 2,200 mg/kg = $\frac{2,200}{35.5}$ mEq = 62.0 mEq

∴ overall diet balance becomes Na + K − Cl = 73.9 + 204.6 − 62.0 = 216.5 mEq

The normal buffering systems within the body will obviously need to temper any major deviation from physiological pH.

Mongin (1980) suggests that -

Diet Na+K-Cl = Diet Cations − Anions + Endogenous acid production + Base excess

The balance of ions in the diet needs to be such that the base excess is close to zero, so that the above equation balances. Alternatively there is a need to produce base excess in order to maintain equilibrium, and this electrolyte imbalance can lead to abnormal physiological conditions. Mongin (1980) concludes that when Na+K-Cl is other than 250 mEq/1000 g of diet, then either acidosis or alkalosis develops and growth will be adversely affected.

Cohen and Hurwitz (1974) indicate that the addition of Na (without Cl) to a diet increases plasma HCO_3^- and pH, while with addition of Cl (without Na) there are reductions in plasma HCO_3^- and pH. Addition of both, as salt, cause little change in pH or plasma HCO_3^-. Diet may also influence the acid-base balance indirectly via an effect on endogenous acid production. Mongin (1981) suggests that this is most evident with protein sources that normally contain a variety of nitrogen:ion balance. For example, Mongin (1981) cites change from 17.4 to 12.1 mEq/100 g when a proportion of soy is replaced by fishmeal. Assuming no other changes in formulation. then substitution of soy with fishmeal would necessitate the inclusion of ions such as bicarbonate in order to maintain electrolyte balance. With animal proteins there may also be the need to consider the contribution of sulfate, since Mongin (1981) states that considerable variation in the growth response to various fishmeals could best be accounted for by estimation of Na+K-Cl-SO_4. Ruiz-Lopez and Austic (1993) compared the relative acidogenicities of several anions using chloride as a standard. Chloride increased blood H^+ concentration, although the effect was most noticeable when high levels (160 – 240 mEq/kg) were fed to young birds. Sulfate was also acidogenic, although there was an indication that this effect was most noticeable on the first day of administration. Dibasic phosphate on the other hand was consistently without effect in changing acid-base parameters in the blood. These authors showed the acidogenic properties of sulfate to depend on source, with values relative to mEq of chloride being approximately 58% when $CaSO_4$ and K_2SO_4 were used, but that potency increased to 84% relative to chloride when sulfate originated from Na_2SO_4. As pointed out by Ruiz-Lopez and Austic (1993) the failure of phosphate to influence acid-base parameters is likely a reflection of the buffering capacity of phosphate, because the pK_2 of phosphoric acid is within the range of normal physiological pH.

In certain situations it may also be necessary to take into account the contribution of divalent ions. For example, feeding calcium chloride will induce acidosis in birds, while feeding NaCl or KCl has little effect (Mongin, 1981). This situation probably develops due to less calcium being absorbed from $CaCl_2$ than occurs with Na from NaCl. Since chloride absorption remains unchanged, and since Ca is excreted as $CaCO_3$, there is the potential net loss of bicarbonate and net gain of Cl. Hurwitz and Bar (1968) also indicate the significance of gut lumen buffering capacity as it influences intracellular ion balance. The bird seems to adjust lumen pH in a very short time period, when confronted with either acidic or alkaline conditions imposed via the diet. Within 10 minutes, pH is normalized from 9.0 or 4.0 to around 7.0. Such buffering must obviously be accomplished by a net shift of electrolytes into the lumen, and so for example, with an acidic lumen pH one assumes a net outflux of ions such as bicarbonate. This buffering will obviously influence the electrolyte balance in the bird.

Electrolyte imbalance causes a number of metabolic disorders in birds, most noteably tibial dyschondroplasia and respiratory alkalosis in layers. Tibial dyschondroplasia (TD) in young broiler chickens, can be affected by the electrolyte balance of the diet. The unusual development of the cartilage plug at the growth plate of the tibia can be induced by a number of factors, although its incidence can be greatly increased by metabolic acidosis induced by feeding products such as NH_4Cl. It seems as though TD occurs more frequently when the diet contains an excess of sodium relative to potassium, and at the same time chloride levels are very high. Unfortunately much of the research involving TD and acid-base balance is confounded with a concommitant effect on body weight. For example, a certain balance of electrolytes may be claimed beneficial in reducing TD, but at the same time the body weight may be greatly reduced and this in itself will reduce TD severity. Great care must be taken in the interpretation of any research data in this area, such that any changes to the diet formulation will hopefully reduce or limit the incidence of TD, while at the same time maintaining normal growth characteristics. TD seems most problematic when high diet chloride levels are used.

5.5.2 Electrolytes and amino acid metabolism

Electrolyte balance can affect the metabolism of a number of basic amino acids, particularly those of lysine and arginine. Lysine and other basic amino acids are known to accumulate in the tissues of animals fed potassium deficient diets where, depending upon the degree of potassium deficit, lysine can become the major amino acid in muscle tissue. Unfortunately, such lysine enrichment is usually associated with dramatically reduced growth due to the potassium deficit. The increase in tissue lysine concentration is approximately equal to the reduction in tissue potassium, suggesting that the basic amino acids are acting in a buffering capacity in order to maintain normal ionic balance. There is known to be a lysine-arginine antagonism in poultry, where an excess of lysine can lead to a metabolic deficiency of arginine, most likely brought about by stimulation of kidney arginase. Various researchers have shown that high levels of dietary potassium can alleviate such adverse effects on growth, while Austic and Calvert (1981) clearly show that the imbalance is accentuated when the diet is high in chloride.

High levels of chloride, regardless of amino acid balance seem detrimental to growth. Using C^{14} labeled lysine, Austic and Calvert (1981) conclude that chloride does not influence lysine degradation *per se*, and that the mechanism relates in some way to electrolyte balance. This concept is also supported by the observation of Austic (1981) that varying K:Cl levels, while influencing the severity of the effects of a lysine:arginine imbalance has little influence on growth of arginine-deficient birds.

During acidosis there is also increased NH_4 loss by the kidneys. For example, feeding $NaHCO_3$ reduces the loss of NH_4 in the urine while feeding HCl has the opposite effect (Austic and Calvert, 1981). Because uric acid production is little affected by ion balance, such changes in NH_4 loss can obviously lead to variability in overall nitrogen balance. In rats, at least, the mechanism is thought to involve acid-base effects on glutaminase activity. Adekunmisi and Robbins (1987) suggest that optimum dietary electrolyte balance varies with diet crude protein level. Growth of chicks fed low protein (14.3%) diets was depressed when electrolyte balance was changed by addition of sodium and potassium. However adding these electrolytes to diets containing 28.6% CP, improved growth rate. As previously suggested by Austic and Calvert (1981) higher levels of cations stimulate uric acid excretion, a situation observed by Adekunmisi and Robbins (1987). Electrolyte imbalance can therefore be expected to be more detrimental when low protein diets are used since reduced nitrogen balance is more problematic. The effect of acid-base balance on amino acid metabolism warrants further investigation, especially since much of the older work on this subject seems to be confounded in terms of nutrient deficiency vs. nutrient balance scenarios. However, in general it seems as though high chloride levels will be detrimental, while higher levels of metabolizable potassium salts may be warranted, especially when higher crude protein diets are to be considered. Adekunmisi and Robbins (1987) conclude that electrolyte balance in the diet will be different for situations involving low crude protein and high levels of synthetic amino acids, compared with formulations with high crude protein aimed at reducing carcass fat content.

5.5.3 Electrolytes and respiratory alkalosis

At high environmental temperatures, birds increase their respiration rate in an attempt to increase the rate of evaporative cooling. Such panting increases CO_2 loss and consequently a degree of alkalosis will develop. Such changes in electrolyte balance may result in reduced growth rate seen in meat birds, and a decline in eggshell quality often seen in high producing laying hens. El Hadi and Sykes (1982) describe the usual pattern of respiratory alkalosis as it develops in laying hens. Panting first started at 35°C, and although there was no increase in body temperature, mild alkalosis (pH 7.55) developed. At 38°C there was moderate alkalosis, while at 41°C the condition was described as severe with blood pH at 7.65. Various attempts have been made to correct this imbalance through the administration of electrolytes via the feed and/or water.

The availability of both calcium and carbonate ions at the uterine mucosa is important for shell synthesis. Acid-base balance can dramatically influence the process of shell formation. This is most clearly seen when birds exhibit respiratory alkalosis during heat stress resulting in thinner eggshells. However, the effects of acid or alkaline conditions in the uterine extracellular fluid, while having a major effect on calcium solubility (precipitation), are not so clearly defined in terms of bicarbonate flux. In fact, it is the availability of bicarbonate *per se* that seems to be the major factor influencing eggshell thickness, and to a large extent, this is influenced by acid-base balance, kidney function and respiration rate.

Normally, shell formation induces a renal acidosis related to the total resorption of filtered bicarbonate. At the same time, shell synthesis induces a metabolic acidosis because the formation of insoluble $CaCO_3$ from HCO_3^- and Ca^{++} involves the liberation of H^+ ions. Such H^+ release would induce very acidic and physiologically destructive conditions, and is necessarily balanced by the bicarbonate buffer system in the uterine extracellular fluid. The release of H^+ ions and the mild acidic conditions also aid in the initial cleavage of calcium from protein-bound transport molecules (Mongin, 1968). While a mild metabolic acidosis is therefore normal during shell synthesis, a more severe situation leads to reduced shell production because of intense competition for HCO_3^- as either a buffer or a shell component. A severe metabolic acidosis can be induced by feeding products such as NH_4Cl, and this results in reduced shell strength. In this scenario, it is likely that NH_4^+ rather than Cl^- is problematic because formation of uric acid in the liver (from NH_4^+) needs to be buffered with HCO_3^+ ions, creating more competition with uterine bicarbonate metabolism. Conversely, feeding sodium bicarbonate, especially when Cl⁻ levels are minimized, may well improve shell thickness. Under commercial conditions, the need to produce base excess in order to buffer any diet electrolytes must be avoided. Likewise it is important that birds not be subjected to severe respiratory excess, as occurs at high temperatures, because this induces reduced blood bicarbonate levels, and in extreme cases, possibly a metabolic acidosis. Under practical conditions, replacement of part of the supplemental dietary NaCl with NaHCO$_3$ may be beneficial in terms of shell production. Acclimatization to heat stress may well be another factor confounding many research results, since temporary acute conditions are more problematic. For example, pullets grown to 31 wks under constant 35° vs. 21°C conditions exhibit no difference in their pattern of plasma electrolytes (Vo et al., 1977). Kohne and Jones (1975) also suggest that if birds are allowed to acclimatize to high environmental temperatures, there is little correlation between plasma electrolytes and shell quality. Certainly temporary acute heat stress and cyclic temperature conditions seem most stressful to the bird.

Respiratory alkalosis can also be a factor in the young bird's response to elevated environmental temperatures. Teeter et al. (1985) studied growth and physiological response of broilers to chronic or acute heat stress situations. Blood pH was elevated by chronic heat stress at 32°C, and further elevated by acute stress at 41°C over a 20 minute period. With chronic heat stress there was some respiratory alkalosis, while with acute heat stress all birds suffered from alkalosis. Including 0.5% NaHCO$_3$ in the diet of chronic heat stressed birds improved weight gain even though blood pH was further elevated. Adding NH$_4$Cl decreased blood pH, but also improved weight gain, while using both NH$_4$Cl and NaHCO$_3$ was synergistic in terms of weight gain and slightly reduced severity of alkalosis. Bottje et al. (1989) suggest that treating heat-stressed broilers with NH$_4$Cl could potentially be deleterious to the bicarbonate buffer system, as any metabolic acidosis associated with NH$_4$Cl catabolism may accentuate HCO$_3^-$ loss due to increased respiratory rate. Bottje et al. (1989) tested this assumption by infusing NH$_4$Cl solution into the crop of heat stressed broilers. As a result of this treatment, acidosis developed, and since equimolor intubation of KCl had no effect, it is suggested that acidosis may relate to NH$_4$ metabolism as previously described (H⁺ liberated during uric acid synthesis). Therefore, while NH$_4$Cl may be beneficial in reducing lactate production under heat stress, this seems to be at the expense of the bicarbonate buffer system.

A confounding factor in electrolyte treatment during heat stress, is the influence on water intake. It seems as though mortality and growth depression can be reduced if birds drink more water, and this does occur in response to some electrolytes. Branton et al. (1986) studied the response of broilers to NH$_4$Cl and NaHCO$_3$ administration during a period of heat stress. NaHCO$_3$ stimulated water intake, while NH$_4$Cl was without effect. These authors concluded that any beneficial effect of electrolyte therapy is via stimulation of water intake, rather than plasma electrolyte balance and/or blood pH *per se*. Teeter and Smith (1986) also showed some alleviation of heat stress in broilers through administration of KCl, but not with K_2CO_3, and that KCl stimulated water consumption, whereas K_2CO_3 depressed water intake. Whiting *et al.* (1991) likewise indicate that adding electrolytes to the drinking water during a period of heat stress is beneficial when water intake is stimulated, and that this effect is independent of cation or anion status of the supplement. Broiler chickens and laying hens obviously differ in their response to, and needs for, electrolyte therapy during heat stress.

5.5.4 Maintaining electrolyte balance

Prevention of electrolyte imbalance should obviously be approached through incorporation of appropriate cations and anions in diet formulations. As suggested by Mongin (1980) electrolyte balance can be accommodated by consideration of Na+K-Cl balance in the diet, and under most dietary situations this seems a reasonable simplification. A balance of around 250 mEq/kg seems a compromise in terms of optimum performance coupled with a minimum of undesirable side effects such as tibial dyschondroplasia or abnormal amino acid metabolism.

While it is true that overall electrolyte balance is of major importance it appears as though this scenario is most critical when chloride or sulphur levels are high. With low diet chloride levels, there is often little response to the manipulation of electrolyte balance, but when diet chloride levels are necessarily elevated then it seems critical to make adjustments to the diet cations such that overall balance is maintained. Alternatively chloride levels can be reduced, although it must be remembered that chickens have requirements around 0.12 – 0.15% of the diet, and deficiency signs will develop with diet levels much less than 0.12%. Therefore care must be taken in meeting the minimum chloride requirements when, for example, $NaHCO_3$ replaces NaCl in a diet. Table 5.8 outlines electrolyte content and electrolyte balance of some major feed ingredients.

TABLE 5.8 Electrolyte content of feed ingredients				
Ingredient	Na	K	Cl	Na+K-Cl(mEq)
	% of ingredient			
Corn	0.05	0.38	0.04	108
Wheat	0.09	0.52	0.08	150
Barley	0.02	0.56	0.18	101
Milo	0.04	0.34	0.08	82
Soybean meal	0.05	2.61	0.05	675
Canola meal	0.09	1.47	0.05	400
Meat meal	0.55	1.23	0.90	300
Fish meal	0.47	0.72	0.55	230
Cottonseed meal	0.05	1.20	0.03	320
Sunflower meal	0.02	1.00	0.03	255

Within the cereals, electrolyte balance for milo is low, while wheat is high relative to corn. Major differences occur in the protein rich ingredients, and relative to soy, all sources are low in electrolyte balance. As shown in Table 5.8, this situation develops due to the very high potassium content of soybean meal. Careful consideration to electrolyte balance must therefore be given when change is made in protein sources used in formulation. For example, the overall balance for a diet containing 60% milo and 25% soy is 210 mEq/kg, while for a diet containing 75% milo and 10% fish meal the balance is only 75 mEq/kg. The milo-fish diet would perhaps need to be supplemented with $NaHCO_3$ if effects of imbalance such as poor growth or TD, were evident.

Assuming that heat stress cannot be tempered by normal management techniques, electrolyte manipulation of the diet may be beneficial. However, this technique should be different for immature birds compared to egg layers. With adult female birds there is need to maintain the bicarbonate buffer system as it relates to eggshell quality. As such, diet or water treatment with sodium bicarbonate may be beneficial, again emphasizing the necessity to meet minimal chloride requirements. For example, Koelkebeck et al. (1992) showed improvement in shell thickness of layers maintained at 24 – 30°C when water was saturated with CO_2 to give pH of 4.7 vs. 7.7 for the control. On the other hand, treatment of respiratory alkalosis in layers with acidifiers such as NH_4Cl, while relieving respiratory distress, may well result in reduced shell quality. For immature birds such as the broiler chicken, treatment with electrolytes is often beneficial, and there seems less need for caution related to bicarbonate buffering. Up to 0.3% dietary NH_4Cl may improve the growth rate of heat stressed birds although as detailed previously it is not clear if this beneficial effect is via electrolyte balance/blood pH or simply via the indirect effect of stimulating water intake. Under commercial conditions, adding salt to the drinking water of heat stressed broilers has been reported to alleviate bird distress and to simulate growth. In this context, Belay and Teeter (1993) show heat distressed broilers to respond well to adding 0.75% KCl to their drinking water by increasing their water consumption by 91%, their evaporative heat loss by 20% and their apparent respiration efficiency by 27%. Ait-Boulashen et al. (1995) likewise showed that giving heat stressed birds 0.6% KCl in their drinking water improved bird performance and tempered body temperature rise.

5.6 SODIUM

Sodium is the chief cation in extracellular fluid, and is required by all plants and animals for normal metabolism. The craving of salt is an innate urge of all animals. Sodium was first shown to be an essential constituent of media for in vitro culture studies, by Ringer (1881). Earlier studies had shown that infusing sodium into patients suffering from cholera (a disease characterized by diarrhea and thus loss of body fluids) produced a beneficial effect (O'Shaughnessy, 1831). Von Leibig, (1874) first reported the unique distribution of sodium and potassium in the body with extracellular fluids being high in sodium while cells were high in potassium.

In the 1920s, a number of important metabolic functions for sodium were demonstrated. These include its role in the regulation of body fluid volume and acid-base balance, movement of sodium into muscle cells during contraction, and the observation that the adrenal gland was important for regulation of sodium retention and the reduced sodium level in blood resulting from adrenal insufficiency. Isolation and identification of the adrenal hormone aldosterone, and the demonstration of its importance in regulating sodium and potassium balance in the body, aided immensely in understanding the functions and metabolism of these two elements.

A deficiency of sodium leads to a lowering of osmotic pressure and a change in acid-base balance in the body. Cardiac output falls, blood pressure is decreased, hematocrit increases, elasticity of subcutaneous tissues decreases, and adrenal function is impaired leading to an increase in blood uric acid levels, which can result in shock and death. A less severe sodium deficiency in chicks can result in retarded growth, soft bones, corneal keratinization, impaired food utilization and a decrease in plasma volume. In layers, reduced egg production, poor growth and cannibalism may be noted. A number of diseases can result in sodium depletion from the body due to gastrointestinal losses such as happens with diarrhea and urinary losses resulting from renal or adrenal damage.

5.6.1 Sodium absorption and homeostasis

Sodium salts are readily absorbed and the body has the ability to conserve its supply by decreasing excretion if intake is low. Moderate increases in diet sodium levels are usually not a problem to poultry, provided that the drinking water is not also high in sodium. Birds will increase their water intake if the diet is high in salt, and thus excrete the excess intake. Toxicity will not develop as long as birds are able to increase their water intake. If excess water is consumed, it can be transferred into the cells and symptoms of water toxicity are noted. If, on the other hand, there is a large negative water loss associated with a sodium loss, extracellular fluid will be depleted and the bird will become seriously dehydrated.

In simple marine animals, body fluids are isotonic with seawater, while in higher aquatic and terrestrial animals, body fluids are either hypotonic or hypertonic to their environment such that the extracellular fluid composition must be maintained against an environmental gradient. Some fish can adapt to changes in an environmental gradient since they have a life cycle which includes living in both fresh and salt water. Chickens, like other farm animals, consume a diet which is hypotonic with respect to sodium, yet they maintain a constant sodium concentration in the body, despite marked variations in sodium intake. Since blood and tissue homeostasis is essential to normal health, the animal has a number of mechanisms that function to preserve homeostasis.

Like most farm animals the sodium content of poultry is approximately 0.1 to 0.14% of body weight. Approximately 30 to 40% of the sodium is found in the skeleton and being firmly bound to the inorganic phase of bone is not readily accessible to the animal to supplement requirements. While sodium makes up approximately 93% of the total cations of the plasma, it is almost completely absent from blood cells. It is for this reason that it is the main basic element governing pH of the plasma. In chickens the sodium content of plasma is around 8.4 mg/ml.

5.6.2 Metabolic functions of sodium

One of the main functions of sodium is to maintain body fluid volume, pH and optimum osmotic relationships. Energy required for nerve impulse transmission is derived from potential energy resulting from the separation of sodium and potassium in the cell wall. Most of the mitochondrial enzymes are activated by the intracellular ions, K^+ and Mg^{++} and inhibited by the extracellular ion, Na+.

A number of anions are present in muscle or tissue cells, such as protein, tricarboxylic acids, organic phosphates including adenosine mono, di- and tri-phosphates, glycerophosphate and creatine phosphate, bicarbonate and some chloride ions. Some anions are readily diffusible through the cell but others are fixed to cytoplasmic structures or otherwise restricted so that they cannot diffuse out of the cell. Such ions electrically attract cations such as H^+, Na^+ and K^+ (and Mg^{++}). Sodium and potassium, in association with these anions, provide the necessary buffer to the cytoplasm for its optimum pH. While it has been shown that both Na^+ and K^+ are readily capable of entering the cell, the cell accumulates K^+ (and some Mg^+), but very little Na^+. It has been demonstrated that the expulsion of Na^+ is a dynamic phenomenon of active transport requiring energy from both ATP and glucose. Under physiological conditions, sodium enters the cell in exchange for potassium at the expense of energy derived from hydrolysis of ATP from the cell membrane. The overall reaction or pump runs in the direction of expelling Na^+ from the cell.

The active transport of Na^+ and K^+ is of major physiological significance. More than a third of the ATP consumed by a resting animal is used to pump these ions. An enzyme that hydrolyzes ATP, only if Na^+ and K^+ are present, along with Mg^{++}, is required in all ATPases. The name Na^+-K^+ ATPase was given to the enzyme. The enzyme is an integral part of the Na^+-K^+ pump and splitting of ATP provides the energy needed for active transport of the ions. Thus, ATPase is the pump in the membrane, with ATP as a substrate and Na^+ and K^+ as co-substrates. These cations may be considered as substrates or products, depending on which side of the membrane they are located and movement across the membrane is equivalent to the conversion of substrate to product. The pump runs in the direction of expelling Na^+ from the cell.

5.6.3 Sodium requirements

Classical earlier studies showed the sodium requirement of young birds to be around 0.15% of the diet, assuming a chloride level in this same region. For laying hens the requirement is around 0.17-0.19% of the diet. With the advent of nipple drinkers in commercial production, it became evident that birds were unwilling or unable to consume normal intakes of water. Consequently diet sodium 'requirements' have been increased. Murakami *et al.* (1997 a,b) show diet sodium level of broilers up to 21 d to be at least 0.25% of the diet. There is a linear relationship between early growth rate and diet sodium, and the limit is usually dictated by manure consistency.

5.6.4 Sodium toxicity

Sodium becomes toxic much above 0.5% of the diet. At around 0.35% sodium, birds will drink much more water, and this is sometimes regarded as a toxicity. High levels of diet sodium adversely influence electrolyte balance and at very high levels can cause water intoxication. There have been reports, mostly from Australia, of a decline in shell quality of birds given saline drinking water. Studies in North America have generally failed to confirm these findings. Damron (1998) for example shows no adverse effect of offering layers water for 6 weeks with up to 800 ppm sodium. Differences in response may relate to strain of birds used since Wideman and Nissley (1992) indicate differences in pullet strain response to receiving water with 10 g NaCl/litre. These authors conclude that susceptible strains have much smaller kidney glomeruli than do other strains that are unaffected by the saline water.

5.7 POTASSIUM

In contrast to sodium, body potassium is primarily within the cells. The blood cells contain approximately 25 times as much potassium as is present in the plasma. Muscle and nerve cells are also very high in potassium, containing over 20 times as much as that present in the interstitial fluid. Muscle usually contains around 4 mg/g, while normal plasmal levels of K are around 100 μg/ml.

5.7.1 Metabolic function

Potassium appears to carry out many of the same functions inside the cell that sodium performs in the plasma and interstitial fluid, namely maintenance of acid-base relationships and proper osmotic balance. Potassium also activates a number of intracellular enzymes, and is required for normal heart activity where it exerts an effect opposite to that of calcium, reducing the contractability of the heart muscle and favoring relaxation.

The main sign of hypokalemia is an overall muscle weakness characterized by weak extremities, poor intestinal tone with intestinal distension, cardiac weakness,

weakness of the respiratory muscles and their ultimate failure. Hypokalemia is apt to occur during severe stress. Plasma protein is elevated, causing the kidney, under the influence of the adrenal cortical hormone, to discharge potassium into the urine. During adaptation to the stress the muscle gradually gains an improved blood flow and begins to retrieve its lost potassium. As liver glycogen is restored, potassium returns to the liver. This may result in temporary prolongation of the hypokalemia. Effects of administration of potassium salts to chickens during and following severe stress periods have not been adequately investigated.

When a low protein diet is combined with a low potassium diet, or during starvation, animals grow slowly but do not show a potassium deficiency. Potassium derived from the metabolized tissue protein replaces that lost in the urine or not supplied by the diet. Under such conditions less potassium is needed. The ratio of potassium to nitrogen in urine is relatively constant, and is at the same ratio as that found in fresh muscle. Thus, tissue nitrogen and potassium are released together from metabolized tissue. If protein is given to a nitrogen starved animal, the animal grows, but may develop a potassium deficiency. Potassium appears to increase membrane permeability. Potassium accelerates the uptake of the free, neutral amino acids such as glycine and it leaves the cell when glycine is entering. Pyridoxal also enhances glycine uptake, and a progressive increase in cellular potassium concentration enhances this effect. In potassium deficiency, the concentration of neutral amino acids in tissues is reduced whereas basic amino acids appear, in part, to replace potassium. Scott and Austic (1976) found that potassium is concerned in the catabolism of lysine. Growth was improved and plasma lysine levels reduced in chicks when potassium was added to a diet in which the excess lysine present caused poor growth due to an amino acid imbalance.

5.7.2 Potassium requirements

Birds deficient in potassium exhibit reduced feed intake and poor growth rate, and eventually death. Requirements as low as 0.17 – 0.20% of the diet have been reported, although more recent studies show values of 0.4-0.6% (Hooge and Cummings, 1995). For adult males, Chavez and Kratzer (1979) suggest 0.06% dietary potassium is adequate for survival, even though some dehydration occurred. In this study, there was a dramatic increase in the half-life of K from 18 → 134d, as diet K was decreased, indicating potassium conservation by the kidneys.

Austic (1983) showed higher potassium requirement for normal vs. hyperuremic birds, suggesting that potassium is needed for uric acid excretion. This situation implies a higher potassium need when diet crude protein is increased, or where amino acid imbalance or excess occurs. There may also be increased need for K during heat stress, a situation that leads to increased K excretion. Smith and Teeter (1987) indicated a 600% increase in K excretion of young broilers exposed to 35 vs. 24°C and that for such birds a dietary equivalent of 1.5-2.0% K was ideal. A similar benefit resulted from including 0.24 – 0.30% K in the drinking water.

5.8 CHLORIDE

Although the physiological significance of chloride has long been recognized, early attempts by Osborne and Mendel, (1918) and others to produce a nutritional deficiency were unsuccessful. The classical experiments by Orent-Keiles and associates (1937) provided the first nutritional evidence for the essentiality of chlorine. Rats fed a diet low in chloride showed retarded growth and signs which differed from those observed with a sodium-deficient diet. Although deficient rats showed no clinical signs, it was possible to induce tetany in a few animals by means of auditory stimuli or mild galvanic shock. Deficient animals had reduced levels of blood chloride, accompanied by increased amounts of carbonate. Dietary carbonate or bicarbonate did not affect these blood changes. The almost complete disappearance of chloride from the urine of deficient rats indicated that animals have a marked ability to conserve body chloride.

5.8.1 Metabolic functions of chloride

Chloride ions have a very weak affinity for combination with protein, enabling it to be a major contributor to the tonicity of ionic strength of the extracellular medium and a predominant matching anion for Na^+. It also enters cells with K^+ as indicated previously. It is very actively transported, especially by gastric mucosal cells in the chloride shift responsible for H^+ concentration of gastric juice. Estimates indicate that only 2 H^+ ions and 2 Cl^- ions are transported across the gastric mucosa for each mole of O_2 consumed. The energy cost of elaborating gastric HCl appears to take precedence over other metabolic considerations.

Leach and Nesheim (1963) produced a chloride deficiency by feeding young chicks a purified diet containing 190 mg Cl^-/kg diet. The chicks showed extremely poor growth rate, high mortality, hemo-concentration, dehydration and a reduced blood chloride level. In addition, deficient chicks had nervous signs, characteristic of chloride deficiency. The addition of 1200 mg Cl^-/kg of basal diet resulted in optimal growth rate and prevented deficiency symptoms. Although excess sodium and potassium did not affect the growth rate of deficient chicks, increasing the levels of these cations in the basal diet increased the incidence of nervous symptoms and mortality. Bromide (676 to 1352 mg/kg) added to the basal diet partially counteracted most of the signs of chloride deficiency except the nervous incoordination. Higher levels of bromide were of no additional value. Iodide (537 to 1074 mg/kg of diet) depressed growth rate and produced mortality and nervous incoordination, which suggested an antagonistic interaction between iodide and chloride. Fluoride (268 mg/kg of diet) had no effect on the development of chloride deficiency. Chloride deficient chicks that are stimulated by a sharp noise or by handling show a typical nervous reaction resembling tetany. They fall forward with their legs extended to the rear. After one or two minutes spontaneous recovery occurs and another spasm cannot be induced for several minutes. The appearance of a chick with nervous signs is shown in Figure 5.14.

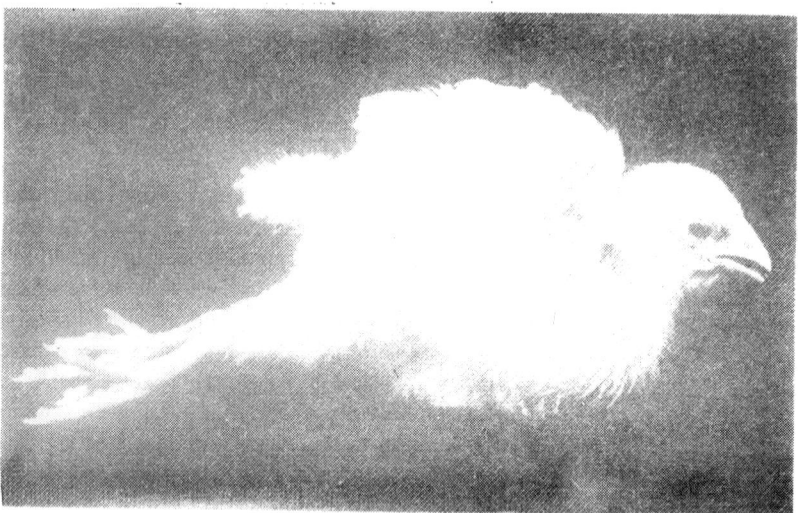

Figure 5.14 Chloride deficient chick showing typical nervous reaction induced by sudden noise or fright. *(Leach and Nesheim, 1963).*

5.8.2 Requirements for chloride

The bird's requirements for chloride must always be balanced against needs and/or diet levels of sodium and potassium. As a general guideline, the levels of diet chloride should exceed those of sodium by 10-15%. There has been surprisingly little research conducted in the last 20 years on chloride requirements. Harms and Wilson (1984) indicated that broiler breeders required only 0.135% dietary chloride for optimal reproductive performance. Christmas and Harms (1982) saw little difference in performance of older laying hens fed 0.14 → 0.28% Cl, although they did observe a reduction in the incidence of eggshell pimpling with higher chloride levels. At very high levels (0.9% chloride) there will be a loss in shell quality (Austic, 1984). Keshavarz (1994) suggests that layers can tolerate up to 200 mEq Cl/kg diet as a supplement to a diet already containing 0.24% Cl$^-$ and 0.16% Na$^+$.

5.9 MAGNESIUM

Magnesium is an important cation necessary for the nutrition of both animals and especially plants, where it is the chelated metal in the porphyrin moiety of chlorophyll. Early studies of the functions of magnesium in animals were concerned mainly with neuromuscular paralysis, which occurs when magnesium salts are intravenously administered. Magnesium was established as an essential element in animal nutrition only about eighty years ago. Although it has been studied extensively, its physiological role in animals, especially in regard to its interactions with other metal ions, is not well established. In 1927 Erdtmann discovered that magnesium activates alkaline phosphatase. Since then, numerous enzymes have been found to be activated by magnesium.

5.9.1 Metabolism and function

Magnesium concentrations are low in newly hatched chicks but rise quickly thereafter. About one half of the total body magnesium is present in the bone representing 0.5 – 0.7% of the bone ash in all animals. Using radiolabelled Mg (half-life 21.8 hrs), it has been found that magnesium equilibrates with a fluid volume which is larger than that of the extracellular fluid. Since the total magnesium composition of the body is much larger than that calculated from the rapidly exchangeable magnesium, one must assume that the bone magnesium is not readily exchangeable with the magnesium present in the extracellular fluid. Nevertheless, bone magnesium may act as a storage reservoir for the bird under most conditions.

Magnesium, like potassium, is concentrated within the cells of the soft tissues. Liver, striated muscle, kidney and brain contain about 430-540 mg/kg, while the blood serum contains only about 10% this amount or approximately 50 mg/liter.

As with calcium, some of the serum magnesium is bound to protein, although serum Mg^{++} does not appear to be affected by parathyroid hormone. All warm-blooded animals have about the same percentage of magnesium bound to protein even though total blood Mg may vary from species to species. The magnesium content of the cerebrospinal fluid is higher than that in serum, although the mechanisms of this accumulation have not been explained. The serum magnesium content of animals increases when the body temperature is artificially lowered.

The egg contains about 25 mg of magnesium with 2.0 mg in the yolk, 4.3 mg in the albumen, and 18.7 mg in the shell and shell membranes. By far the major portion of magnesium in eggs occurs in eggshells and during incubation from 1 to 1.8 mg of the shell magnesium is transferred to the embryo. Thus the shell seems to be a reservoir for both calcium and magnesium for use by the embryo.

Most enzymes activated by magnesium are metal-enzyme complexes as opposed to metalloenzymes in which the specific metal is tightly bound to a protein. The catalytic functions of magnesium, as with other metals, have been determined in *in vitro* studies of enzyme activity. Since the enzymes contain some activity without the addition of the metal and the activity is only increased by the metal ion, it is difficult to determine how important *in vitro* enzyme studies are to the actual *in vivo* occurrences in the cell. Magnesium activates the numerous enzymes which split and transfer phosphate groups such as the phosphates and the enzymes concerned in reactions involving ATP. Since ATP is required in numerous different functions such as muscle contractions, protein, nucleic acid, fat and coenzyme synthesis, glucose utilization, and oxidative phosphorylation, it is clear that magnesium is important in almost all functions of the body. In its *in vitro* activation of phosphate transfer from ATP to phosphate receptors, the action of magnesium can usually be replaced by manganese. It is not known whether this also occurs *in vivo*. The common soluble magnesium salts are readily absorbed from the small intestine. It has been shown that vitamin D_3 has no effect on magnesium absorption.

5.9.2 Magnesium requirements and signs of deficiency

Magnesium was first shown by LeRoy (1926) to be essential for normal growth in mice. Kruse, *et al.* (1932) subsequently induced magnesium deficiency in rats and described the classical syndrome, which included vasodilation manifested by erythema and hyperemia followed by pallor and cyanosis about 12 days later. Subsequently the animals exhibited signs of increasing neuromuscular hyperirritability, culminating in generalized seizures. Many died during the first seizure, while others survived for longer periods before another seizure occurred. Chronic deficiency in animals surviving for a long time was manifested by alopecia, trophic skin lesions, hematomas of the ear lobes and swollen hyperemic gums. Many signs of magnesium deficiency were found to be similar to hypocalcemic tetanies, including the lower sensitivity threshold.

Newly hatched chicks fed a diet devoid of magnesium live only a few days. They grow slowly when fed diets low in magnesium, are lethargic, and often pant and gasp. When disturbed, they exhibit brief convulsions and go into a comatose state, which is sometimes temporary, but often fatal. Mortality is often high on diets only marginally deficient in magnesium even though growth of survivors may approach that of control animals. Plasma magnesium levels are markedly depressed by the magnesium deficiency. Investigations at Purdue University showed that the magnesium content of the blood of chicks receiving a diet containing 122 mg magnesium per kg was only 0.47 mg/100 ml of blood whereas this increased to 0.72 mg/100 ml when the magnesium content of the diet was raised to 250 mg/kg, the approximate level required for maximum growth. Higher levels of magnesium in the diet raised the blood magnesium levels still higher. A level of 4,000 mg magnesium per kg of diet resulted in a blood magnesium level of 2.4 mg/100 ml of blood. Mahoney *et al.* (1992) noted a 80% reduction in growth of broilers fed 200 vs. 600 ppm Mg. In trying to explain the metabolic consequences of such a deficiency, these workers suggested a reduced role as co-factor in cAMP production, rather than altered thyroid status, as has been suggested by others.

The levels of calcium and phosphorus in the diet have a marked effect upon magnesium requirements. Increasing either the calcium or the phosphorus content of the diet increases the magnesium requirement of chicks. In rats, a high calcium and normal magnesium intake is accompanied by alkaline urine, calciuria and urinary calculi. The serum magnesium concentration of these animals is low while the serum calcium is increased.

A deficiency of magnesium in the diet of laying hens results in a rapid decline in egg production, blood hypomagnesemia and a marked withdrawal of magnesium from bones. Egg size, weight of shell and magnesium content of yolk and shell, are decreased due to magnesium deficiency. An increase in the calcium content of the diet of laying hens accentuates the effects of a deficiency. Magnesium seems to play a central role in eggshell formation, although it is not clear if there is a need related to structural integrity *per se*, or the fact that Mg simply gets deposited as a co-factor associated with calcium deposition. There is one peak of Mg concentration in the core layer, and another immediately underneath the outer shell surface. A normal shell contains around 0.65% Mg while feeding a Mg deficient diet (200 ppm) reduces shell thickness and Mg content declines to around 0.25%. With a Mg deficiency, eggs spend comparable time in the shell gland, and so for whatever reason there is impaired calcium deposition. Waddell *et al.* (1991) indicate that both plasma Ca and Mg naturally decline during periods of active shell calcification. These workers suggest that the majority of ATP-ase dependent transfer can only occur in the presence of magnesium, which acting as a co-factor, coincidentally ends up in the eggshell. Consequently the thicker the shell, the more Mg deposited, and vice versa. In support of this supposition, Waddell *et al.* (1991) suggest that galliform birds are less affected by DDE (organopesticide) thinning of the shell than are non-galliforms such as raptors, because Mg-dependent ATP-ase systems are less affected by this compound. Birds such as raptors have little Mg-dependant shell calcification systems, and their alternate enzyme systems are particularly susceptible to products such as DDE. Requirements for most classes of chicken seem to be around 500-600 ppm Mg, a level that is usually achieved with contributions by natural feed ingredients.

5.9.3 Magnesium toxicity

Magnesium salts were employed as cathartics as early as the 16th century (LaWall, 1927). Epsom salt ($MgSO_4 \cdot 7H_2O$), was isolated from water obtained from springs at Epsom in the UK in 1695. The external use of magnesium sulfate solutions, except for bathing at the Epsom 'Spa,' began in the early 1900s. Magnesium sulfate solutions were used, not because of their astringent properties, but because their local anesthetic properties produced relief to patients suffering from erysipelas. Stanley *et al.* (1992) fed up to 8.5 g $MgSO_4$/litre drinking water as a means of flushing broilers immediately prior to processing. Such treatment is claimed to reduce coliform bacteria in intestinal contents.

Lee and Britton (1980) showed that 0.9% Mg fed to broilers was cathartic and dramatically reduced early growth rate, while increasing the incidence of leg disorders. There was an indication that the leg condition was somewhat ameliorated by increasing the chloride level of the diet. Lee *et al.* (1980) described bone lesions as rachitic with a widened and lengthened growth plate. Tibias were usually short, thick and deviated to the left or right. These authors observed a decrease in size of the parathyroids suggesting altered calcium metabolism. In feeding layers 0.8 or 1.2% Mg, Hess and Britton (1997) described loss in egg production and body weight as a consequence of reduced feed intake. Decline in shell quality was associated with a 30% decrease in plasma calcium and a 100% increase in plasma Mg. That plasma P was increased by up to 80% suggests that the bird was mobilizing more medullary bone in an attempt to meet demands for calcium.

Common feed ingredients contain moderate levels of Mg, with corn at around 1,000 ppm and soybean meal at 2,600 ppm. Corn-soy diets will therefore normally contain 1,100-1,200 ppm Mg. Magnesium toxicity can therefore only occur if magnesium salts are incorrectly dosed, or if it is a contaminant of another mineral source. The usual culprit is dolomitic limestone, which can contain up to 10% magnesium. In very unusual circumstances, drinking water can contain sufficient Mg to cause diarrhea in birds.

5.10 MANGANESE

Bertrand and associates were the first to show that manganese occurs in relatively constant amounts in the tissues and organs of both plants and animals, and that manganese is especially concentrated in the reproductive organs. Kemmerer, *et al.* (1931) were probably the first to demonstrate manganese to be an essential element in nutrition. A diet composed exclusively of milk caused poor growth and poor reproduction in mice, which could be corrected by supplementing the diet with manganese. Others soon showed that manganese also is required by the rat and that high mortality, testicular degeneration and poor lactation accompany manganese deficiency. Interest in manganese nutrition was greatly stimulated by the discovery that a deficiency of this element was largely responsible for a crippling disease of chickens known as perosis or slipped tendon. Bone is the richest source of manganese in the body, at 3-4 μg/g tissue, followed by liver at around 2 μg/g. Interestingly both the pituitary and pineal glands are relatively high in manganese.

5.10.1 Metabolic functions of manganese

The absorption of manganese from the intestinal tract is poor. Hence, it is questionable how much of the manganese found in the various feedstuffs is available to the bird. Absorption and excretion of manganese appears to be dependent upon formation of natural chelates especially with bile salts. Marked changes have been noted in the distribution of manganese in the body with artificial chelation. Manganese is excreted in the feces mainly via the bile and is probably reabsorbed as bile-bound manganese. While the rate of excretion of manganese is affected by dietary concentration, it does not appear to be unduly influenced by other dietary ions or by changes in acid-base balance.

The availability of manganese in different mineral salts is likely a reflection of differences in absorption. Using $MnSO_4$ as a standard, Smith *et al.* (1995) suggest MnO to be 70-80% available, while the carbonate is only 40% available. Excess

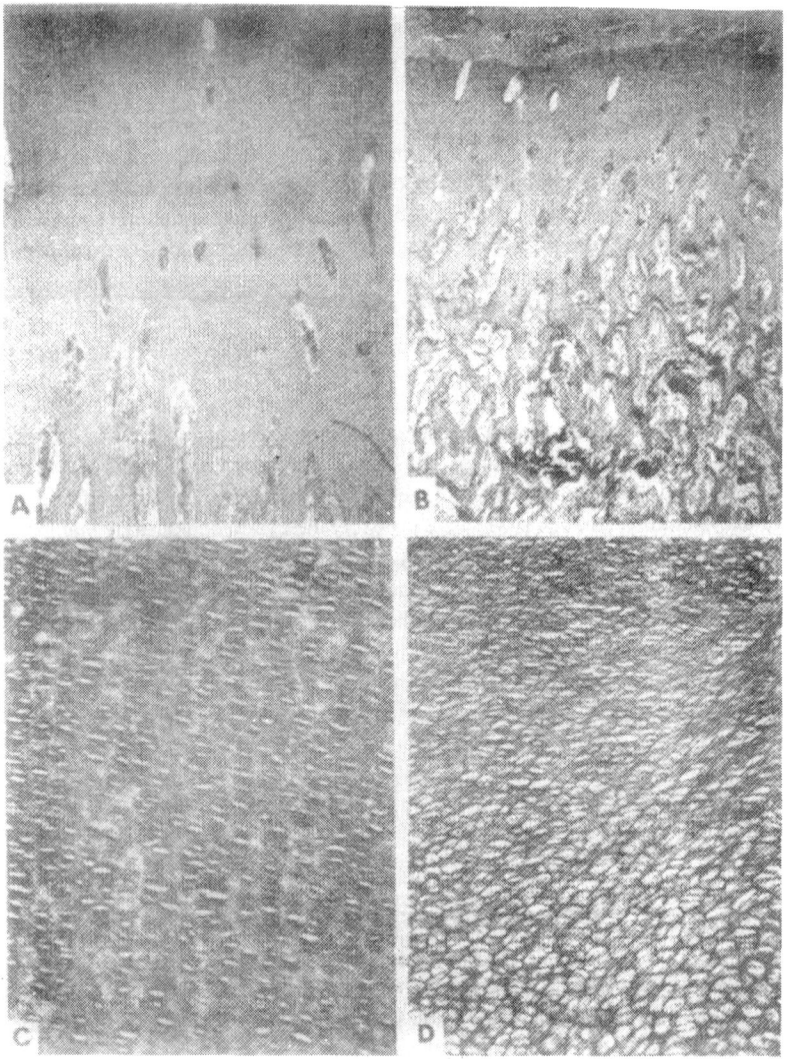

Figure 5.15 areas of endochondral bone formation from chicks receiving adequate (A&C) and deficient (B&D) amounts of manganese.

A. Epiphyseal growth plate and metaphysis of normal chick. H&E, x38.
B. Epiphyseal growth plate and metaphysis of Mn-deficient chick. H&E, x38
C. Epiphyseal growth plate of normal chick. H&E, x205.
D. Epiphyseal growth plate of Mn-deficient chick. Alcian blue-Pas, x205.

phosphorus seems to be antagonistic to Mn absorption, and more so than the effect of calcium. However the effect is quite small, since it takes some 0.2% extra available phosphorus in the diet to reduce Mn absorption by just 10%. High levels of Mn impair Fe absorption, although the converse interaction does not seem to be significant. Liver and bone Mn are very responsive to diet concentrations, with a 3-5% increase in concentration for each 100 ppm increase in diet Mn.

Manganese plays a critical role in bone formation, and such activity has been extensively studied by Leach and co-workers. In manganese deficient chicks the chondroitin sulfate content of the epiphyseal cartilage is markedly reduced. The photomicrographs shown in Figure 5.15, illustrate the lack of intracellular matrix in the cartilage. The epiphyseal plate of the manganese deficient chick (B), is markedly reduced in width compared to a normal chick (A). Under higher magnification, the cells are more closely packed and disorganized (D) for the deficient chick, as compared to those of the control (C). Lack of intracellular cartilage is observed in leg and wing bones in manganese deficient chicks.

According to Leach (1967) the enzymatic steps in the synthesis of chondroitin sulfate involve: (a) synthesis of a specific protein associated with the mucopolysaccharide; (b) xylation of the serine residues for protein-polysaccharide linkage formation; (c) addition of two galactose residues to the xylose to complete the protein-polysaccharide linkage; (d) polymerization of UDP-N-acetyl-galactosamine and UDP glucuronic acid to form the polysaccharide; (e) conversion of UDP-N-acetyl glucosamine to UDP-N-acetyl-galactosamine; and (f) sulfation of the galactosamine portion of the polysaccharide molecule. Manganese appears to be required for the galacto-transferase required in step (c) and the polymerase in step (d). This is one of the few cases in which a biochemical function of an element can be closely linked with the pathology associated with a deficiency.

Liu *et al.* (1994) suggest that while normal cartilage proteoglycan is 90% composed of chondroitin sulfate sidechains, with Mn deficiency there are either fewer or smaller carbohydrate side chains. The deficient bird also has less proteoglycan *per se* in the cartilage. Leach and Gross (1983) also describe defects to the eggshell in Mn deficient layers. In addition to there being less shell mass, the egg takes on a more rounded shape, with translucent areas around the equator. Microscopy of these shell defects reveal irregular mammillary knobs due to fusion of several smaller mammillary cores during the early phases of shell formation (Figure 5.16). The eggshells also have reduced hexosamine and hexuronic acid content, which is consistent with the role of Mn in polysaccharide synthesis.

Manganese has also been reported to be effective in the *in vitro* activation of several enzymes, including arginase, cysteine desulfhydrase, thiaminase, carnosinase, deoxyribonuclease, enolase, intestinal prolinase and glycyl-L-leucine dipeptidase.

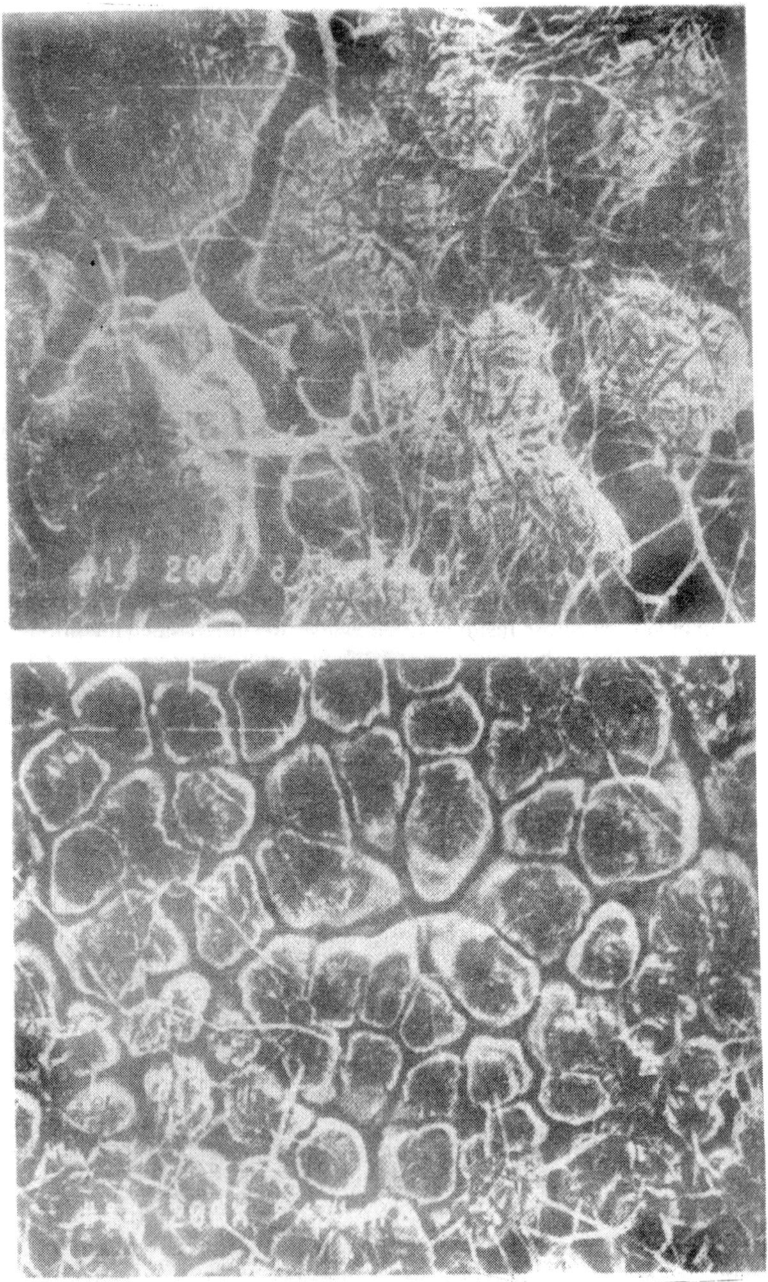

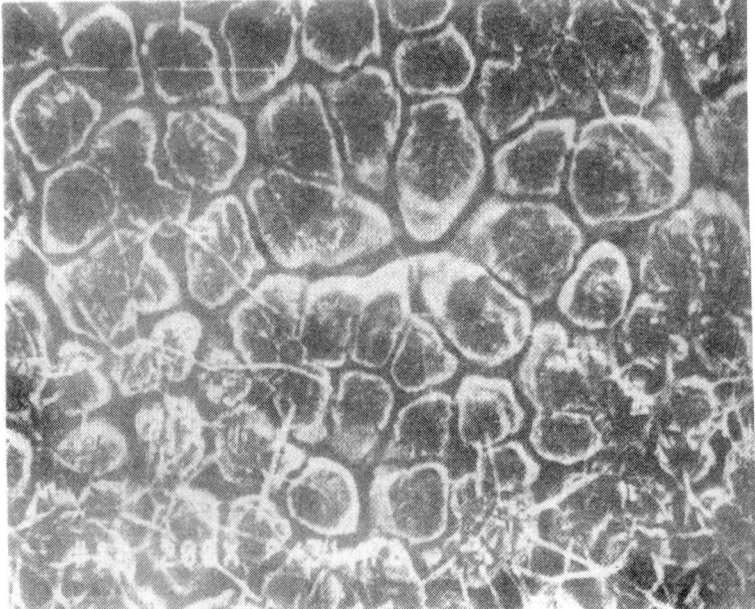

Figure 5.16 Top photograph is an SEM picture of the interior of an eggshell from a manganese deficient hen. Note larger but fewer mammillary knobs when compared to egg in bottom photograph (X200)

Reprinted with permission from Leach and Gross,(1983)

It is also thought to be required for: (1) oxidative phosphorylation in mitochondria; (2) fatty acid synthesis (as a manganese chelate of acetoacetyl-S-coenzyme A); and (3) acetate incorporation into cholesterol.

5.10.2 Manganese requirements and signs of deficiency

Manganese requirement is around 60 mg/kg diet, even for modern broiler strains growing quite rapidly (Collins and Moran, 1999). Halpin and Baker (1986) suggest that when using purified diets the young bird's requirement is only around 14 mg/kg diet. However when more conventional diets are fed, requirement increases to around 60 mg/kg, likely because of natural antagonists to Mn, such as phytic acid, fiber and calcium. Southern and Baker (1983) suggest than the Mn content of bone and bile are probably more sensitive indicators of the bird's Mn status, than are either liver Mn or simply weight gain. Toxic levels seem to be around 3,000 mg/kg, when a mild anemia develops.

The most dramatic manganese deficiency syndrome is perosis which occurs in young chicks. It is characterized by enlargement and malformation of the tibiometatarsal joint, twisting and bending of the distal end of the tibia and the proximal end of the tarsometatarsus, thickening and shortening of the leg bones and slippage of the gastrocnemius or Achilles tendon from its condyles (Figure 5.17). Higher intakes of calcium and or phosphorus, will aggravate the condition. This is due to reduced absorption of magnesium by precipitated calcium phosphate in the intestinal tract. In laying hens, reduced egg production, markedly reduced hatchability and egg shell thinning are often noted.

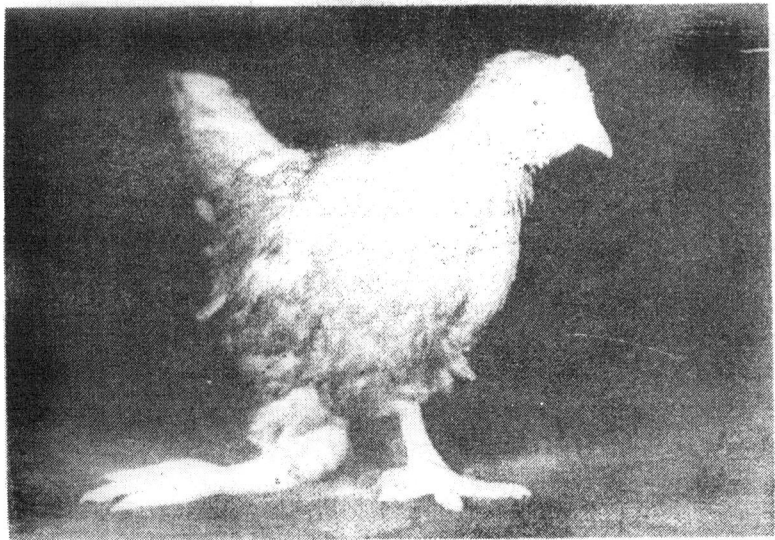

Figure 5.17 Perosis in chicken fed a manganese deficient diet.

A manganese deficient breeder diet can result in a condition in chick embryos referred to as chondrodystrophy. This condition is characterized by shortening and thickening of the legs and shortened wings; a parrot beak brought about by a disproportionate shortening of the lower mandible; globular contour of the head, due to anterior bulging of the skull; edema usually occurring just above the atlas joint of the neck and extending posteriorly; protruding abdomen, apparently due to a relatively large amount of unassimilated yolk; and retarded growth of down and feathers. In the young chick nervous symptoms may also be noted, which are characterized by a star-gazing posture similar to that observed with a thiamin deficiency. The appearance of a manganese deficient chick is shown in Figure 5.18.

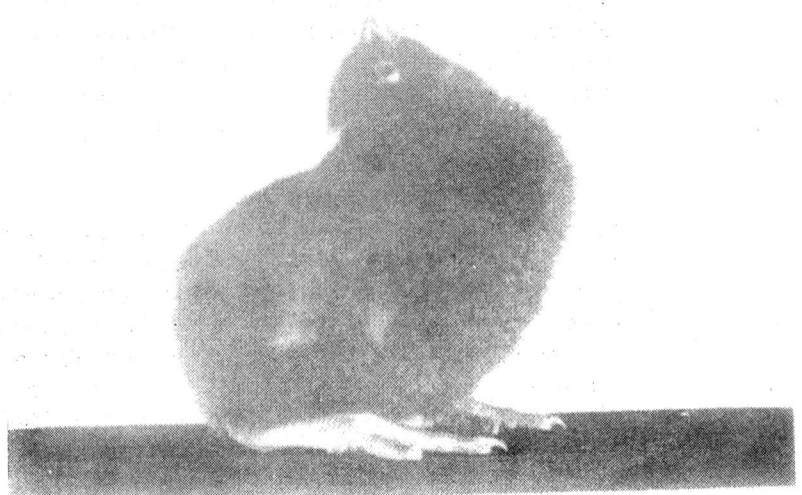

Figure 5.18 Characteristic star-gazing posture of a manganese deficient day-old chick.

According to Erway *et al.* (1970), in ataxic manganese deficient hatchlings, the otoliths of the inner ear are defective or absent. Otoliths are formed from many small crystalline otoconia embedded in an apparently amorphous matrix rich in mucopolysaccharides. Chondrodystrophy in chick embryos and the disproportionate growth at the site of the otolithic matrix, resulting in abnormal development of the inner ear, both appear to be caused by faulty synthesis of mucopolysaccharides.

5.11 ZINC

The nutritional importance of zinc was first demonstrated for mice and rats in 1934. In 1940, Keilin and Mann, isolated and purified carbonic anhydrase which catalyzes the breakdown of carbonic acid to CO_2 and H_2O, and showed that it was a metalloenzyme containing 0.33% zinc. Nutritional interest in zinc was markedly increased when it was shown that a deficiency resulted in parakeratosis in swine. Shortly thereafter, it was shown that a zinc deficiency was responsible for the poor growth and abnormal bone development, reported for chicks fed purified diets.

Zinc is found in every tissue in the body and tends to accumulate in bones rather than the liver as do many of the trace elements. High concentrations are also found in skin and feathers. It is found in several important enzymes like carbonic anhydrase, pancreatic carboxypeptidase, lactate dehydrogenase, and alkaline phosphatase, as well as being an activator of several enzyme systems. Most tissues contain around 30 ppm Zn assuming a normal diet intake of Zn and other trace minerals.

5.11.1 Zinc metabolism

Many studies have been made in an attempt to determine the primary metabolic defects responsible for the pathology of zinc deficiency. The skin lesions and corneal changes noted in zinc deficient animals are similar, in many respects, to those occurring in animals deprived of other nutrients such as vitamin A, riboflavin, biotin, pantothenic acid, pyridoxine, or essential fatty acids. Thus, zinc may be concerned in the metabolism of one or more of these nutrients.

Crystalline preparations of carbonic anhydrase contain 0.3% zinc. This enzyme plays an important role in the acid-base equilibrium of the body and release of carbon dioxide in the lungs. It is also involved in the hydration of carbon dioxide in gastric mucosa, a reaction necessary for neutralization of the excess alkalinity remaining from secretion of hydrogen ions in the production of gastric hydrochloric acid. Carbonic anhydrase also plays a role in the calcification of bone and in the formation of eggshells. High concentrations of this enzyme have been reported in the shell gland of the oviduct in laying hens.

Interestingly, the negative impact of saline drinking water on shell quality is counteracted to some extent by also supplementing such water with zinc. Balnave and Zhang (1993) suggest that saline drinking water reduces the level of carbonic anhydrase, a Zn-dependent enzyme, in the uterine mucosa. With Zn supplementation, carbonic anhydrase (a calcium binding protein) levels are increased, leading to less shell defects. Kidd et al. (1996) describes the role of zinc in enzymes involved in most aspects of the immune system.

5.11.2 Zinc requirements and signs of deficiency

As with some other trace minerals, diet composition can influence apparent Zn requirement. In semi-purified diets it is difficult to show a bird response to levels much above 25-30 mg/kg diet, whereas in practical corn-soy diets requirement values are increased to 60-80 mg/kg. Such variable Zn needs likely relate to phytic acid content of the diet, because this ligand is a potent chelator of zinc. If phytase enzyme is used in diets, then presumably the need for supplemental zinc will be reduced.

Zinc requirement may also be influenced by source of supplemental zinc. Wedekind and Baker (1990) suggest that zinc oxide is only 40% as potent as is zinc sulfate for young birds. In young chicks, the signs of zinc deficiency include: retarded growth, shortening and thickening of leg bones and enlargement of the hock joint, scaling of the skin (especially on the feet), very poor feathering, reduced feed utilization, loss of appetite and in severe cases, mortality. Some of these effects of zinc deficiency are shown in Figure 5.19.

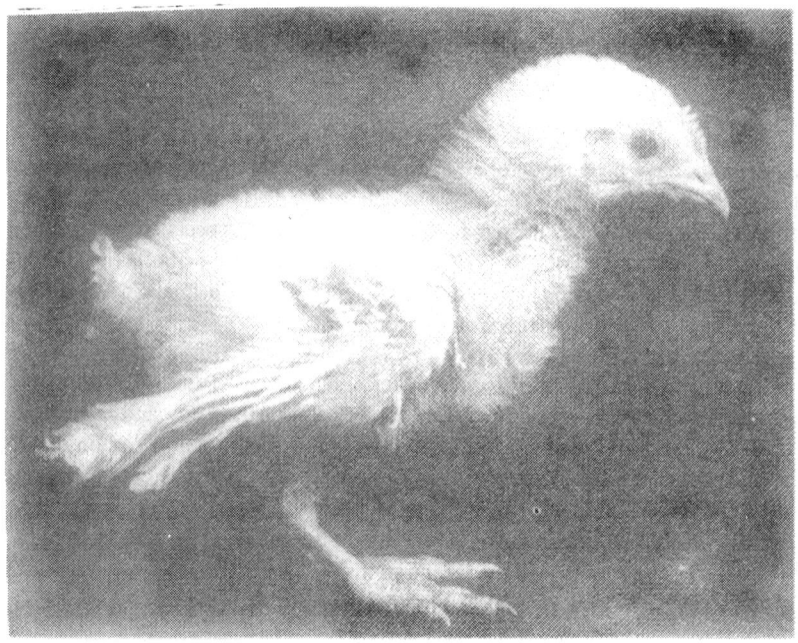

Figure 5.19 Four week old chick fed a zinc deficient diet. Note retarded growth, lack of feathering, short legs and dermatitis of feet.

Dewar *et al.* (1982) suggest that growth depression and other clinical signs due to Zn deficiency are a consequence of anorexia. These workers also recorded deranged crop epithelial tissue where there was heterophil infiltration, and areas of epithelial degeneration and erosion. The authors compare this epithelial degeneration to similar changes reported by other workers regarding foot pad degeneration. There is also degeneration of epithelial tissue in the mouth, a factor which may relate to the apparently enhanced taste sensitivity of Zn deficient animals.

It is often difficult to induce Zn deficiency in birds held in conventional galvanized cages. If zinc-coated (galvanized) feeders, waterers and cages are used, or if the diet is prepared in galvanized equipment, considerable amounts of zinc may be ingested from these sources. The use of stainless steel or plastic-coated equipment is essential to induce a severe zinc deficiency. Emmert and Baker (1995) also suggest that onset of signs of Zn deficiency will be greatly influenced by prior nutrition and Zn reserves of the bird. Deficiency signs are seen within 5d for birds previously fed marginal levels of Zn, while it takes at least 8d to show the same signs in birds previously receiving more generous Zn supplements.

Extensive studies with laying hens at the University of Wisconsin showed that egg production was decreased by zinc deficiency. However, the effects observed on hatchability of eggs and development of the embryo were the most striking consequences. Chicks hatched from hens fed zinc deficient diets were weak and could not stand, eat or drink. They had an accelerated respiratory rate and showed labored breathing. If the chicks were disturbed, the symptoms were aggravated and the chicks often died. Retarded feathering and frizzled feathers were found. The chicks could be helped somewhat by zinc chloride injections after hatching. Embryonic development was markedly affected; the major defect being grossly impaired skeletal development. Zinc deficient embryos showed micromelia, curvature of the spine, and shortened fused thoracic and lumbar vertebrae. Toes often were missing and in extreme cases the embryos had no lower skeleton or limbs. Some embryos were rumpless, and occasionally the eyes were absent or underdeveloped. A typical zinc deficient embryo is shown in Figure 5.20.

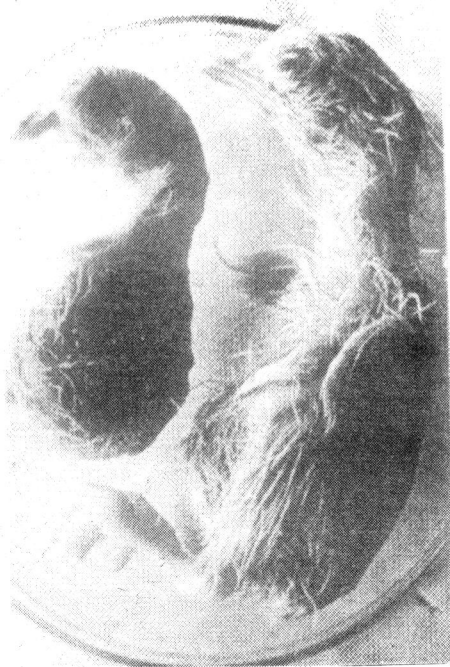

Figure 5.20 Zinc deficient embryo. Note absence of legs and wings. Larger chick is normal. Courtesy of E. W. Kienholz, M.L. Sunde and W.G. Hoekstra.

In other animals the effects of zinc deficiency are similar to those described for the chicks. In swine, a dermatitis called parakeratosis is a particularly important zinc deficiency condition seen under practical conditions. The condition is characterized by skin lesions, retarded growth, listlessness, vomiting and scouring.

5.11.3 Zinc toxicity

High levels of zinc are anorexic, and this has led to its application in force-molting or 'pausing' of egg production in older birds. Using up to 20,000 mg Zn/kg diet, birds will reduce their feed intake from around 100g to 10 g/d within 4-5 days. Feed intake will remain low while zinc feeding continues and then gradually return to normal once the special diet is removed. A complication today, is that virtually all of this dietary Zn ends up in manure and so poses an environmental hazard. Layers do accumulate vast quantities of Zn with such high level feeding, yet within 20-30 d of consuming a normal diet, base line levels return, suggesting body clearance.

Dewar *et al.* (1983) suggest that prolonged (2-6 weeks) feeding of 2-6,000 mg Zn/kg diet causes gizzard erosion, while the highest concentration also results in aneurysms. Up to 2,000 mg Zn/kg diet seems to have little effect on performance of broiler breeders or their offspring. Jensen (1975) suggests that 2-4,000 mg Zn/kg diet can lead to muscular dystrophy due to an induced selenium deficiency.

5.12 IRON

Centuries ago the Greeks recognized anemia and learned to treat it by administering rusty water. In 1664, Syndenham showed that administration of salts of iron would restore the pink color in the cheeks of people suffering from chlorosis. Mangahinis, in 1746 discovered that iron was a constituent of blood, while Froddisch, in 1832, showed that the iron content of the blood of anemic people was lower than that of healthy individuals. Zinoffsky (1886), refined pure crystals of horse hemoglobin that contained 0.33% iron, a level which later workers showed to be similar in a wide range of animals. MacMunn (1885) described the cytochrome enzymes which contain iron, and later the catalyses and peroxidases were also shown to contain iron. Iron is also present in serum protein as transferrin, which plays a role in the transfer of iron to various parts of the body.

Hemoglobin, as well as the iron containing enzymes, contain divalent or trivalent iron, chelated in the form of a porphyrin complex called heme. This is linked to a protein component, which varies with each enzyme. The cytochromes are involved in the activation of oxygen and electron transport, while the catalyses and peroxidases play a role in catalyzing hydrogen peroxide decomposition.

Two flavoproteins enzymes, NADH-cytochrome reductase and xanthine oxidase, also contain iron, as does an oxygen carrying compound, myoglobin, present in muscle. Cytochromes and other iron containing enzymes are essential for cell metabolism, and myoglobin, which is necessary for the functioning of the muscles, including the heart muscles, and these appear to have priority claim on the dietary supply of iron. Hence, the first sign of an iron deficiency is a hypochromic, microcytic anemia, resulting from insufficient iron for normal hemoglobin synthesis.

5.12.1 Iron absorption and metabolism

The iron content of the body represents about 0.005% of body weight. Over 90% of the iron is present in complex forms bound to porphyrins in two different ways. Some contain iron as an integral part or chelate of heme or porphyrin units, while others contain iron that is not chelated in the porphyrin ring. About 57% of the total iron is in the blood hemoglobin, and 7% in the myoglobin.

Bone marrow is one of the last reserves to be depleted of iron, and also one of the last to normalize in recovery from depletion. Thus, bone marrow iron is regarded as the most valuable clinical criterion of body iron stores and is used to confirm states of body depletion or body overload. Hematocrit is one of the main parameters used in assessing iron requirements or iron status of birds (Aoyagi and Baker, 1995). There are considerable amounts of iron in the egg, and Cao *et al.* (1996) suggest that each egg, which contains around 1.5 mg Fe, represents almost 25% of labile liver reserves.

Under normal physiological conditions, the excretion of iron is quite minimal. Most of the iron in feces represents unabsorbed dietary iron. Usually, the only loss of body iron occurs when blood is lost either through an external wound or into the gastrointestinal tract through bleeding or desquamation. Because of the negligible loss of iron under normal conditions, the body has ingenious regulatory mechanisms for prevention of iron absorption. Researchers have used double tracer techniques (using Fe^{59} and Fe^{55}) to simultaneously determine the absorption of iron and iron turnover. It appears that iron is taken up by the intestinal mucosa, stored there temporarily, and then gradually released for hemoglobin synthesis over time. A mucosal block has been suggested, which occurs when the mucosal cells become saturated with iron. The mucosal block theory is an attempt to explain the exclusion of uptake of dietary iron to avoid accumulations of harmful amounts. In addition to limiting the Fe uptake, this provides a mechanism for insuring that the mucosal cells act as a storage reservoir for iron in the face of limited and variable quantities in the diet.

A schematic outline of iron metabolism is shown in Figure 5.21. It is apparent from this outline that absorbed iron, iron from the catabolism of hemoglobin (either directly or via the reticuloendothelial system) and iron from the death of cells through-

out the body is transported as a compound called transferrin. Plasma will usually take up about two or three times as much iron as is already present,
demonstrating that transferrin is always capable of taking up the iron resulting
from metabolism of iron containing compounds in the body.

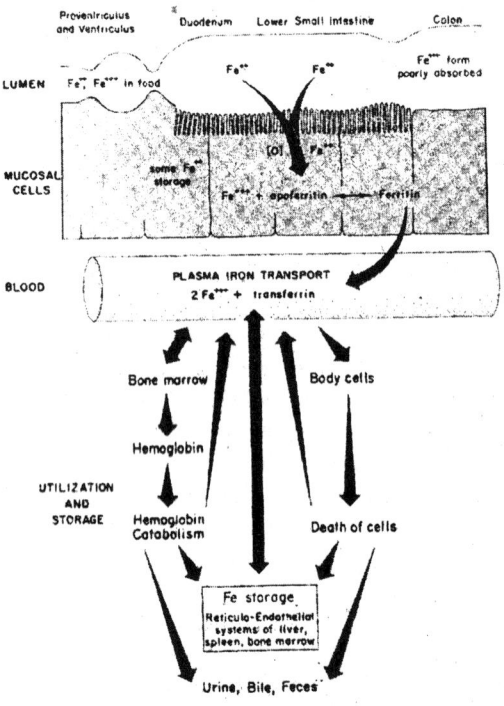

Figure 5.21 Iron metabolism

Ferritin, one of the storage forms of iron, is a brown iron containing protein, which
in the crystallized state may contain up to 23% of iron. The odorless, iron-free
protein apoferritin, is a globulin. The iron of ferritin is in the ferric state in the
form of ferric hydroxide micelles with an average composition of $(FeO$
$OH)_8FeOPO_3H_2$. Hemosiderin was originally regarded as the main storage form
of iron but it is now apparent that ferritin and hemosiderin are equally important.
Hemosiderin is a colloidal ferric hydroxide phosphate. It exists in the tissues as
a brownish yellow, granular pigment. The iron in hemosiderin is stainable while
that in ferritin is not. Hemosiderin may contain as much as 35% iron, which has
magnetic properties similar to the iron in ferritin. Hemosiderin represents body
iron present in excess of the binding capacity of the apoferritin and seems to be
a secondary storage form of iron.

Iron is sometimes used to detoxify gossypol in cottonseed meal. Ferrous salts react with gossypol in a 1:1 molar ratio, forming an iron-gosspol complex, which markedly decreases the toxicity of the gossypol for growing chickens and also largely prevents the olive green yolk discoloration, which occurs in eggs in cold storage from hens receiving gossypol. Addition of ferrous salts to the diet does not prevent the pink discoloration of eggs produced by the cyclopropenoid fatty acids present in cottonseed meal. It has been shown that gossypol reduces the metabolizable energy content of cottonseed meals. This reduction in metabolizable energy is also prevented by adding sufficient ferrous salts to the diet to complex with the gossypol present in the cottonseed meal.

Although egg yolk is one of the richest sources of iron in the human diet, its presence can be problematic when eggs are boiled during food preparation. When eggs are subjected to prolonged boiling, the high temperature causes some breakdown in the cysteine present in the egg albumen. This releases hydrogen sulfide gas, which penetrates the yolk membrane and reacts with the iron of the yolk, producing a greenish-black iron sulfide, a discoloration which most people find objectionable. Reducing the boiling time to the minimum needed to produce hardboiled eggs and cooling the eggs immediately in cold water largely prevents the development of this greenish-black discoloration.

5.12.2 Iron requirement, deficiency and toxicity

Working with laying hens, Mark and Austic (1991) suggest a minimal Fe requirement of 35-45 mg/kg diet for maintaining normal hematocrit. The need for optimum hatchability is somewhat higher, at around 55 mg/kg diet. Aoyagi and Baker (1995) suggest a need for 85 mg Fe/kg diet when young birds are fed semi-purified diets, based on hemoglobin status. Heart hypertrophy was observed in birds fed less than 55 mg/kg.

Iron deficiency causes a severe anemia with a reduction in packed cell volume. In colored feathered strains there is also loss of pigmentation in the feathers. The bird's requirement for RBC synthesis takes precedence over metabolism of feather pigments, although if a fortified diet is introduced, all subsequent feather growth is normal. It is postulated that iron may be needed, not only for the red feather pigments, which are known to contain iron, but that iron may also function in an enzyme system involved in the pigmentation process. New Hampshire chickens lose not only the red, iron containing pigment, but also the black melanin, which is a normal protein of feather pigmentation in this breed. When a diet containing iron is fed to the deficient chick, the new feathers contain first a band of black pigment, followed by a normal deposition of the red pigment. As the feathers continue to grow the black melanin pigment is distributed throughout the feathers in the normal pattern.

Huff *et al.* (1979) indicated that ochratoxin at 4-8 µg/g diet causes an iron deficiency characterized by hypochronic microcytic anemia. Aflatoxin also reduces iron absorption. With high levels of iron salts there can be formation of insoluble phosphates in the digesta, leading to reduced phosphorus absorption and subsequent incidence of rickets. Insoluble iron phosphates produce a colloidal suspension that may also adsorb vitamins and other trace minerals. Such problems will not occur unless supplements are at least 10x normal inclusion.

5.13 COPPER

While Boutigny (1883) had demonstrated that copper was present in animal tissues, it was not until the late 1920's that University of Wisconsin workers showed that both copper and iron were necessary for hemoglobin formation in rats. Although copper is not a constituent of hemoglobin it is present in certain plasma proteins that are concerned with the release of iron from cells in the plasma. Thus a deficiency of copper results in the animal being unable to absorb iron, mobilize it from the tissues, and utilize it in hemoglobin synthesis.

Copper is also a component of other blood proteins, one being erythrocuprein, found in erythrocytes where it is important in oxygen metabolism. The element also plays a role in many enzyme systems, such as cytochrome oxidase, which is important in oxidative phosphorylation. Copper also occurs in certain pigments, especially turacin, a pigment of feathers. It is present in most body cells, being particularly concentrated in the liver which is the main body storage site.

Interest in copper nutrition was markedly increased in the 1930's when it was demonstrated that certain diseases of sheep and cattle were shown to be due to a copper deficiency. Studies into these ruminant problems led to extensive mapping of copper deficient areas around the globe. In all copper deficient locations the situation was similar as follows: (a) sheep and cattle failed to thrive unless supplied with extra copper; (b) blood and liver of the copper deficient animals contained copper levels which were markedly below normal; and (c) the forages and the soils contained low levels of copper.

5.13.1 Copper metabolism, requirements and signs of deficiency

A deficiency of copper manifests itself as anemia, emphasizing its role in iron metabolism. Iron absorbed as Fe^{++} is usually transported as Fe^{3+}, a conversion which requires ferroxidase enzyme, a component of which, is copper. Copper is also important for normal bone formation and in particular cartilage formation. Lilburn and Leach (1980) showed that cartilage from copper deficient chicks oxidized less glucose than normal, and at a rate comparable to that seen in situations of tibial dyschondroplasia. There are similarities in cartilage structure for birds suffering from TD or copper deficiency.

Interaction between copper and other minerals such as zinc are most problematic during absorption. A large proportion of copper is absorbed from the duodenum, and in the mucosa is found attached to a protein carrier. Because zinc also binds aggressively to the same carrier, excess of zinc for example can induce a deficiency of copper. When molybdenum intake is high, there is a need for extra dietary copper. Corn distillers solubles, whey and groundnut meal are the most concentrated sources of copper within the commonly used feed ingredients.

Copper deficiency results in a wide range of signs in different animal species, and indeed, in the same species different situations are noted. However, anemia is a common sign noted for all animals, as is growth depression, bone disorders, depigmentation of hair, wool, fur and feathers, demyelination of the spinal cord, fibrosis of the myocardium, and diarrhea.

Young chicks will become lame in 2 to 4 weeks when fed a copper deficient diet. Bones will be fragile and easily broken, epiphyseal cartilage becomes thickened, and vascular penetration of the thickened cartilage is markedly reduced. These bone lesions for chickens are quite different from those seen with other farm animals and resemble the bone changes noted with birds suffering from a vitamin A deficiency. The bones of pigs and dogs fed a copper deficient diet show a diffuse osteoporosis accompanied by a cessation or destruction of the calcified cartilaginous matrix. These disorders were shown to be the result of a specific copper deficiency and not the result of anemia. Iron deficiency, resulting in an equally severe anemia, failed to produce similar bone changes. A copper deficiency resulting in severe ataxias in young ruminants now referred to as enzootic neonatal ataxia, is a fairly common occurrence in many parts of the world. Two types of ataxia are noted, namely a common acute form in newborn lambs, and a delayed type, for which clinical symptoms are not noted for several weeks and sometimes several months after birth. In both conditions, spastic paralysis, incoordination of the hind legs and a stiff and staggering gait, are observed. Although the disease is not characterized as such with poultry, copper deficient chicks have also been shown to suffer from ataxia and spastic paralysis.

Both copper and iron deficiencies have been reported to result in loss of feather pigmentation (achromotrichia) in New Hampshire chickens. A syndrome consisting of achromotrichia, alopecia and dermatitis has been reported as the most readily noted signs of a copper deficiency in rabbits, while a lack of pigment in black wooled sheep, along with loss of wool crimp, is also a common occurrence. While these conditions have been studied for quite some time, the complete clinical picture of a copper deficiency has, as yet, not been elucidated. The copper containing enzyme polyphenoloxidase, is known to catalyze production of melanin from L-tyrosine, and the lack of wool crimp has been reported to be due to the need for copper in the normal oxidation of cysteine to the S-S- bond required for maintaining the proper protein structure of wool.

Studies by Missouri workers in the 1960's showed that a copper deficiency with chickens could produce a dissecting aneurysm of the aorta along with various bone deformities that closely resembled lathyrism. Similar results have been noted with swine. There is some evidence that β-aminoproprionitrile (BAPN), which has been shown to experimentally produce lathyrism, may act as a chelate in tying up trace minerals that may prevent lathyrism. Chicks hatched from copper deficient hens have been shown to have no amino oxidase in the aorta or liver. If such chicks are fed a copper deficient diet the enzyme is still not detectable even up to 4 weeks of age, while the same type of chicks fed a copper supplemented diet show high amine oxidase levels after the third day of life. Kim and Hill, (1966) reported that amino oxidase increases the incorporation of lysine into elastins (desmosines) of the aorta. Hence, the role of copper in elastin formation in the chicken appears to be in meeting the requirement for this element by amino oxidase, which in turn is involved in the oxidative deamination of the epsilon amino group of lysine. A copper deficiency apparently can result in a reduction in the number of oxidized lysine residues available to condense for the formation of desmosine in cartilage. BAPN has been shown to inhibit amino oxidase formation.

5.13.2 Copper toxicity and high inclusions as a growth promoter

Jensen and Maurice (1979) indicated the growth rate of chicks to be depressed at 500-700 mg/kg dietary Cu. Interestingly the apparent toxicity could be alleviated by administering 0.4% extra DL-methionine even though the diet was apparently adequate in this amino acid. The authors conclude that methionine and/or a protein are combining with copper, either in the digesta, the intestinal mucosa or the liver, and so rendering it less toxic to the bird. Alternatively one can conclude that high levels of copper increase the bird's need for sulfur amino acids. Wideman et al. (1996) describe a case of proventriculitis in young broilers that was caused by feeding 200 ppm Cu. High levels of dietary copper can also act as a pro-oxidant, potentially destroying the fat and fat-soluble components of the diet (Miles et al., 1998).

While there are obvious toxic effects of copper, the mineral is still used periodically as a growth promoter, at 200-250 mg/kg diet (Ewing et al. 1998). The exact mechanism for such enhanced growth has not been elucidated. Certainly the excreta color of the bird changes markedly, and it is presumed that there will be some changes to the gut microflora. Aoyagi and Baker (1995) suggest that the beneficial effect of copper may result from improved digestion of hemicellulose. After feeding 250mg Cu/kg diet, they recorded a 15% increase in hemicellulose digestion (22→33%) when feeding corncobs, where diet AMEn increased from -200 kcal/kg to +117 kcal/kg. In explaining their results, Aoyagi and Baker (1995) suggest that excess copper stimulates clearing of liver copper into bile through exocytosis of hepatocellular lysosymes. A side effect of such action is increased bile secretion of glucosidases, which could be available for carbohydrate digestion. When feeding much in excess of 50 ppm copper, most of the mineral will end up in the excreta, which is of concern regarding potential pollution.

5.14 MOLYBDENUM

For decades molybdenum had been recognized as a toxic element when consumed in excessive amounts. The first indication of it being an essential nutrient was obtained in 1953 with the work of Richert and Westerfield who showed that xanthine oxidase, which is important in purine metabolism, was a metallo-enzyme containing molybdenum. It was later shown that the element was also a component of aldehyde and sulphite oxidase. In addition to being a component of xanthine oxidase, molybdenum participates in the reaction of cytochrome C and also plays a role in the reduction of cytochrome C by aldehyde oxidase.

As discussed in the previous section (5.13), there is an important interaction between molybdenum and copper. Studies with rats have shown that feeding molybdate, in the presence of sulfate, results in a growth depression that could be overcome by supplementing the diet with copper. It was later reported that methionine was as effective as copper in overcoming the growth depression noted by adding molybdenum to the diet.

Molybdenum requirement of most classes of poultry, is around 0.03 mg/kg and toxicity occurs at around 250 mg/kg. Requirements are affected by the SO_4 level of the diet, which seems to reduce the availability of dietary molybdate. The feeding of molybdenum-deficient diets to chicks has been reported to cause reduced growth, especially when these diets contain a low level of added sodium tungstate. Tungstate competitively inhibits the utilization of molybdenum for the formation of xanthine dehydrogenases. Leach et al. (1962) showed in repeated experiments with chicks, that increased growth was obtained by molybdenum supplementation of a purified diet of low zinc content (45 mg Zn/kg) containing isolated soybean protein, but not in chicks receiving this diet supplemented with zinc at 60 mg/kg of diet. No increase in growth was observed with molybdenum supplementation of a low zinc purified diet containing vitamin-free casein instead of isolated soybean protein. The isolated soybean protein diet was found to contain 1.05 – 1.09 mg Mo/kg while the casein diet contained only 0.17-0.2 mg Mo/kg. Thus the results indicated that most, if not all, of the molybdenum in isolated soybean protein is unavailable to the chick. The available molybdenum requirement of chicks fed a purified diet containing vitamin-free casein was found to be not more than 0.11 mg/kg. The chicks used for this study were obtained from dams fed a diet of low molybdenum content and both received demineralized drinking water.

A more severe molybdenum deficiency was obtained in chicks by adding sodium tungstate to the isolated soybean protein diet. The deficiency was overcome largely by molybdenum supplementation, except when the tungsten was fed at

2000 mg/kg of diet, which appeared to cause a toxicity that was not due to competitive inhibition of molybdenum. No correlation was observed in these experiments between the degree of growth retardation and the level of liver xanthine dehydrogenase, indicating that the growth retardation due to molybdenum deficiency was not caused by interference with the activity of this enzyme. The effect of molybdenum on growth rate and xanthine dehydrogenase activity in chicks is shown in Table 5.9.

TABLE 5.9 Effect of Tungstate on the molybdenum requirement of chicks		
Treatment	Avg. wt @ 4 wks	Liver xanthine dehydrogenase activity
	(g)	mm O_2/266 mg Fresh tissue/20 min
Basal	344 (39)*	30.7
+500 mg tungstate (W)/kg	360 (38)	8.8
+1000 mg W/kg	315 (38)	5.3
+2000 mg W/kg	155 (22)	8.7
+500 mg W/kg and 0.5 mg molybdenum (Mo)/kg	339 (40)	32.6
+1000 mg W/kg and 1.0 mg Mo/kg	333 (39)	28.3
+2000 mg W/kg and 2.0 mg Mo/kg	222 (39)	28.7
*Figures in parentheses are survivors of duplicate lots of 10 male and 10 female depleted chicks per lot (Leach et al., 1962)		

Payne (1977) and Payne and Bains (1975) describe two deficiency situations in broilers, that they claimed were caused by molybdenum deficiency. In Australian breeders, poor hatchability and weak chicks led to an investigation of molybdenum status. Chicks had clubbed down and characteristic ginger hairs in the neck and head region. The chicks were responsive to dosing with 40 µg of molybdenum. The similarity in characteristics of the hatchlings, with those seen in situations of riboflavin deficiency may be due to both nutrients being integral parts of several flavoprotein enzymes. Payne and Bains (1975) reported that femoral head necrosis and 'scabby-hip' syndrome were related to molybdenum deficiency.

It is not common practice to add molybdenum to a diet although it is conceivable that deficiencies could be induced by excess of other minerals and/or sulfates.

5.15 SELENIUM

I t has long been recognized that cattle grazing on certain pastures suffer from a syndrome characterized by stiffness in the joints, loss of hair and hoof deformities. The condition was generally referred to as alkali disease, and some 50 years ago, selenium toxicity was discovered as the cause. In the mid 1950s selenium was found to be an essential nutrient. Because selenium is required in very small amounts, equivalent to just 0.05 – 0.2 ppm, natural feedstuffs often supplied adequate quantities. However, selenium responsive conditions continue to occur in the 1950s, and this lead to mapping of North America for selenium deficient soils. In general the Eastern USA has soil that is selenium deficient, and especially areas bordering the Great Lakes. In contrast to this, numerous small isolated regions of the mid-western USA were found to contain very high levels of selenium. This mapping of soil selenium levels provided the first logical basis for differential selenium nutrition of animals and man based on geographical location. Today the situation is slightly more complex, due to the active transport of feed ingredients throughout the world.

Attention was focused on selenium status of animals after Schwarz and Foltz (1957) showed that Se was an essential nutrient. During the early 1950's Schwarz and associates at the National Institute of Health in Maryland, found that brewers yeast contained an unknown factor that prevented liver necrosis in vitamin E deficient rats. Researchers at Cornell, using a similar basal diet, found that it would prevent exudative diathesis in vitamin E deficient chicks. Schwarz and co-workers in 1957 reported that the unknown factor in brewer's yeast was selenium and Scott and associates at Cornell, shortly thereafter, showed that selenium would prevent exudative diathesis in chicks. In mammals, a deficiency of selenium can result in White Muscle Disease, a situation where muscle degeneration occurs, usually in young animals. Gill et al. (1980) describe White Muscle Disease in chicks, where both inter- and intra-cellular lipid content increases, and muscle fibers are displaced by adipocytes.

5.15.1   Selenium absorption, transport and excretion

Selenium has properties that are similar to those of sulfur and tellurium, and is often found in association with sulfur in inorganic and organic compounds. While selenium does replace sulfur in some of these compounds, in others it is found complexed to sulfur by coordinate covalent bonding. Common forms of selenium are selenic acid, selenous acid, selenates and selenites. These are the analogues of sulfuric acid, sulfurous acid, sulfates and sulfites. Some plants and microorganisms have been shown to be able to replace the sulfur in cystine and methionine with selenium, thereby producing selenocystine and selenomethionine.

Selenomethionine is absorbed from the digestive tract by an active transport mechanism similar to that involved in the transport of methionine, while inorganic selenite and selenocystine are not actively transported. It has been shown that selenium uptake appears to be greater in chicks that are deficient in selenium as compared to those with normal intakes of the element. Selenium uptake by erythrocytes is very rapid after an animal is dosed with selenium.

Selenium binding proteins are found in the plasma, the most important being glutathione peroxidase. Another selenium-binding protein is present in association with the lipoprotein fraction of the plasma. Selenium intake in excess of that bound by these protein, appears to be methylated, which takes place in two steps: either the formation of dimethyl selenide, or its further conversion to a trimethyl selenonium ion, which is water-soluble and represents the normal excretory product of a moderate excessive intake of the element. If intake of selenium exceeds that of the body's ability to convert it to the trimethyl selenonium ion, then dimethyl selenide, being a volatile compound is excreted via expired air, imparting a garlic like odor. High levels of dietary copper or zinc seem to interfere with selenium uptake. Jensen (1975) indicated that the growth depression and mortality caused by feeding 800 ppm Cu or 2,000 ppm Zn, could be alleviated by feeding 0.5 ppm Se. The cause of mortality was similar to that of selenium deficiency.

5.15.2 Early studies on pancreatic fibrosis

Early research in the 1960's with selenium focused mainly on studies investigating the effects of selenium on various vitamin E deficiency diseases of poultry rats and other farm animals. It was discovered that selenium or vitamin E would prevent exudative diathesis, and that selenium spared the requirement for vitamin E in the prevention of muscular dystrophy in chicks but would not prevent the condition unless the diet contained a minimum level of vitamin E. Selenium was not effective in the prevention of encephalomalacia.

Thompson and Scott (1970) reported that chicks from selenium depleted hens fed a selenium deficient purified diet, failed to grow normally and died of exudative diathesis before 4 weeks of age, even though the diet contained an adequate level of vitamin E. Further experiments revealed that mortality was due to severe pancreatic degeneration. Gries and Scott (1972) describe the condition in detail. It was assumed that the degenerated pancreas failed to produce lipase, resulting in the lack of monoglycerides, which are needed for the formation of lipid bile salt micelles, necessary for vitamin E absorption. Adding bile salts and monoglycerides to the selenium deficient diet resulted in vitamin E being absorbed and exudative diathesis being prevented. However, such chicks still developed pancreatic degeneration before they were 30 days of age. Adding selenium to the test diet at 0.1 ppm cured the selenium deficiency, thus allowing the pancreas to return to normal within 7 to 10 days.

5.15.3 Metabolic functions of selenium

i) Association with glutathione peroxidase and exudative diathesis.

Rotruck *et al.* (1973) discovered that selenium was an integral part of the enzyme glutathione peroxidase. This discovery allowed for a clearer understanding of the precise roles of vitamin E and selenium in prevention of vitamin E/selenium diseases.

Selenium spares vitamin E in at least three ways: 1) It preserves the integrity of the pancreas which in turn allows normal fat digestion, normal lipid bile salt micelle formation and thus normal vitamin E absorption; 2) Selenium is an integral part of glutathione peroxidase (Figure 5.22) which converts reduced glutathione to oxidized glutathione while at the same time destroying peroxides by converting them to harmless alcohols. It thus prevents the attack by peroxides on the polyunsaturated fatty acids of the lipid membranes of cells. This greatly reduces the amount of vitamin E required for maintenance of these membranes; 3) Selenium aids in the retention of vitamin E in plasma.

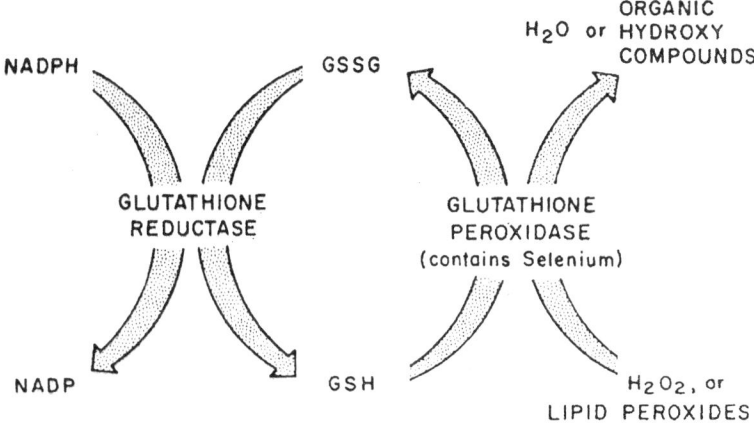

Figure 5.22   Important reactions showing mechanism whereby glutathione peroxidase destroys peroxides.

Vitamin E reduces selenium requirement in at least two ways: 1) by maintaining blood selenium in an active form or by preventing its loss from the body, and 2) by preventing a chain reactive autoxidation of the membrane lipids within the membrane itself. This occurrence inhibits the production of hydroperoxides, thus reducing the amount of selenium–containing glutathione peroxidase needed to destroy the peroxides formed in the cells.

As previously described in Chapter 4, both vitamin E and selenium can be involved in prevention of exudative diathesis. Noguchi *et al.* (1973) showed that the glutathione peroxidase level of plasma is high in chicks receiving adequate levels of selenium but in deficient chicks it drops almost to zero some two days before the onset of exudative diathesis. Protection against the disease was directly proportional to the level of glutathione peroxidase in the plasma.

Both vitamin E and glutathione peroxidase are required for protection of hepatic mitochondria and microsomes from ascorbic acid induced peroxidation. Hepatic mitochondria and microsomes from selenium and vitamin E deficient chicks undergo marked peroxidation upon incubation with ascorbic acid. Dietary selenium or vitamin E alone produced no significant decrease in peroxidation levels. However no peroxidation was noted in the mitochondria and microsomal membranes from chicks receiving both vitamin E and selenium.

ii) Preventing peroxidation of sub-cellular membranes

Scott and co-workers examined the role of selenium in preventing oxidation of hepatic microsomes. An experiment was undertaken with a test diet containing taurocholic and oleic acids and 100 IU of vitamin E per kg of diet. Six graded levels of selenium as sodium selenite, were added to the basal diet. The results, after 5 weeks on the experiment are shown in Figure 5.23 (Scott *et al.* 1982). Oxidation as measured by the TBA value of hepatic microsomes, decreased with increasing levels of selenium, reaching a minimum level at 0.08 ppm Se. This value is similar to that reported by Thompson and Scott (1970), to be the level of selenium required for protection of the pancreas from fibrotic degeneration.

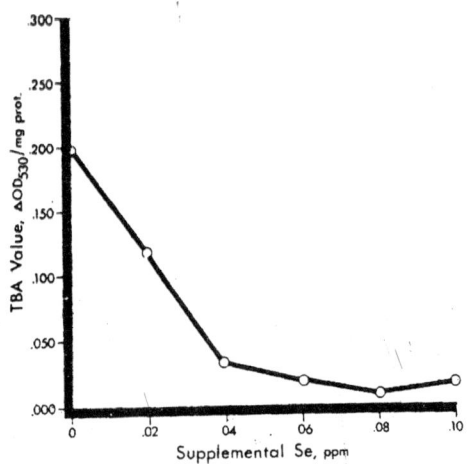

Figure 5.23 Dietary selenium requirement for prevention of peroxidation of hepatic microsomes.

5.15.4 Mode of action of selenium in preventing exudative diathesis and lipid membrane peroxidation

i) Exudative diathesis

A schematic representation of a chick capillary cell is shown in Figure 5.24. According to the hypothesis put forth to explain the action of vitamin E and selenium in preventing exudative diathesis, plasma glutathione peroxidase represents the first line of defense against peroxidation of the unsaturated lipids of the capillary plasma membrane. In the presence of adequate dietary selenium any peroxides inside the cell are immediately destroyed by glutathione peroxidase. With sufficient dietary vitamin E, exuative diathesis is prevented by the action of vitamin E within the lipid portion of the membrane itself.

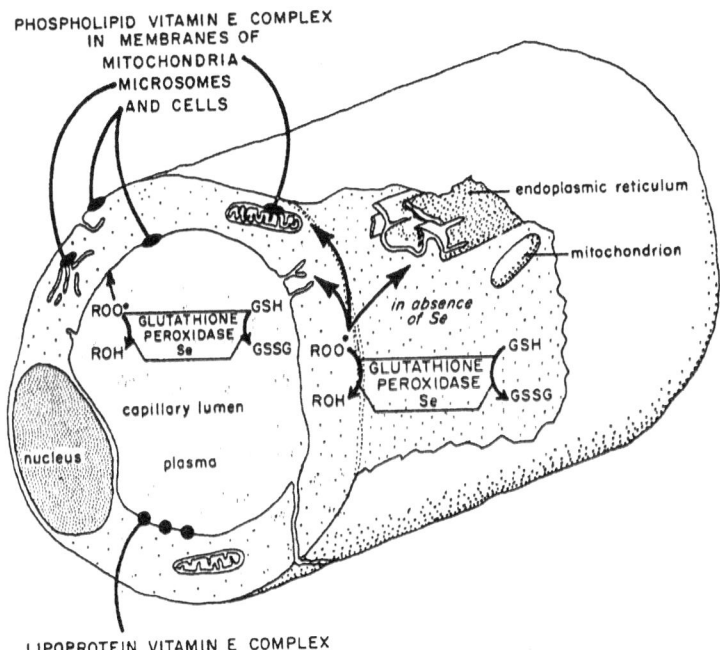

Figure 5.24 Diagramatic representation of the protective actions of glutathione peroxidase and vitamin E in prevention of exudative diathesis.

ii) Protection against lipid peroxidation

King et al. (1975) showed that microsomal NADPH – cytochrome P450 reductase activity initiates lipid peroxidation in biological membranes because the enzyme generates superoxide anion radicals when catalyzing NADPH oxidation. The investigations indicated that the superoxide *per se* was not the radical species responsible for the lipid peroxidations in the microsomes but that the oxidative attack on the membrane lipids was most likely due to hydroxyl free radicals produced by subsequent reactions of superoxide. Fridovich (1975) indicated that superoxide dismutase is present in all respiring cells and is essential for survival of aerobic cells, providing a defense against oxidation.

King *et al.* (1975) observed that superoxide itself is not reactive with lipids or with radical scavengers and hence cannot be the radical which initiates lipid peroxidation. Their results also indicate that xanthine oxidase, which forms superoxide anion during its activity under aerobic conditions, does not form singlet oxygen. However, if the hydrogen peroxide generated by the superoxide dismutase is not destroyed it may react with superoxide ion in the presence of ferric ion to produce a hydroxyl free radical.

Removal of the H_2O_2 by glutathione peroxidase would markedly inhibit 'OH radial formation. McCay *et al.* (1976) have provided evidence using *in vitro* microsomal systems, that this destruction of hydrogen peroxide is responsible for the effect of glutathione peroxidase in protecting microsomal membranes. A hypothetical representation is shown in Figure 5.25.

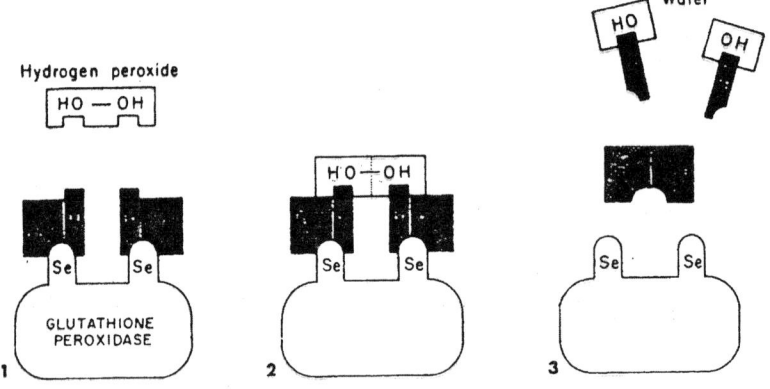

Figure 5.25 A schematic representation of the mechanism of the glutathione peroxidase reaction with GSH and hydrogen peroxide.

A schematic representation showing the sites of action of glutathione peroxidase and vitamin E in protecting lipid membranes is presented in Figure 5.26. This scheme shows that both vitamin E and selenium are required for prevention of the reactions which result in disruption of the membrane lipids of the vital organelles of the animal body. In vitamin E or selenium deficient mitochrondria and microsomes, these peroxides move into all segments of the cell, reacting with membranes and sulfhydryl-containing enzymes, causing severe damage to the cell and its vital processes. Since mitochrondria and microsomes (ribosomes, etc.) act to produce antibodies and other defense mechanisms, it is clear that adequate vitamin E and selenium nutrition are important not only for prevention of overt signs of deficiency but also for preservation of the organelles responsible for building the defense mechanisms against disease and other stresses.

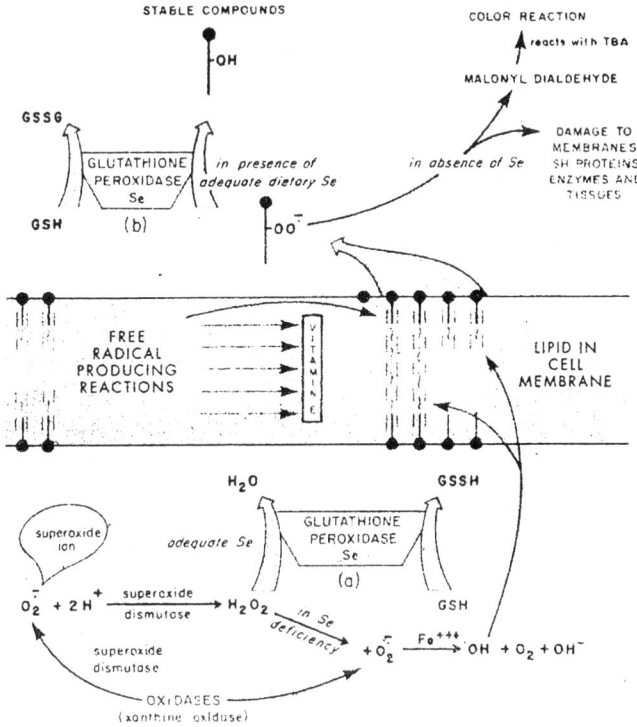

Figure 5.26 Protection of lipid membranes by vitamin E and glutathione peroxidase. Vitamin E in lipid membrane shields polyunsaturated lipids from free radical attack. Glutathione peroxidase in cytosol (a) prevents formation of membrane-destructive •OH; and (b) destroys any hydroperoxides which may form.

5.15.5 Selenium content of feed ingredients

The selenium values presented in Table 5.10 show wide variation among feedstuffs, and among different samples of the same material, depending upon geographical location. This is due to the wide variation in selenium content of the soil. Even though the biological availability of the selenium in fish meals is poor, they represent the best natural sources of selenium among the common poultry feedstuffs. The variability in selenium content of corn and soybean meal is indicated by the listing of these feedstuffs from different regions. A more detailed listing of the selenium content of foods and feedstuffs from various points in the United States and other parts of the world is summarized by Scott (1973a).

TABLE 5.10 Selenium content of poultry feedstuffs

Feed material	Selenium content (µg/g)	Feed material	Selenium content (µg/g)
Bakery by-product	0.40	Oyster shell	0.01
Barley: Eastern	0.10	Phosphates, dicalcium	0.20
Midwestern	0.30	Phosphates, defluorinated rock	1.4
Blood meal	0.01	Poultry by-product meal	1.2
Brewer's dried grains	0.70	Soybean meal:	
Corn: Yellow	0.025	Midwestern U.S.A.	0.10
Nebraska and S Dakota	0.38	Nebraska	0.54
Distiller's dried solubles	0.50	Wheat:	
Gluten meal, 60% protein	1.15	Nebraska, S. Dakota	1.20
Cottonseed meal	0.06	Eastern U.S. and Central Canada	0.06
Fish meals	1.5	Durum, Western Canada	2.22
Hominy feed	0.10	Shorts, Western Canada	0.6
Limestone	0.17	Whey, dried	0.08
Flax meal	1.0	Yeast:Brewers dried	1.1
Meat and bone meal	0.29		
Oats	0.06		

The value of a feedstuff as a source of selenium depends on the biological availability as well as the selenium content. Biological evaluation of feedstuffs (Cantor *et al*, 1975) showed that the selenium in most feedstuffs of plant origin was highly available, ranging from 60 to 90%, but was less than 25% available in animal products. Selenium in pure selenium compounds showed the following relative availabilities:

selenite > selenate > selenomethionine > selenide > elemental selenium.

5.15.6 Selenium requirements

In view of the potential toxicity of selenium, very rigid levels of diet supplementation are put forth by federal governments in most countries. By and large the amount of selenium supplementation permitted in layer and breeder diets is 0.2 to 0.3 ppm. This will also readily meet the requirement of the growing chick, which has been stated as approximately 0.15 to 0.2 ppm. Cantor and Scott (1974) found that egg production in laying hens was maximized by the addition of 0.1 ppm of selenium to the respective diets. This level of supplementation also resulted in a level of, 0.035 to 0.138% respectively, for the selenium content of eggs from the negative control versus the selenium supplemented diet. Davis and Fear (1996) indicate a linear relationship between diet Se and that appearing in the egg. Both yolk and white increase by about 10-12 nmol/g for each 1 ppm Se added to the diet. Hassan (1986) describes the importance of knowing the Se status of breeders when defining the Se requirement of chicks. Feeding low levels of Se to chicks caused reduced levels of glutathione peroxidase, regardless of dam nutrition, although onset of exudative diathesis was delayed in chicks from dams fed Se fortified diets.

Studies by Latshaw *et al.* (1977) and Combs and Scott (1979) further confirmed the importance of selenium for egg production and hatchability. Cunningham *et al.* (1987) suggest that it is possible to select birds for high vs. low selenium requirement, and because of larger heritability estimates in females, a sex-link gene is likely involved.

5.15.7 Selenium toxicity

The toxic levels of selenium (10-20 ppm and above) are approximately 100-fold higher than the nutritional requirements for selenium. One of the mechanisms by which selenium exerts its toxic effects in animals appears to be through its competition with sulfur compounds or via its strong affinity for sulfur in the formation of sulfur-selenium complexes. Selenium toxicity can be divided into three categories in terms of the enzymes affected: (1) those enzymes which are relatively unaffected by selenite, such as glucose, lactate and pyruvate oxidases of brain, and 1-tyrosinase, xanthine oxidase and alcohol oxidase of the liver; (2) those enzymes inhibited by selenium, which appear to destroy an active part of the enzymes. These include succinic dehydrogenase, choline oxidase, tyraminase and d-proline oxidase; and (3) enzymes, which are inactivated directly upon addition of selenite, which includes 1-proline oxidase, where selenium inhibits by combining with the active group of the enzyme.

In chickens excessive levels of selenium cause reduce growth rate, egg production, and hatchability and cause embryonic abnormalities. Ort and Latshaw (1978) showed reduced egg production and hatchability for breeders fed 7 ppm Se, while at 9 ppm egg production was affected. An interesting abnormality in embryos was a swollen head, due to fluid accumulation and tissue hypertrophy (Fig. 5.27).

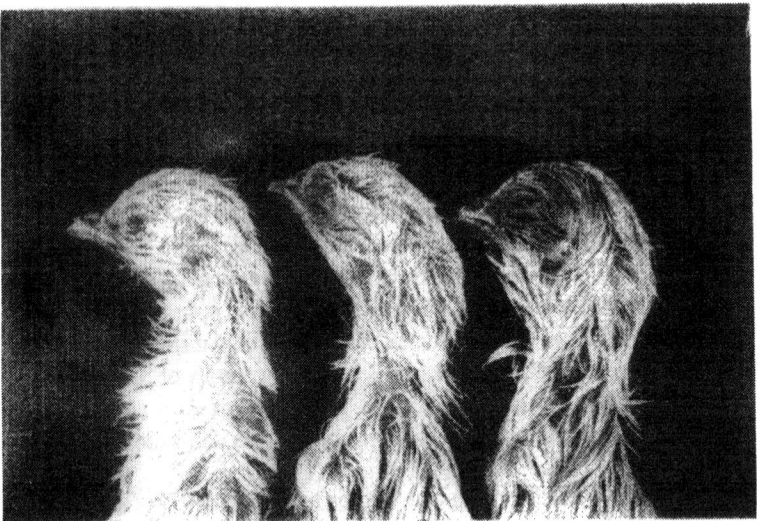

Figure 5.27 Enlarged neck and head of dead-in-shell 21d embryos as a result of selenium toxicity *(Ort and Latshaw, 1978; courtesy Dr. D. Latshaw).*

5.16 IODINE

In the third millenium B.C. the Chinese Emperor Shen-nung mentioned that seaweed was effective in preventing goiter. After the discovery of the element, Coindet (1820) a Swiss physician, recommended iodine as a remedy for goiter.

5.16.1 Metabolic functions of iodine

Iodine is present in very small amounts in the body, and although the element is widely distributed throughout tissues the only known function is its role in the synthesis of the two hormones triiodothyronine and tetraiodothyronine (thyroxine), produced in the thyroid gland. The structures of thyronine, thyroxine (T4) and triodothyrine (T3), are shown in Figure 5.28.

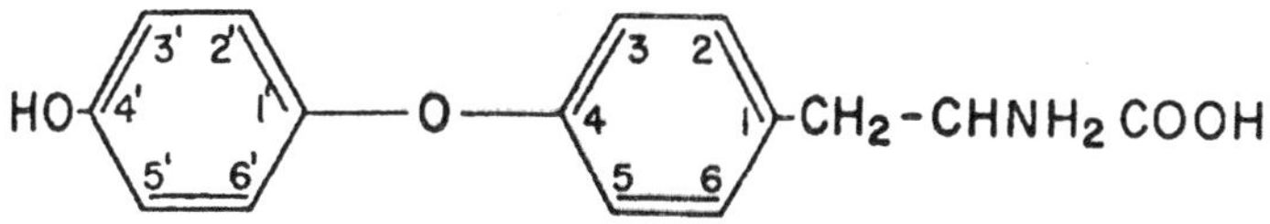

Thyronine

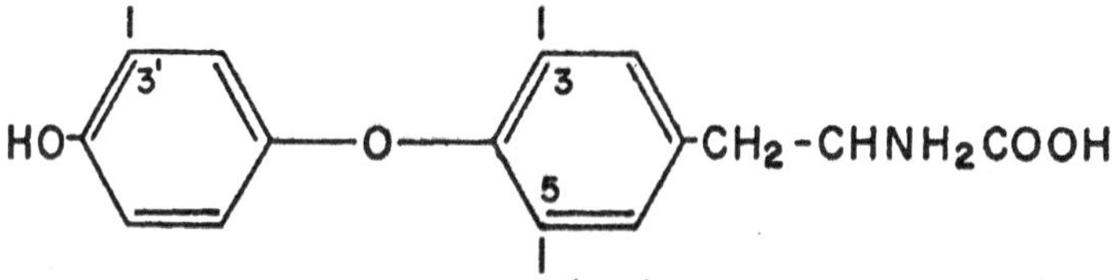

L-Triiodothyronine (T_3)

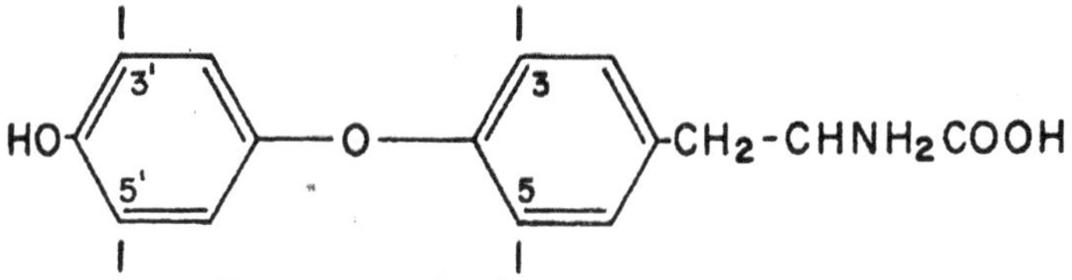

Thyroxine (T_4)

Figure 5.28 The structures of thyronine [4-(4'-hydroxyphenoxy)-phenylalanine], 3,5,3'- triiodothyronine and thyroxine [3,5,3',5'-tetraiodothyronine].

Ingested iodine is absorbed readily from the gastro-intestinal tract into the blood stream, primarily in the intestine, although there is some absorption in the stomach. Free iodine, or iodate, undergoes reduction to iodide before absorption. From the blood stream iodide diffuses into the extracellular fluid similar to mechanisms for chloride. Although the thyroid gland contains most of the iodine in the body, some is concentrated in the kidney with even smaller concentrations present in the salivary glands, stomach, and portions of the small intestine, skin, feathers and ovary. The iodide trapped by the thyroid gland is quickly converted to organic iodine in synthesis of thyroxine. The thyroid hormones accelerate reactions in most organs and tissues in the body, thus resulting in increased metabolic rate, accelerated growth, and increase in oxygen consumption of the whole organism. The thyroid gland secretes predominately thyroxine (T4) and also some triiodothyronine (T3). Some T4 is deiodinated to T3 in the peripheral tissues, where it is conjugated with sulfate in the liver and kidney, and released into the circulation as the sulfate ester, ST_3. Hydrolysis of ST_3 results in free triiodothyronine in the cell, where it influences energy metabolism as well as other functions.

Several systems help to maintain a constant level of thyroid hormones. A thyroxine bound protein which migrates with the α-globulins, is referred to as thyroxine-binding protein (TBP) or thyroxine-binding globulin (TBG). Although there is a thyroxine-binding pre-albumin protein (TBPA), the α-globulin TBG forms a complex with most of the thyroxine present in the serum at physiological concentrations, which is closely associated with retinol-binding protein.

Functions of the thyroid hormones include (a) controlling the rate of energy metabolism or level of oxidation of all cells in the body; (b) influencing physical as well as mental development and differentiation or maturation of tissues; (c) affecting other endocrine glands, especially the hypophysis and the gonads; (d) influencing neuromuscular functioning; (e) affecting circulatory dynamics; (f) influencing rate of feathering; and (g) influencing the metabolism of the feed nutrients, including various minerals and water. Many of the above functions are interrelated and all probably are based upon the primary function of the thyroid which is that of controlling the rate of cellular oxidation.

5.16.2 Signs of iodine deficiency

An iodine deficiency results in a decreased output of thyroxine from the thyroid gland, which in turn stimulates the anterior pituitary to produce and release increased amounts of thyroid stimulating hormone, (TSH). This increased production of TSH results in a stimulation, with subsequent enlargement, of the thyroid gland, termed a goiter. This enlarged gland is an attempt by the thyroid to increase the secretory surface of the thyroid follicles by hypertrophy and hyperplasia of these follicles. Enlarged thyroids of iodine deficient chicks are shown in Figure 5.29.

Lack of thyroid activity or inhibition of the thyroid by administering thiouracil or thiourea, causes hens to cease laying, become obese, and also results in the growth of abnormally long lacy feathers. Administration of thyroxine or iodinated casein, reverses these effects on egg production with eggshell quality returning to normal levels. The iodine content of an egg is markedly influenced by the hen's intake of iodine. Eggs from a breeder fed an iodine deficient diet, will exhibit reduced hatchability and delayed absorption of the yolk sac.

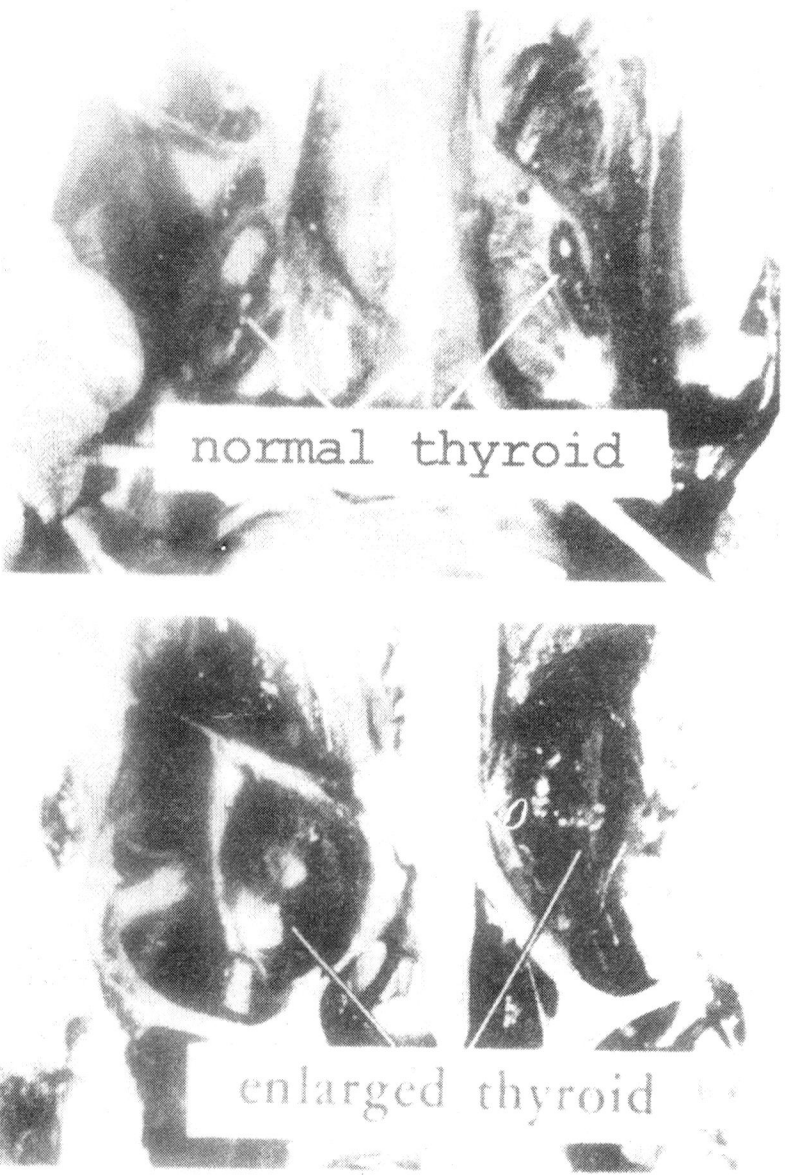

Figure 5.29 Enlarged thyroids from an iodine deficient chick as compared with the smaller thyroids from a chick fed a diet supplemented with iodine.

5.16.3 Iodine requirements

Iodine requirements are around 350 µg/kg diet. Some studies have shown iodine requirements as low as 75 µg/kg diet, although in such situations thyroid status is not maintained long term. While breeders may require only 35 µg/kg diet for their reproductive process, normal thyroid histology of the embryo necessitates higher intakes of iodine by the breeders. The iodine stores in the hen are difficult to deplete. Rogler *et al.* (1959) fed diets containing just 10-19 µg I/kg diet for over a year, without affecting the hen's thyroid size. Even if such breeders were reared on an iodine deficient diet, it was still difficult to influence their thyroid status as adults. Iodine is present in most feedstuffs in trace amounts, but is relatively rich in products of marine origin. The iodine content of plants is closely related to the iodine content of the soil.

High levels of dietary iodine (in excess of 300 mg/kg) can result in reduction of egg production within a week after feeding such a diet. While the fertility of eggs produced from breeders fed high iodine diets is not significantly reduced, early embryonic mortality, reduced hatchability and delayed hatching time have been reported. May and Vardaman (1978) fed broilers up to 500 ppm I and while serum iodine increased from 3 to 1,200 ppm, there was little effect on growth and feed efficiency.

5.17 OTHER TRACE MINERALS

5.17.1 Chromium

Jacobsen (1913) demonstrated that when olive oil or gelatin were fed to fasting men, there was no increase in blood glucose levels. However, when glucose or starch (carbohydrate) were fed, blood glucose levels increased above normal levels and then gradually returned to normal at a rate of about 4% of the excess glucose removed per minute from the blood. This rate of return of excess blood glucose to normal, is now referred to as the glucose tolerance curve. In 1955, Mertz and Schwarz observed that rats fed a low vitamin E, low selenium diet showed a slow rate of removal of excess blood glucose and that the problem could be overcome by adding to the diet dried yeast and several other natural foods. After a number of experiments, and then only by chance, they discovered that the glucose tolerance factor (GTF) in brewer's yeast was trivalent chromium (Cr^{+++} or CrIII, Schwarz and Mertz, 1959). Subsequent studies showed that chromium enhanced the *in vitro* incorporation of glucose into epididymal fat tissues and to a lesser extent acetate into fat, reactions which were enhanced by the addition of insulin. Hence, the primary role of chromium appeared to be its involvement in the initial steps of glucose utilization, with its activity being closely linked to that of insulin.

While there has been little work done investigating the chromium requirement for poultry, several workers have reported that the reduction in growth, noted in chicks following the feeding of vanadium, could be alleviated with the addition of chromium to the diet (Hill and Matrone, 1970; Hafez and Kratzer, 1976). However, the decrease in egg albumen quality noted with diets containing vanadium, could not be reversed by supplementing the diet with chromium (Jensen and Maurice, 1980). Chromium is not a particular toxic element, and most practical diets usually contain sufficient levels to meet any dietary needs of poultry.

5.17.2 Fluorine

In 1972, fluorine was added to the list of essential elements when it was demonstrated that the growth rate of rats on a fluorine-free purified diet, could be increased up to 30% by addition of the element. However, the importance of fluorine in the prevention of dental caries had been demonstrated many years previously. Fluorine can be a very toxic element resulting in reduced appetite, and pitted and worn teeth, in certain farm animals. There is little evidence that fluorine is a required element for poultry.

5.17.3 Vanadium

A vanadium deficiency has been observed in rats and chicks fed vanadium free purified diets. Chicks fed such diets containing less than 10 μg of vanadium/kg showed reduced growth of tail and wing feathers. There is little information showing the vanadium content of feedstuffs. However, it has been shown that fish products are relatively good sources of the element. Vanadium, at relatively low dietary levels, is known to result in growth depression in chicks and to reduce the Haugh unit value of eggs. There is little likelihood that practical poultry diets require vanadium supplementation to meet any dietary requirements for poultry. Vanadium toxicity is more likely due to potential contamination of feed phosphates. Older hens are most susceptible where there is characteristic thinning of the albumen, and loss of hatchability.

5.17.4 Silicon

Rats and chicks both respond to silicon supplementation of purified diets. Silicon has been reported to be essential for normal skeletal development. It is believed that silicon functions as a biological cross-linking agent, forming bridges with other nutrients that give strength, structure and resilience to certain tissues. In deficient rats and chicks, bone abnormalities occur as the result of a reduction in mucopolysaccharide synthesis in the formation of cartilage. It is also suggested that silicon is involved in other functions involving mucopolysaccharides, such as the growth and maintenance of arterial walls and the skin. Silicon is widely distributed in many feedstuffs, and there is little chance of a deficiency showing up in practical poultry diets.

5.17.5 Nickel

Physical symptoms of nickel deficiency have been reported in rats, pigs and chicks under laboratory conditions. Chicks were shown to develop skin pigmentation changes, dermatitis and swollen hocks. It is thought that nickel may play a role in nucleic acid metabolism. Any requirement for poultry should be readily met by concentrations of the element in practical diets.

5.17.6 Tin

In 1970, it was reported that rats fed a purified, trace element free diet, showed a significant improvement in growth with the addition of tin to the diet, thus suggesting that tin was an essential element for mammals. Tin is found in extremely low concentrations in feedstuffs and its importance in the nutrition of farm animals is of questionable significance today.

5.17.7 Arsenic

Arsenic is widely distributed throughout the tissues and fluids of the body, especially the skin, nails and feathers. In recent years there is work showing that it plays a physiological role in the rat. The element is very toxic at low dietary levels, and is of questionable importance for farm animals.

5.18 WATER

While water can hardly be classified as an inorganic element it is perhaps the most important chemical in the body. Water is essential for almost all body functions, being the basic substance of blood and extracellular and intercellular fluids acting in the transport of nutrients, metabolites and waste products to and from all cells in the body. Because of its high specific heat and its evaporative properties, it is extremely important in the regulation of body temperature. Water also plays an important role in homeostasis by participating in reactions and physiological changes which control pH, osmotic pressure, electrolyte concentrations and other functions necessary for life. While chickens can survive for weeks without feed, they can only survive for days without water. Starved birds may lose all their fat, about half of their protein, and about 40% of their body weight and still survive, but a 10% to 20% loss of their body water will result in death.

The water content of the body of a one week old chick is around 85%, and this gradually decreases as the animal accumulates body fat, eventually reaching a level of around 55% for a normal mature hen. Of this body water, approximately 70% is intracellular and 30% extracellular, whilst 75% of the latter is present in the interstitial space and the remaining 25% is found in plasma. Water balance and metabolism are related to the maintenance of a dynamic equilibrium within and between these compartments.

5.18.1 Water intake

The bird obtains most of its water by drinking, although some will be present in feed and variable quantities will arise from body metabolism. Drinking water intake increases with age, although its consumption per unit weight decreases with age. For growing pullets, water intake decreases from 0.45 g/g body weight at 1 wk of age to 0.13 at 16 wk of age (Medway and Kare, 1959). Brake *et al.* (1992) described daily water intake (ml) in broilers to 21 d by the equation: 9.73 + 6.142 x d age. Because water intake is closely correlated with feed intake, factors affecting feed intake indirectly influence water consumption. Although the texture of poultry diets does not appear to affect water consumption, high levels of various dietary constituents such as molasses and salt are known to stimulate water consumption. Differences in environmental temperature significantly affect water consumption by the fowl. Laying birds housed at 31°C will consume twice as much water as birds housed at 15°C. Since feed intake decreases with increased environmental temperature, the ratio of water:feed ingested by poultry is greatly increased at these temperatures. May and Lott (1992) indicate that with daily cyclic temperatures of 24-35°C, the water intake pattern of broilers closely follows ambient temperature. Compared to birds kept at constant 24°C that consume water at about 4% of body weight depending upon age, during heat stress this value increases to 6% of body weight. Budgell (1970) describes three hypotheses to explain the relationship between water intake and environmental temperature: (a) stimulation of water intake at high temperatures due to local dryness of oropharyngeal receptors; (b) systemic dehydration; and (c) alteration in brain temperature. At cold environmental temperatures, water intake may be reduced although birds usually show little aversion to water as cold as 0°C. Metabolic body water, created from increased fat metabolism, may be of significance in contributing to the body water pool at low environmental temperatures. Table 5.11 shows the average water intake values for chickens.

TABLE 5.11 Daily ad-lib water consumption of poultry (litres/1,000 birds)		20°C	32°C
Leghorn pullet	4 wk	50	75
	12 wk	115	180
	18 wk	140	200
Laying hen	50% prod.	150	250
	90% prod.	180	300
Non-laying hen		120	200
Broiler breeder pullet	4 wk	75	120
	12 wk	140	220
	18 wk	180	300
Broiler breeder hen	50% prod	180	300
	80% prod	210	360
Broiler chicken	1 wk	24	40
	3 wk	100	190
	6 wk	240	500
	9 wk	300	600

At high environmental temperatures, birds will drink more water in order to meet the demands for evaporative cooling. However as water temperature increases, birds seem to drink less water, and there are reports that birds are able to differentiate water samples that differ by only 2°C. At high environmental temperatures (>28°C), it is conceivable that birds are not consuming enough water in relation to metabolic needs, and so this may contribute to reduced growth or egg production. For example, Deyhim and Teeter (1991) indicate improved performance of heat stressed broilers by including salt in the drinking water where survival rate closely paralleled the change in water consumption. It is possible that the temperature of water *per se* may limit water intake at high environmental temperatures. Herrick (1971) states that water at body temperature is more readily consumed during cold weather, and cold water increases consumption during warm weather. As water and feed intake are closely correlated, stimulation of water intake may increase feed intake at these temperatures. While broiler chickens will drink fairly continuously throughout the day, the water intake of layers is greatly affected by oviposition and the photoperiod (Figure 5.30).

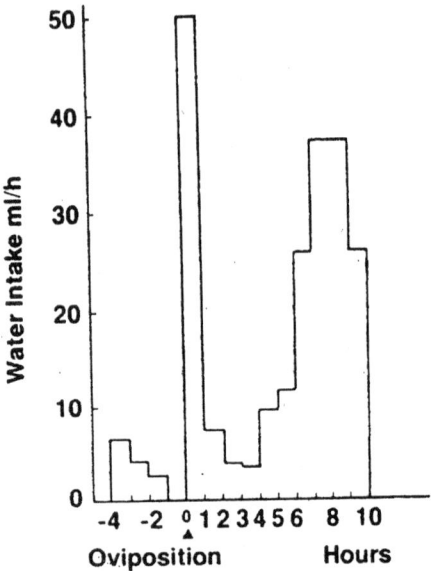

Figure 5.30 Water consumption of laying hens in relation to time of oviposition.
(from Mongin and Sauveur, 1974)

Water is also supplied as a component of the feed, because most ingredients contain about 10% water. Water is created in the body as a by-product of the catabolism of various metabolites, where different amounts of water are produced from the oxidation of fat, carbohydrate and protein. The oxidation of one gram of these nutrients yields 1.18, 0.6 and 0.5 g of water respectively. Total metabolic water can be more easily estimated from energy intake because about 0.135 g of water is produced per kilocalorie of energy consumed (Kerstens, 1964). Thus for a bird consuming 300 kcals ME per d, approximately 40 g of metabolic body water is produced and enters the body pool. This water represents about 15% of total water intake by the fowl. Some exotic birds weighing less than 50 g (therefore with high metabolic rates) are known to be capable of surviving without drinking water for many days on a diet of dry seeds (Wagner, 1964).

5.18.2 Water output

Birds do not urinate as such because the urine is mixed with the feces in the distal large intestine. The excreta of birds can therefore be quite wet, although urine *per se* is much more concentrated than that produced by mammals. The quantity of water excreted in the feces and urine depend upon the water intake. Broiler chickens produce excreta containing about 60-70% moisture while that produced by the laying hen contains up to 80% moisture. Dicker and Haslam (1972) showed that laying hens produce about 12 ml urine daily per kg body weight. The fact that this value is doubled in birds with exteriorized ureters, suggests that considerable water resorption occurs in the large intestine. Two types of urine are produced, a fraction of low concentration produced following eating and drinking corresponding to an elevated glomerular filtration rate, and another urine fraction of higher osmolarity occurring when kidney filtration rate is low. The lining of the coprodeum and urodeum, as well as the rectum, are suited to water resorption and retrograde urine flow into the rectum has been demonstrated, hence water resorption will occur and will be of the order of 25-30 ml/d for the adult fowl as long as urine is hypotonic to extra-cellular fluid (Dicker and Haslam, 1972). For the laying hen at least, the quantity of water excreted in the feces is about four times that excreted as urine. Undoubtedly this loss is subject to considerable variation commensurate with the amount and hydrophilic nature of the digesta. Belay and Teeter (1993) indicate considerable variation in urine output in response to increased environmental temperature. Broilers subjected to heat distress at 35°C vs. 24°C showed a 133% increase in water loss that was associated with only a 78% increase in water intake. The increased water loss was due to greater output of hypo-osmotic urine.

Birds also lose water by evaporation from respired air. Evaporation is one of four physical routes by which the fowl can control its body temperature. Some 575 calories of heat are required to vaporize one gram of water. Evaporative heat loss takes place through the body surface and the respiratory tract. The fowl has no sweat glands, and consequently evaporation via the skin is limited. Such losses overwhelmingly occur via the moist surface layer of the respiratory tract to the inspired air which is saturated with water vapor at body temperature. Evaporative rate is therefore proportional to respiratory rate. Heat lost through evaporation represents only about 12% of total heat loss in the broiler chicken housed at 10°C, but this increases dramatically through 26-35°C where it may contribute as much as 50% of total heat loss from the body. High environmental humidity will reduce the efficiency of evaporative heat loss through the respiratory system.

5.18.3 Water balance

Under normal physiological conditions, water intake and output for adult birds are controlled to maintain a constant level of water in the body. A positive water balance is found in the growing bird related to deposition in developing tissue. Young birds have a greater proportion of body water than do mature birds. Water balance is achieved by the maintenance of equilibrium between the three water compartments of the body, i.e. intracellular, extracellular and plasma. The total volume of water is relatively constant under the conditions already described, although the fluid in the different compartments constantly interchanges. The concentration of water in these compartments is the same relative to osmotically active electrolytes, and a net shifting of water only occurs when an imbalance in osmolarity between two compartments occurs. Such changes in osmolarity may be due to loss of either water or electrolytes. Fluid transfer from the capillary to the extracellular fluid will only occur when the hydrostatic pressure in the former is greater than the osmotic pressure of the extracellular fluid. Barragry (1974) states that the principal cause of water or fluid shift between the extra- and intracellular fluids is a change in composition of the former, although a simple loss of extracellular fluid does not markedly affect the fluid within the cell, because its ionic composition remains relatively unchanged despite the fact that its volume is reduced. Water movement across the cell membrane is initiated by changes in the concentration of the intra- and extracellular fluids, such that the initial equilibrium with respect to osmolarity is achieved. By using tritiated water, the rate of water turnover in the body in terms of radioactive half-life may be measured. Chapman and Mihai (1972) determined the half-life of body water in laying birds, non-laying birds and roosters to be 3.5, 5 and 7 d respectively. These values suggest that factors other than egg production *per se* influence the rate of water turnover in hens. Chapman and Mihai (1972) showed the laying bird to have a greater body water flux (pool size x turnover rate) than the non-laying bird (419 as opposed to 195 ml/d). Even accounting for the water content of the egg, body water flux in the laying hen is significantly greater than in the non-laying hen and may relate to an increased reservoir of soluble metabolites necessary for egg production. This scenario parallels the normal observation that the laying hen consumes more water than does the non-layer, and that this difference is much larger than can be accounted for by the egg and its synthesis. Body water flux in the laying bird is also greater than that recorded for the adult male birds. Water turnover rates may be affected by age. Lopez *et al.* (1973) recorded values of 8.2 and 6.1 d for the half-life of body water in 7 year old hens and 5 month old pullets, respectively. These authors suggested that this age difference might be due to an increased utilization of body water by the young birds for their greater anabolic needs.

5.18.4 Dehydration

Birds become dehydrated because of excess water loss, or less commonly due to water deprivation. As with most animals the most common cause of water loss is diarrhea. When the body loses water at a rate exceeding intake, circulatory fluid volume is decreased resulting in decreased hydrostatic and increased osmotic pressure. Movement of extracellular fluid into the plasma compensates for this depletion. The greater susceptibility of the young animal to dehydration may be associated with the fact that older animals contain greater quantities of extracellular fluid in relation to their size.

Acidosis often develops in cases of diarrhea, due to the losses of alkaline digestive secretions. It has already been noted that feed and water intake are closely related. If feed intake is decreased, the accumulation of ketone bodies resulting from fat metabolism may aggravate any existing acidosis. Acidosis may contribute to hyperkalemia by stimulating kidney potassium resorption in exchange for hydrogen ions thus elevating circulating levels of this element. Because of the dangers of hyperkalemia to the myocardium, the administration of potassium containing fluids to the dehydrated animal (e.g. with excessive diarrhea) is a potentially dangerous procedure.

With drinking water supplied *ad libitum* in commercial poultry units, dehydration due to insufficiency of drinking water should not occur. The drastic effect of partial or complete deprivation of drinking water to the fowl is well documented. Ross (1960) observed that chicks offered water during three 30 minute periods each day, consumed as much water as control *ad libitum* watered birds, but grew only 90% as well. This difference in growth was attributed to differences in feed intake. With birds of 8, 12 and 18 wk of age, Mulkey and Huston (1967) recorded a 45% loss of body water prior to death due to water deprivation. With 48-72 h periods of water deprivation in the laying bird, Adams (1973) observed a reduction in egg production from 65 to 15% over a 2 wk period. Under conditions of complete water starvation, Bierer *et al.* (1966) found laying birds to survive about 8 d while non-laying birds survived some 15d longer. Early death in the layers was attributed to toxemia.

Whatever the reason for dehydration in the bird, the intracellular and extracellular fluids and plasma, to some extent, share the water deficit. Depending on the severity of water deficit, circulation is affected, resulting in increased body temperature and metabolic acidosis. In extreme cases, subsequent death is often a result of bradycardia, circulatory failure, toxemia, and damage to the nervous system or cardiac failure in cases of hyperkalemia.

5.18.5 Water restriction

In certain situations, it is necessary to restrict the quantity of water consumed by birds, usually in an attempt to prevent excessively wet manure. This most commonly occurs with broiler breeding stock that is fed limited quantities of feed in order to control growth. Under these conditions, high water:feed intake occurs due either to physical satiety needs by the bird and/or boredom. In extreme situations it may also be necessary to limit the water intake of adult egg layers, although this is usually a last resort situation when all other management attempts at reducing water:feed intake have failed. Poultry seem to adapt readily to reduced water intake which is usually imposed through limiting time that water is available. As little as two 1 h watering periods each day (8-10 h light) is sufficient to achieve desired growth and there are rarely signs of excessive thirst when water becomes available.

As boredom/satiety is often considered to be a factor in the imbalance of water and feed in feed-restricted breeders, it is generally assumed that water intake will be most problematic on the off-feed days of a skip-a-day feed program. Bennett and Leeson (1989) suggest that most water is voluntarily consumed on feed days (Table 5.12). When given free access to water, birds do not consume an excessive quantity of water relative to restricted time access watering, since average intake is 153 ml/d vs. around 140 ml/d. However, it is obvious that birds consume excessive quantities on the feed day, and this is much more than occurs with restricted time watering, and so water:feed ratio will be increased. Under practical conditions, it is water:feed intake over a relatively short period of item (5-6 hours) that will likely influence water loss, and so the occurrence of wet manure. These data do show, however, that water intake on feed-days rather than off-feed days may contribute most to wet litter. Hocking (1993) suggests that over-drinking of feed-restricted breeders may be an extension of foraging activity and act as a dearousal activity. Hocking (1993) observed that birds subjected to water-restriction spent more time scratching and pecking the litter, but that when given water only 2-8 times daily, they exhibited no unusual signs of thirst when water was reintroduced.

TABLE 5.12 Water consumption of 13 week old growing breeder pullets (ml/bird/day)			
	Water restriction		Free choice water
	Daily	Only on "feed-day"	
Water intake on "feed-day"	175	182	270
Water intake on "off-feed day"	108	109	36
Average	141	145	153
Bennett and Leeson, (1989)			

SELECTED REFERENCES

Adams, A.W., 1973. Consequences of depriving laying hens of water a short time. Poultry Sci. 52:1221-1223.

Adekunmisi, A.A. and K.R. Robbins, 1987. Effects of dietary crude protein, electrolyte balance, and photoperiod on growth of broiler chickens. Poultry Sci. 66:299-305.

Ait-Boulashen, A., J.D. Garlich, and F.W. Edens, 1995. Potassium chloride improves the thermotolerance of chickens exposed to acute heat stress. Poultry Sci. 74:75-87.

Al-Batshan, H.A., E. Scheideler, B. Black, J. Garlich and K. Anderson, 1994. Duodenal calcium uptake, femur ash and eggshell quality decline with age and increase following molt. Poultry Sci. 73: 1590-1596.

Aoyagi, S. and D.H. Baker, 1995. Effect of high copper dosing on hemicellulose digestibility in cecectomized cockerels. Poultry Sci. 74:208-211.

Aoyagi, S. and D.H. Baker, 1995. Iron requirement of chicks fed a semipurified diet based on casein and soy protein concentrate. Poultry Sci. 74:412-415.

Austic, R.E. and C.C. Calvert, 1981. Nutritional interrelationships of electrolytes and amino acids. Fed. Proc. 40:63-67.

Austic, R.E., 1981. Importance of electrolytes in animal nutrition. Proceedings of the 17th Annual Guelph Nutrition Conference for Feed Manufacturers. April 28 & 29, 1981, Toronto, Ontario. pp. 114-121.

Austic, R.E., 1983. Variation in the potassium needs of chickens selected genetically for variation in blood uric acid concentrations. Poultry Sci. 62:365-370.

Austic, R.E., 1984. Excess dietary chloride depresses eggshell quality. Poultry Sci. 63:1773-1777.

Balnave, D. and D. Zhang, 1993. Responses of laying hens on saline drinking water to dietary supplementation with various zinc compounds. Poultry Sci. 72:603-606.

Barragry, T.B., 1974. Some aspects of fluid and electrolyte imbalances in animals. Irish Vet. J. 28 (8):153.

Bélanger, L.F. and D.H. Copp, 1972. The skeletal effects of prolonged calcitonin administration in birds under various conditions. In Calcium, Parathyroid Hormone and the Calcitonins (Talmadge, R.V. and P.L. Munson, eds.) Excerpta Medica, Amsterdam, p. 41

Belay, T. and R.G. Teeter, 1993. Broiler water balance and thermobalance during thermoneutral and high ambient temperature exposure. Poultry Sci. 72:116-124.

Bennett, C.D. and S. Leeson, 1989. Water usage of broiler breeders. Poultry Sci. 68:617-621.

Berthet-Colominas, C., A. Miller and S.W. White, 1979. Structural study of the calcifying collagen in turkey leg tendons. Mol. Biol. 134:431-445.

Bierer, B.W., T.H. Eleazer and B.D. Barnett, 1966. The effect of feed and water deprivation on water and feed consumption, body weight and mortality in broiler chickens of various ages. Poultry Sci. 45:1045-1051.

Bottje, W.G., T.J. Raup and S. Wang, 1989. Effect of ammonium chloride on the bicarbonate buffer system in heat stressed broilers. Br. Poultry Sci. 30:899-905.

Brake, J.D., T.N. Chamblee, C.D. Schultz, E.D. Peebles and J.P. Thaxton, 1992. Daily feed and water consumption of broiler chicks from 0-21 d. J. Appl. Poultry Res. 1:160-163.

Branton, S.L., F.N. Reece and J.W. Deaton, 1986. Use of ammonium chloride and sodium bicarbonate in acute heat exposure of broilers. Poultry Sci. 65:1659-1663.

Brown, D.M., D.Y.E. Perez and J. Jowsey, 1970. Effects of ultimobranchialectomy on bone composition and mineral metabolism in the chicken. Endocrinol. 87:1282.

Budgell, P., 1970. The effect of changes in ambient temperature on water intake and evaporative water loss. Psychon. Sci. 20:275-278.

Bussolati, G. and A.G.E. Pearse, 1967. Immunofluorescent localization of calcitonin in the "C" cells of pig and dog thyroid. J. Endocrinol. 37:205.

Cao, J. et al., 1996. Effect of iron concentration age and length of iron feeding on feed intake, and tissue iron concentration of broiler chicks. Poultry Sci. 75:495-504.

Candlish, J.K., 1971. The formation of mineral and organic matrix of fowl cortical and medullary bone during shell calcification. Br. Poultry Sci. 12:119.

Cantor, A.H. and M.L. Scott, 1974. The effect of selenium in the hen's diet on egg production, hatchability, performance of progeny and selenium concentration in eggs. Poultry Sci. 53:1870.

Cantor, A.H., M.L. Scott and T. Noguchi, 1975. Biological availability of selenium in feedstuffs and selenium compounds for prevention of exudative diathesis in chicks. J. Nutr. 105:96.

Chah, C.C., 1972. A study of the hens nutrient intake as it relates to egg formation. M.Sc. Thesis, Univ. Guelph, Guelph, Ontario Canada N1G 2W1.

Chapman, T.E. and A.L. Black, 1967. Water turnover in chickens. Poultry Sci. 46:761-765.

Chapman, T.E. and D. Mihai, 1972. Influence of sex and egg production on water turnover in chickens. Poultry Sci. 51:1252-1256.

Chavez, E. and F.H. Kratzer, 1979. Potassium deficiency in the adult male chicken. Poultry Sci. 58:652-658.

Christmas, R.B. and R.H. Harms, 1982. Performance of laying hens when fed various levels of sodium and chloride. Poultry Sci. 61:947-950.

Cipera, J.D., 1980. Source of carbon for the biosynthesis of eggshell carbonate in the hen. Comparison of six 14C labeled compounds as sources of carbon in eggshells, albumen, and yolk. Poultry Sci. 59:1529.

Clunies, M., J. Emslie and S. Leeson, 1992. Effect of dietary calcium level on medullary bone calcium reserves and shell weight of Leghorn hens. Poultry Sci. 71:1348-1356.

Cohen, I. and S. Hurwitz, 1974. The response of blood ionic constituents and acid-base balance to dietary sodium, potassium and chloride in laying fowls. Poultry Sci. 53:378-383.

Collins, N.E. and E.T. Moran, Jr., 1999. Influence of supplemental manganese and zinc on live performance and carcass quality of broilers. J. Appl. Poultry Res. 8:222-227.

Combs, G.F., Jr. and M.L. Scott, 1979. The selenium needs of laying and breeding hens. Poultry Sci. 58:871.

Combs, G.F., Jr., A.H. Parsons and M.B. Ross, 1979. Calcium homeostasis in pullets of two lines selected for differences in eggshell strength. Poultry Sci. 58:1250.

Copp, D.H., 1970. Endocrine regulation of calcium metabolism. Ann. Rev. Physiol. 32:61.

Couch, J.R., 1955. Cage layer fatigue. Feed Age 5:55-57.

Cunningham, D.L., G.F. Combs, J.A. Saroka and M.W. LaVargua, 1987. Response to divergent selection for early growth of chickens fed a diet deficient in selenium. Poultry Sci. 66:209-214.

Damron, B.L., 1998. Sodium chloride concentrations in drinking water and eggshell quality. Poultry Sci. 77:1488-1491.

Davis, R.H. and J. Fear, 1996. Incorporation of selenium into egg proteins from dietary selenite. Br. Poultry Sci. 37:197-211.

Dewar, W.A., I.R. Sibbald and P.A.L. Wight, 1982. The contributions of anorexia to reduced growth in zinc deficient chickens. Br. Poultry Sci. 23:129-134.

Dewar, W.A., P.A.L. Wight, R.A. Pearson and M.J. Gentle, 1983. Toxic effects of high concentrations of ZnO in the diet of the chick and laying hen. Br. Poultry Sci. 2:397-404.

Deyhim, F. and R.G. Teeter, 1991. Sodium and potassium chloride drinking water supplementation effects on acid-base balance and plasma corticosterone in broilers reared in thermoneutral and heat distressed environments. Poultry Sci. 70:2551-2553.

Dicker, S.E. and J. Haslam, 1972. Effects of exteriorization of the ureters on the water metabolism of the domestic fowl. J. Physiol. 224:4515-4517.

Edwards, H.M., A.B. Carlos, A.B. Kasim and R.T. Toledo, 1999. Effects of steam pelleting and extrusion of feed in phytate phosphorus utilization in broiler chickens. Poultry Sci. 78:96-101.

El Hadi, H. and A.H. Sykes, 1982. Thermal panting and respiratory alkalosis in the laying hen. Br. Poultry Sci. 23:49-57.

Emmert, J.L. and D.H. Baker, 1995. Zinc stores in chickens delay the onset of zinc deficiency symptoms. Poultry Sci. 74:1011-1021

Erway, L., L.S. Hurley and A.S. Fraser, 1970. Congenital ataxia and otolith defects in mice. J. Nutr. 100:643.

Etches, R.J., 1987. Calcium logistics in the laying hen. J. Nutr. 117:619-628.

Ewing, H.P., G.M. Pesti, R.I. Bakalli, M. Fernando and J. Menten, 1998. Studies on feeding of cupric sulfate, cupric citrate and copper oxychloride to broiler chickens. Poultry Sci. 77:445-448.

Fidler, J.W., K. Schuh, E.C. Naber and JD. Latshaw, 1980. Induction of glutathione peroxidase activity by selenium in the chick. Poultry Sci. 59:135-140.

Fridovich, I, 1975. Superoxide dismutases. Ann. Rev. Biochem. 44:147.

Garlich, J., C. Morris and J. Brake, 1982. External bone volume, ash, and fat-free dry weight of femurs of laying hens fed diets deficient or inadequate in phosphorus. Poultry Sci. 61:1003-1006.

Gill, T.A., G.B. Sundeen, J.F. Richards and D.B. Bragg, 1980. The effects of dietary selenium and vitamin E on avian White Muscle Disease as measured by both chemical and physical parameters. Poultry Sci. 59:2088-2097.

Gries, C.L. and M.L. Scott, 1972. Pathology of selenium deficiency in the chick. J. Nutr. 102:1298.

Grunder, A.A., R.B. Guyer, E.G. Buss and C.O. Clagett, 1980. Calcium binding proteins in serum: quantitative differences between thick and thin shell lines of chickens. Poultry Sci. 59:880-884.

Hafez, Y.S.M. and F.H. Kratzer, 1976. The effect of diet on the toxicity of vanadium. Poultry Sci. 55:918.

Halpin, K.M. and D.H. Baker, 1986. Manganese utilization in the chick: Effects of corn, soybean meal, fish meal, wheat bran and rice bran on tissue uptake of manganese. Poultry Sci. 65:995-1003.

Harms, R.H. and H.R. Wilson, 1984. The chloride requirement of the broiler breeder hen. Poultry Sci. 63:835-837.

Harms, R.H. and A.S. Arafa, 1986. Changes in bone fragility in laying hens. Poultry Sci. 65:1814.

Harms, R.H., D.R. Sloan and G.D. Butcher, 1999. Changes in the laying cycle as a result of a phosphorus deficiency. J. Appl. Poultry Res. 8:191-194.

Hassan, S., 1986. Effect of dietary selenium in the prevention of exudative diathesis in chicks, with special reference to selenium transfer via eggs. J. Vet. Med. Assoc. 33:689-697.

Herrick, J.B., 1971. Water quality for livestock and poultry. Feedstuffs 43:28.

Hess, J.B and W.M. Britton, 1997. Effects of dietary magnesium excess in WL hens. Poultry Sci. 76:703-710.

Hill, C.H. and G. Matrone, 1970. Chemical parameters in the study of in vivo and in vitro interactions of transition elements. Fed. Proc. 29:1474.

Hocking, P.M., 1993. Welfare of broiler breeder and layer females subjected to food and water restriction. Br. Poultry Sci. 34:53-64.

Hodges, R.D., 1974. Histology of the Fowl. London, New York and San Francisco: Academic Press, pp. 444-450.

Hooge, D.M. and K.R. Cummings, 1995. Dietary potassium requirements of poultry explored. Feedstuffs. Sept. 4. P 12.

Houpt, T.R., 1970. In: Dukes Physiology of Domestic Animals, 8th Edition. Cornell Univ. Press. Ithaca, N.Y.

Huff, W.E., C.F. Chang, M.F. Warren and P.B. Hamilton, 1979. Ochratoxin A induced iron deficiency anemia. Appl. Env. Microbiol. 37:601-604.

Hurwitz, S. and A. Bar, 1968. Regulation of pH in the intestine of the laying fowl. Poultry Sci. 47:1029-1030.

Hurwitz, S., A. Bar and A. Meshorer, 1973. Field rickets in turkey poults: plasma and bone chemistry, bone histology, intestinal calcium-binding protein. Poultry Sci. 52:1370-1374.

Jensen, L.S., 1975. Precipitation of a selenium deficiency by high dietary levels of copper and zinc. Proc. Soc. Exp. Biol. Med. 149:113-116.

Jensen, L.S. and D.V. Maurice, 1979. Influence of sulfur amino acids on copper toxicity in chicks. J. Nutr. 109:91-97.

Jensen, L.S. and D.V. Maurice, 1980. Dietary chromium and interior egg quality. Poultry Sci. 59:341.

Kerstens, R., 1964. Investigation of the production of heat and water vapor and the influence of environment on the growth rate of broiler chicks. Funki Information, Funki, Ltd. Acrhus, Denmark.

Keshavarz, K., 1989. The balance between osteoporosis and nephritis. Egg industry. July 1989, pp. 22-25.

Keshavarz, K., 1994. Laying hens respond differently to high dietary levels of phosphorus as monobasic and dibasic calcium phosphate. Poultry Sci. 73:687-703.

Keshavaz, K., 2000. Nonphytate phosphorus requirement of laying hens with and without phytase on a phase feeding program. Poultry Sci. 79:748-763.

Kidd, M.T., P.R. Ferket and M.A. Qureshi, 1996. Zinc metabolism with special reference to its role in immunity. Wld. Poultry Sci. J. 52:309-324.

Kim, C.S. and C.H. Hill, 1966. Interrelation of dietary copper and amine oxidase in the formation of elastin. Biochem. Biophys. Res. Commun. 24:395.

King, M.M., E.K. Lai and P.B. McCay, 1975. Singlet oxygen production associated with enzyme-catalyzed lipid peroxidation in liver microsomes. J. Biol. Chem. 250:6496.

Koelkebeck, K.W., P.C. Harrison, and C.M. Parsons, 1992. Carbonated drinking water for improvement of eggshell quality of laying hens during summertime months. J. Appl. Poultry Res. 1:194-199.

Kohne, H.J. and J.E. Jones, 1975. Acid-base balance, plasma electrolytes and production performance of adult turkey hens under conditions of increasing ambient temperature. Poultry Sci. 54:2038-2045.

Kratzer, F.H., J.B. Allred, P.N. Davis, B.J. Marshall and P. Vohra, 1959. The effect of autoclaving soybean protein and the addition of ethylenediaminetetraacetic acid on the biological availability of dietary zinc for turkey poults. J. Nutr. 68:313.

Latshaw, J.D., J.F. Ort and C.D. Diesem, 1977. The selenium requirements of the hen and effects of a deficiency. Poultry Sci. 56:1876.

Leach, R.M., Jr. and M.C. Nesheim, 1963. Studies on chloride deficiency in chicks. J. Nutr. 81:193.

Leach, R.M., Jr., 1967. Studies on the role of manganese in chondroitin sulfate synthesis. Poultry Sci. 46:1284.

Leach, R.M. and J.R. Gross, 1983. The effect of manganese deficiency upon the ultrastructure of the eggshell. Poultry Sci. 62:499-504.

Lee, S.R, and W.M. Britton, 1980. Magnesium toxicity: effect on phosphorus utilization by broiler chicks. Poultry Sci. 59:1989-1994.

Lee, S.R., W.M. Britton and G.N. Rowland, 1980. Magnesium toxicity: Bone Lesions. Poultry Sci. 59:2403-2411.

Leeson, S., R.J. Julian and J.D. Summers, 1986. Influence of prelay and early-lay dietary calcium concentration on performance and bone integrity of Leghorn pullets. Can. J. Anim. Sci. 66:1087-1096.

Lent, A.J. and R.F. Wideman, 1994. Hypercalciuric response to dietary supplementation with DL-methionine and ammonium sulfate. Poultry Sci. 73:63-74.

Lilburn, M.S. and R.M. Leach, 1980. Metabolism of abnormal cartilage cells associated with TD. Poultry Sci. 59:1892-1896.

Liu, A.C., B.S. Heinrichs and R.M. Leach, 1994. Influence of manganese deficiency on the characteristics of proteoglycans of avian epiphyseal growth plate cartilage. Poultry Sci. 73:663-669.

Lopez, G.A., R.W. Phillips and C.F. Nockels, 1973. The effect of age on water metabolism in hens. Proc. Soc. Exp. Biol. Med. 142:545.

Mahoney, C.P., F.A. Alster and L.B. Carew, 1992. Growth, thyroid function and serum macromineral levels in Mg deficient chicks. Poultry Sci. 71:1669-1679.

May, J.D. and B.D. Lott, 1992. Feed and water patterns of broilers at high environmental temperatures. Poultry Sci. 71:331-336.

May, J.D. and T.H. Vardaman, 1978. Effect of a high level of dietary iodine on resistance of broilers to mycoplasma synoviae. Poultry Sci. 57:65-69.

McCay, P.B., D.O. Gibson, K.L. Fong and K.R. Hornbrook, 1976. The effect of glutathione peroxidase activity ion lipid peroxidation in biological membranes. Biochim. Biophys. Acta.

Medway, W. and M.R. Kare, 1959. Water metabolism of the growing domestic fowl with special reference to water balance. Poultry Sci. 38:631-637.

Mertz, W. and K. Schwarz, 1959. Relation of glucose tolerance factor to impaired intravenous glucose tolerance of rats on stock diets. Am. J. Physiol. 196:614.

Miles, R.D., S.F. O'Keefe, P.R. Henry, C.B. Ammerman and X.G. Luo, 1998. The effect of supplementation with CuSO4 or Cu2(OH)3Cl on broiler performance, relative copper bioavailability and dietary prooxidant activity. Poultry Sci. 77:416:425.

Mongin, P., 1968. Role of acid-base balance in the physiology of egg-shell formation. Wld. Poultry Sci. J. 24:200-230.

Mongin, P., 1980. Electrolytes in nutrition. 3rd Int. Minerals Conf. Orlando, Florida. Jan. 16, 1980. pp 1-16.

Mongin, P., 1981. Recent advances in dietary anion/cation balance in poultry. Recent Adv. Anim. Nutr. 109-119. Publ-Butterworths, London.

Mongin, P. and B. Sauveur, 1974. Voluntary food and calcium intake by the laying hen. Br. Poultry Sci. 15:349-359.

Mongin, P. and B. Sauveur, 1979. The specific calcium appetite of the domestic fowl. In Food Intake Regulation in Poultry. pp 171-179. Ed. Boorman and Freeman. Publ. Br. Poultry Sci. Edinburgh.

Mongin, P. and B. Sauveur, 1979. Plasma inorganic phosphorus concentration during egg-shell formation. Br. Poultry Sci. 20:401-412.

Mork, T.A. and R.E. Austic, 1981. Iron requirements of White Leghorn hens. Poultry Sci. 60:1497-1503.

Mueller, W.J., 1966. Effect of rapid temperature changes on acid-base balance in shell quality. Poultry Sci. 45:1109.

Mulkey, G.J. and T.M. Huston, 1967. The tolerance of different stages of domestic fowl to body water loss. Poultry Sci. 46:1564-1569.

Murakami, A.E. et. al. 1997a. Effect of level and source of sodium on performance of male broilers to 56 days. J. App. Poultry Res. 6:128-136.

Murakami, A.E., et al. 1997b. Estimation of the sodium and chloride requirements for the young broiler chick. J. Appl. Poultry Res. 6:155-162.

Namkung, H. and S. Leeson, 1999. Effect of phytase enzyme on dietary AMEn and ileal digestibility of nitrogen and amino acid in broiler chicks. Poultry Sci. 78:1317-1320.

Noguchi, T., A.H. Cantor and M.L. Scott, 1973. Mode of action of selenium and vitamin E in prevention of exudative diathesis in chicks. J. Nutr. 103:1502.

Ort, J.F. and J.D. Latshaw, 1978. The toxic level of sodium selenite in the diet of laying chickens. J. Nutr. 108:1114-1120.

Payne, C.G. and B.S. Bains, 1975. Femoral degeneration and scabby hip syndrome in chicks. Vet. Rec. 97:436-437.

Payne, G.G., 1977. Involvement of molybdenum in feather growth. Br. Poultry Sci. 18:427-432.

Rao, K., D.A. Roland, J.L. Adams and W.M. Durboraw, 1992. Improved limestone retention in the gizzard of commercial Leghorn hens. J. Appl. Poultry Res. 1:6-10.

Roberson, K.D., C.H. Hill and P.R. Ferket, 1993. Additive amelioration of TD in broilers by supplemental calcium or feed deprivation. Poultry Sci. 72:798-805.

Rogler, J.C., H.E. Parker, F.N. Andrews and C.W. Carrick, 1959. The effects of an iodine deficiency on embryo development and hatchability. Poultry Sci. 38:398.

Rojas, S.W. and M.L. Scott, 1969. Factors affecting the nutritive value of cottonseed meal as a protein source in chick diets. Poultry Sci. 48:819.

Roland, D.A., 1987. Recent developments with D3 concerning eggshell pimpling, bone splintering and body storage. Proc. Maryland Nutr. Conf., pp. 109-115.

Roland, D.A. and R. Gordon, 1997. Phosphorus, calcium optimization requires new approach. Feedstuffs. April 7, 1997 p14.

Ross, E., 1960. The effect of water restriction on chicks fed different levels of molasses. Poultry Sci. 39:999-1002.

Rotruck, J.T., A.L. Pope, H.E. Ganther, A.B. Swanson, D.G. Hafeman and W.G. Hoekstra, 1973. Selenium: Biochemical role as a component of glutathione peroxidase. Science 179:588.

Roush, W.B., M. Mylet, J.L. Rosenberger and J. Derr, 1986. Investigation of calcium and available phosphorus requirements for laying hens by response surface methodology. Poultry Sci. 65:964-970.

Rowland, G.N. and T. Foutz, 1990. Production induced osteopenia. Proc. Av. Skeletal Dis. Symp., San Antonia, TX.., July 22.

Ruff, C.R. and B.L. Hughes, 1985. Bone strength of height-restricted broilers as affected by levels of calcium, phosphorus, and manganese. Poultry Sci. 64:1628-1636.

Ruiz-Lopez, B. and R.E. Austic, 1993. The effect of selected minerals on the acid-base balance of growing chicks. Poultry Sci. 72:1054-1062.

Sauveur, B. and P. Mongin, 1978. Interrelationships between dietary concentrations of sodium, potassium and chloride in laying hens. Br. Poultry Sci. 19:475.

Schwarz, K. and C.M. Foltz, 1957. Selenium as an integral part of factor 3 against dietary necrotic liver degeneration. J. Am. Chem. Soc. 79:3292.

Schwarz, K. and W. Mertz, 1959. Chromium (III) and the glucose tolerance factor. Arch. Biochem. Biophys. 85:292.

Scott, J.T., C.R. Creger, F.M. Farr and S.S. Linton, 1977. Skeletal effects in the prelay bird when fed a high calcium diet. Nutr. Rep. Int. 15:139-144.

Scott, M.L., 1973. The selenium dilemma. J. Nutr. 103:803.

Scott, R.L. and R.E. Austic, 1976. Influence of potassium on lysine catabolism in the chick. Poultry Sci. 55:2089

Sebastian, S., S.P. Touchburn and E.R. Chavez, 1998. Implications of phytic acid and supplemental microbial phytase in poultry nutrition: a review. Wld. Poultry Sci. J. 54:27-47.

Sebastian, S., S.P. Touchburn, E.R. Chavez and P.C. Lagne, 1996. The effects of supplemental microbial phytase on the performance and utilization of dietary calcium, phosphorus, copper and zinc in broiler chickens fed corn-soybean diets. Poultry Sci. 75:729-736.

Shafey, T.M., 1993. Calcium tolerance of growing chickens: effect of ratio of dietary calcium to available phosphorus. Wld. Poultry Sci. J. 49:5-18.

Smith, M.O. and R.G. Teeter, 1987. Potassium balance of 5-8 week old broiler exposed to constant heat and cycling high temperature stress. Poultry Sci. 66:487-492.

Smith, M.O., I.L. Sherman, L.C. Miller and K.R. Robbins, 1995. Relative biological activity of manganese from Mn proteinate, MnSO4 and MnO in broilers reared at elevated temperatures. Poultry Sci. 74:702-707.

Southern, L.L. and D.H. Baker, 1983. Excess manganese ingestion in the chick. Poultry Sci. 62:642-646.

Stanley, V.G., D.M. Hutchingson, A.H. Reine, D. Carrier and A.A. Hinton, 1992. Magnesium sulfate effects on coliform bacteria in the intestines, ceca and carcasses of broiler chickens. Poultry Sci. 71:76-80.

Teeter, R.G. and M.O. Smith, 1986. High chronic ambient temperature stress effects on broiler acid-base balance and their response to supplemental ammonium chloride, potassium chloride and potassium carbonate. Poultry Sci. 65:1777-1781.

Teeter, R.G., M.O. Smith, F.N. Owens and S.C. Arp, 1985. Chronic heat stress and respiratory alkalosis: occurrence and treatment in broiler chicks. Poultry Sci. 64:1060-1064.

Thompson, J.N. and M.L. Scott, 1970. Impaired lipid and vitamin E absorption related to atrophy of the pancreas in selenium-deficient chicks. J. Nutr. 100:797.

Vo, K.V., M.A. Boone and A.K. Torrence, 1977. Electrolyte content of blood and bone in chickens subjected to heat stress. Poultry Sci. 57:542-544.

Vohra, P. and F.H. Kratzer, 1964. Influence of various chelating agents on the availability of zinc. J. Nutr. 82:249.

Waddell, A.L., R.G. Board, V.D. Scott and S.G. Tullett, 1991. Role of magnesium in egg shell formation in the domestic hen. Br. Poultry Sci. 32:853-864.

Wagner, M.J., 1964. Thirst in the regulation of body water. Florida St. Univ. Tallahassee, 1963, Pergamon Press.

Waldroup, P.W. and M.H. Adams, 1994. Evaluation of the phosphorus provided by animal proteins in the diet of broiler chickens. J. Appl. Poultry Res 3:209-218.

Wedekind, K.J. and D.H. Baker, 1990. Zinc bioavailability in feed grade sources of zinc. J. Anim. Sci. 68:684-689.

Whiting, T.S., L.D. Andrews and L. Stamps, 1991. Effects of sodium bicarbonate and potassium chloride drinking water supplementation. Poultry Sci. 70:53-59.

Wideman R. F. et al., 1996. Excess dietary copper triggers enlargement of the proventriculus in broilers. J. Appl. Poultry Res. 5:219-230.

Wideman, R.F. and A.C. Nissley, 1992. Kidney structure and responses of two commercial SCWL strains to saline in the drinking water. Br. Poultry Sci. 33:489-504.

Wilson, J.H., 1991. Bone strength of caged layers as affected by dietary calcium and phosphorus concentrations, reconditioning, and ash content. Br. Poultry Sci. 32:501-508.

Zhang, B. and C.N. Coon, 1997. The relationship of calcium intake, source, size, solubility in vitro and gizzard limestone retention in laying hens. Poultry Sci. 76:1702-1706.

Non-Nutritive Feed Addititives

Feed for broilers and laying hens is formulated to contain an optimum nutrient concentration obtainable at reasonable cost for desirable growth, production and efficiency of feed utilization. To ensure that dietary nutrients are ingested, digested, protected from destruction, absorbed, and transported to the cells of the body, certain non-nutritive feed additives are sometimes used in addition to this optimum concentration and balance of nutrients. Other feed additives have been used to alter the metabolism of the chicken in an effort to produce better growth or more desirable finished products. Following is a list of the most common type of feed additives.

1)   Pellet binders affect texture and firmness of pelleted feeds,

2)   Flavoring agents have been used in an effort to improve the palatability of feed,

3)   Enzymes have been shown, under certain conditions, to improve the digestibility of specific nutrients,

4)   Antibiotics and arsenicals have been used at low levels to help protect feeds from microbial destruction and to prevent production of toxic products by the intestinal microflora,

5)   Antifungals have been used to prevent growth of harmful molds and fungi in feeds and/or in the digestive tract of the chicken,

6)   Anticoccidials are routinely used in broiler feeds and also (usually at lower levels) in diets for rearing replacement pullets,

7)   Worming drugs are periodically added to feeds for protection against intestinal parasites,

8)   Antioxidants are used to protect polyunsaturated fatty acids and the fat soluble vitamins from destruction by peroxidation,

9)   Carotenoids are added to many feeds to improve pigmentation of broilers or egg yolks,

10) Probiotics and yeasts can be used to influence the intestinal microflora,

11) Odor and fly control agents that influence manure composition.

6.1 PELLET BINDERS AND PELLETABILITY

Diets for meat birds are almost universally steam pelleted. This expensive process involves application of steam to the mash diet which is then forced, under great pressure, through dies with holes that dictate pellet diameter. Pellets are cut to desired length, and then may be gently broken to produce crumbled diets for young birds. Some feeds, and especially corn soybean mixtures, are notoriously difficult to pellet, since the resultant product is easily broken during normal transfer and transportation. Pellet quality is often assessed as Pellet Durability Index, which is a measure of the proportion of intact pellets remaining after a predetermined time of physical agitation and shaking. The index can range from a low of 50-60 for corn-soy diets, to a high of 90 for diets containing significant amounts of wheat.

The advantages to using pelleted feed are greatly reduced physical separation of ingredients and ease of flow in mechanical equipment. For the bird, there is potential for increased feed intake of low energy diets and/or reduced energy expended in consuming feed. The bird also has less chance to select particles of individual ingredients from the diet which can lead to nutrient imbalance. Consequently, there is a desire to produce as firm a pellet as possible, such that it will withstand the rigors of transport to the feed trough.

The gluten proteins in wheat are what give it its unique dough-making characteristics, and these same proteins help to hold pellets intact during manufacture. The best pellet quality is invariably produced in wheat based diets, and in some instances wheat or products such as wheat shorts may be included in a diet simply to aid the pelleting process, rather than merely to supply nutrients.

When wheat is unavailable, other pelleting agents may be considered. Different products are used at quite different inclusion levels and such levels should be clearly specified. When wheat or wheat by products are used at less than 10% of the diet, then a binder will often be necessary if high pellet durability is desired. The two major types of binders have lignosulfonate or colloidal clays as the base product, with inclusions levels of around 5-12 kg/tonne. There have been reports of colloidal clay type products binding some B vitamins in the gut, and so making them unavailable to the bird. The colloidal clay products may also aid in reducing apparent moisture content of the bird's excreta and more recently some forms of clay have been shown to have activity in binding aflatoxin. The lignosulfonate pellet binders often contain 20-30% sugars and so contribute to diet energy level. Studies show lignosulfonate binders to have ME values of 900-2200 kcal/kg depending upon sugar content. Because these binders are often used at 1-1.2% of the diet, energy contribution is meaningful at 10-25 kcal/kg of diet.

Pelleting rate is also influenced by ingredient selection. Adding 1-2% fat usually increases the pelleting rate, because fat acts as a lubricant at the die. However, with much more than 4% fat in the mash mixture, it is increasingly difficult to maintain pellet durability. Today high fat diets are produced by adding 2-3% fat in the mash diet, with the remainder added post-pelleting. Most mineral supplements will slow the pelleting rate, because they increase friction at the die. Defluorinated rock phosphate is sometimes used in poultry diets, ostensibly as a source of phosphorus, but also because it increases rate of pelleting up to 10% compared to diets containing most other phosphate sources.

6.2   FLAVORING COMPOUNDS

Compared to other farm animals, the chicken does not have an acute sense of taste or smell. Chickens have only about 24 taste buds in comparison to 9,000 in humans and cattle which have around 25,000. Birds seem better able to differentiate the taste of compounds in water, where they will consistently select water containing sucrose, for example, compared to some bitter tasting compounds. This fact may be of importance in the taste perception of water medications.

Many studies have been conducted to determine whether or not chickens accept or reject certain feedstuffs or feed mixtures on the basis of taste. Kare (1965) identified numerous chemical agents which are so objectionable that they cause a decrease in normal feed consumption by chickens. However, no flavoring agent has yet been found which will increase feed consumption above that normally obtained with well-balanced poultry feeds composed largely of conventional ingredients.

However, it is possible that certain natural feedstuffs are relatively unsuitable for chickens because they are not palatable. Chickens tend to avoid diets high in barley and rye in comparison to similar diets containing corn. Healthy chickens will gradually increase consumption of many feeds initially avoided and often normal growth is ultimately obtained with such feeds.

Whether chickens avoid certain feedstuffs on the basis of taste, lack of eye appeal or because of adverse effects upon metabolism or sense of well-being is unknown. Relatively few studies have been conducted with flavoring agents for poultry in the last 30 years and for this reason, care must be taken in extrapolating data from other species. For example, sucrose octaacetate solution is reported to be readily accepted by birds, but universally rejected by humans. There seems little scope for use of flavoring agents with broiler chickens for stimulating feed intake. However, there may be some potential with breeders for isolation of agents that are distasteful to birds, as an aid in limiting their feed intake. Flavoring agents may be beneficial in masking any unpalatable ingredients, and for maintaining a constant feed flavor during formulation changes. Flavors may also be useful tools in masking any undesirable changes in drinking water during medication. It is conceivable that use of a single flavor agent in both feed and medicated water may prevent some of the refusals seen with medicated water.

6.3   ENZYMES

There has been considerable interest in the use of exogenous feed enzymes over the last 10-15 years. Enzymes are added to feeds in order to augment low levels of natural endogenous enzymes or to add novel systems not naturally produced by the bird. The most common enzyme products currently used are those for digestion of complex carbohydrates and for the release of phosphorus from phytic acid. Protease, lipase and carbohydrase enzymes have been used for many years in various manufacturing industries, but it has only been in the last 10-15 years that they have been developed specifically for use in animal feeds. Of the 3,000 or so enzymes known to biochemists, only 30-35 are used for industrial purposes. This latter consideration is important, because to be effective in poultry feeds, these exogenous enzymes must be active at the pH level of the gut where substrates become available and must not be inactivated by prior pH changes as occur in

the gizzard. Likewise, exogenous enzymes must stand the rigor of ingredient processing and feed preparations. In this respect, the harsh conditions generated during
pelleting and expanding of feed, often dictate the need for novel post-processing
application.

Exogenous enzymes theoretically have most application in diets for very young
birds because their natural production is low relative to that seen in the bird by
14-21d (see Chapter 1). It is likely that the digestion of fats, carbohydrates and
proteins can be improved in young birds less than about 14d of age when appropriate enzymes are added to the diet. Currently most exogenous enzymes are not
applicable for this application, since they are designed to cleave more complex
molecules such as arabinoxylans and β-glucans. When lipase is added to the diet
of young chicks there is a 5-7% increase in fat digestion, and corresponding increase
in diet metabolizable energy.

The initial interest in enzymes as feed additives arose as an attempt at improving
the digestibility of ingredients such as rye and barley. These cereals contain complex
carbohydrates that imbibe water in the digesta, producing a thick viscous medium and very wet excreta. Studies involving digesta viscocity resulted in a greater
appreciation of indigestible carbohydrates, previously called crude fiber and now
generally referred to as non-starch polysaccharides (NSP's). These NSP's are essentially indigestible fiber which add little to the nutrient value of an ingredient, and
may in fact reduce overall nutrient availability by providing a hostile environment
to endogenous enzymes in the intestine. High levels of NSP's are found in grains
such as wheat, barley and epecially rye. There is also potential to improve the
utilization of protein ingredients, such as soybean meal, although again this may
essentially revolve around improved utilization of carbohydrates that are normally undigested by the bird. Phytase is a different type of enzyme that degrades the
normally indigestible phytic acid molecule. Use of exogenous phytase therefore
improves phosphorus digestion and concurrently reduces phosphorus excretion
by the bird. Lipase enzymes are also receiving some attention, because it is known
that young birds have difficulty in digesting saturated fats as are commonly found
in cheaper animal fat blends. A major limitation with many enzymes is their susceptibility to heat and so instability during pelleting.

6.3.1   β-glucans and arabinoxylans

As previously described, the main concern with cereals is their NSP content, and
especially β-glucan in barley and arabinoxylans or pentosans in wheat. Table 6.1
shows average NSP content of some cereal grains.

TABLE 6.1 NSP content of cereals			
Cereal	β-glucans	Pentosans	Total
	(g/kg DM)		
Dehulled rice	0	0	0
Sorghum	1	28	29
Maize	1	43	44
Wheat	5	61	66
Triticale	7	70	77
Barley	33	76	109
Rye	12	89	101
Modified from Choct and Annison (1990)			

Barley is very high in β-glucans, while both wheat and barley are high in pentosans, the chemical structure of which is previously shown in Figure 2.25. These carbohydrates are normally difficult to digest, and as they pass through the small intestine they imbibe water, making a highly viscous medium. This increased viscosity reduces the normal physical transport of other digested nutrients to the epithelium of the gut, which effectively reduces absorption. The more viscous digesta also reduces the chance of contact between substrates and corresponding endogenous enzymes and digestion enhancers such as bile salts. The increased digesta viscosity is noticeable in the excreta, which becomes stickier and quickly leads to litter moisture problems. The major effect of NSP's, therefore, is reduced energy availability to the birds and there is a direct relationship between NSP and AMEn.

Dehulled rice has virtually no NSP's (Table 6.1) and this correlates with an AMEn:GE ratio of close to 1.0. Wheat is intermediate in NSP's and yields an AME:GE of around 0.8, while rye and barley are notoriously high in NSP's and have the lowest AME yield of GE at around 0.65. There is also a direct relationship between intestinal viscosity and overall diet digestibility. Viscosity caused by NSP's is, therefore, the major problem to be overcome by enzymes designed for barley and wheat. Of these two cereals, wheat is by far the most commonly used worldwide, both as the grain and as the by-product and so improvement in the digestion of wheat is of commercial importance. Our recent data with several commercial enzymes show reduced digesta viscosity at 2 and 6 weeks of age in broilers and in most situations an improvement in AMEn of the diets that contained 65-70% wheat (Figure 6.1).

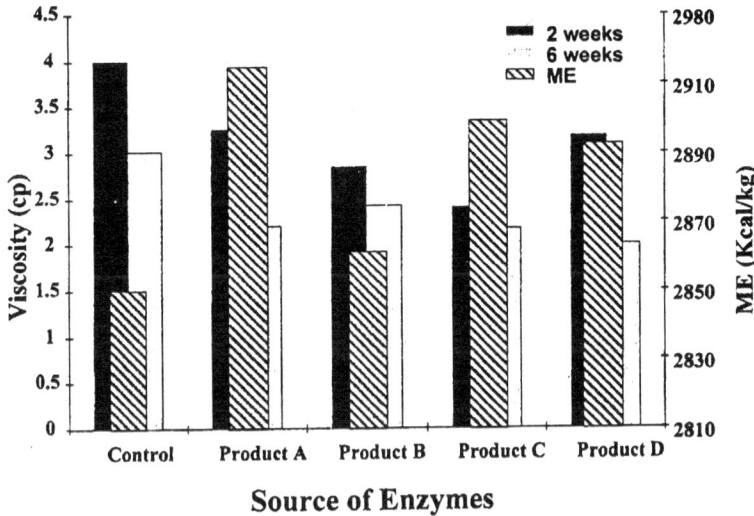

Figure 6.1 Effect of dietary enzymes on metabolizable energy of the diets and viscosity of intestinal content of male broiler chickens.

Rye is perhaps the most problematic cereal in terms of intestinal viscosity, and for this reason rye is very rarely used in poultry diets. However, in the past, rye genes have been incorporated into wheat (which is genetically very similar to rye) for improvements in yield and pest/drought resistance. It is now interesting to note that it is wheat varieties that have these rye genes that produce the most problems with intestinal viscosity and reduced nutrient availability. If a range of wheat samples is tested and ranked for intestinal viscosity there is usually a clear differentiation for those with, versus those without, rye gene insertion. Because there are obviously differences in NSP content of various wheat samples, then enzymes are expected to have variable results depending upon the seed variety used. We have shown variable response to barley, dependent on the β-glucan content of the variety tested (Table 6.2). In this study, the β-glucanase enzymes generally improved AMEn and nitrogen utilization when diets contained barley with a high level of β-glucan. However, with a low β-glucan barley, a number of negative results are seen. Prior to using β-glucanase or pentosanase-type enzymes, it would be advisable to assay the cereal for potential substrate, the presence of which dictates the need for enzyme addition.

Barley type	Enzyme source	Metabolizable energy (kcal/kg)	Apparent nitrogen retention (mg/bird/day)
TABLE 6.2 Effect of enzyme addition on metabolizable energy of diets containing barley			
High β-glucan	None	3232c	119b
	Product A	3351ab	229ab
	Product B	3272bc	180ab
	Product C	3462a	353ab
	Product D	3406ab	394a
	Product E	3335abc	311ab
	± SD	94	160
Low β-glucan	None	3271a	200a
	Product A	3134ab	28ab
	Product B	3086b	-183b
	Product C	3025b	-160b
	Product D	3110b	59ab
	Product E	2994b	-98b
	± SD	110	186
Adapted from Leeson and Proulx (1994)			

About 70-75% of NSP's are depolymerised by exogenous enzymes, and these yield energy available to the bird. However, even with 2% arabinoxylans in wheat, their total digestion would yield at most, 100 kcal AMEn/kg. When arabinoxylanase enzymes are used, the improved AMEn can be as high as 600 kcal/kg (Annison and Choct, 1993) and so release of sugars *per se*, from NSP, represent only a minor advantage to using such enzymes. The NSP's obviously impair digestion of other major dietary nutrients and so the major advantage to enzyme addition is full expression of endogenous enzyme mechanisms.

6.3.2   Oligosaccharides and proteases

Almost all poultry diets contain soybean meal and surprisingly, this ingredient is not that well utilized by poultry. The AMEn of soybean meal is very low in relation to its gross energy, mainly because of indigestible oligosaccharides such as raffinose, cellobiose, etc. (Figure 2.25). The microbes in the cecum of the pig make better use of these unusual carbohydrates, and this is why much higher AMEn values are determined for soybean meal with pigs. Soybean meal produced by extraction with ethanol, rather than hexane, has these NSP's removed, and AMEn is almost equivalent to that of corn. Enzymes designed to improve carbohydrate digestibility of soybean meal therefore have great potential in poultry nutrition. Data in Table 6.3 shows variability in analyses of soybean meal samples.

TABLE 6.3 Range in composition of soybean samples				
Origin	Protein	Trypsin inhibitor	Lectin	Oligosaccharides
	(%)	(mg/g)		(mg/kg)
Brazil	46.6-49.2	1.5-2.5	0.09-0.38	55.7-59.0
China	43.2-46.1	1.0-6.8	0.34-2.28	57.9-64.4
Europe	43.4-49.3	1.6-3.5	0.01-0.13	57.9-64.4
India	48.2-49.9	1.5-3.2	0.20-1.24	48.4-59.7
USA	48.2-49.4	2.2-3.3	0.02-0.05	57.1-66.1
Adapted from Bedford (1996)				

Table 6.4 indicates improvement in performance of broilers fed enzymes designed specifically for corn soybean meal diets. In this study, the treatment involved a 4% reduction in diet AMEn and amino acids, and use of enzymes resulted in comparable performance to birds fed the control diet. These authors concluded that the enzyme improved digestibility of the diet by about 4%. Other enzyme manufacturers are currently claiming a 7% improvement in utilization of soybean meal.

TABLE 6.4 Performance of broilers fed corn-soy diets to 49d				
	Standard diet		-4% ME & CP/AA	
Parameters	Control	+Enzyme	Control	+Enzyme
Weight gain (g)	3140	3270	3063	3124
Feed intake (g)	5344	5467	5379	5430
Feed:gain	1.70	1.67	1.76	1.74
Adapted from Pack and Bedford (1997)				

6.3.3 Phytase

Phosphorus is a very expensive nutrient, and in many countries there are now concerns about the phosphorus content of manure as it impacts the environment. Most of the phosphorus in plants occurs as phytic acid, being about two thirds of the total plant phosphorus. Poultry have virtually no endogenous phytase activity, and so there is little digestion of phytate phosphorus. The phytic acid molecule has six phytic acid residues and these can have a high affinity for several cations (Figure 5.12) and one mole of phytic acid can bind 3 to 6 moles of calcium. These mineral complexes are insoluble at the pH of the gut, and so render both phosphorus and calcium unavailable to the bird. Zinc and copper can also be strongly bound by phytate and, under certain conditions, various amino acids may also form insoluble phytate protein complexes.

Phytase (which is usually a microbial enzyme) catalyzes the hydrolytic cleavage of the phosphorus acid esters of inositol, liberating phosphorus, which can then be absorbed. Other minerals and amino acids that are bound may also be made available for absorption. Phytase activity is expressed as phytase units or FTU per unit of feed. Microbial phytase, produced by fermentation, is much more potent than naturally occurring plant phytase. The phytate phosphorus and phytate activity of a number of plant products is shown in Table 6.5. Most cereals, and vegetable protein supplements are relatively low in phytase content, with the exception of wheat by products. The relative activity of natural wheat phytase as compared to microbial phytase has been reported to be between 50 and 60%. Because calcium, as well as phosphorus, is liberated from the phytic acid molecule by phytase, then both mineral levels need to be reduced if phytase is used during formulation.

TABLE 6.5 Phytate phosphorus content and phytase activity of some common feed ingredients			
Ingredient	Phytate Phosphorus		Phytase activity (FTU/kg)
	%	% of Total P	
Cereals and by-products:			
Corn	.24	72	15
Wheat	.27	69	1193
Sorghum	.24	66	24
Barley	.27	64	582
Oats	.29	67	40
Wheat bran	.92	71	2957
Oilseed meals:			
Soybean meal	.39	60	8
Canola meal	.70	59	16
Sunflower meal	.89	77	60
Peanut meal	.48	80	3
Cottonseed meal	.84	70	NA
From BASF Technical Symposium (1996)			

If phytase is used in formulation, there are a number of different approaches to account for increased phytate availability. Where few ingredients are used, then the available phosphorus level of these ingredients can be increased accordingly. Alternatively, the specification for available phosphorus in the diet can be reduced or phytase enzyme can be included as an ingredient with specifications for available phosphorus and calcium. Each 500 units of phytase activity are equivalent to about 1g of phosphorus as provided by sources such as dicalcium phosphate.

Adding 500 units/kg of feed therefore provides about 0.10% available phosphorus in the diet.

Currently there are two problems with using phytase, namely cost and degradation during pelleting. Most phytases are denatured to some degree at around 65°C, and so any pelleting or feed processing involving the high temperatures used to control salmonella in feed mean that phytase enzymes must be added post-processing. In many countries it is still economical to use phosphates rather than phytase enzyme. However, this situation may change as phytase costs are reduced or there are economical incentives to reduced manure phosphorus levels. Future research may also confirm that phytase enzymes increase the availability of nutrients other than just phosphorus and calcium, because positively charged molecules, such as lysine, can complex with the negatively charged phytate molecule. In a recent study, we showed improved AMEn (2%) and digestibility of a number of amino acids (1-2%) when phytase was added to broiler starter diets (Namkung and Leeson, 1999).

6.3.4 Lipases

Fats are utilized with varying efficiency in poultry diets, the major variables being bird age and degree of saturation. Young chicks (<21d) have difficulty digesting saturated fats, mainly due to limited production of lipase enzyme and secondly to inefficient recycling of bile salts which are an important emulsifying agent. Table 6.6 shows fat digestion, soap formation and diet AMEn when lipase enzyme is used in a broiler diet. Adding lipase caused a linear increase in fat digestion and diet AMEn. Concurrently, there was a reduction in fat present in the excreta as indigestible soaps. These soaps occur quite readily when minerals such as calcium bind with saturated fatty acids. At the present time, the lipase enzymes available seem to depress feed intake. The lipase used in our study was an extract from porcine pancreas, and may therefore be contaminated with hormones such as cholecystokinin, which is known to depress feed intake.

TABLE 6.6 Response of the young broiler chick to exogenous lipase			
Lipase enzyme (%)	Fat digestion	Excreta soap	Diet AMEn (kcal/kg)
	%		
0	76.6	18.0	2736
0.21	78.9	16.1	2793
0.43	84.0	15.0	2844
0.64	89.8	11.2	2800
0.85	90.1	11.5	2810
1.07	86.5	9.8	2899
Linear effect	**	**	**
Adapted from Marzooqui and Leeson (unpublished data)			

6.4   ANTIBIOTICS AND GROWTH PROMOTERS

Antibiotics represent a group of chemical compounds produced biologically by certain plants or microorganisms, usually a fungus, which possess bacteriostatic or bacteriocidal properties. Some antibiotics are particularly effective against gram negative bacteria. Other antibiotics are most effective against gram positive bacteria while some, termed broad spectrum antibiotics, are effective against a wide range of both gram positive and gram negative bacteria. Certain chemotherapeutic agents, such as arsenicals and nitrofurans have been found to possess bacteriostatic or bacteriocidal properties and yet, at the effective levels, are not toxic to chickens or other host animals.

Although most of these drugs are used to combat diseases in man and animals, it was discovered in 1949 that the presence of antibiotics at very low levels in the feed of chicks (approximately 5-10 ppm) usually produced improved growth when fed in diets containing adequate quantities of all known nutrients. The initial spectacular results of 20-25% improved growth rate were initially thought to be due to residues of vitamin B_{12} in the crude antibiotic extracts. In fact, the early products were marketed as sources of B_{12} because no regulations existed for routinely adding antibiotics to poultry feeds.

The growth promoting benefits of antibiotics in poultry appear to be involved with decreasing the negative effects of highly variable disease conditions, which have come to be recognized as the environmental disease level. Such disease may be in many different forms at various degrees of severity. It may be confined to the gastrointestinal tract or may be a systemic infection, localized or general. It is obvious, therefore, that no single mode of action could possibly explain the growth promoting effects of antibiotics under wide ranges of environmental conditions. Research on the subject to date strongly indicates that the amount and kind of antibiotic which produce beneficial results, and the magnitude of improvement over the basal unsupplemented controls, depends to a great extent upon the type and severity of the disease challenge. Thus, the modes of action of antibiotics may differ widely.

Antibiotics may produce one or more of the following effects:

1.   They may favor the growth of nutrient-synthesizing microbes or inhibit that of nutrient destroying microorganisms. Many research studies with diets having a borderline deficiency of a vitamin or an amino acid, suggest that a dietary antibiotic acts by sparing the requirement for the deficient nutrient. Thus, the antibiotic apparently was effective in reducing the destruction of the limiting nutrient or by causing increased synthesis or efficiency of utilization of the specific nutrient. However, it is difficult to see how this action of antibiotics can explain improvements in growth when diets contain adequate amounts of known nutrients.

2.   Antibiotics may inhibit the growth of organisms that produce excessive amounts of ammonia and other toxic nitrogenous waste products in the intestines. Visek (1978) has shown that antibiotics significantly decrease hydrolysis of 14°C urea in the intestinal tract of rats and reduce the production of urease by intestinal microorganisms. Free ammonia and other nitrogenous compounds, such as trimethylamine, may be sufficiently toxic to reduce growth.

3.   Antibiotics may improve availability or absorption of certain nutrients. Antibiotic supplementation of poultry diets improves the absorption of nutrients such as calcium, phosphorus and magnesium. Antibiotic feeding may also cause development of an appreciably thinner intestinal wall than is found in animals fed diets containing no antibiotic. It has been suggested that the thickened intestinal wall may result from irritation by toxins of *Clostridium* species or other toxin-producing microorganisms, that are eliminated from the intestinal tract upon feeding a low level of an antibiotic.

4.   Antibiotics may improve feed or water consumption, or both. It is impossible to determine definitely if increased feed consumption is a primary effect or is simply due to the better state of health brought about by an antibiotic. It is also possible that any feed intake effect is secondary to an effect upon water intake. Studies by many workers have shown a fairly constant relationship between feed intake and water intake in chickens. Because antibiotics are effective in changing the intestinal microflora, they may often affect water consumption by affecting water absorption and retention in the intestinal tract (for example, by prevention of diarrhea). The ceca of antibiotic-fed chickens usually are larger and filled with a greater quantity of moist excreta than are the ceca of chickens fed the same diet without an antibiotic.

5.   Antibiotics in many instances prevent or cure actual pathological disease, which occur either in the intestinal tract, or systemically. Low level feeding of an antibiotic such as zinc bacitracin, penicillin, a tetracycline or combinations of these will usually control minimal disease challenge, which may be encountered in poultry operations. This effect is mainly confined to the intestinal tract. Certain intestinal diseases such as ulcerative enteritis may require high levels of antibiotics to provide control. For such diseases the unabsorbed antibiotic, zinc bacitracin, is as effective as the absorbable antibiotics.

Once the invasion of the blood stream by pathogenic microorganisms has occurred, high levels of absorbable antibiotics are needed which are specifically effective against the microorganisms responsible for the disease. To promote high blood levels, the antibiotics should be administered along with a potentiator or in low calcium diets.

Some workers have concluded that the major site of action of the antibiotics is in the blood and internal tissues. However, it is evident, in view of the growth-promoting effects of the non-absorbable antibiotics, that the beneficial effects of antibiotics are also upon the microflora of the intestinal tract. Fevier *et al.* (1955) reported that antibiotics, copper sulfate and 3-nitro-4-hydroxyphenylarsonic acid all caused growth stimulation in swine (8-13%) and all inhibited *in vitro* deaminases of the intestinal microorganisms. They found less ammonia in the portal vein in the presence of the antibacterials and degradation of choline was also inhibited.

6.   Antibiotics may reduce the maintenance cost associated with turnover of the intestinal epithelium. Visek (1978) suggests that up to 20% of the nutrient requirements for maintenance are directed to epithelial resupply. Because antibiotics cause a thinning of the epithelium, there is up to a 40% reduction in this maintenance component. Visek (1978) concludes that for a 1,000 g broiler, gaining at 50 g/d, reduced maintenance needs for epithelial regeneration caused by feeding antibiotics, could account for the 4-5% improvement in growth often seen with these products.

The routine use of antibiotics in poultry feed is now coming under close scrutiny due to the concern about bacterial resistance. If any antimicrobial is used for a sufficiently long time period, some bacteria will attain resistance and so proliferate in the bird. For this reason feed-borne 'growth promoters' tend to become less efficacious over time, and shuttling of products is now a common industry practice. Shuttling involves use of different antibiotics every six months in a broiler operation. Concurrently or alternatively, different antibiotics may be used at different times for the same flock of birds.

While bacterial resistance is of ongoing concern to the poultry industry, transfer of the resistance factor from one microbe to another is becoming of greater concern in human medicine. Although the situation is far from clear, there is potential for antibiotic resistant bacteria in chickens to transfer resistance to similar (or other) strains naturally resident in humans. This issue was first raised in the UK, when in the 1960's an outbreak of Salmonellosis in dairy calves was transmitted to humans. In treating the calves, the salmonella became resistant to 8 antibiotics commonly available at that time, and treatment of humans with these same antibiotics was ineffective. This problem led to the Swann Committee Report, which was the starting point of general concern about antibiotic use in animal nutrition. Interestingly, the report suggested the banning of subtherapeutic compounds concurrently used in human medicine, although their use as therapeutics was permissible under veterinary supervision. These same concepts are cause for concern today, some 35 years after the report was issued.

There has never been any conclusive documentation of antibiotic use in poultry feeds causing specific bacterial resistance. Group 1 compounds are most efficacious long term, while chloramphenicols in Group 6 show fairly rapid bacterial resistance:

Group   1.   eg. Virginiamycin, Flavomycin, Zn bacitracin
          2.   eg. Lincomycin, Erythromycin
          3.   eg. Penicillin, Tetracycline
          4.   eg. Ampicillin
          5.   eg. Sulfonamide, Streptomycin, Neomysin
          6.   eg. Chloramphenicol

Arsenic containing compounds have long been used in human medicine as antibacterials, and in some countries arsenicals in the feed are still used for growth promotion in chickens. The use of arsenic and its compounds, in a wide variety of applications, dates back to antiquity. Hippocrates (460-377 BC) used realgar (arsenic sulfide) in the treatment of ulcers. However, its poisonous properties were not known until the Middle Ages when poisoning with arsenic became the standard method used, particularly by women, to dispose of their adversaries or of unwanted suitors. The early alchemists considered arsenic as the key to the Philosopher's Stone with which they might convert base metals into gold. In the early 1900's Ehrlich reported on his studies with hundreds of organic arsenic compounds, of which number 606 became the most important because of its effectiveness against syphillis. Antibiotics have now almost completely replaced the arsenicals in the treatment of this disease. Thus, arsenic has proved to be useful in many ways, but highly dangerous and poisonous when misused.

The growth stimulating effect of 3-nitro-4-hydroxyphenylarsonic acid was discovered by Morehouse and Mayfield (1946) in studies on the effects of various aryl arsonic acids on coccidiosis infection in chickens. Since then, other arsonic acid derivatives, notably para-amino-phenylarsonic acid (arsanilic acid) and its sodium salt (sodium arsanilate) have been shown to possess growth stimulating properties.

Feeding arsenicals will result in accumulation of some arsenic in the tissues and eggs of birds. Using 0.01% arsanilic acid usually results in liver and egg arsenic levels approaching 10% of the upper limits established as toxic for humans. However, arsenicals may be toxic to birds if used improperly. Abbot et al. (1954) found that arsanilic acid was not toxic at 500 mg per kg of diet but depressed growth slightly at 1,000 mg per kg. At the level of 1,500 mg per kg, symptoms appeared which were similar to those observed in thiamin deficiency. At levels of 2,000 mg per kg of diet and above, excessive mortality occurred. Sweet, et al. (1954) observed that arsanilic acid as well as sulfaquinoxaline and oxytetracycline alone, or in combination, caused delayed blood clotting time in chicks which was restored by addition to the diet of alfalfa or menadione. When 0.1% arsanilic acid was inadvertently fed to turkey breeders for a period of three weeks, egg production and hatchability were significantly reduced, with no apparent effect on fertility. Two weeks after the level had been restored to 0.01% of arsanilic acid, egg production and hatchability returned to normal. The arsanilic acid at this level had no detrimental or beneficial effects upon egg production, hatchability or fertility. Arsenic compounds seem to offer some protection against toxicity of selenium.

6.5 ANTIFUNGALS, MOLD INHIBITORS AND TOXIN BINDERS

During their normal metabolism, a number of molds and fungi produce toxins that are either retained in their cells, or excreted on the growing medium. Such toxins are generally referred to as mycotoxins, and these can be very hazardous to chickens. Unfortunately mycotoxins are now virtually ubiquitous in poultry diets, and with ever decreasing levels of testing sensitivity, they are isolated as common contaminants of most grains and some vegetable protein ingredients. We still do not know the causes of high levels of mold growth occurring in pre-harvest grains. Certainly such aerobic molds are more prevalent in hot humid conditions, and insect damage to the standing crop seems to provide a route of entry for the mold. Unfortunately, visual inspection of harvested grains can be misleading in regard to mycotoxin content. Likewise, merely because grains appear moldy, does not mean to say that they are contaminated with harmful toxins. In storage, the major factors affecting mold growth are again, temperature and humidity. The higher the temperature, the greater the chance for mold growth. However, such mold growth rarely occurs in grains containing less that 14-15% moisture. Unfortunately, many grain silos are not waterproof, or grains are not aerated, such that pockets of moisture cause microclimates ideal for mold growth. The molds of greatest concern are *Aspergillus* species which produce aflatoxin and *Fusarium* species which can produce a range of toxins including the tricothecenes.

Once mycotoxins are formed, they are virtually indestructible unless the feed or ingredient is subject to extreme processing conditions. For example, corn contaminated with aflatoxin can be partially detoxified by treating under pressure with hot, moist ammonia. Feed additives can however, be used to prevent subsequent mold growth (antifungals) or to bind existing mycotoxins.

6.5.1 Mold inhibitors

There is little doubt that the best control over mold growth in stored grains or mixed feeds is achieved by limiting the moisture available to the microbes. Molds and fungi will not grow on a medium that contains much less than 15% moisture. At 13% moisture, it is unusual to find any subsequent mold growth. Unfortunately, it is very difficult to ensure that all pockets of feed and grain are adequately dry. With the large tonnage of grain stored at feed mills, pockets of moisture develop in warm conditions, especially where cool night time temperatures cause condensation inside silos. Likewise in manufactured feed, small pockets of moisture inside a storage tank or transfer system can provide enough water to initiate mold growth. These relatively small pockets of mold growth are problematic, because any resultant mycotoxins are detrimental to the bird at levels of ppm (tricothecenes) or even ppb (aflatoxin).

In situations where moisture control in grain or mixed feed is logistically difficult, then the development of mold growth can be prevented or delayed by including mold inhibitors in the feed. Many inhibitors are composed of organic acids, such as propionic or acetic. Adding these acids at up to 0.25% of the diet, simply lowers diet pH and prevents mold growth. Most acids are efficacious and their effect remains as long as the acid is not volatilized. Variable results can sometimes be seen with mold inhibitors, and this may relate to inherent buffering capacity of various ingredients. While corn and soy are neutral or slightly acidic (pH 6.2-7.0), fish meal can be very acidic at around pH 5.3. Perhaps the major variable is mineral content, because limestone and phosphates will act as natural buffers, with formation of calcium proprionate which has greatly reduced antifungal properties. Diets for laying hens that contain high levels of limestone would therefore need more organic acid as an antifungal, than would a low calcium broiler grower diet. Organic acids are very corrosive to metallic poultry equipment. In some countries gentian violet is used as an antifungal and this has the added advantage of limited bacteriocidal activity.

6.5.2   Toxin adsorbants

While antifungals and organic acids can help control subsequent mold growth in feed, they have no effect on any mycotoxins already present. As previously suggested, it is virtually impossible to inactivate these complex molecules, although there is some potential for binding them to inert carriers, such that they pass unchanged through the digestive tract. Perhaps the most well known adsorbent is activated charcoal, which has been used for centuries as a cure for poisoning in humans. Activated charcoal at 200 g/tonne has been reported to be moderately effective in alleviating the toxic effects of up to 500 ppb aflatoxin. Of more interest today are the various aluminosilicates and clay loam products whose chemical structure allow the capture of aflatoxin and perhaps other mycotoxins. Such products have been used as anticaking agents and pellet binders, but are now finding application as mycotoxin adsorbants. Adding up to 0.5 – 1.2% aluminosilicate/clay products has been shown to greatly reduce the toxicity of up to 3 ppm aflatoxin and 8-10 ppm T2 tricothecene toxin. Variability in the efficacy of these inorganic adsorbants may relate to differences in physical and chemical structures, since efficacy depends entirely on physical sequestering of the toxin molecule. Studies have shown that clays with identical chemical composition and mined just 1 km apart, have vastly different binding characteristics.

6.6   ANTICOCCIDIALS

Anticoccidials are used to prevent the parasitic disease of poultry known as coccidiosis. Coccidial oocysts cycle and spread through infected excreta, and so the need for anticoccidial compounds is most important in litter reared birds. Anticoccidials impair oocyst growth or reproduction in some way, although their mode of action may have some influence in the bird.

Sulfur compounds were one of the first products used to treat or prevent the disease. Most sulfur anticoccidials prevented the oocyst from metabolizing B vitamins, regardless of their supply in the digesta. They had little effect on the bird's B vitamin status, but were toxic at 1-2x normal inclusion. Sulfaquinoxaline induced a 5-10x increase in the bird's vitamin K requirement. Chemical anticoccidials were introduced in the 1970's and were very efficacious for a number of years. Amprolium® was a very widely used product where mode of action was to induce a specific deficiency of thiamin in the oocyst. In most instances, thiamin deficiency will not occur in birds, although cases have been reported of combinations of Amprolium® and poorly processed fish meal that is high in thiaminase enzyme, leading to thiamin deficiency in young birds. Amprolium® is still used today in juvenile breeders, since it allows some degree of oocyst immunity to develop.

Nicarbazin® was another very successful chemical anticoccidial that has regained popularity in recent years in diets for very young birds. Nicarbazin seems to accentuate the undesirable effects of extreme heat stress, and if inadvertently added to layer or breeder diets at normal anticoccidial levels, can cause loss in reproductive performance. Nicarbazin fed to brown egg birds turns their eggshells white within 48 hrs although this is completely reversible when the product is withdrawn from the feed. Even low levels of Nicarbazin can cause some loss in shell color and mottling of egg yolks.

The most successful and efficacious group of anticoccidals have been ionophore compounds. As their name implies, these compounds influence transmembrane movement of mono- and/or divalent cations. Oocysts absorb greater quantities of ions such as Na^+ or K^+, and in order to maintain osmotic balance concurrently increase their uptake of water. This rapid influx of water ruptures the cell wall of the single cell oocyst. Ionophores have little effect on ion balance of poultry and, in general, mineral nutrition is unaffected. Monensin has perhaps been one of the most successful ionophore anticoccidials whose primary mode of action is via transmembrane flow of sodium.

Ionophores can have an adverse effect when used in conjunction with low protein (methionine) diets. When low protein diets, or feed restriction are employed for birds less than 21d of age, alternatives to ionophores should be considered in an attempt to alleviate potential growth depression, loss of uniformity, and/or poor feathering. However, with normal diet protein levels, the ionophores do not have a measurable effect on TSAA requirement. Ionophores and monensin in particular do impart some growth depression in young birds, although this seems to be completely overcome with compensatory growth during the withdrawal or finisher period. For monensin, a 5-7d withdrawal is optimum for compensatory gain, assuming that no major coccidiosis challenge will occur during this time.

There has also been some controversy surrounding the relationship between wet litter and certain ionophore compounds. Lasalocid, in particular, has been associated with wet litter and, as such, recommendations are often given for reducing diet sodium levels when this anticoccidial is used. Under such conditions, adjustment of chloride levels is often ignored, and as a consequence performance is sub-optimal. The whole area of ionophores and water intake has not been fully resolved other than the fact that birds fed monensin do seem to produce drier manure. Ionophores can be toxic to non-target animals, with the horse and dog being most susceptible. In these animals, there is a change in ion balance of heart tissue, and resultant arrythmia can lead to sudden death. Older turkeys, if they have not previously received an ionophore, are also susceptible to ionophore toxicity.

6.7   WORMING COMPOUNDS

Any bird that is grown in a non-cage environment is likely to be exposed to parasitic worms. In many instances, such a challenge can be prevented or minimized with the use of antihelminthic agents. Products based on piperazine and hygromycin have been used most commonly over the last 15-20 years. Piperazine used in diets for laying birds has been shown to result in discoloration of the yolk. When administered at 28d intervals, one report indicated about a 4% incidence of discolored yolks, which appeared as irregular areas of olive to brownish discoloration. Such yolk discoloration is most pronounced in summer months especially after prolonged storage at regular egg cooler temperatures. The mottling of yolks seen with another commercial product has been compared to the mottling seen with calcium deficient birds, suggesting a similar mode of action. However, we are unaware of any published reports relating worming compounds to calcium deficiency and problems with shell quality.

6.8 ANTIOXIDANTS

Antioxidants are added to feed in order to prevent the oxidation of lipids and lipid soluble nutrients such as vitamins A, D and E and carotenoids. Fats that oxidize in the feed, or the bird's body, can lead to encephalomalacia and exudative diathesis, and there is growing evidence that resultant free radicals compromise the immune system. Oxidative rancidity of a fat or oil initiates at the C-H bond adjacent to the C=C bond. The greater the degree of unsaturation therefore, the greater the susceptibility to oxidation. These reactions are autocatalytic, and result in the formation of peroxides, free radicals and perhaps polymers which are indigestible to the bird (Figure 6.2).

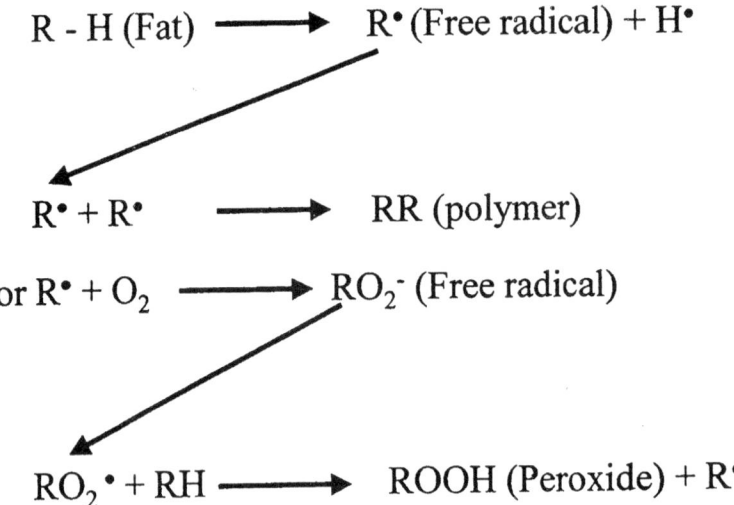

$$R - H \text{ (Fat)} \longrightarrow R^{\bullet} \text{ (Free radical)} + H^{\bullet}$$

$$R^{\bullet} + R^{\bullet} \longrightarrow RR \text{ (polymer)}$$

$$\text{or } R^{\bullet} + O_2 \longrightarrow RO_2^{-} \text{ (Free radical)}$$

$$RO_2^{\bullet} + RH \longrightarrow ROOH \text{ (Peroxide)} + R^{\bullet}$$

Figure 6.2 Schematic of Fat Oxidation.

The reaction is autocatalytic because of the continued regeneration of the very reactive $R^{\bullet}$ free radical. An antioxidant will essentially sacrifice itself, and attach to free radicals and restabilize the fat. The antioxidant accepts the unpaired electron within its molecule, yet this reduced configuration is stable, and so the reaction is stopped. Most antioxidants are quinones some with an H-N grouping, which are stable when reduced. The formula for ethoxyquin, a common feed antioxidant, is shown in Figure 6.3.

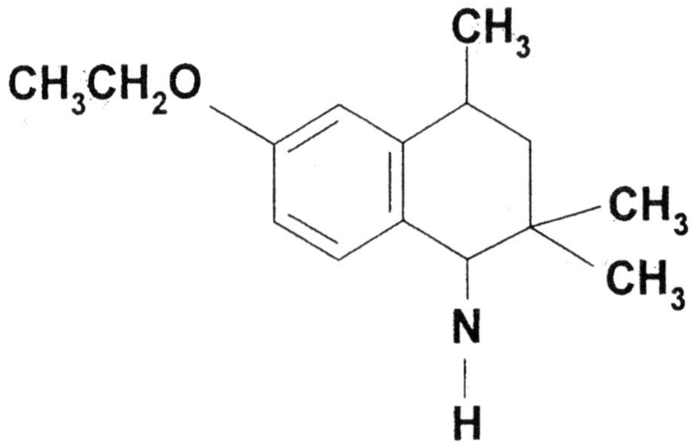

Figure 6.3 Composition of ethoxyquin.

Oxidation occurs most frequently and most quickly with multiple points of unsaturation and so, for example, fish oils are much more prone to oxidation than is tallow. In human foods, oils are routinely hydrogenated so as to nullify the unsaturated bonds making the fat less prone to rancidity, especially during repeated heating.

The rancid taste and smell of oxidized fat is due to formation of breakdown products such as aldehydes, ketones and hydroxy acids which have characteristic organoleptic properties. Antioxidants can prevent oxidation occurring, or at least slow down the process. However once started, the process of oxidation is difficult to stop and so antioxidants must be added to ingredients or diets as early in the manufacturing process as is possible. For fats, oils and animal proteins, addition should be at point of manufacture, rather than upon delivery at the feed mill. Fats for example, may require 400-500 mg antioxidant/kg for protection, while vitamin premixes more commonly contain 100-150 mg/kg. Addition of an antioxidant should therefore be based on anticipated oxidative stress, time of storage and environmental temperature.

6.9 CAROTENOIDS

Pigments are routinely added to the diets in order to provide poultry products with an esthetically pleasing color for the consumer. Interestingly, the acceptable color can vary dramatically in different geographical locations and so nutritionists are faced with the challenge of either augmenting or tempering the inclusion of products such as xanthophylls in poultry diets. These pigments serve no nutritional role for poultry or humans. Most pigments are derivatives of β-carotene that itself has no pigmenting value. Carotenoids of interest in poultry nutrition include cryptoxanthin, zeaxanthin, lutein, canthaxanthian and β-apo-8-carotenoic acid. The first three of these products are usually referred to as xanthophylls.

Alfalfa, clover and pasture grasses contain, in addition to the chlorophyll which gives them the green color, a number of yellow and red pigments which are referred to collectively as xanthophylls. When the chlorophyll is removed or destroyed, as for example when maple leaves are exposed to frost in autumn, the yellow and red xanthophylls, no longer masked by the green color of the chlorophyll, change the leaves from the deep green of summer to the reds and yellows of autumn.

Yellow pigments from corn, forage crops and other synthetic sources are deposited in the fat and skin of broilers and in the yolks of eggs. If free-range birds are maintained on green pastures, they consume such a large supply of xanthophylls from the grasses and clovers that the skin, shanks and beaks of the broilers are a bright orange color while yolks of layers are orange-red. These colors are perceived by consumers to associate with 'natural' and 'freshness' of the various products. These same colors can be copied by using synthetic dietary pigments. The xanthophyll content of some common ingredients is shown in Table 6.7. Marigold petals are the most concentrated source of xanthophylls and are used routinely in some countries. Paprika and other peppers are also regaining some popularity as dietary pigments.

TABLE 6.7 Xanthophyll content of selected ingredients	
Ingredient	**Xanthophyll (mg/kg)**
Marigold petal meal (*Tagetes erecta*)	6,000-10,000
Algae (*Cholella pyrenoidosa*)	4,000
Seaweed (*Fucus serratus*)	920
Seaweed (*Fucus vesiculosus*)	350
Dried kao haole meal - Hawaii (called ipil-ipil in Philippines) (*Leucaena leucocephalaLam de Wit*)	660
Dehydrated clover meal	490
Red peppers	440
Dehydrated alfalfa leaf meal (20% protein)	400-550
Dehydrated alfalfa meal (17% protein)	185-350
Corn gluten meal (41% protein)	90-180
Corn gluten meal (60% protein)	330
Paprika	275
Acidulated soybean soapstock	168-260
Dried chili peppers	185
Dried carrots	65
Yellow corn	20-25

The various xanthophylls differ in their ability to impart color, and to some extent, this situation is a reflection of the level of incorporation. About 10% of a dietary zeaxanthin is absorbed and deposited in the body, while for some of the synthetic products such as β-apo-8-carotenoic acid ester, incorporation rate may be as high as 30-40%. Lutein, which is found in grasses, tends to impart a yellow color in poultry, while zeaxanthin found in corn, produces an orange-red color. In the laying hen, the xanthophylls tend to accumulate in the ovary. Natural xanthophylls are unstable and effective levels will decline over time, due to oxidation during storage. Such oxidation can be reduced by adding antioxidants to the feed.

Yolk color and skin pigmentation are commonly measured on the Roche Scale, of 1-15, with the highest number corresponding to the color of an orange. A wheat-based diet without any added pigments will likely produce eggs with a Roche color of 3-4. With 25% corn, the color will be around 6-7 while at 70% corn a value of 9-10 is achievable. Adding 2.5% dehydrated alfalfa meal to any diet will increase Roche color by 1-2. Figure 6.4 shows the Roche color score obtained by feeding various levels of xanthophylls and red-orange pigments such as canthaxanthin.

There is little response in yolk color with xanthophyll levels much in excess of 30-35 mg/kg diet, at which level a color of around 9-10 is achieved. In order to attain higher color scores, it is necessary to add products such as canthaxanthin. In fact, a mixture of the two carotenoids is commonly used, since alone, the products give unacceptable color tones. The xanthophylls produce a simple yellow color and alone the canthaxanthins an unacceptable orange-red. A mixture of the two, usually in at least a 4:1 (xanthophyll:canthaxanthin) mix provides color tones acceptable in many markets.

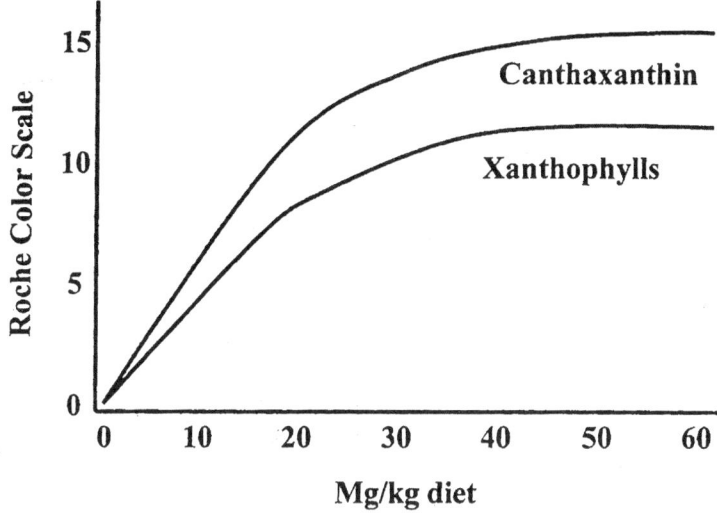

Figure 6.4 Effect of dietary carotenoids on egg yolk color score.

Pigments are destroyed by oxidation, and so addition of antioxidants such as ethoxyquin to feed, and general feed management used for fat protection also apply to preservation of pigments. Coccidiosis, malabsorption and certain mycotoxins will all reduce pigment absorption. Pigmentation in the young meat bird is directly proportional to pigments fed throughout growth. For the laying hen however, yolk color is a consequence of pigments consumed in the layer feed and also the transfer of pigments accumulated in the skin and shanks when the bird was immature. This transfer of pigments to the ovary occurs regardless of diet pigments, and is responsible for the "bleaching" effect on the shanks and beak of yellow skinned birds over time. Because many of the naturally carotenoid-rich ingredients are low in energy, it is difficult to achieve high levels of pigmentation of meat birds without using synthetic sources. Canthaxanthin, astaxanthin and β-apo-8-carotenoic acid (where allowable in poultry diets) can be used to impart the spectrum from yellow to orange/red coloration in either skin or egg yolk.

6.10   PROBIOTICS, YEASTS AND COMPETITIVE EXCLUSION PRODUCTS

Probiotics, yeasts and the more recently introduced competitive exclusion products are aimed at promoting the growth of beneficial gut microbes or in some way rendering others less pathogenic. Unlike antibiotics, the probiotics and yeast are living organisms, and their mode of action relies on replication and survival in the gastro-intestinal tract. Probiotics can be classified into two major types, namely viable microbial cultures and microbial fermentation products. Most research has centered on *Lactobacilli* species, *Bacillus subtilis* and some *Streptococcus* species. Similar to the situation with antibiotics, the mode of action is still unclear although the following have been suggested: (a) beneficial change in gut flora with reduction in the population of *E. Coli*; (b) lactate production with subsequent change in intestinal pH; (c) production of antibiotic-type substances; (d) reduction of toxin release (suppression of *E. Coli*). With these potential diverse routes of activity, it is perhaps not too surprising that research results are inconsistent. In most instances, the feeding of live cultures modifies the gut microflora of birds usually with increases of *Lactobacilli* at the expense of coliforms. A healthy animal has a preponderance of lactic acid producing bacteria, and so it is only under situations of stress, when coliforms often increase in numbers, that probiotics will be of measurable benefit. In this context, there is interest in the use of live cultures administered orally to day-old chickens as a means of preventing harmful bacteria such as salmonella from predominating in the gut.

With potential instability of *Lactobacillus* species in most textured feeds, there has been recent interest in probiotics based on *Bacillus subtilis* species, because they possess viable spores that have greater stability than do most lactic acid producing cultures. Regardless of somewhat inconclusive results, it appears that probiotic use is increasing, and that the animal industry looks to such products as substitutes for conventional antibiotics.

Yeasts, or single-celled fungi, have been used in animal feed and the human food industry for many years. Brewer's yeast was a common feed ingredient in diets for monogastric animals prior to the identification of all the B vitamins. Today some nutritionists still incorporate these inactivated microbes as a source of so-called unidentified growth factor. More recently there has been an interest in the use of live yeast cultures. Most often these cultures contain the yeast themselves and the medium upon which they have been grown. Such yeast cultures are usually derived from *Saccharomyces* species, in particular, *Saccharomyces cerevisiae*. As with other probiotics, their mode of action in enhancing animal performance is not well understood. Yeasts may beneficially alter the inherent gut microflora, possibly through controlling pH. The presence of living yeast cells may also act as a reservoir for free oxygen, which could enhance growth of other anaerobes. At the present time there does not seem to be any move to manipulate yeast for specific purposes related to animal nutrition. To some extent, this relates to scant knowledge on their mode of action. Should more facts be uncovered in this area, so-called designer yeast may be considered.

Lactobacillus species are one of the most important probiotic strains. These bacteria produce large amounts of lactic acid from monosaccharides and disaccharide substrates, and the resultant lower pH is fatal to many other bacteria. The chicken's intestine normally contains a complement of *Lactobacilli*, starting in the crop region. However, under conditions of stress or major bacterial challenge, the *Lactobacilli* population will decline. To be effective the probiotics must remain viable over a wide range of pH, and ideally will initially colonize the crop. As feed passes through the crop, then resident *Lactobacilli* can seed the digesta. A review of probiotics in poultry nutrition is given by Jernigan and Miles (1985).

A major limitation in using yeasts and probiotics such as *Lactobacillus* species, is that they are destroyed by the heat processing as occurs during pelleting. An alternative approach is to provide cell components that effectively compete with pathogens for sites of attachment in the intestine. Many bacteria use fimbrae to attach to the chicken's intestinal wall. Mannanoligosaccharide (MOS) sugars derived from yeast cell walls, provide the bacteria with an alternative binding site. The MOS-bacteria complex can then pass undigested through the intestine (Parks *et al*, 2000).

6.11   ODOR AND FLY CONTROL

Intensive poultry production systems result in a range of air pollutants, some of which can cause complaints from neighbors because of odor. Ammonia production is common to all poultry facilities, while other noxious gases can arise from liquid manure systems. Ammonia is problematic to both birds and humans and chronic exposure to levels as low as 10-15 ppm can cause disruption of moist epithelial tissues. Most of this ammonia arises as a consequence of bacterial degradation of uric acid in the excreta. There are a number of feed additives claiming to bind ammonia and/or suppress bacterial enzyme systems hat degrade uric acid and other nitrogenous compounds. Products such as Deodorase® that contain sarsaponin, an extract from the Yucca plant seems to reduce ammonia release from manure. When added to the diet at just 100-150g/tonne, there are reports of 20-30% reduction in atmospheric ammonia within confinement houses.

In some countries, systemic larvacides are registered, for use in the control of flies, especially in laying hen facilities. Early studies utilized products containing methoprene, and while initially effective in controlling fly emergence, resistance quickly developed. Diflubenzuron was another insect growth regulator used as a feed additive, but again resistance developed and the product also accumulated in the birds fat depots. Most research has centered on cyramizine, which is a metabolite of another insect growth regulator. Commonly called Larvadex® the compound has been shown to dramatically reduce fly populations in layer facilities, when fed at just 1-2 ppm. Cyramizine does not accumulate in appreciable quantities in the bird's fat depots, resistance is slow to develop and there is little effect on bird performance even at 1000 ppm.

6.12   TOLERANCES, TOXICITY AND FEED WITHDRAWAL OF ADDITIVES

Many feed additives are toxic if used at higher than recommended inclusion rates, and may be harmful to non-target species. For example, some additives designed for chicken diets are toxic to turkeys. In chickens, toxicity can manifest itself as slightly reduced growth rate or egg production with no change in mortality or morbidity patterns. Toxicity of additives may therefore be difficult to detect. Some additives are incompatible with others and care should be taken in following the manufacturer's directions not only as far as the level of inclusion in the feed is concerned, but also instructions as to when an additive can be fed or if any interactions occur with other compounds. There are usually specific government regulations concerning the use of drugs in feed, and withdrawal periods required or recommended prior to the marketing of poultry products.

SELECTED REFERENCES

Abbot, O.J., H.R. Bird and W.W. Cravens, 1954. Effects of dietary arsanilic acid on chicks. Poultry Sci. 33:1245.

Annison, G. and M. Choct, 1993. Enzymes in poultry diets in: Enzymes in Animal Nutrition. Proc 1st Symp. Switzerland Oct. 13-16, 1993. pp 61-68.

Bedford, M.R., 1996. The effect of enzymes on digestion. J. Appl. Poultry Res. 5:370-378.

Choct, M. and G. Annison, 1990. Anti-nutritive activity of wheat pentosans in broiler diets. British Poultry Science 31:811-821.

Fevier, R., A. Francois, M. Michel, R. Pero and E. Salmon-Legagneur, 1955. Antibiotics and growth. Compt. Rend. Acad. Agric., France 41:698.

Jernigan, M.A. and R.D. Miles, 1985. Probiotics in poultry nutrition – A review. Wld. Poultry Sci. J. 41:99-107.

Kare, M.R., 1965. Special Senses in: Avian Physiology, 2nd Ed., P.D. Sturkie, Ed. Compstock Publ. Associates, Ithaca, New York.

Leeson, S. and J. Proulx, 1994. Enzymes and barley metabolizable energy. J. Appl. Poultry Res. 3:66-68.

Morehouse, N.F. and O.J. Mayfield, 1946. The effect of some aryl arsonic acids on experimental coccidiosis infection in chickens. J. Parasitol. 32:20.

Namkung, H. and S. Leeson, 1999. Effect of phytase enzyme on dietary AMEn and ileal digestibility of nitrogen and amino acids in broiler chicks. Poultry Sci. 78:1317-1320.

Pack, M. and M. Bedford, 1997. Feed enzymes for corn-soybean broiler diets. Wld. Poultry 13, No. 9, pp. 87-93.

Parks, C.W., J.L. Grimes, P.R. Ferket and A.S. Fairchild, 2000. The case for mannano-ligosaccharides in poultry diets. An alternate to growth promotant antibiotics. in: Biotechnology in the Feed Industry Ed. Lyons and Jacques. Publ. Alltech Inc., KY.

Sweet, G.B., G.L. Romoser and G.F. Combs, 1954. Further observations on the effect of sulfaquinoxaline, p-aminophenylarsonic acid and oxytetracycline on blood clotting time of chicks. Poultry Sci. 33:430.

Visek, W.J., 1978. The mode of growth promotion by antibiotics. J. Anim. Sci. 46:1447-1469.

Factors Affecting Nutrient Needs

T he nutrient requirements of poultry have been well established due, not only to the rapid growth of the industry in the past five decades, but also due to the fact that the chick is a very good experimental animal for basic nutritional studies. The chick requires 13 vitamins, 13 to 16 inorganic elements, 13 amino acids and one essential fatty acid. Countless studies during the past 50 years have resulted in the determination of precise requirement values for most nutrients, including metabolizable energy.

The classical procedure for determining nutritional requirements for a specific nutrient was to feed graded levels of the nutrient in question in a purified diet, lacking in the nutrient under study. The requirement determined would then be accepted as the minimum amount of the nutrient required to produce the best weight gain, feed efficiency etc. and the lack of any signs of a nutritional deficiency. For most nutrients, such a requirement has been firmly established and is reproducible under standard conditions of environment and diet composition. The requirements determined with purified diets under ideal environmental conditions are referred to as minimum requirement values. In all commercial situations and in many experimental situations these minimum nutrient levels are inadequate for optimal bird performance. This dichotomy is due to environmental and disease challenge and the fact that nutrients in conventional ingredients are not digested and absorbed at 100% efficiency, as often occurs in simple purified diets. The factors that can influence the bird's need for nutrients are:

1. Genetic make-up of the bird,

2. Energy content of the diet (a major factor influencing feed intake),

3. Environment temperature (another factor influencing feed intake as well as acid-base balance),

4. Type of housing (cage, wire or litter floor),

5. Nutrient availability from particular feedstuffs,

6. Influence of intestinal pH and transit flow on the destruction or sequestering of dietary nutrients,

7. Presence of dietary oxidizing fats, especially in the presence of catalyzing minerals and lack of antioxidants,

8. Influence of intestinal parasites,

9. Beneficial or detrimental intestinal bacteria,

10. Fungal toxins in feedstuffs (eg. Aflatoxins and other mycotoxins),

11. Nutrients made unavailable to the bird through colloids in ingredients, or adverse interactions with other nutrients in the intestinal tract.

12. Nutrient destruction in feed or drinking water by nitrites, sulfites or other chemicals,

13. Destruction of nutrients by ultraviolet light,

14. Positive or negative effects of enzymes found in ingredients,

15. Decreased absorption due to damage to absorptive cells, lack of digestible fat, or bile,

16. Competition for absorption due to nutrient imbalances or lack of factors needed for active nutrient absorption,

17. Influences of intestinal bacteria in nutrient biosynthesis,

18. Presence of antimetabolites in certain feedstuffs,

19. Nutrient interrelationships (eg. lysine:arginine)

20. Influence of hormones in the bird, and from animal byproduct ingredients,

21. Effect of disease and environmental stress factors,

22. Restricted feeding – imposed either as a management tool or an effect due to limitations of feeder space.

Considering all of the factors that can influence nutrient requirements, it is readily apparent that minimum nutrient requirements, as established with purified diets under ideal environmental conditions, can fall short of meeting the requirements of a bird in a different environment and exposed to variable feed ingredients and stress factors. Hence, the nutrient requirements established in a temperate zone are usually not suitable for birds reared in a tropical environment.

While most of the interrelationships listed above have been discussed at some length in previous chapters, it is appropriate to summarize briefly some of the more important factors known to influence nutrient requirements. Among the more important topics are interrelationships between: 1) protein and energy; 2) nutrition and disease; 3) various types of stress; 4) factors influencing the quality of meat and eggs.

7.1 WELL KNOWN INTERRELATIONSHIPS

A number of nutrient interrelationships are well known and the manner in which they affect requirements has been relatively well established. These include: a) energy:protein ratio; b) interaction of calcium, phosphorus and vitamin D_3; c) niacin, tryptophan relationship; d) choline, methionine, folic acid and vitamin B_{12} relationship in methyl group metabolism and transmethylation reactions; e) involvement of vitamin E, selenium and cystine in the prevention of exudative diathesis and muscular dystrophy in chicks; f) chelation effects of certain amino acids and minerals in the transport of specific nutrients; g) numerous trace mineral interrelationships such as copper and zinc, zinc and cadmium, copper and molybdenum, and selenium and arsenic; h) amino acid interrelationships such as lysine:arginine, leucine, isoleucine and valine and specific amino acid imbalances and antagonisms. Discussions of the above interrelationships have been covered in previous chapters.

7.2 NUTRITION AND GENETICS

The physiological and metabolic makeup of an animal's body is controlled by genetic material passed on by its parents. All animals have specific enzyme systems whose function is to regulate the many chemical reactions taking place in the body. Of interest is the fact that all higher animals have metabolic activities that are relatively uniform among and between species. Thus, the nutrients that must be supplied in feed for the chicken, through to man, are essentially the same. While genetic variations in nutrient requirements are noted between animals species, these are more of a quantitative rather than a qualitative nature. Although man, monkeys, guinea pigs, certain birds and fish require dietary vitamin C, most other animals do not. This is an unusual example of variation between species that is not generally found within species.

Most nutritionists accept the fact that our major poultry species differ in nutrient requirements. For example, we differentiate specifications for broilers versus laying hens. However, if we look more closely at these values, surprisingly small differences are seen relative to the phenotypic strain differences and relative weight of these birds at maturity. Even for avian specie as phenotypically diverse as quail and turkeys we see comparable values for amino acids, minerals and vitamins. Based on this simple comparison, it is questionable if meaningful differences in nutrient requirements exist within commercially available strains of Leghorns or broilers.

The body and egg composition of most poultry species are quite similar, and so it is perhaps logical not to expect any major species differences in nutrient needs. For example, the amino acid profile of most muscles in the chicken are quite similar and, in fact, across species there is little difference in the constituents of poultry muscles. It is also important to realize that most commercial species of poultry have been selected using similar criteria. For example, with broilers we have been primarily interested in weight gain, feed efficiency, mortality for obvious reasons, and more recently, carcass composition. For commercial layers, the selection emphasis has been on egg size, eggshell quality, egg numbers and feed intake, and more recently on egg components related to yield for processing. It is this change in emphasis of selection related to both meat and egg processing that fuels the question of these 'new birds' having different nutrient requirements. Certainly it is very difficult to identify such 'new strains' as being different on the basis of any biochemical profiling or even DNA fingerprinting. The DNA profiles of most types of bird are remarkably similar and, for example, within all the strains of commercial Leghorn, it is difficult to isolate a specific strain banding. The DNA fingerprint of birds as phenotypically different as a Leghorn and a Barred Rock hen are virtually indistinguishable, suggesting a common basis for genetic background and diversity.

However, this is not to say that genetic diversity does not exist for nutrient requirements, and in fact, such variance is well documented (Nesheim, 1975; Sorensen, 1985; Pym, 1990). Within these extensive reviews is convincing evidence for meaningful variance in maintenance energy requirement, and the need for many amino acids and trace minerals. However, as previously discussed, because there is a common (economically driven) theme for selection of most commercial specie types, we are not likely to see such variance expressed. Most commercial selection programs are obviously going to ignore birds that are inefficient in any way, when such an inefficiency can occur through a need for more nutrients.

The fact that there is genetic variance related to the need for many nutrients does, however, create the interesting opportunity of developing birds that can survive and perform well on lower planes of nutrition. Falconer (1977) selected mice for growth rate on a regular diet or on this diet either restricted in quantity or diluted by 50%. Two lines were developed from this and the most interesting results arose when diets were switched for the two groups. Mice selected for growth rate on the restricted diet did as well as the control mice when fed the control diet. However, mice selected on the control diet did not grow well when fed the diluted or restricted diets. Falconer (1977) concluded that some, but not all genes, were common to the two strains of mice. For example, type A genes would affect growth on a good diet, type B genes influenced growth on a poor diet, whereas type C genes were influential in either environment. This type of study clearly shows the potential for genetic selection, and subsequent success, under conditions of differing nutrient intake. Currently, however, this concept is of academic interest only, because virtually all commercial strains are selected under conditions of ideal or adequate nutrition.

There have been relatively few reports of genetic-nutrition interactions in chickens. If such differences exist, it is assumed that birds may vary with respect to:

a. ability to metabolize energy or digest other nutrients,

b. maintenance nutrient requirements,

c. differential deposition of nutrients per unit of egg mass,

d. differential utilization of nutrients for growth,

e. response to selected metabolites or antinutrients.

There are few indications of differences within bird strains with respect to ability to metabolize energy. Spratt and Leeson (1987) indicated that broiler breeders were less able to metabolize diet energy relative to Leghorn strain birds. However, this difference was only some 2.3%, and so when comparing any such effects with light vs. heavy strains of laying hen they are expected to be quite minimal. There have been no reports of differential strain effect on maintenance energy requirement. However, observations of Morrison and Leeson (1978) and Leeson and Morrison (1978) suggest that differences in feed efficiency observed with various groups of Leghorns may relate to differences in maintenance energy requirement. Birds classified as efficient or inefficient produced a comparable egg mass, and were of similar body weight and/or weight gain characteristics. However, they did show markedly different feed efficiency, and this in part was related to a major difference in maintenance energy requirement (Morrison and Leeson, 1978). In subsequent studies Leeson and Morrison (1978) indicated major differences in feather cover of such efficient and inefficient strains of bird. Regression analysis of this data suggested that feed efficiency deteriorated by around 0.04 for each 1 g loss in feather cover. Depending upon environmental conditions, such differences may have an effect on feed efficiency.

If different strains of bird deposit different amounts of any nutrient into the egg (per unit of egg mass) then presumably such birds will have different nutrient requirements. Leeson *et al.* (1979a,b) showed convincing evidence of differential deposition of vitamins into the egg by Leghorn and Rhode Island Red breeders. In these studies pure strains of White Leghorn and Rhode Island Red birds were fed corn-soy diets devoid of selected synthetic vitamins. The brown egg Rhode Island Red seems to respond more quickly and more severely to diets devoid of selected synthetic vitamins.

Different strains of layers certainly show differential responses to certain pathogens, although there is less specific data related to the response of such strains to various antimetabolites and/or pharmaceuticals. Perhaps the most interesting situation is the fishy taint seen in brown eggs when these birds are fed rapeseed/canola that contain appreciable quantities of glucosinolates and sinapine. The problem does not occur with White Leghorns, and seems to relate to the presence of an autosomal gene in some strains of brown egg bird that suppresses production of trimethylamine oxidase, resulting in trimethylamine (TMA) accumulation in the egg. Sinapine content of rapeseed seems to accentuate production of TMA. There are also indications of brown egg birds responding adversely to pharmaceutical products such as the anticoccidial, Nicarbazin®. In this situation, high levels of nicarbazin inadvertently added to diets of brown egg layers, results in almost immediate loss in shell color.

7.2.1 Variations in requirements for specific nutrients

Quantitative requirements have been reported to vary between breeds or strain of chickens. Heavy breeds seem to require more vitamin E to prevent encephalomalacia than do White Leghorns and Leghorns may deposit more thiamin in eggs than do heavy breeds. Workers at Cornell were able to select two strains of White Leghorns that differed in their response to riboflavin and lysine. Also breed differences have been reported for pantothenic acid, pyridoxine and choline. However, in all these cases the quantitative difference was relatively small and, for practical purposes, special diets to account for such small differences are not warranted. Size of bird will also have a noticeable effect on the requirement for certain nutrients. The heavy broiler breeder will be partitioning a greater percentage of her nutrient intake into maintenance as compared to the smaller high egg output strains of White Leghorn. Also the physiological makeup of the dwarf bird with its slightly lower body temperature and reduced metabolic rate accounts for the small differences in nutrient requirements for this bird as compared to normal sized birds.

7.2.2 Specific metabolic variations

In man, a number of individual metabolic variations have been described and many of these variations have an effect on nutrient requirements. An example is phenylketonuria, a condition in which the conversion of phenylalanine to tyrosine is diminished because of limited synthesis of the enzyme phenylalanine hydroxylase. While a number of such disorders have been discovered in man and some farm animals, few are known to exist or have been discovered in chickens. This situation is due mainly to the fact that most nutritional studies involve replicated groups of birds rather than individuals.

However, there are specific inherited metabolic abnormalities that have been detected in chickens, including hens that lay eggs almost devoid of riboflavin regardless of the level found in the diet. Likewise the conversion of methionine to cystine has been reported to be less efficient in Australorps vs. White Leghorns. An abnormal uric acid metabolism in a selected strain of birds produced by Cornell workers was later reported to be a defect in uric acid transport in the kidney of these birds. While in the future some of these metabolic abnormalities noted in chickens might prove to be of practical significance there is presently little commercial interest in their identification and subsequent strain maintenance.

Some strains of birds respond differently to certain antimetabolites. Carnaghan et al. (1967) and Smith and Hamilton (1970) reported marked differences in the susceptibility of birds to aflatoxin, with brown egg breeds being more susceptible than are White Leghorns. It has been reported that a bird's susceptibility to Hemorrhagic Fatty Liver Syndrome is influenced by genetics (Ivy and Nesheim, 1973).

7.2.3 Genetic selection as a nutrition research tool

Genetic selection for traits may be useful in solving particular nutrition or metabolic problems. This approach has been used to advantage in developing a chick assay for vitamin D_3. A strain of chicks was selected that had bone ash of approximately 30% when fed a diet containing 100 IU D_3 /kg diet. The error variance for bone ash in these chicks was less than one third of that seen in unselected chicks. The use of these birds to improve the precision of the vitamin D_3 assay demonstrated the application of genetic selection in helping to quantitate nutrient requirements.

In studying possible genetic differences in arginine metabolism in chicks, workers at Cornell developed a strain with a relatively high requirement for arginine. Birds with an apparently elevated requirement for arginine grow at only 50% of normal rate and have high mortality when fed normal levels of arginine. Later studies demonstrated that the chicks with a high arginine requirement metabolized lysine slowly because they had a low level of the enzyme lysine-α-ketoglutarate reductase in their livers. Chicks from the high arginine requirement strain when fed a diet high in lysine had a build up of lysine in their blood and tissues. This resulted in increased activity of the enzyme arginase, subsequently resulting in excessive degradation of arginine. Other studies have shown that selected strains of chicks convert tryptophan to niacin at different rates.

7.3 NUTRITION, DISEASE AND STRESS

The development of the poultry industry during the past half-century has been due in part, to the ability of the chicken to accommodate many of the stresses imposed on them by modern production techniques. Such stressors include genetic selection for increased rate of growth and egg numbers, environmental and management changes, increased disease challenges and exposure to a wide array of pharmaceuticals and vaccines needed to maintain flock health.

The metabolic changes in chickens associated with response to external stressors are:

1. Enlargement of the anterior pituitary gland, probably due to the increased production of adrenocorticotropic hormone (ACTH),

2. Adrenal hypertrophy with increased output of corticosterone,

3. Atrophy of the thymus, Bursa of Fabricius and the spleen. The regression of the Bursa of Fabricius is the most sensitive indicator of stress in young birds. In adult animals the Bursa disappears due to the influence of gonadal steroids.

4. Changes in the circulating leukocytes, with a decrease in lymphocytes and an increase in heterophils,

5. Slower growth or weight loss.

Chronic stress, if not too great, will result in the animal adapting completely and showing almost normal growth. However, if multiple stressors are encountered simultaneously, the animal may be less able to adapt. Hence, the animal may adversely react to conditions in which individual stresses may be minimal but in combination with other factors, the bird reacts negatively.

According to this theory, an animal may live and grow moderately well even though the diet is slightly deficient in a required nutrient. However, if this same bird is exposed to coccidia for example, it may succumb to the disease even though the disease challenge is not severe enough to cause mortality in birds fed a nutritionally adequate diet. There are many different stresses that birds can be exposed to. A well managed poultry enterprise obviously is one that does everything possible to minimize the number and degree of stresses upon the flock.

7.3.1 Parasites and nutrition

The intestinal tract of a chicken provides an ideal habitat for microorganisms including bacteria and protozoa which may be parasitic. The presence of microorganisms in the digestive tract cause a number of anatomical changes, the most notable being a longer and heavier tract than is found in germ-free chickens. There are differences in the epithelial cells, the amount of lymphatic tissue of the lamina propria and pH of the duodenal contents of conventional versus germ-free chickens. Also, there is a difference in bile acid secretion with greater amounts occurring in the conventionally reared birds. The lower part of the small intestine, and especially the ceca, contain more volatile fatty acids as well as such compounds as ammonia and pharmacologically active amines in the conventional bird while these are virtually missing in the germ-free animal. The cecal contents of the conventional bird also contain a wide array of the B-vitamins although these seem to contribute little to the vitamin requirements of the bird (Coates *et al.*, 1968).

Protozoans and particularly coccidia have marked effects on the digestive physiology of the host. They have been shown to result in significant damage to the intestinal wall, and so reducing the absorption of a number of nutrients (Turk, 1974). Crompton and Nesheim (1976) reviewed the work reported on the effect of coccidia on vitamin A requirements. Chicks fed diets low in vitamin A showed higher mortality together with reduced liver storage of vitamin A and reduced pigmentation. There are a number of other studies demonstrating alteration in the absorption of amino acids and certain minerals when birds harbour coccidial oocysts. In essence, coccidia, due to capillary cell damage, reduce the absorption of most dietary nutrients.

7.3.2 Nutrition and other diseases

It has been shown experimentally that low levels of dietary vitamin A appear to accentuate the severity of lesions caused by infection with mycoplasma and infectious bronchitis. It has also been demonstrated that high levels of dietary vitamin A will reduce the severity of lesions and mortality due to coccidiosis. Work with mice has shown that animals fed synthetic diets were far more susceptible to an avirulent culture of salmonella than were mice fed a more practical type diet. This phenomenon implies that natural feedstuffs may contain unknown nutritional factors which aid in overcoming environmental stress and infectious disease. The often reported observation that high levels of dietary protein accentuate mortality of chicks suffering from a disease challenge, has been suggested to be the result of an associated increased need for vitamins (for protein catabolism) which negatively impact the bird's immune system.

While many studies indicate definite relationships among nutrition, disease and other stresses, there is little information available concerning possible metabolic mechanisms to explain such interactions. Much is known about the various mechanisms of the body in preventing and fighting disease. For example, the epidermis and mucous membranes of the respiratory systems are the first line of defense against disease. Keeping these membranes healthy goes a long way to inhibiting pathogenic organisms from gaining access to the blood stream and subcutaneous tissues. Again it is quite likely that vitamin A plays a significant role in maintaining the integrity of the cells of the mucous membranes, and hence is probably one of the major mechanisms by which vitamin A increases an animal's resistance to infectious disease.

7.3.3   Effects of nutrient deficiencies upon antibody production

Gamma globulins, antibodies and leukocytes in the blood are capable of reacting with infectious agents and, hopefully, rendering them harmless. Since all of these components of the immune system are composed of amino acids and require certain vitamins for the enzyme systems necessary for their synthesis, marked dietary deficiencies of such nutrients can reduce the levels of these protective systems.

The white blood cells and phagocytes of the reticuloendothelial system also play a role in fighting disease by engulfing microorganisms which are then destroyed by lysosomal enzymes. Folic acid deficiency causes a marked reduction in the number of white blood cells because this vitamin appears to be needed for their synthesis. A deficiency of folic acid not only weakens the animal because of resultant anemia, but also because of associated loss in the number of white blood cells. The adrenal cortex has a marked effect on the resistance of an animal to a number of diseases. Vitamin C, folic acid and vitamin B_{12} are known to be concerned with the functioning of this gland.

Dibner *et al.* (1998) suggest that nutrition of the chick in the first 24-36 hr can have a measurable effect on bursa weight, biliary immunoglobin levels and resistance to an oral challenge of coccidiosis. Klasing (1988) suggests that a period of feed deprivation increases the bird's cellular and humoral response to novel antigens such as sheep red blood cells. On the other hand, it is not clearly established whether or not the voracious appetite of the broiler in any way compromises the bird's immune response. There has been more recent interest in the role of some dietary fatty acids on immune competence. Fritsche *et al.* (1991) conclude that antibody titres in chicks are higher when the diet contains fish oil rather than other fat sources such as lard, corn oil, or canola oil. It seems as though ω-3 fatty acids may enhance cell-mediated cytotoxicity.

The immune response seems to initiate a series of changes in the metabolism of all nutrients. During acute infection, carbohydrate utilization and gluconeogenesis increases dramatically due to changes in metabolism induced by hormonal change (Klasing, 1992). There is a concomitant reduction in β-oxidation of fats. The inflammatory response also influences protein metabolism, as characterized by loss of muscle tissue. Klasing (1992) suggests that cytokines stimulate nitrogen excretion. Any amino acids lost from the muscle are used for gluconeogenesis and leukocytic protein synthesis to help production of immune cells and immunoglobulins in particular. Perhaps the biggest change in nutrition of the animal due to disease challenge is caused simply by reduced feed intake. However, a challenge with organisms such as *E. coli* has been shown to reduce the bird's need for nutrients such as methionine and lysine. Klasing (1992) suggests that this latter phenomenon is due to the fact that reduced growth rate causes a greater quantitative reduction in the need for these nutrients compared to the increased requirement associated with enhanced gluconeogenesis.

7.4 NUTRITION AND EGG QUALITY

Egg quality encompasses a wide range of physical and chemical properties that interrelate to ultimately produce a high quality egg. These are: 1) shell quality, 2) albumen quality, 3) nutritional composition, 4) freedom from defects such as blood spots, mottling, etc., 5) yolk pigmentation, and 6) perhaps egg size. Most of these parameters can be influenced by a wide range of dietary situations and nutrient interrelationships.

7.4.1 Eggshell quality

White or brown shelled eggs are preferred in different markets. Shell color is dependent on the quantity of pigments secreted from the shell gland during the final stages of calcification and is generally independent of normal bird nutrition. Shell color has no effect on the nutrient composition of the egg. However, inadvertantly feeding the anticoccidial Nicarbazin® causes almost complete loss of pigmentation of brown shelled eggs. Figure 7.1 shows the effect of feeding 80 ppm Nicarbazin® to layers over 2 three day periods. The eggs are from an individual bird, and arranged left-to-right and top-to-bottom for sequential production. Nicarbazin® was fed

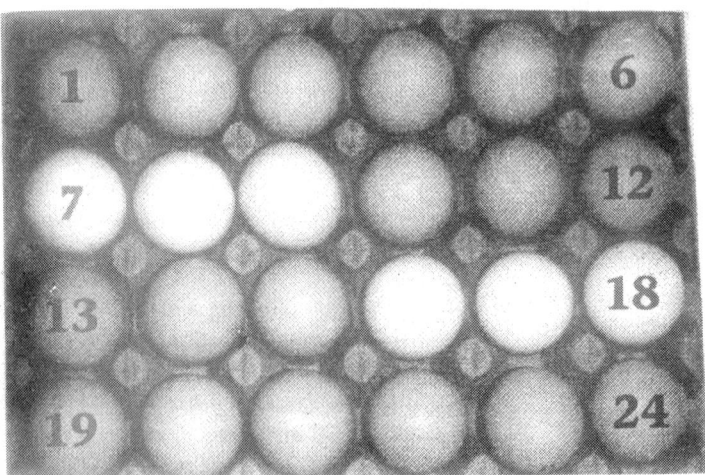

Figure 7.1 Depigmentation of brown shelled eggs due to feeding 80ppm Nicarbazin®. Day 1-6 eggs arranged sequentially on top row etc. Nicarbazin fed on days 6,7 and 8; and on days 15,16 and 17.

on days 5-7, leading to production of 3 white shelled eggs. Removal of Nicarbazin®
caused resumption of normal shell pigmentation. Feeding Nicarbazin® in the following week, again for 3 days, caused the same reversible effect. Feeding high levels
of chlorotetracycline antibiotics causes a characteristic yellow coloring of white
shelled eggs.

Eggshell thickness is the most important feature of shell quality and as detailed
in Chapters 4 and 5 the major nutrients involved are calcium, phosphorus and vitamin D_3. When shell quality (thickness) problems persist, it is common practice
to feed more calcium, vitamin D_3 or a combination of these nutrients. Unfortunately
feeding an excess of these nutrients can cause excessive particulate calcium deposits
on the shell (Figure 7.2). These extra calcium deposits may be reason for down-
grading in some markets, and are also prone to separation from the shell surface
causing a potential route of entry by bacteria.

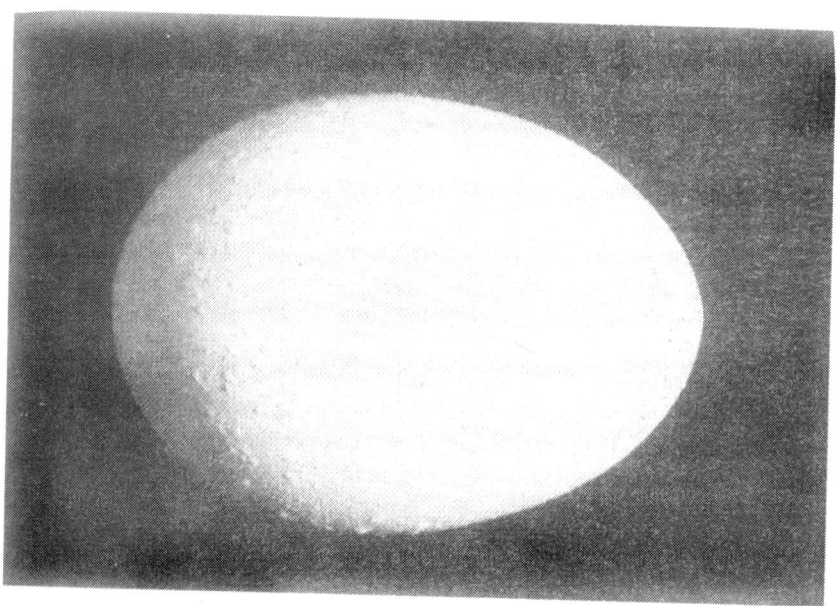

Figure 7.2 Severely pimpled egg shell due to feeding high levels
of calcium or vitamin D_3 *(with permission from Dr. S. Gillingham)*

7.4.2 Albumen quality

The grade of table eggs depends to a major degree on the firmness or gel structure of the albumen. The protein in egg albumen most associated with the gel structure is ovomucin. This protein fraction of eggs is apparently heterogeneous and is composed of two or more fractions which may vary markedly in carbohydrate composition (Smith et al., 1974). There is a positive correlation between Haugh units and ovomucin content of fresh eggs. Those eggs with a firm albumen that have high Haugh unit values have greater quantities of ovomucin. Eggs examined in the isthmus of the oviduct have similar quantities of ovomucin even though eggs may be laid with varying albumen quality. Major changes in the ovomucin content of eggs seem to occur in the shell gland, likely due to plumping with water and solutes. Few studies have examined directly the influence of nutrition of the hen on the ovomucin content of eggs. It has generally been difficult to demonstrate effects of feeding on albumen quality.

Dietary vanadium causes a decrease in albumen quality but similar effects of feeding vanadium can be produced by injecting small amounts of ammonium vanadate directly into fresh eggs. Feeding ammonium chloride causes an increase in albumen height and the amount of thick white. Austic (1977) found that feeding hens a diet containing ammonium chloride increased the Haugh units of freshly laid eggs and also caused an increase in the ovomucin content of the eggs. The mechanism responsible for these effects is not known although the influence of ammonium chloride may be mediated through slight changes in egg pH. Although ammonium chloride feeding can increase albumen quality, it also causes a reduction in blood pH and reduced egg shell thickness.

7.4.3 Egg defects caused by nutritional problems

Blood spots are one of the most significant defects in eggs that cause considerable economic loss. These are usually seen as blood clots on the surface of the yolk which are the result of rupture of a small blood vessel as the yolk is released from the ovarian follicle. The clots may be very small or may be large enough to cause discoloration of the entire egg. Although blood spots do not adversely affect the nutritional value of eggs, they are very objectionable to consumers.

The major nutritional factor known to affect blood spot formation is vitamin A deficiency, which usually causes a marked increase in their incidence in eggs. The quantity of vitamin A required to minimize blood spotting is essentially the same as that required for maximum egg production. Thus higher than normal vitamin A levels do not seem to further reduce the incidence of blood spots in eggs. A marginal deficiency of vitamin K has been shown to decrease blood spotting, possibly because the blood released during ovulation may be diffused throughout the egg rather than forming a small clot that is easily seen upon candling. Thus some vitamin K antagonists have been shown to reduce blood spots, whereas high levels of alfalfa meal in laying rations have been reported to increase the incidence of blood spots.

The feeding of Nicarbazin® to hens results in a characteristic mottling of the yolk as shown in Figure 7.3. Yolk mottling has also been reported from feeding a combination of the worming drugs piperazine, phenothiazine and dibutyltin dilaurate to laying hens. Individually, these drugs seem to have no effect on egg yolks.

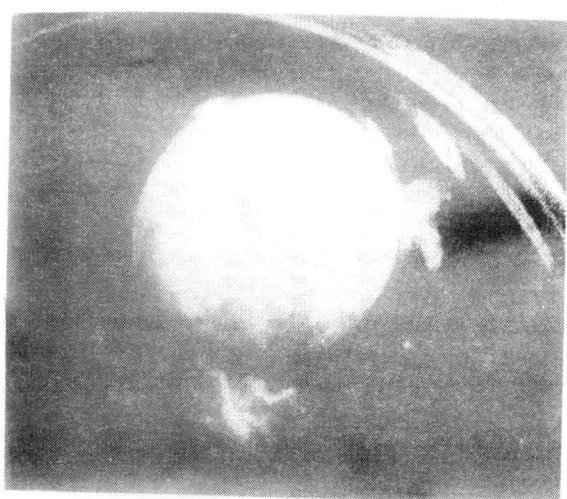

Figure 7.3 A severely mottled egg yolk from a hen receiving a high dietary level of Nicarbazin®

Cottonseed oil contains two substances responsible for poor internal egg quality. The cyclopropene fatty acids, malvalic and sterculic acids, cause a pink discoloration of the white in eggs when hens are fed cottonseed oil (see also section 10.2). Small amounts of gossypol can cause severe bluish green discoloration of yolks along with severe mottling. The effect of gossypol is particularly evident in eggs stored for a few days after they are laid. All cottonseed oil products and meals, therefore, should be kept out of rations for hens to avoid these conditions, unless the cottonseed meals are known to be low in gossypol. Egg yolks from a hen receiving gossypol are shown in Figure 7.4. Mottling is shown on the left, while the picture on the right shows complete yolk discoloration due to the gossypol condition. When it is encountered, the xanthophyll pigments in the feed should also be checked.

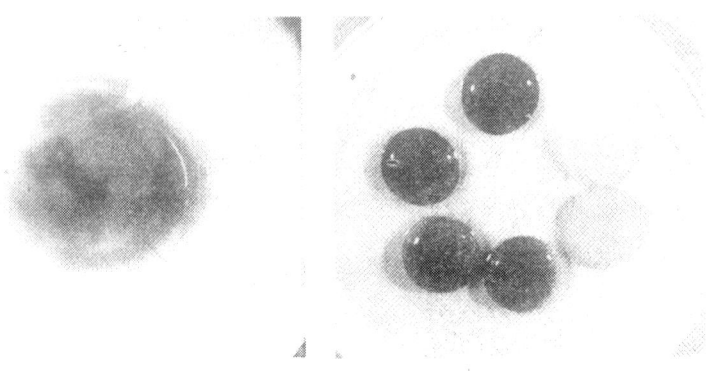

Figure 7.4 Left: Mottled yolk from hen fed gossypol. Right: Effect of feeding graded levels of gossypol on yolk color.

7.4.4 Nutrition and egg size

The size of an egg is controlled by many factors, including genetics, stage of sexual maturity, age, some drugs, and some dietary nutrients. The most important nutritional factors known to affect egg size are protein and amino acid adequacy of a diet and linoleic acid.

Since about 50% of the dry matter of an egg is protein, the supply of amino acids for protein synthesis is critical for egg production. When the supply of one of several amino acids is low, egg protein with an altered amino acid composition will not be synthesized. This has the effect of reducing egg size or completely stopping egg production. Often a reduced egg size is the only consequence observed with a marginal protein or amino acid deficiency.

A striking reduction in egg size can be produced by a linoleic acid deficiency. In a severe deficiency, eggs laid by mature hens may weigh only about 40 grams compared with a weight of 60 grams for eggs from control hens. Under practical conditions, the linoleic acid content may be marginal in diets containing low levels of corn and no added fat. Improvements in egg size related to linoleic acid have been observed when hens are fed diets composed primarily of barley, wheat or milo as grain sources. Linoleic acid deficiency is discussed in detail in Chapter 4

Other unrecognized dietary factors may be responsible for improvements in egg size. Hens fed highly purified diets usually lay eggs somewhat smaller than those produced by hens fed practical diets. Whether this results from an unidentified factor in the practical diet or from an unrecognized nutrient deficiency in the purified diet remains to be determined. Birds fed 5-8% canola or rapeseed meal often lay eggs 1-2 g smaller than normal, and this may be related to a slight depresson in feed intake.

Efforts to increase egg size by treating hens with thyroid hormone or with diethyl-stilbestrol usually have had no effect, or have actually decreased egg size. High and low levels of antibiotics have had little or no effect upon egg size. Nicarbazin® in the diet of laying hens has been shown to cause a marked decrease in egg weight by decreasing the size of the yolk. Gossypol at high levels has quickly brought egg production to a stop, and the eggs decrease in size as the hens go out of production.

While tranquilizers have been suggested to improve egg weight, high levels of reserpine decreases egg size. Exposure of hens to grains treated with fumigants such as carbon tetrachloride and ethylene dibromide have been reported to cause a marked decline in egg weight.

Many experiments have demonstrated that pullets of the same chronological age lay eggs of comparable size. Thus, if sexual maturity is delayed during the rearing period, the first eggs laid by pullets reared in such a manner will be larger than the first eggs of pullets maturing at a younger age. Sexual maturity can be delayed by feeding diets very low in energy, by physical restriction of energy intake, or by feeding deficient levels of protein or an essential amino acid.

SELECTED REFERENCES

Austic, R.E., 1977. Role of the shell gland in determination of albumen quality. Poultry Sci. 56:202-210.

Carnaghan, R.B.A., C.N. Herbert, D.S.P. Patterson and D. Seveasy, 1967. Comparative biological and biochemical studies in hybrid chicks. 2. Susceptibility to aflatoxin and effects on serum protein constituents. Br. Poultry Sci. 8:279.

Coates, M.E., J.E. Ford and G.F. Harrison, 1968. Intestinal synthesis of vitamins of the B-complex in chicks. Br. J. Nutrition 22:493.

Crompton, D.W.T. and M.C. Nesheim, 1976. Host-parasite relationships in domestic birds. Advances in Parasitol. 14:95. Academic Press, New York.

Dibner, J.J., C.D. Knight, M.L. Kitchell, C.A. Atwell, A.C. Downs and F.J. Ivey, 1998. Early feeding and development of the immune system in neonatal poultry. J. Appl. Poultry Res. 7:425-436.

Falconer, D.S., 1977. Nutritional influences on the outcome of selection. Proc. Nutr. Soc. 36:47-51.

Fritsche, K.L., N.A. Cassity and S-C Huang, 1991. Effect of fat source on antibody production and lymphocyte proliferation in chickens. Poultry Sci. 70:611-617.

Ivy, C.A. and M.C. Nesheim, (1973). Factors influencing the liver fat content of laying hens. Poultry Sci. 52:281.

Klasing, K.C., 1988. Influence of acute starvation or acute excess intake on immunocompetence of broiler chicks. Poultry Sci. 67:626-634.

Klasing, K.C., 1992. Interactions between nutrition and infectious disease in broiler chickens. Proc: Multi-State Poultry Mtg. May 20, Indianapolis.

Leeson, S. and W.D. Morrison, 1978. Effect of feather cover on feed efficiency in laying birds. Poultry Sci. 57:1094-1096.

Leeson, S., B.S. Reinhart and J.D. Summers, 1979a. Response of White Leghorn and RIR breeder hens to dietary deficiencies of synthetic vitamins. 1. Egg production, hatchability and chick growth. Can. J. Anim. Sci. 59:561-567.

Leeson, S., B.S. Reinhart and J.D. Summers, 1979b. 2. Embryo mortality and abnormalities. Can. J. Animal Sci. 59:569-579.

Morrison, W.D. and S. Leeson, 1978. Relationship of feed efficiency to carcass composition and metabolic rate in laying birds. Poultry Sci. 57:735-739.

Pym, R.A.E., 1990. Nutritional Genetics. In Poultry Breeding and Genetics. Ed. R.D. Crawford, Publ. Elsevier, N.Y.

Smith, J.W. and P.B. Hamilton, 1970. Aflatoxicosis in the broiler chicken. Poultry Sci. 49:207.

Smith, M.B., T.M. Reynolds, C.P. Buckingham and J.F. Back, 1974. Studies on the carbohydrate of egg-white ovomucin. Aust. J. Biol. Sci. 27:349.

Sorensen, P., 1985. Influence of diet on response to selection for growth and efficiency. In Poultry Genetics and Breeding. Ed. W.G. Hill, J.M. Manson and D Hewitt. Brit. Poult. Sci. Symp. #18.

Spratt, R.S. and S. Leeson, 1987. Determination of ME of various diets using Leghorn, Dwarf and regular broiler breeder hens. Poultry Sci. 66:314-317.

Turk, D.E., 1974. Intestinal parasitism and nutrient absorption. Federation Proc. 33:106.

Feed Ingredients and Feed Formulation

There are surprisingly few feed ingredients used in poultry diets today. By far the major ingredients are corn and soybean meal, which together often account for 70-80% of the components of a feed. Other ingredients vary depending upon local availability, but again there are few viable choices. Wheat and byproducts such as wheat shorts together with milo are the other major cereal choices, and most diets will contain some supplemental fat of either animal or vegetable origin. Alternates to soybean meal are canola meal, sunflower meal, corn gluten meal and cottonseed meal. Many diets today contain some meat meal, because currently it is inexpensive due to its exclusion from ruminant diets. Poultry by-product meal is another animal protein available in regions where there is a major broiler industry. In total therefore we have just over ten ingredients that constitute the major portion of most poultry diets. The largest producers of these ingredients are N. America, Brazil and Asia.

In formulating diets, it is essential to know the bird's nutrient needs, and consequently the concentration of these nutrients in the various ingredients. Many nutrients are determined by direct chemical analyses, and so procedures are relatively inexpensive and rapid as well as being accurate and precise. Consequently such nutrients as fat, calcium, sodium and crude protein are routinely determined. Where a measure of digestibility is required, there is currently no alternative to using live birds in a bioassay procedure. Determination of metabolizable energy and digestible amino acids therefore becomes expensive, takes considerable time to accomplish, and having a biological component, is less repeatable. Because of the time factor involved in these complex bioassays they are rarely used to prescreen ingredients prior to formulation, but rather to establish trends that over time are used to adjust ingredient matrix data.

Tables 8.1 - 8.5 show the nutrient levels for ingredients of importance in nutrition of the chicken.

Table 8.1 Major nutrients

Ingredient	Crude protein (%)	Digestible protein (%)	Metabolizable energy (kcal/kg)	Crude fat (%)	Crude fiber (%)	Calcium (%)	Available phosphorus(%)	Linoleic acid (%)
Cereals and by-products								
Yellow Corn	7.9	7.2	3340	3.8	2.5	0.01	0.13	1.9
Wheat	14.0	12.1	3140	1.5	2.9	0.05	0.20	0.5
Barley	11.5	9.3	2795	2.0	8.0	0.10	0.20	0.9
Milo	9.0	7.9	3263	2.5	2.7	0.02	0.15	1.1
Wheat bran	15.8	11.7	1540	4.8	12.0	0.10	0.65	1.7
Wheat shorts	15.1	14.3	2870	4.2	3.6	0.07	0.30	1.8
Rice bran	13.0	7.7	1900	1.7	12.0	0.06	0.90	3.4
Rice polishings	11.0	8.5	2750	15.0	2.4	0.06	0.18	3.3
Bakery by-product	10.6	9.8	3200	9.8	2.4	0.05	0.13	2.9
Molasses (cane)	3.0	2.1	1962	-	-	0.50	0.03	-
Vegetable proteins								
Canola meal	37.5	34.0	2000	1.8	11.9	0.66	0.47	0.4
Soybean meal (48%)	47.0	43.5	2540	0.5	3.0	0.20	0.37	0.4
Full-fat soybeans	37.5	33.4	3880	20.0	2.0	0.15	0.28	9.0
Corn gluten meal	60.0	54.4	3770	2.5	2.5	0.10	0.20	1.2
Cotton seed meal	41.0	33.2	2350	0.5	14.0	0.15	0.48	0.2
Peanut meal	47.0	35.7	2205	1.0	13.0	0.20	0.30	0.3
Sesame meal	44.0	30.6	1984	5.0	5.0	0.20	0.75	2.0
Sunflower meal	46.8	35.6	2205	2.9	11.0	0.30	0.50	1.8
Lupins	34.5	29.8	3000	6.3	16.0	0.20	0.20	3.0
Flaxseed	22.0	18.1	3500	34.0	6.1	0.25	0.17	5.2
Animal proteins								
Meat Meal	50.0	45.0	2500	6.0	2.5	8.00	4.00	0.6
Fish meal (60%)	60.0	55.4	2720	2.0	1.0	6.50	3.50	0.3
Poultry by-product meal	60.0	52.5	2950	8.0	2.0	3.50	2.10	2.4
Feather meal	82.0	71.4	3000	2.5	1.5	0.20	0.75	0.1

TABLE 8.2 Total amino acid composition

Ingredient	Methionine %	Cystine %	Lysine %	Histidine %	Tryptophan %	Threonine %	Arginine %	Isoleucine %	Leucine %	Phenylalanine %	Valine %
Cereals and by-products											
Yellow Corn	0.2	0.1	0.2	0.2	0.1	0.4	0.4	0.5	1.0	0.5	0.4
Wheat	0.2	0.2	0.5	0.2	0.2	0.4	0.7	0.3	0.9	0.6	0.5
Barley	0.2	0.2	0.4	0.3	0.2	0.4	0.5	0.5	0.8	0.6	0.6
Milo	0.1	0.2	0.3	0.3	0.1	0.3	0.4	0.5	1.5	0.5	0.5
Wheat bran	0.1	0.1	0.6	0.3	0.3	0.4	1.0	0.6	0.9	0.5	0.7
Wheat shorts	0.2	0.2	0.6	0.2	0.2	0.5	0.9	0.7	1.0	0.6	0.7
Rice bran	0.2	0.1	0.5	0.3	0.2	0.4	0.5	0.4	0.8	0.4	0.6
Rice polishings	0.2	0.1	0.5	0.2	0.1	0.3	0.6	0.3	0.7	0.4	0.7
Bakery by-product	0.2	0.2	0.3	0.3	0.1	0.3	0.5	0.4	0.8	0.6	0.5
Molasses (cane)	-	-	-	-	-	-	-	-	-	-	-
Vegetable proteins											
Canola meal	0.7	0.6	2.2	1.1	0.5	1.7	2.2	1.4	2.7	1.5	1.9
Soybean meal (48%)	0.7	0.8	3.2	1.3	0.7	2.0	3.6	2.6	3.7	2.5	2.5
Full-fat soybeans	0.5	0.6	2.4	0.9	0.5	1.5	2.7	2.0	2.8	1.9	1.9
Corn gluten meal	1.6	0.9	0.9	1.4	0.3	1.7	2.2	2.4	8.1	3.2	2.6
Cotton seed meal	0.5	0.6	1.7	1.0	0.5	1.3	4.6	1.3	2.4	2.2	1.9
Peanut meal	0.4	0.7	1.6	1.2	0.5	1.5	4.9	2.0	3.0	2.7	2.8
Sesame meal	1.5	0.6	1.4	1.2	0.8	1.7	5.1	2.3	3.2	2.3	2.5
Sunflower meal	0.8	0.7	1.6	1.0	0.9	1.6	3.3	1.8	2.4	1.9	2.2
Lupins	0.3	0.6	1.7	0.9	0.4	1.2	4.5	1.4	2.4	1.3	1.4
Flaxseed	0.4	0.4	0.9	0.4	0.3	0.8	2.1	1.0	1.3	1.0	1.1
Animal proteins											
Meat meal	0.7	0.6	3.6	0.7	0.5	1.7	3.0	1.3	3.3	1.6	2.4
Fish meal (60%)	1.8	1.1	5.3	1.6	0.6	2.9	4.0	4.1	5.0	2.7	3.6
Poultry by-product meal	1.3	2.0	3.4	1.0	0.4	2.2	3.5	2.1	4.5	1.8	3.0
Feather meal	0.6	5.5	1.7	0.5	0.6	4.5	6.4	4.3	6.5	4.3	7.4

TABLE 8.3 Available amino acid composition

Ingredient	Methionine %	Cystine %	Lysine %	Histidine %	Tryptophan %	Threonine %	Arginine %	Isoleucine %	Leucine %	Phenylalanine %	Valine %
Cereals and by-products											
Yellow Corn	0.18	0.08	0.16	0.18	0.07	0.33	0.36	0.44	0.8	0.42	0.33
Wheat	0.16	0.18	0.40	0.18	0.17	0.32	0.56	0.26	0.81	0.54	0.42
Barley	0.16	0.16	0.31	0.26	0.16	0.30	0.41	0.41	0.73	0.53	0.48
Milo	0.09	0.17	0.23	0.26	0.07	0.24	0.28	0.42	1.30	0.40	0.40
Wheat bran	0.08	0.07	0.42	0.24	0.24	0.28	0.79	0.48	0.72	0.41	0.55
Wheat shorts	0.16	0.14	0.48	0.16	0.15	0.40	0.71	0.56	0.84	0.49	0.57
Rice bran	0.15	0.07	0.39	0.24	0.14	0.28	0.40	0.31	0.54	0.30	0.46
Rice polishings	0.16	0.08	0.42	0.18	0.07	0.26	0.51	0.27	0.57	0.31	0.52
Bakery by-product	0.17	0.16	0.19	0.24	0.08	0.21	0.40	0.32	0.71	0.51	0.40
Vegetable proteins											
Canola meal	0.63	0.45	1.76	0.93	0.38	1.30	1.98	1.04	2.40	1.30	1.55
Soybean meal (48%)	0.64	0.64	2.88	1.07	0.51	1.76	3.21	2.30	3.20	2.10	2.20
Full-fat soybeans	0.42	0.50	2.00	0.74	0.42	1.27	2.30	1.72	2.20	1.70	1.70
Corn gluten meal	1.44	0.81	0.80	1.14	0.21	1.60	2.10	2.30	7.90	3.10	2.40
Cotton seed meal	0.35	0.42	1.19	0.69	0.36	0.91	3.70	0.95	1.72	2.00	1.70
Peanut meal	0.33	0.55	1.28	0.96	0.38	1.20	4.00	1.80	2.70	2.30	2.40
Sesame meal	1.30	0.54	1.30	1.00	0.60	1.43	4.60	2.00	2.80	2.10	2.30
Sunflower meal	0.72	0.55	1.30	0.80	0.65	1.20	2.64	1.28	1.90	1.55	1.75
Lupins	0.27	0.54	1.40	0.81	0.26	1.00	4.10	1.20	2.20	1.10	1.20
Flaxseed	0.33	0.30	0.72	0.32	0.34	0.65	1.76	0.72	1.10	0.76	0.95
Animal proteins											
Meat Meal	0.60	0.35	2.68	0.56	0.37	1.36	2.50	1.00	2.60	1.30	1.90
Fish meal (60%)	1.62	0.80	4.70	1.40	0.48	2.50	3.60	3.70	4.50	2.30	3.20
Poultry by-product meal	1.07	1.20	2.70	0.80	0.29	1.76	3.00	1.70	3.80	1.40	2.40
Feather meal	0.47	2.40	1.10	0.35	0.41	3.10	5.00	3.60	5.00	3.50	6.10

Table 8.4 Vitamin composition

Ingredient	Vit B$_{12}$ mcg/kg	Vit E mg/kg	Pantothenic acid mg/kg	Niacin mg/kg	Choline equiv. mg/kg	Riboflavin mg/kg	Thiamin mg/kg	Biotin mg/kg	Folic Acid mg/kg	VitA activity 10³IU/kg	Xanthophyll mg/kg
Cereals and by-products											
Yellow Corn	–	19	5	21	660	1.3	4.4	0.07	0.02	2.40	20
Wheat	–	13	12	55	2200	1.1	4.8	0.11	0.40	–	3.5
Barley	–	20	7	61	1210	2.2	5.5	0.20	0.51	–	–
Milo	–	11	11	41	660	1.1	3.7	0.29	0.02	–	1.3
Wheat bran	–	13	28	187	3674	3.1	7.9	0.11	1.78	–	–
Wheat shorts	–	21	17	92	3580	2.0	15.6	0.11	0.66	–	–
Rice bran	–	55	22	286	1254	2.4	22.8	0.42	2.20	–	–
Rice polishings	–	85	57	528	1320	1.8	19.3	0.62	0.20	–	–
Bakery by-product	–	10	10	20	1100	1.0	7.2	0.12	0.30	–	–
Molasses (cane)	–	5	40	56	1200	4.0	2.8	0.09	0.18	–	–
Vegetable proteins											
Canola meal	1.1	4	9	159	6450	1.2	4.0	0.28	0.55	–	–
Soybean meal (48%)	–	2	14	20	2860	3.1	2.4	0.40	0.70	–	–
Full-fat soybeans	–	40	10	15	2174	2.4	1.8	0.31	0.53	–	–
Corn gluten meal	–	22	3	48	330	1.5	0.2	0.40	0.20	3.2	–
Cotton seed meal	–	12	7	38	3080	3.7	3.5	0.50	0.28	7.5	273
Peanut meal	–	3	52	165	1980	5.3	7.0	0.40	0.59	–	–
Sesame meal	–	7	6	13	1500	3.1	3.0	4.4	0.50	–	–
Sunflower meal	–	11	40	290	4300	3.3	2.0	1.8	0.60	–	–
Lupins	–	2	2	35	3100	2.8	5.3	0.04	0.40	–	–
Flaxseed	–	18	4	40	3200	4.5	7.0	0.10	0.70	–	–
Animal proteins											
Meat Meal	70	1	4	44	1650	4.4	1.1	0.09	0.44	–	–
Fish meal (60%)	185	5	8	55	2860	4.8	0.7	0.22	0.24	–	–
Poultry by-product meal	100	5	8	45	3000	8.0	0.6	0.30	0.75	–	–
Feather meal	66.0	–	8	16	1320	2.0	0.1	0.04	0.22	–	–

Table 8.5 Mineral composition

Ingredients	Chloride %	Magnesium %	Sodium %	Potassium %	Iron %	Manganese (mg/kg)	Copper (mg/kg)	Zinc (mg/kg)	Selenium (mg/kg)
Cereals and by-products									
Yellow Corn	0.04	0.15	0.05	0.38	0.01	4	3	29	0.04
Wheat	0.08	0.16	0.09	0.52	0.01	48	7	40	0.51
Barley	0.18	0.12	0.02	0.56	0.01	16	7	40	0.35
Milo	0.08	0.17	0.04	0.34	0.01	14	9	26	0.03
Wheat bran	0.30	0.15	0.06	1.24	0.02	115	12	89	0.95
Wheat shorts	0.10	0.26	0.07	0.85	0.01	104	9	99	0.81
Rice bran	0.07	0.85	0.10	1.35	0.02	425	14	30	0.20
Rice polishings	0.10	0.65	0.11	1.17	0.02	310	8	30	0.12
Bakery by-product	0.48	0.20	0.52	0.60	0.02	30	7	41	0.30
Molasses (cane)	0.65	0.40	0.30	3.50	0.02	50	20	35	0.08
Vegetable proteins									
Canola meal	0.05	0.51	0.09	1.47	0.02	61	7	44	0.92
Soybean meal (48%)	0.05	0.27	0.05	2.54	0.01	27	36	52	0.11
Full-fat soybeans	0.04	0.21	0.03	1.50	0.01	20	27	41	0.09
Corn gluten meal	0.06	0.05	0.10	0.03	0.04	7	28	66	0.31
Cotton seed meal	0.03	0.39	0.05	1.20	0.01	18	16	40	0.05
Peanut meal	0.55	0.04	0.07	1.10	0.03	29	6	80	0.12
Sesame meal	0.05	0.50	0.04	1.20	0.04	48	4	27	0.06
Sunflower meal	0.03	0.75	0.02	1.00	0.10	15	3	100	0.25
Lupins	0.01	0.13	0.10	1.00	0.01	70	4	30	0.18
Flaxseed	0.05	0.30	0.08	1.20	0.02	74	17	91	0.12
Animal proteins									
Meat meal	0.90	1.00	0.55	1.23	0.04	18	8	98	0.40
Fish meal (60%)	0.55	0.21	0.47	0.32	0.06	25	8	119	1.83
Poultry by-product meal	0.40	0.18	0.36	0.28	0.05	20	6	79	0.92
Feather meal	0.41	0.20	0.70	0.30	0.05	15	12	7	0.72

8.1 CEREALS

a) Corn

Yellow corn is the major cereal used in most poultry diets. It is very high in energy contribution, and so usually provides the single largest source of energy in a diet. Corn is usually sold by grade where the lower the number denotes a better quality. As grade declines, there are more damaged and broken kernels, and the bulk density (bushel weight) declines. The standard is #2 grade which has a bushel weight of 54 lbs. or about 70 kg/hl. This grade of corn will have no more than 5% damaged kernels and 3% broken kernels or foreign material. As bushel weight declines, there is loss in energy by about 10 kcal/kg for each kg/hl decline.

The energy value of corn is contributed by the starchy endosperm which is composed mainly of amylopectin, and the germ which contains most of the oil. Most corn contains 3-4% oil, although newer varieties are now available which contain up to 6-8% oil, and so contribute proportionally more energy. These high oil corn varieties also contain 2-3% more protein, and proportionally more essential amino acids. The protein in corn is mainly as prolamin (zein),and as such,its amino acid profile is not ideal for poultry. This balance of amino acids, and their availablility is most important when low protein diets are formulated because under these conditions the corn prolamin can contribute up to 50-60% of the diet protein. Corn is also quite high in the yellow/orange pigments, usually containing around 5 ppm xanthophylls and 0.5 ppm carotenes. These pigments ensure that corn-fed birds will have a high degree of pigments in their body fat and in egg yolks.

Depending upon the growing season and storage conditions, molds and associated mycotoxins can be a problem. Aflatoxin contamination is common with insect damaged corn grown in hot humid areas, and there is little that can be done to rectify the horrendous consequences of high levels of this mycotoxin. There is an indication of aluminosilicates partially alleviating the effects of more moderate levels of aflatoxin. If aflatoxin is even suspected as being a problem, corn samples should be screened prior to blending and mixing. Zearalenone is another mycotoxin that periodically occurs in corn. Because the toxin ties up vitamin D_3, skeletal and egg shell problems can occur. With moderate levels of contamination, water soluble D_3 via the drinking water has proven beneficial. Mold growth can be a serious problem in corn that is transported for any length of time. With corn shipped at $\geq 16\%$ moisture and subjected to $\geq 25°C$ during shipping, mold growth often occurs. One solution to the problem is to add organic acids to the corn. However, it must be remembered that while organic acids will kill molds, and prevent re-infestation, they have no effect on any mycotoxins already present.

If corn is to be fed in mash diets, there seems to be an advantage to grinding to as uniform a particle size as possible, and to a size of about 0.7 - 0.9 mm. This size is often referred to as "medium" ground. Birds fed fine or coarse ground corn seem to exhibit lower digestibility values. Corn presents some problems to the manufacture of pelleted diets, and often good pellet durability in diets containing ≥ 30% corn can only be obtained by inclusion of pellet binders.

b) Wheat and Wheat by-products

Wheat is commonly used in many countries as the major energy source in poultry diets. There is often confusion regarding the exact type of wheat being used, because wheats are described in a number of different ways. Traditionally wheats were described as being winter or spring varieties and these were traditionally grown in different regions because of prevailing climate and soil conditions. Wheats are sometimes referred to as white or red, depending upon seed coat color, and finally there is the classification of hard vs soft. In the past, most winter wheats were white and soft, while spring wheats were hard and red. In terms of feeding value, the main criterion is whether wheat is soft or hard, because this will have an effect on the composition, especially protein. Because of developments in plant breeding, the color and time of planting can now be more variable. Hard wheats have a greater proportion of protein associated with the starch and contain more protein that is also higher in lysine. The proteins in hard wheat are useful in bread making, while the soft wheats are only used for manufacture of cookies and cakes. Durum wheat, used in manufacture of pasta is a very hard wheat. The physical hardness of these wheats is due to the strong binding between starch and the more abundant protein.

The composition of wheat is usually more variable than that of other cereals. Even within the hard wheats, protein level can vary from 10 - 18%, and this may relate to varietal differences and variance in growing conditions. Most hard wheats will not have to be dried after harvest, although drying conditions and moisture content of wheat at harvest appear to have little effect on feeding value. Growing conditions seem to have a major effect on wheat nitrogen content, and although high temperature can result in a 100% increase in nitrogen level, the relative proportion of both lysine and starch tends to be decreased.

Depending upon the growing region, frost damaged or sprouted wheat is sometimes available to the feed industry. Frost damage effectively stops starch synthesis, and so kernels are small and shrunken. While 100 kernel weight should be around 27g, with severe frost damage, this can be reduced to 14 - 16g. As expected the metabolizable energy level of this damaged wheat is reduced, and under these conditions there is a very good correlation between bulk density and metabolizable energy. For non-frosted wheat however, there does not seem to be the same relationship between energy level and bushel weight.

While wheats are much higher than corn in protein content, and provide only slightly less energy, there are some potential problems from feeding much more than 30% in a diet, especially for young birds. Wheat contains about 5 - 8% of pentosans which can cause problems with digesta viscosity, leading to reduced overall diet digestibility and wet manure. Component arabinoxylans are linked to other cell wall components, and these are able to adsorb up to 10 times their weight as water. Unfortunately, birds do not produce adequate quantities of xylanase enzymes, and so these polymers increase the viscosity of the digesta. The 10 - 15% reduction in the ME of wheats seen with most young birds (< 10 d age) likely relates to their inability to handle these pentosans. Variability in pentosan content of wheats *per se* likely accounts for most of the variability of results seen in wheat feeding studies. Another factor is our inability to predict feeding value based on simple proximate analyses. These adverse effects on digesta viscosity seem to decrease with increased storage time for wheats. Problems with digesta viscosity can be controlled to some extent by limiting the quantity of wheat used, especially for young birds, and/or by using exogenous xylanase enzymes (see Chapter 6).

Wheats also contain α-amylase inhibitors, thought to be albumin proteins, found predominantly in the starch. These inhibitors seem to be destroyed by the relatively mild temperatures employed during pelleting. Compared to corn, wheat is also very low in levels of available biotin. Whereas it is sometimes difficult to induce symptoms of biotin deficiency in birds fed corn diets devoid of synthetic biotin, problems soon develop if wheat is fed. While newly hatched chicks have liver biotin levels of around 3,000 ng/g, this number declines to 600 ng/g within 14 d in the wheat fed bird. Adding just 50μg biotin/kg diet almost doubles the liver biotin reserve, while adding 300μg/kg brings levels back to that seen in the day old chick. There is also concern that wheat causes a higher incidence of necrotic enteritis in broiler chicks. It seems that wheat provides a more suitable medium for the proliferation of certain pathogenic bacteria. The problem is most severe when wheat is finely ground, and the incidence of necrotic enteritis can be tempered by grinding wheat through a roller mill. Fine grinding of wheat can also cause beak impaction in young birds. The proteins in wheat tend to be sticky, and so they adhere to the beak and mouth lining of the bird. Severe beak impaction with feed tends to reduce feeding activity, increase feed deposited in open bell drinkers, and provides a medium within the mouth that is ideal for bacterial and fungal growth. These problems can be resolved by coarse grinding of wheat.

Using wheat in diets for meat birds does however improve pellet durability. The same proteins that enhance the baking characteristics of hard wheats, also help to bind ingredients during pelleting. Adding ≥ 25% to a diet has the same effect as including a pellet binder in diets that are difficult to pellet.

Wheat by-products result as inedible waste material during flour manufacturing. There is considerable variation in the classification of various wheat by-products, and names for the same product differ in different countries. Traditionally wheat was passed through a series of grinders of decreasing sieve size, producing so-called middlings, most of which became flour. The non-usable portion of this flour stream was often termed wheat middlings as opposed to wheat shorts which were a by-product of the extraction of bran. Today, only three major animal feed ingre dients are available (although again nomenclature may vary in different countries). Bran is from the outer seed coat, and is obviously high in fiber, and apart from specialized applications, is little used in poultry nutrition. After extraction of flour, bran and wheat germ (also for human consumption) the remaining product is now most commonly referred to as wheat shorts. Shorts are therefore by-products remaining from extraction of the other three distinct components (flour, bran and germ). In N. America the term red dog was sometimes used, although this is now commonly included in the shorts. Red dog represented the very finest particles of bran, endosperm and germ.

The main characteristics of wheat bran are high fiber, low bulk density and low metabolizable energy. Bran is however quite high in protein, and amino acid profile is comparable to that seen with whole wheat. Bran has been claimed to have a growth promoting effect for birds which is not directly related to any contribution of fiber to the diet. Such growth promotion is possibly derived from modification of the gut microflora. The energy value of bran may be improved by up to 10% by steam pelleting, while the availability of phosphorus is increased by up to 20% under similar conditions. Bran would only be considered where limits to growth rate are required, and where physical feed intake is not a problem. High bran diets promote excessively wet manure, and transportation costs of bran diets are increased in proportion to the reduced bulk density of the diet.

Because wheat shorts are most commonly an end point for various wheat milling by-products, composition can be quite variable. If shorts contain much more than 5% crude fiber, it is an indication of a greater proportion of bran-type residues, and so the energy value will be correspondingly reduced. Shorts are higher in protein than is whole wheat, but provide about 20% less energy, and therefore should be priced accordingly. Higher fiber content wheat shorts are obviously worth proportionally less. Sometimes wheat shorts are combined with bran to produce wheat mill-run.

c)   **Barley**

Barley is a medium energy protein ingredient, falling between oats and wheat in most characteristics. Young birds are less able to digest barley, although this may be a consequence of β-glucan content. The protein content of barley is usually around 11 - 12%, although much higher levels of 14 - 16% are sometimes encountered. These high protein barleys often contain no more essential amino acids than normal. The lysine content of barley within the range of 10 - 14% CP is described by the equation $0.13 + 0.024\% \times CP$. The metabolizable energy level of barley is highly correlated with bulk density, and there is a strong negative correlation with fiber.

Barley contains moderate levels of trypsin inhibitor, whose mode of action relates to sequestering of arginine, although by far the major problem with barley is its content of β-glucans. Most barley samples will contain 4 - 9% β-glucan, although with dry growing conditions that induces rapid maturation and early harvest, the content can increase to 12 - 15%. As previously described for wheat, the main problem of these β-glucans is the bird's inability to digest the molecule, resulting in the formation of a more viscous digesta. This increased viscosity slows the rate of mixing with digestive enzymes and also adversely affects the transport of nutrients to the absorptive mucosal surface. The rate of diffusion to the intestinal microvilli is a function of the thickness of the unstirred boundary layer, and this increases with increased digesta viscosity. Motility of the digesta will also indirectly affect the thickness of the unstirred boundary layer, which in turn affects the rate of absorption of all nutrients. The adverse effect of β-glucans is most pronounced with dietary fats and fat soluble compounds. Adding synthetic β-glucanase enzymes to diets containing more than 15 - 20% barley seems to resolve many of these problems, the usual outward sign of which is wet litter. Unfortunately the description and units of measurement of exogenous enzymes is not standardized, and so it is often difficult to compare products. Early studies show that any product should provide at least 120 units of β-glucanase/kg diet.

Enzymes seem to be less efficacious as the birds get older. For younger birds however, the efficacy of β-glucanase enzymes is well established, and many nutritionists consider barley plus enzymes as being equivalent in feeding value to wheat. These values can be used as a basis for economic evaluation of enzymes. While β-glucans are most often regarded as being problematic to birds, there seems to be one advantage to their inclusion in the diet. Feeding β-glucans reduces blood cholesterol in birds, and this likely positive effect is reversed by the use of synthetic β-glucanases. The mode of action of β-glucans may well be simply via sequestering of fats and bile acids in the digesta.

d)   Milo (Sorghum)

The feeding value of milo is essentially 95 - 96% that of corn, although in many markets it is priced at less than this. The starch in milo is intimately associated with the protein, and this leads to slightly reduced digestibility, especially in the absence of any heat processing. The major concern with milo, is the content of tannins, which are a group of polyphenols having the property of combining with various proteins. Birds fed tannins therefore exhibit reduced growth rate and in some instances an increased incidence and severity of skeletal disorders. Tannins that can be hydrolyzed are characterized by having a gallic acid unit combined by ester linkages to a central glucose moiety. Condensed tannins on the other hand are based on flavan-3-ols (catechin). Because tannins in milo are essentially condensed tannins, studies involving tannic acid (hydrolyzable) as a source of tannin may be of questionable value. The tannins are located in the outer seed coat and the underlying testa layer. Generally, the darker the seed coat, the higher the tannin content, although the tannins in the testa layer may be more indicative of general tannm content in the milo.

So-called bird resistant milos are usually very high in tannin, and are characterized by a darker seed coat color. These higher levels of tannin can result in up to 10% reduction of dry matter and amino acid digestibility. There is a good correlation between tannin content and AMEn, and as a generalization the following formula can be used: AMEn = 3900 - 500 (% tannin), kcal/kg. Tannins are most detrimental when fed to young birds, and especially when protein content of the diet is marginal. Feeding more protein or higher levels of certain amino acids seems to temper any growth retardation. The fact that methionine supplementation can overcome detrimental effects of tannins on growth rate, without alleviating problems with digestibility, suggests that birds can compensate for inferior digestibility by increasing their feed intake. Tannins also seem to increase the incidence of leg problems, especially in broiler chickens. The exact mechanism is unknown, although because bone mineral content is little affected, it is assumed to relate to inadequate development of the organic matrix, especially in the region of the growth plate. There seems no advantage to increasing supplemental levels of any minerals or vitamins when high tannin milos are necessarily used.

e) Rice by-products

Rice by-products are the result of dehulling and cleaning of brown rice, necessary for the production of white rice as a human food. Rice by-products are one of the most common cereal by-products available to the feed industry, with world production estimated at around 50 M tonnes. The by-product of preparing white rice, yields a product called rice bran, which itself is composed of about 30% by weight of rice polishing and 70% true bran. In some regions the two products are separated, being termed polishing and bran. Alternatively, the mixture is sometimes called rice bran, whereas in other areas the mixture may be called rice pollards. The polishings are very high in fat content and low in fiber, while the true bran is low in fat and high in fiber. The proportions of polishing and true bran in a mixed product will therefore have a major effect on its nutritive value. In the following discussion, rice bran refers to the mixture of polishing and true bran. The composition of any sample of mixed rice bran can be evaluated from consideration of fiber content.

Because of a high oil content (6 - 10%) rice bran is very susceptible to oxidative rancidity. Raw bran held at moderate temperatures for 10 - 12 weeks can be expected to undergo some rancidity. Rice bran should be stabilized with products such as ethoxyquin at around 250 ppm. Rice bran can also be stabilized by heat treatment. Extrusion at 130°C greatly reduces chances of rancidity, and of the development of free fatty acids.

When high levels of raw rice bran are used (≥ 40%) there is often growth depression and a reduction in feed efficiency, likely associated with the presence of trypsin inhibitor and high levels of phytic acid. Trypsin inhibitor, which seems to be a relatively low molecular weight structure, is destroyed by moist heat, although phytic acid is immune to this process. The phosphorus content of rice bran is assumed to be only 10% available for very young birds. However, phosphorus availability may increase with age, and if this happens it could create an imbalance of the calcium:phosphorus ratio. This latter effect is suggested as the reason for improved growth response in older birds fed rice bran when extra calcium is added to the diet.

f) Bakery by-product

Bakery meal is a by-product of the bakery and confectionary industries, and so considerable quantities are often available in large urban areas. Unfortunately the composition of bakery by-product can vary considerably, because of variation in raw ingredients used, and also the potential inclusion of inert fillers. The meal can vary considerably in fat content and also in fiber and ash depending upon fillers used to improve flow characteristics of high fat meals. If soybean hulls are used, the meal will be high in fiber, whereas when limestone is used ash and calcium levels are elevated. The AMEn will obviously be less as the fiber and/or ash content increase:

AMEn (kcal/kg) = 4000 - [100(% fiber) + 25 (% ash)]

Quality control procedures necessarily involve monitoring fiber and ash content. Bakery by-product meal can also be very high in sodium content, because of inherently high salt content of some raw ingredients such as potato chips. Because of subsequent problems with water intake, the meal should be checked periodically for sodium content.

g) Molasses

Molasses is a by-product of the sugar refining industry, where either sugar beet or sugar cane are used as raw materials. Because of a high water content and concomitantly low energy value, it is only used extensively in poultry diets in areas close to sugar refineries. The molasses usually available for animal feeding is called final or blackstrap molasses, which is the product remaining after all sugar has been extracted for human consumption. Depending upon local conditions, high-test and type A and B molasses are sometimes available. The high-test product is basically unrefined cane or beet juice that has had its sugars inverted to prevent crystallization. Type A and B molasses are intermediate to final molasses. The energy level of molasses decreases as more and more sugar is extracted. Molasses is usually quantitated with a Brix number, measured in degrees, and these numbers relate very closely to the sucrose concentration in the product. Both cane and beet molasses contain about 46 - 48% sugar.

Although molasses contains relatively little energy and protein, it can be used to advantage to stimulate appetite and to reduce dustiness of feed. For example, feed intake is usually increased in birds such as young Leghorn pullets, if molasses is poured directly onto feed in the feed trough. It is doubtful that molasses improves taste of feed under these conditions, rather it presents a novel feed texture to the bird. A major problem with molasses is a very high potassium content, at 2.5 - 3.5%, which has a laxative effect on birds. While most birds perform well on balanced diets containing up to 20% molasses, inclusion levels much above 4% will likely result in increased manure wetness.

8.2 VEGETABLE PROTEINS

a) Soybean meal

Soybean meal has become the world wide standard against which other protein sources are compared. The amino acid profile is excellent for poultry and when combined with corn or sorghum, methionine is usually the only limiting amino acid. The protein level in soybean meal can be variable, and this may be a reflection of seed variety and/or processing conditions involved in fat extraction. Traditionally the higher protein meals are produced from de-hulled beans, whereas the lower protein (44% CP) meals invariably contain the seed hulls, and are higher in fiber and lower in metabolizable energy. Whereas fat content of the seed is dictated early in seed development, protein is deposited almost to the end of maturity, therefore growing and harvesting conditions tend to have more of an effect on protein content of the seed.

During processing, soybeans are dehulled (about 4% by weight) and then cracked prior to conditioning at 70°C. The hot cracked beans are then flaked to about 0.25 mm thickness so as to enhance oil extraction by a solvent, usually hexane. Hexane must be removed from the meal because it is a highly combustible material and also a potent carcinogen.

Soybeans contain a number of natural toxins for poultry, the most problematic being trypsin inhibitor. As with most types of beans, the trypsin inhibitors will disrupt protein digestion, and their presence is characterized by compensatory hypertrophy of the pancreas. Apart from reduced growth rate and egg production, presence of inhibitors is diagnosed by a 50 - 100% increase in size of the pancreas. Fortunately, the heat treatment employed during processing is usually adequate to destroy trypsin inhibitors and other less important toxins such as hemaglutinins (lectins). In developing countries, trypsin inhibitor levels are sometimes controlled by simply fermenting or germinating beans, where after 48 hrs of treatment, protein digestibility is almost equivalent to that seen in conventionally heated beans. Trypsin inhibitor levels are usually assayed indirectly by measuring urease activity in processed soybean meal. Urease is of little consequence to the bird, although the heat sensitivity characteristics of urease are similar to those of trypsin inhibitors, and urease levels are easy to measure. Residual urease in soybean meal has therefore become the standard in quality control programs. Urease is assessed in terms of change in pH during the assay, where acceptance values range between 0.05 and 0.2. Higher values mean there is still residual urease (trypsin inhibitor) and so the test is useful to indicate undercooked meal. However, while low values indicate the inhibitors have been destroyed, there is no indication of potential overcooking, which can destroy lysine and reduce ME value. For this reason other tests are sometimes used. A fairly easy test to accomplish is protein solubility in potassium hydroxide. Dale and co-workers at the University of Georgia have shown a good correlation between the amount of protein soluble in 2% KOH, and chick growth determined in a bioassay. Heating tends to make the protein less soluble, and so high values suggest under cooking, while low values mean overcooking. Values of $\geq 85\%$ solubility indicate underprocessing and $\leq 70\%$ mean the sample has been over-processed. The assay is influenced by particle size of soybean meal and time of reaction, and so these must be standardized within a laboratory.

Over the last few years there has been growing concern about some of the less digestible carbohydrates in soybean meal. The α-galactoside family of oligosaccharides cause a reduction in metabolizable energy with reduced fiber digestion and quicker digesta transit time. Birds do not have an α -1:6 galactosidase enzyme in the intestinal mucosa. Soybean meal usually contains about 6% sucrose, 1% raffinose and 5% stachyose, none of which are well digested by the bird. Adding raffinose and stachyose to isolated soybean protein to mimic levels seen in soybean meal, causes a significant reduction in metabolizable energy. The solution to the problem relates to change in soybean processing conditions or use of exogenous feed enzymes. Extracting soybeans with ethanol, rather than hexane, removes the oligosaccharides, while there are now some galactosidase enzyme products available which are designed specifically to aid digestion of vegetable proteins.

As with the manufacture of soybean meal, soybeans must be heat processed in some way to destroy the trypsin inhibitors and also to improve overall protein digestibility. Feeding raw soybeans, or improperly processed soybeans will cause poor growth rate or reduced egg production and egg size. If processing conditions are suspect the bird's pancreas should be examined, because if trypsin inhibitors are still present, pancreas size can be expected to increase by 50 - 100%. While processed beans should be periodically tested for trypsin inhibitor or urease levels, a simple on-going test is to taste the beans. Under-heated beans have a characteristic nutty taste, while over-heated beans have a much darker color and a burnt taste. The problem with overheating is potential destruction of lysine and other heat sensitive amino acids.

b) Canola meal

Canola is a widely grown crop in western Canada and production is increasing in other parts of the world. Production increases have been influenced by the marked increase in the demand for canola oil as well as the ability of this high protein oilseed to grow in more northern climates not suitable for the production of soybeans. While canola is derived from the original rapeseed varieties, its composition has been altered through genetic selection. The level of goitrogens and erucic acid, two of the more detrimental constituents of the original rapeseed cultivars, have been markedly reduced. Erucic acid levels are now negligible while goitrogen levels are down to less than 20 µg/g. These levels are low enough to be of little or no problem to poultry. Varieties containing such levels of toxins are classified as canola. Canola still has enough goitrogen activity to result in significant increases in thyroid weight, although this does not appear to be a problem affecting the performance of poultry. The tannin levels in canola can also be relatively high at up to 3% for some cultivars. Again research has shown that the canola tannins have little influence on the utilization of the protein in diets containing appreciable levels of the meal. Canola meal also contains significant quantities (1.5%) of sinapine. While this compound poses no problem to most classes of poultry, a significant percent of brown egg birds produce eggs with a fishy and offensive odor when fed canola sinapines. One of the end products of the degradation of sinapine in the intestinal tract is trimethylamine and it is this compound which is involved in the production of fishy flavored eggs. A proportion of today's brown egg laying birds lack the ability to produce trimethylamine oxidase, and consequently the trimethylamine is deposited into the egg. Even 1% sinapine can produce off-flavored eggs. It should be pointed out that eggs produced by broiler breeders and most other medium or heavy weight birds, producing brown shelled eggs, have no problem with the utilization of sinapine containing diets.

While canola meal has been accepted by the feed industry as a high quality feedstuff for poultry, there continues to be isolated reports of increased leg problems with broilers and smaller egg size with layers. Leg problems resulting from feeding canola may be due to its having a different mineral balance than does soybean meal. The addition of dietary K, Na and in some cases Cl have, under certain conditions, altered bird performance. Canola is also high in phytic acid and thus there is speculation that the high level of this compound may be tying up zinc and so affecting bone development. The smaller egg size reported with canola meal diets seems to be a direct result of lower feed intake. Canola levels should therefore be limited in diets for very young laying hens, or at least until feed intake plateaus at acceptable levels.

Within the past few years there are reports which suggest that the high level of sulfur in canola meal may be responsible for some of the leg problems and reduced feed intake noted with canola meal diets. Canola meal contains up to 1.4% sulfur while soybean meal contains around .44%. Of the sulfur in soy, 75% is contributed by the amino acids compared to around 20% for a similar comparison for canola meal. High levels of dietary sulfur have been reported to complex intestinal calcium and lead to increased calcium excretion. This could explain the reports suggesting low availability of calcium in canola meal and possibly a factor in enhanced leg problems reported with canola diets. While lower weight gain has at times been reported with canola diets, feed:gain is little affected. This suggests that the reduction in gain was not the result of poorer diet quality but rather a direct effect on appetite, resulting in reduced feed intake.

c) Corn Gluten Meal

Corn gluten meal is a by-product of the wet milling processes of corn for the manufacture of high fructose corn syrup. Removing the energy yielding starch component and the germ yields a concentration of the original protein components. Corn gluten meal is very high in protein (60%) and as such is compared with the animal proteins during formulation. Corn gluten meal is very deficient in lysine, although with appropriate use of synthetic lysine, the product is very attractive where high nutrient density is required. Gluten meal is also very high in xanthophyll pigments (up to 300 mg/kg) and is a very common ingredient where there is a need to pigment poultry products.

d) Cottonseed Meal

Cottonseed meal is not extensively used in diets for poultry, although for obvious economic reasons it is often considered in cottonseed producing areas. A high fiber content and potential contamination with gossypol are the major causes for concern. Gossypol is a yellow polyphenolic pigment found in the cottonseed gland. In most meals, the total gossypol content will be around 1%, although of this only about 0.1% will be free gossypol. The remaining bound gossypol is fairly inert, although unfortunately binding can have occurred with lysine during processing, making both the gossypol and the lysine unavailable to the bird. So-called glandless varieties of cottonseed are virtually free of gossypol.

Birds can tolerate fairly high levels of gossypol before there are general problems with performance, although at much lower levels there can be discoloration of the egg yolk and albumen. Characteristically the gossypol causes a green-brown-black discoloration in the yolk depending upon gossypol levels, and length of egg storage. As storage time increases, the discoloration intensifies, especially at cool temperatures (5°C) where there is more rapid change in yolk pH. Gossypol does complex with iron, and this activity can be used to effectively detoxify the meal. Adding iron at a 1:1 ratio in relation to free gossypol greatly increases the dietary inclusion rate possible in broiler diets and also the level at which free gossypol becomes a problem with laying hens. Because most cottonseed samples contain around 0.1% free gossypol, detoxification can be accomplished by adding 0.5 kg ferrous sulfate/tonne of feed. With addition of iron, broilers can withstand up to 200 ppm free gossypol, and layers up to 30 ppm free gossypol without any adverse effects.

If cottonseed meal contains any residual oil, then cyclopropenoid fatty acids may contribute to egg discoloration. These fatty acids are deposited in the vitelline membrane, and alters its permeability to iron that is normally found only in the yolk. This leached iron complexes with conalbumen in the albumen, producing a characteristic pink color. Addition of iron salts does not affect this albumen discoloration, and the only preventative measure is to use cottonseed meals with very low residual fat content.

e) Peanut (Groundnut) Meal

The peanut is an underground legume and because of warm moist conditions in the soil, is very susceptible to fungal growth, with *Aspergillus* contamination being of most concern. Grown essentially for their oil, peanuts yield a solvent extracted meal containing 0.5 - 1% fat with about 47% protein. As with soybeans, peanuts contain a trypsin inhibitor that is destroyed by the heating imposed during oil extraction. Potential aflatoxin contamination is the major problem with groundnut meal. Being a potent carcinogen, aflatoxin causes rapid destruction of the liver, even at moderate levels of inclusion. Peanut meal that is contaminated with aflatoxin can be treated by ammoniation which seems to remove up to 95% of the toxin. Alternatively, products such as sodium-calcium aluminosilicates can be added to the diet containing contaminated groundnut, because these minerals bind with aflatoxin preventing its absorption.

f) Sesame meal

Sesame meal is very deficient in available lysine, and this is sometimes used to advantage in formulating lysine deficient diets for research purposes. Sesame also contains high levels of phytic acid which can cause problems with calcium metabolism leading to skeletal disorders or poor eggshell quality. If diets contain ≥10% sesame, then the diet should be formulated to contain an extra 0.2% calcium.

g) Sunflower Meal

Sunflowers are grown in cooler climates, being harvested for either oil extraction or increasingly as a source of wild bird seed. The extracted meal is very low in energy and quite deficient in lysine and also in available threonine. For meat birds the high fiber-low energy characteristics are problematic, and so maximum inclusion relates to the bird's ability to increase feed intake in order to maintain energy intake. Pelleting significantly improves feed intake of young birds fed 10% sunflower meal, and there is also an indication of improved metabolizable energy with some form of heat processing.

h) Lupins

Low alkaloid lupins are being increasingly used as an alternative feedstuff for poultry in certain areas of the world. These new cultivars have been reported to contain low levels of the toxic alkaloids (less than .01%) normally found in wild varieties. Low alkaloid lupin seeds are often referred to as sweet lupins and can either be white, yellow or blue seeded varieties. The high level of fiber in the seeds (12 to 18%) results in low metabolizable energy values compared to soybean meal. Mature lupin seeds contain little or no starch, the bulk of their carbohydrate being oligosaccharides (sugars) and non-starch polysaccharides. Many reports suggest that sweet lupins are comparable to soybeans with respect to protein quality although they are slightly lower in methionine and lysine.

i) Flaxseed

Flax is grown essentially for its oil content, although in Europe there is still some production of the fibrous plant material for linen production. Fat-extracted flax, which is commonly called linseed meal, has traditionally been used for ruminant feeds. Over the last few years there has been interest in feeding full-fat flax seeds to poultry, because of its contribution of linolenic acid. Flax oil contains about 50% linolenic acid ($18:3\omega3$) which is the highest concentration of this fatty acid outside of marine oils. It has recently been shown that $18:3\omega3$, and its desaturation products docosahexaenoic acid and eicosapentaenoic acid are important in human health, and especially for individuals at risk from chronic heart disease. Feeding flax seeds to poultry results in direct incorporation of linolenic acid into poultry meat and also into eggs. Feeding laying hens 10% flax results in a 10 fold increase in egg linolenic acid content. Linolenic acid enriched eggs therefore provide an attractive alternative to consumption of oily fish. Linolenic acid is essentially responsible for the characteristic smell of fish oils, and undoubtedly flax oil does have a "paint-type" smell.

8.3 ANIMAL PROTEINS

a) Meat Meal

Most meat meals are by-products of beef and swine processing, and can be of variable composition. For each 1 tonne of carcass meat prepared for human consumption, about 300 kg is discarded as inedible product, and of this about 200 kg ends up in meat meal. In the past, meat meal referred to only soft tissue products, while meat and bone meal also contained variable quantities of bone. Today, meat meal most commonly refers to animal by-products with bone where protein level is around 50% and calcium and phosphorus are at 8 and 4% respectively. Because the mineral comes essentially from bone, the calcium phosphorus ratio should be around 2:1, and deviations from this usually indicate adulteration with other mineral sources. Variation in calcium and phosphorus content is still problematic, and the potential for overfeeding phosphorus is a major reason for upper limits on inclusion level. Meat meals usually contain small residues of fat, and the best quality meals will be stabilized with antioxidants. Recent evidence suggests that the metabolizable energy content of meat meal, and other animal protein by-products, is higher than the most common estimates used in the past. In bioassays, ME values determined at inclusion levels of 5 - 10% are much higher than those determined at more classical levels of 40 - 50% inclusion. The reason for the higher values is unclear, although it may relate to synergism between protein or fat sources, and these are maximized at low inclusion levels. Alternatively, with very high inclusion levels of meat meal, the high calcium levels involved may cause problems with fat utilization due to soap formation, and energy retention will be reduced. The ME value shown in Table 8.1 reflects this higher energy estimate. A more recent concern with meat meal is microbial content, and especially potential for contamination with salmonella. Due to increasing awareness and concern about microbial quality, surveys show that the incidence of contamination has declined, but remains at around 15%.

b) Fish meals

Because of the decline in commercial fisheries directed at human consumption, fish meals are now almost exclusively produced from smaller oily fish caught specifically for meal manufacture. Menhaden and anchovy are the main fish species used for meal manufacture, with lesser quantities of herring meal produced in Europe. Fish meal is usually an excellent source of essential amino acids, while energy level is variable and dependent upon residual oil content. Because of variable oil and protein content, expected ME value can be calculated based on knowledge of their composition in the meal

$$ME \text{ (kcal/kg)} = 3000 \pm (\text{Deviation \% fat} \times 8600) \pm (\text{Deviation \% CP} \times 3900).$$

where standard fat content is 2%, and CP is 60%. Therefore a 4% fat, 63% CP sample is expected to have an ME of 3289 kcal/kg, while a 1% fat, 58% CP sample will have an ME closer to 2836 kcal/kg. The ash content of fish meal will be predominantly calcium and phosphorus and the latter can be considered approximately 90% available, as is any phosphorus from quality animal proteins. All fish meals should be stabilized with an antioxidant.

Potential problems in feeding fish meal are taint of both eggs and meat, and gizzard erosion in young birds. With inadequately heat-treated fish meal there is also the potential problem of excessive thiaminase activity. Depending upon geographical location, taint in eggs and meat can be detected by consumers when birds are fed much more than 2 - 3% fish meal. Problems of taint will be more acute with high fat samples, and of course the problems are most acute if fish oil *per se* is used. Even at levels as low as 2.5%, some brown egg birds produce tainted eggs which may be related to the trimethylamine content of fish meal, and the genetic predisposition of certain birds failing to produce sufficient trimethylamine oxidase. Excess trimethylamine is shunted to the egg, producing a characteristic fishy taint (see canola meal). The trimethylamine content of fish meal is around 50 - 60 mg/kg, and assuming a 2.5% inclusion level, and maximum feed intake of these brown egg layers of 115g/day, means that the bird is taking in about 0.2mg/day. Each affected egg contains around 0.8 mg, and so even at 80% egg production, it is obvious that the diet contains sources of trimethylamine other than fish meal, or that there is microbial synthesis in the intestine.

A proportion of chicks fed almost any level of fish meal develop gizzard lesions (see Chapter 10 for more detailed description), although there is a strong dose relationship. Affected birds have signs ranging from small localized cracks in the gizzard lining, through to severe erosion and hemorrhage which ultimately leads to total destruction of the lining. The hard lining is required for physical processing of feed, and also acts as a barrier for the sensitive underlying mucosa against the degrading effects of acid and pepsin produced by the proventriculus. Because of disrupted protein degradation, the affected birds show very slow growth rate. The condition is most common when fish meal is included in the diet, although similar signs are seen with birds fed high levels of copper (250 ppm) or vitamin K deficient diets, or simply induced by starvation. Gizzard erosion was initially thought to be associated with histamine levels in fish meal. Feeding histamine to birds simulates the condition, as does feeding a semi-purified diet containing histidine that has been heat-treated. Fish meals contain histamine, and following microbial degradation during precooking storage, bacteria possessing histidine decarboxylase will convert variable quantities of histidine to histamine. Histamine has the effect of stimulating excessive acid production by the proventriculus, and it is this acid environment that initiates breakdown of the gizzard lining. More recently, a compound termed gizzerosine has been isolated from fish meal, and this acts like histamine in stimulating acid secretion. Gizzerosine is formed by heating histidine and a protein during manufacture of fish meal. The most common components are lysine and histidine. Gizzerosine is almost 10 x as potent as histamine in stimulating proventricular acid production and some 300 x more potent in causing gizzard erosion.

c) Poultry by-product meal(PBM)

As with meat meal, poultry by-product meal is produced essentially from waste generated during poultry meat processing. Because only one species is used, PBM should be a more consistent product than is meat meal, and certainly calcium and phosphorus levels will be lower. Variability in composition relates to whether or not feathers are added during processing, or kept separate to produce feather meal. PBM and feathers are best treated using different conditions, because feathers require more extreme heat in order to hydrolyze the keratin proteins. PBM with feathers may therefore mean that either the feather proteins are undercooked or that the offal proteins are overcooked. Overcooking usually results in a much darker colored product. PBM contains more unsaturated fats than does meat meal, and so if much more than 0.5% remains in the finished product, it should be stabilized with an antioxidant.

There is current interest in ensiling various poultry carcasses and/or poultry by-products prior to heat processing. Ensiling allows for more control over microbial contamination prior to processing, and allows the potential to better utilize smaller quantities of poultry carcasses on-farm or from sites more distant to the PBM processing plant. Ensiling is also being considered as a means of handling spent layers prior to production of PBM. Poultry carcasses or offal do not contain sufficient fermentable carbohydrate to allow lactic acid fermentation which will quickly reduce pH to about 4.2, and stabilize the product. These lactic acid producing mircrobes can therefore be encouraged to proliferate by adding, for example, 10% molasses or 10% dried whey to ground carcasses. These mixtures quickly stabilize at around pH 4.2 - 4.5, and can be held for 10 - 15 d prior to manufacture of PBM. Carcasses from older birds may require slightly higher levels of these carbohydrates, and because of their inherently high fat content may be mixed with products such as soybean meal in order to improve handling characteristics. Ensiled whole carcasses, as are currently produced with spent fowl, may present problems with availability of feather proteins for reasons outlined previously in terms of ideal processing conditions for tissue versus feathers. In the future, this problem may be resolved by adding feather degrading enzymes to the ensiling mixture.

d. Feather meal

Feather meal can be an excellent source of cystine and a good source of crude protein where this is needed to meet regulatory requirements. However, its use is severely limited by deficiencies of several amino acids, including methionine, lysine and histidine. Feather meal usually contains about 4.5 - 5.0% cystine, and this should be around 60% digestible. The energy value of feather meal is quite high, being around 3300 kcal ME/kg, and Dale and co-workers at the University of Georgia suggests TMEn of feather meal is highly correlated with its fat content (2860 + 77x% fat, kcal/kg). Variability in quality is undoubtedly related to control of processing conditions. Feathers are partially dried and then steam treated to induce hydrolysis, and within reason, the higher the temperature and/or processing time, the better the chance of complete hydrolysis. Obviously extreme processing conditions will cause destruction of heat-labile amino acids such as lysine. Feather meal also contains an amino acid called lanthionine, which is not normally found in animal tissues. Total lanthionine levels can therefore be used in assaying meat meal type products for potential contamination with feathers. Lanthionine can occur as a breakdown product of cystine, and there are some research results which indicate a very good correlation between high lanthionine levels and poor digestibility of most other amino acids. In most feather meal samples, lanthionine levels should be at 20 - 30% of total cystine levels. A potential problem in using lanthionine assays in quality control programs, is that it is readily oxidized by performic acid, which is a common step used in preparation of samples for amino acid analysis and particularly where cystine levels are of interest. Treating feathers with enzyme mixtures that presumably contain keratinase enzyme, has been shown to improve overall protein digestibility and bird performance. More recently it has been shown that a pre-fermentation with bacteria such as *Bacillus licheniformis* for 5 d at 50ºC, produces a feather lysate that is comparable in feeding value to soybean meal when amino acid balance is accounted for.

8.4 FATS AND OILS

F ats provide a concentrated source of energy, and so relatively small changes in inclusion levels have meaningful effects on diet ME. Depending upon the demands for pellet durability, 3 - 4% is the maximum level of fat that can be mixed with the other diet ingredients. To this, 2 - 3% can be added as a spray-on coat to the formed pellet. Fats also provide varying quantities of the essential nutrient linoleic acid. Unless a diet contains considerable quantities of corn, it may be deficient in linoleic acid, because all diets should contain a minimum of 1% linoleic acid. A major problem facing the feed industry at the moment is the increasing use of restaurant grease in feed grade fats. These greases are obviously of variable composition in terms of fatty acid profile and their content of free fatty acids. Also, dependent upon the degree of heating that they have been subjected to, these greases can contain significant quantities of undesirable break-down products. In order to ensure adequate levels of linoleic acid, and to improve palatability and reduce dustiness of diets, all diets require a minimum of 1% added fat, regardless of other economic or nutritional considerations.

Feed grade fats will always contain some non-fat material, that is generally termed moisture, impurities and unsaponifiables (M.I.U). Because these impurities impart no energy or little energy, they act as diluents. The feeding value of fats can obviously be affected by oxidative rancidity that occurs prior to, or after feed preparation. Rancidity can influence the organoleptic qualities of fat, as well as color and texture, and can cause destruction of other fat soluble nutrients, such as vitamins, both in the diet and the body stores. Oxidation is essentially a degradation process that occurs at the double-bond in the glyceride structure. Because presence of double-bonds infers unsaturation, then naturally the more unsaturated a fat, the greater the chance of rancidity. The initial step is the formation of a free radical when hydrogen leaves the α-methylenic carbon in the unsaturated group of the fat. The resultant free radical then becomes very susceptible to attack by atmospheric oxygen (or mineral oxides) to form unstable peroxide free radicals. These peroxide free radicals are themselves potent catalysts, and so the process becomes autocatalytic and rancidity can develop quickly. Breakdown products include ketones, aldehydes and short chain fatty acids which give the fat its characteristic rancid odor. Animal fats develop a slight rancid odor when peroxide levels reach 20 meq/kg while for vegetable oils problems start at around 80 meq/kg. Oxidative rancidity leads to a loss in energy value, together with the potential degradation of the bird's lipid stores and reserves of fat soluble vitamins. Fortunately we have some control over these processes through the judicious use of antioxidants.

Fat composition will influence overall fat utilization because different components can be digested with varying efficiency. It is generally recognized that following digestion, micelle formation is an important prerequisite to absorption of fat into the portal system (Chapter 1). Micelles are complexes of bile salts, fatty acids, some monoglycerides and perhaps glycerol. The conjugation of bile salts with fatty acids is an essential prerequisite for transportation to and absorption through the microvilli of the small intestine. Polar unsaturated fatty acids and monoglycerides readily form this important association. However, micelles themselves have the ability to solubilize non-polar compounds such as saturated fatty acids. Fat absorption is, therefore, dependent upon there being an adequate supply of bile salts and an appropriate balance of unsaturates:saturates. Taking into account the balance of saturated to unsaturated fatty acids, can therefore be used to advantage in designing fat blends.

Concern is often raised about the level of free fatty acids in a fat, because it is assumed these are more prone to peroxidation. Acidulated soapstocks of various vegetable oils contain the highest levels of free fatty acids, which can reach 80 - 90% of the lipid material. Free fatty acids are more problematic when the fat is predominantly saturated and is fed to young birds. Hydrogenation of fats also becomes an issue with the general use of these fats in restaurants, and the fact that restaurant grease is now a common, and sometimes the major component of feed grade fat blends. Hydrogenation results in a high level of trans oleic acid (40 - 50%) and such treated vegetable oils have physical characteristics similar to those of lard. There seems to be no problem in utilization of these hydrogenated fats by poultry with ME values of restaurant greases being comparable to that of vegetable oils. The long-term effect of birds eating trans fatty acids is unknown at this time. It seems obvious that the use of a single value for fat ME during formulation is a compromise. Table 8.6 gives different ME values for birds younger or older than 21 d.

Tallow has traditionally been the principle fat source used in poultry nutrition. However, over the last 20 years, there has been less use of pure tallow and greater use of blended oils. Being highly saturated, it is not well digested by young chickens. The digestibility of tallow can be greatly improved by the experimental addition of bile salts suggesting this to be a limiting feature of young chicks. However, the use of such salts is not economical and so inclusion of pure tallow must be severely restricted in diets for birds less than 15 - 17d of age. Poultry fat is perhaps the best animal type fat for use in poultry diets. There is current interest in the use of fish oils in diets for humans and animals since its unusual component of long chain fatty acids is thought beneficial for human health. Feeding moderate levels of fish oils to broiler chickens has been shown to increase the eicosapentaenoic acid content of meat. However, with dietary levels in excess of 1%, a distinct fish type odor is often present in both meat and eggs, which is due mainly to the contribution of the omega-3 fatty acids.

TABLE 8.6 Composition of fat sources

| Ingredient | Metabolizable energy (kcal/kg) | | Fat | M.I.U.[5] | Fatty acid profile (%) | | | | | | | |
	1[1]	2[2]	%	%	12:0	14:0	16:0	18:0	16:1	18:1	18:2	18:3
Tallow	7400	8000	98	2		4.0	25.0	24.0	0.5	43.0	2.0	0.5
Poultry fat	8200	9000	98	2		1.0	20.0	4.0	5.5	41.0	25.0	1.5
Fish oil	8600	9000	99	1		8.0	21.0	4.0	15.0	17.2	4.4	3.0[3]
Vegetable oil	8800	9200	99	1		0.5	13.0	1.0	0.5	31.0	50.0	2.0
Coconut oil	6500	7800	99	1	50.0[4]	20.0	6.0	2.5	0.5	4.0	2.1	0.2
Palm oil	7200	8000	99	1		2.0	42.4	3.5	0.7	42.1	8.0	0.4
Vegetable soapstock	7800	8100	98	2		0.3	18.0	3.0	0.3	29.0	46.0	0.8
Animal-Vegetable blend	8200	8600	98	2		2.1	21.0	15.0	0.4	32.0	26.0	0.6
Restaurant grease	8100	8900	98	2		1.0	18.0	13.0	2.5	42.0	16.0	1.0

[1]ME for young birds up to 3 weeks of age
[2]ME for birds after 3 weeks of age
[3]Contains 25% unsaturated fatty acids ≥ 20:4
[4]Contains 15% saturated fatty acids ≤ 10:0
[5]Moisture, impurities, unsaponifiables

A range of vegetable oils is available as an energy source, although under most situations, competition with the human food industry makes them uneconomic for animal feeds. Most vegetable oils provide around 8700 kcal ME/kg and are ideal ingredients for very young birds. If these oils are attractively priced as feed ingredients, then the reason(s) for refusal by the human food industry should be ascertained i.e, contaminants. Coconut oil is a rather unusual ingredient in that it is a very saturated oil, being more saturated than tallow. It contains 50% of saturated fatty acids with chain length less than 12:0. In many respects, it is at the opposite end of the spectrum to fish oil in terms of fatty acid profile. There has been relatively little work conducted on the nutritional value of coconut oil, although due to its saturated fatty acid content it will be less well digested, especially by young birds. Palm oil production is now only second to soybean oil in world tonnage. Palm oil is produced from the pulpy flesh of the fruit, while smaller quantities of palm kernel oil are extracted from the small nuts held within the body of the fruit. Palm oil is highly saturated, and so will have limited usefulness for very young birds. Also, soapstocks produced from palm oil, because of their free fatty acid content, will be best suited for older birds. There is potential for using palm and coconut oils as blends with more unsaturated oils and soapstocks, so as to benefit from potential fatty acid synergism.

An increasing proportion of feed fats is now derived from cooking fats and oils, and the generic product is termed restaurant grease. Their use has increased mainly due to problems of alternate disposal. Traditionally restaurant greases were predominately tallow or lard based products and this posed some problems in collection and transportation of solid fats. In recent years due to consumer concerns about saturated fats, most major fast food and restaurant chains have changed to hydrogenated vegetable cooking fats and oils. The fats are hydrogenated to give them protection against high temperature cooking. Today, restaurant greases contain higher levels of oleic acid, and much of this will be trans-oleate. Assuming there has not been excessive heating, and that the grease has been cleaned and contains a minimum of M.I.U, then the energy value will be comparable to that of poultry fat.

8.5 MINERAL SUPPLEMENTS

The bird's need for calcium, phosphorus, sodium and trace minerals will be accomodated by supplements containing concentrated sources of these nutrients. Calcium and phosphorus are usually fed as limestone and dicalcium phosphate respectively, while sodium needs are met by the addition of salt. The trace minerals are usually added to diets as a composite premix. Composition of such mineral supplements are shown in Table 8.7.

Table 8.7 Composition of mineral supplements					
Ingredient					
Calcium, Phosphorus		**%Ca**		**%P**	
Limestone		38.0		-	
Oyster shell		38.0		-	
Monocalcium phosphate		17.0		25.0	
Dicalcium phosphate		23.0		20.0	
Defluorinated rock phosphate		34.0		19.0	
Salt		**%Na**		**%Cl**	
Plain salt		39.0		60.0	
Iodized salt		39.0		60.0(I,70 mg/kg)	
Cobalt iodized salt		39.0		60.0(I,70 mg/kg; Co, 40 mg/kg)	
Sodium bicarbonate		27.0			

Trace Minerals	Form	% Major mineral	Trace Minerals	Form	% Major mineral
Cobalt	oxide	71.0	Zinc	oxide	78.0
	chloride	24.0		chloride	48.0
	sulphate	21.0		sulphate	36.0
	carbonate	46.0		carbonate	52.0
Copper	oxide	79.0	Selenium	sodium selenite	46.0
	chloride	37.0		sodium selenate	42.0
	sulphate	25.5			
	carbonate	55.0			
Iron	oxide	77.0	Iodine	potassium iodine	77.0
	chloride	34.0		calcium iodate	65.0
	sulphate	32.0			
	carbonate	40.0			

a) Calcium and phosphorus

There has been considerable controversy concerning the relative potency of limestone vs oyster shell as sources of calcium, especially for the laying hen. Perhaps of more importance than the source of calcium, is particle size. Usually the larger the particle size, the longer the particle will be retained in the upper digestive tract. This means that the larger particles of calcium are released more slowly, and this may be important for the continuity of shell formation, especially in the dark period when birds are reluctant to eat. Oyster shell is a much more expensive ingredient than limestone, but it offers the advantage of being clearly visible in the diet to the egg producer and so there is less chance of omission during feed manufacture. Birds also have some opportunity at diet self selection if oyster shell is given, and this may be of importance in maintaining optimum calcium balance on egg-forming versus non egg-forming days. Limestone should be in as large a particle size as can be readily manipulated by the bird's beak. Dolomitic limestone contains at least 10% magnesium, and this complexes with calcium or competes with calcium for absorption sites. The consequence of feeding dolomitic lime-stone is induced calcium deficiency, usually manifested by poor skeletal growth or egg shell quality.

A considerable number of inorganic phosphorus sources are used around the world. Most naturally occurring phosphate sources are unavailable to the bird unless they are heat treated during processing. Insoluble phosphate sources are unlikely to be available to the bird, however, solubility is not a guarantee of subsequent availability. Solubility tests are therefore only useful in screening out insoluble sources. Tests for biological availability are much more complex, because they necessarily require a chick bioassay during which growth and bone ash are measured. The phosphorus in most phosphate sources, with the exception of soft phosphate, can be regarded as close to 100% available. Rock phosphate and curaco phosphate are the major exceptions because these products may only be 60 - 65% available to the bird. Some rock phosphates contain various contaminants, the most common being vanadium. At just 7 - 10 ppm of the diet, vanadium will cause loss in internal egg quality. At slightly higher levels (15 - 20 ppm), there is a change in the shell structure where the shell takes on a somewhat translucent appearance, and appears more brittle. Rock phosphates can also contain as much as 1.5% fluorine. Because fluorine can influence calcium metabolism, there are often regulations governing the maximum permissable levels in feed. Only de-fluorinated rock phosphates are recommended although it must be remembered that this product usually contains about 5% sodium. Most mineral sources are detrimental to the pelleting process because they create significant friction at the pellet die. With phosphates, there is a distinct advantage to using rock phosphates rather than mono-or dicalcium phosphate in terms of pelleting efficiency. Numerous studies show a 10% increase in pellet throughput and energy saving with rock phosphates. However because of shorter dwell time in the steam conditioning chamber, pellet quality will deteriorate unless changes are made to the production system.

b) Sodium

Most diets contain supplemental salt, usually in the form of sodium chloride. Where iodine is not added as a separate ingredient, iodized salt must be used. In most countries the various salt forms are differentiated by color, with common salt being a natural white color, and iodized salt being red. Blue cobalt iodized salt is often used in diets for swine and ruminants, and this can be used without any problems for poultry. Because high levels of sodium chloride can lead to increased water intake, then a substitution of sodium bicarbonate for a portion of this chloride salt has been shown to be beneficial. Under these conditions, up to 30% of the supplemental salt can be substituted with sodium bicarbonate without loss in performance, and such birds often produce drier manure. For inclusions of sodium bicarbonate above 30%, care must be taken to balance the chloride levels. Chloride contributed by ingredients such as choline chloride and lysine-HCl should be accommodated during formulation.

c) Trace minerals

Trace minerals are available in a variety of forms, and periodically problems arise due to lack of knowledge of the composition, and/or stability of mineral salts. Most research into mineral availability has been conducted with the so-called reagent-grade form of minerals, which are very pure and of known composition and purity. Unfortunately, the feed industry cannot afford the luxury of such purity, and so obviously, feed grade forms are used.

One of the most important factors to ascertain prior to formulation is the state of hydration of a mineral. Many mineral forms contain bound water which obviously dilutes the effective mineral concentration. For example, hydrated cupric sulfate (white crystal) contains about 40% copper, whereas the more common pentahydrate (blue) contains 26% copper. It should also be emphasized that the various processing conditions used in manufacturing will likely reduce the biological availability.

Because feed manufacturers are often concerned about space in the diet during formulation, there is a trend towards making very concentrated mineral and vitamin premixes. In considering concentration of mineral sources, oxides appear attractive, since they invariably contain the highest mineral concentration. Oxides however are potent oxidizing agents, and if stored with premixed vitamins for any length of time, can cause the destruction of vitamins that are susceptible to oxidation. Since oxides are generally less available than other mineral salts, they should not be used exclusively in mineral premixes.

Trace minerals are sometimes used as chelated compounds. Chelates are mixtures of mineral elements bonded to some type of carrier such as an amino acid or polysaccharide. These carriers, or ligands, have the ability to bind the metal, usually by covalent bonding through amino groups or oxygen. The chelate usually has a ring structure with the divalent or multivalent metal held strongly or weakly through two or more covalent bonds. The uptake of chelated minerals is claimed to be more consistent, and less affected by adverse environments in the gut lumen. Bioavailability of minerals from chelates should also be consistent, because of standardization during manufacture, versus less standard conditions with some supplies of inorganic salts. There are also claims of chelated minerals being used more effectively at the cellular level, following absorption. There are few classical supporting claims for these suppositions, and so enhanced performance of meat birds and layers is discussed in terms of stimulation of various biological processes by the mineral and/or that the chelated mineral enters certain pools with greater affinity or efficiency.

8.6 SYNTHETIC AMINO ACIDS

Synthetic sources of methionine and lysine are now used routinely in poultry diets, and tryptophan and threonine will likely be used more frequently as future prices decline. In most situations, the use of synthetic amino acids is an economic decision, and so their price tends to shadow that of soybean meal, which is the major protein (amino acid) source used world wide. By the year 2002, lysine use in N. America is estimated at just over 100,000 tonnes while that for methionine will be around 80,000 tonnes, of which 40 - 75% are used in poultry diets.

Lysine is usually produced as the hydrochloride salt, and consequently, the commercial products have 79% lysine activity on a weight basis. Tryptophan may become a limiting nutrient as crude protein levels of diets are reduced. Tryptophan levels in ingredients and feed are much more difficult to assay than are the other common amino acids, and in part, this situation leads to variability in research results aimed at quantitating the response to tryptophan. This amino acid is most likely to be considered when diets contain appreciable quantities of meat or poultry by-product meal. Methionine is available in a number of forms and also as an analogue. Over the years there has been considerable research into the potency and use of these various sources. With the exception of lysine and threonine, which are not involved in transamination processes, it is possible to replace amino acids with their keto acid analogues. The bird produces the corresponding amino acid by transamination involving mainly non-essential amino acids such as glutamic acid. Such transamination can occur in various tissues, and some bacteria in the intestine may also synthesize amino acids prior to absorption. The question of the relative potency of products such as methionine hydroxy analogue (eg. Alimet®) often arises in selection of methionine sources.

8.7 FEED FORMULATION

Formulation is the mathematical exercise of establishing a blend of ingredients that meet the bird's nutrient requirements. In order to accomplish this task, the nutritionist must:

a) decide which nutrients are essential for the bird

b) establish requirement values for these nutrients using some quantifiable units

c) establish which ingredients are available for feed production

d) quantify nutrient levels and cost of these ingredients

e) establish the mathematical blend of ingredients that meet the bird's nutrient needs as previously established.

As will be discussed later in this section, there are also a number of practical feed mixing and manufacturing factors that have to be considered, but essentially the above basic steps must be repeated each time a diet is manufactured.

In most situations the solution to the formulation will be a least-cost diet. Depending upon the number of ingredients considered, there can be a number of possible solutions so as to meet the bird's nutrient requirements. However, if the cost of each ingredient is included in the input data, then the potential solutions (that all meet the bird's nutrient needs) can be ranked according to cost. The cheapest diet, or the least-cost diet, is the solution provided by the formulation program. Figure 8.1 shows an example formulation for a broiler starter diet.

The formulation report is divided into two sections. The upper portion (Fig 8.1) shows the actual quantity of ingredients used, while the lower section details the nutrient profile of the diet in relation to requirements. Most formulation reports provide a great deal of information about the diet, and especially economic considerations.

The ingredients used are listed in order of quantity in the diet. Corn represents about 50.8% of the diet, soybean meal 28% etc., and these total 100%, and in this exercise quantities total 1,000 kg. The cost of each ingredient is shown with units in $/100 kg. Corn therefore is at $125/tonne. The low and high range columns indicate the price spread at which the ingredient usage rate will remain unchanged. Therefore the high range of $150 for corn, indicates that the quantity of corn used (50.8%) will not change until the price of corn reaches $150/tonne. The range for soybean meal is $228.4 - 324.7/tonne.

The top right-hand column shows ingredient minimum and maximum levels. These values are dictated prior to formulation, and override all other mathematical calculations. In this formulation, there is a 10% minimum and a 10% maximum imposed on wheat shorts. This effectively gives the program no option but to use 10% wheat shorts - for the broiler starter this is to ensure good pellet quality. There is a 5% maximum imposed on meat and bone meal. In this situation, the maximum is due to potential variability in the ingredient, and so the 5% max is something of an insurance value. Fat has a 1% minimum, meaning that regardless of cost, and nutrient contribution, there must be 1% fat added to this diet. The vitamin-mineral premix is forced into the diet at 1%, because this is the level necessary to provide all its component nutrients.

Detailed between the two major components of the report, is information on rejected ingredients, namely corn gluten meal and calcium phosphate. Both ingredients are unused, because they are too expensive in relation to the selected ingredients. For example corn gluten meal has a current cost of $41/100kg, and the report indicates that it will not be considered unless the price declines to $28.84/100kg.

Rounded Amount	Ingredient Num	Ingredient Name	Percent of Mix	Cost/ 100 Kg	Range Low	Range High	Ingredient Min.	Ingredient Max.
508.42	1	Corn	50.872	12.50		15.00		
280.55	30	Soy 48	28.055	24.50	22.84	32.47		
100.00	21	Wheat Shorts	10.000	10.00			10.0	10.0
46.23	57	Meat & Bone	4.623	32.00	21.92	34.03		5.0
39.91	71	A-V Fat	3.991	30.00	20.39	63.43	1.0	
10.00	95	Vitamin-Min	1.000	100.00			1.0	1.0
8.92	80	Limestone	0.892	3.50		40.44		
3.51	83	Salt	0.351	10.00		869.63		
2.20	60	Alimet	0.190	300.00	21.41	642.34		
0.26	61	L-Lysine	0.026	200.00	36.77	307.58		
1000.00	Total Weight		$185.99 per Tonne					
	14	Corn Gluten Meal	41.00	28.84				5.0
	81	Dicalphosphate	45.00	37.44				

Num	Restriction[1]	Unit	Min.	Actual	Max.	Nutrient Cost
1	Weight	kg	1.00	1.00	1.00	
2	ME Poultry	kcal/kg	3000.00	3000.00		0.04599
5	Crude Protein	%	22.00	22.00		0.12216
8	Calcium	%	0.90	0.90	0.97	0.23446
10	Av. Phos.	%	0.40	0.40		2.09374
11	Methionine	%	0.50	0.54		
12	Meth and Cyst	%	0.85	0.85		2.84406
13	Lysine	%	1.20	1.20		2.30624
14	Arginine	%		1.47		
15	Tryptophan	%		0.28		
17	Leucine	%		1.79		
18	Isoleucine	%		1.12		
21	Threonine	%		0.88		
22	Valine	%		1.08		
24	Linoleic Acid	%	1.00	1.72		
25	Vit A	IU/kg	8000.00	8800.00		
26	Vit D3	IU/kg	1500.00	3300.00		
27	Vit E	IU/kg	11.00	58.75		
28	Vit K	mg/kg	1.50	3.30		
29	Choline	mg/kg	900.00	2197.79		
33	Folic Acid	mg/kg	0.90	1.39		
34	Biotin	mg/kg	0.20	0.39		
35	Niacin	mg/kg	20.00	78.07		
38	Xanthophyll	mg/kg		12.72		
39	Manganese	mg/kg	55.00	110.38		
40	Iron	mg/kg	30.00	60.11		
41	Copper	mg/kg	5.00	22.77		
42	Zinc	mg/kg	50.00	114.20		
43	Selenium	mg/kg	0.30	0.45		
44	Sodium	g/kg	2.10	2.10	2.10	
45	Potassium	g/kg		8.86		
48	Chloride	g/kg	2.20	2.69		
50	Dry Matter	%		89.16		
	Not all nutrients listed					

Figure 8.1 Least Cost Formulation

The remaining lower portion of the formulation report (Fig 8.1) details the nutrient profile of the diet. The nutrients of interest are listed in the left hand column, together with units of measurement. Minimum and maximum levels are dictated prior to formulation. In this exercise there is a minimum requirement for crude protein of 22% and for metabolizable energy of 3000 kcal/kg. In most situations it is unnecessary to specify a maximum nutrient level, because working against cost, the solution is unlikely to provide more than is necessary. In this formulation, there is only a maximum given for calcium (0.97%) because there is concern about maintaining the calcium:phoshorous levels.

Not all essential amino acid levels are dictated, because it is very unusual to see deficiencies of amino acids other than those specified, especially when a crude protein minimum is used.

The actual level of nutrients provided are shown in the next column. The actual levels will always be equal to, or exceed, the minimum levels. If any nutrient is deficient, then the formula becomes infeasible ie: a solution cannot be made with the ingredients selected. For an infeasible solution, the options are to seek more ingredients or to re-evaluate the minimum nutrient levels demanded. The final column shows a nutrient cost, indicating that this specific nutrient is a pressure point on economics. The highest value is shown for methionine + cystine at $2.84/0.1%. Therefore reducing the need for this nutrient by 0.1% will reduce feed cost by $2.84/tonne. However, reducing the methionine + cystine level will likely lead to reduced performance, and so the nutritionist is faced with the final decision. Most formulation programs have an option known as parametrics: this allows the operator to view price changes of the diet in relation to variable nutrient levels or ingredient use. For example, it is possible to see price changes in a diet using lysine levels of from 1.1 to 1.3% in increments of say 0.01%. Likewise, it is possible to determine price changes that occur as a result of changing the inclusion level of an ingredient such as wheat shorts.

8.8 DIET SPECIFICATIONS AND DIET INGREDIENT COMPOSITION

K nowledge about nutrition of the chicken is ultimately used in preparing diets. From a consideration of information about the bird's nutrient needs, together with comparable data on ingredient composition and nutrient availability, it is possible to prepare diet specifications. Tables 8.8 - 8.15 provide examples of such specifications for pullets, layers, broilers and broiler breeders. There are hundreds of possible ingredient combinations which will produce these specifications, although world-wide there are more likely to be 20-30 major variations, since ingredient usage is limited. Examples of diets are shown in the following tables using corn or wheat as the major cereal choice. The actual number of nutrients needed to be considered in these specifications is also quite small. The vitamins and trace minerals will be accommodated by addition of appropriate premixes, and so the only minerals of major importance are calcium, phosphorus and sodium. If acid-base balance is a consideration, then chloride, potassium and perhaps sulfur levels will be included in diet specifications. Tables 8.8, 8.10, 8.12 and 8.14 list all essential amino acids. However, the most important amino acids are usually lysine, methionine and cystine, because they are first limiting for most ingredient combinations. There is no substitute for consideration of metabolizable energy specifications, and in practice the levels of most other nutrients will be tied to this specification. If for

TABLE 8.8 Diet specifications for growing egg-strain pullets			
	Chick Starter (0-8 wk)	Chick Grower (8-15 wk)	Pre-lay (15-17 wk)
Approximate protein level (%)	18	15	17
Amino acids (% of diet)			
Arginine	1.05	0.80	0.80
Lysine	0.93	0.72	0.70
Methionine	0.45	0.34	0.40
Methionine + cystine	0.75	0.60	0.70
Tryptophan	0.19	0.16	0.17
Histidine	0.33	0.28	0.30
Leucine	1.16	0.95	1.00
Isoleucine	0.62	0.51	0.55
Phenylalanine	0.58	0.48	0.51
Phenylalanine + tyrosine	1.13	0.93	1.00
Threonine	0.60	0.52	0.50
Valine	0.69	0.67	0.67
Metabolizable energy (kcal/kg)	2950	2850	2850
Calcium (%)	1.0	0.85	2.0
Available phosphorus (%)	0.44	0.39	0.43
Sodium (%)	0.18	0.18	0.18

Table 8.9. Examples of Chick Starter and Grower Diets (kg)						
Ingredients	1	2	3	4	5	6
Corn	709.5	---	374.0	737.0	–	392.0
Wheat	—	796.5	372.5	—	822.0	392.0
Soybean meal (48%)	238.0	150.0	200.0	205.0	120.0	158.0
Fat	10.0	10.0	10.0	10.0	10.0	10.0
Ground limestone	15.0	15.0	15.0	15.0	15.0	15.0
Calcium phosphate (20% P)	15.0	15.0	15.0	20.0	20.0	20.0
Salt	2.5	2.5	2.5	2.5	2.5	2.5
Vitamin:mineral premix[1]	10.0	10.0	10.0	10.0	10.0	10.0
Methionine	0.88	1.25	1.10	0.8	1.0	0.8
Calculated analyses						
Crude protein (%)	17.6	17.6	17.7	16.2	16.6	16.1
Digestible protein (%)	16.0	16.0	16.1	14.8	14.9	14.7
Crude fat (%)	3.8	2.3	3.1	3.9	2.3	3.2
Crude fiber (%)	2.5	2.8	2.6	2.5	2.8	2.6
Metabolizable energy (kcal/kg)	3045	2970	3010	3059	2800	3030
Calcium (%)	0.94	0.95	0.95	1.04	1.06	1.05
Available phosphorus (%)	0.41	0.43	0.42	0.50	0.53	0.51
Sodium (%)	0.17	0.19	0.18	0.16	0.19	0.18
Methionine (%)	0.41	0.40	0.40	0.37	0.35	0.34
Methionine + cystine (%)	0.66	0.68	0.67	0.61	0.61	0.58
Lysine (%)	0.90	0.88	0.90	0.80	0.80	0.78

[1]Use additional choline if premix does not contain this vitamin

TABLE 8.10 Diet specifications for layers			
	Feed intake/day (g)		
	120	100	90
Approximate protein level (%)	14.0	17.0	19.0
Amino acids (% of diet)			
Arginine	0.60	0.75	0.82
Lysine	0.56	0.70	0.77
Methionine	0.31	0.37	0.41
Methionine + cystine	0.53	0.64	0.71
Tryptophan	0.12	0.15	0.17
Histidine	0.14	0.17	0.19
Leucine	0.73	0.91	1.00
Isoleucine	0.50	0.63	0.69
Phenylalanine	0.38	0.47	0.52
Phenylalanine + tryosine	0.65	0.83	0.91
Threonine	0.50	0.63	0.69
Valine	0.56	0.70	0.77
Metabolizable energy (kcal/kg)	2700	2800	2850
Calcium (%)	3.00	3.50	3.60
Available phosphorus (%)	0.35	0.40	0.42
Sodium (%)	0.17	0.18	0.19

TABLE 8.11 Examples of layer diets (kg)			
Ingredients	1	2	3
Corn	596.0	---	300.0
Wheat	----	682.0	360.0
Barley	---	---	---
Soybean meal (48%)	280.0	195.0	222.0
Fat	20.0	20.0	15.0
Limestone	78.0	78.0	78.0
Calcium phosphate (20% P)	11.5	11.5	11.5
Salt	3.5	2.5	2.5
Vitamin:mineral premix[1]	10.0	10.0	10.0
Methionine	1.0	1.0	0.75
Calculated analyses			
Crude protein (%)	18.6	17.9	17.8
Digestible protein (%)	17.0	16.0	16.1
Crude fat (%)	4.4	3.2	3.3
Crude fiber (%)	2.3	3.3	2.8
Metabolizable energy (kcal/kg)	2860	2768	2800
Calcium (%)	3.30	3.3	3.3
Available phosphorus (%)	0.41	0.43	0.41
Sodium (%)	0.19	0.19	0.18
Methionine (%)	0.42	0.37	0.36
Methionine + cystine (%)	0.70	0.66	0.54
Lysine (%)	1.02	0.96	0.95

[1]Use additional choline if premix does not contain this vitamin

TABLE 8.12 Broiler diet specifications				
	Pre-starter	Starter	Grower	Finisher/Withdrawal
Approximate protein level (%)	23	22	20	18
Amino acids (% of diet)				
Arginine	1.40	1.20	1.10	0.95
Lysine	1.35	1.20	1.10	0.95
Methionine	0.52	0.48	0.44	0.37
Methionine+Cystine	0.95	0.82	0.73	0.64
Tryptophan	0.22	0.20	0.17	0.14
Histidine	0.42	0.40	0.32	0.28
Leucine	1.50	1.40	1.10	1.00
Isoleucine	0.85	0.75	0.55	0.47
Phenylalanine	0.80	0.75	0.60	0.53
Phenylalanine+tyrosine	1.50	1.40	1.10	1.00
Threonine	0.75	0.70	0.60	0.55
Valine	0.90	0.80	0.65	0.58
Metabolizable energy (kcal/kg)	3000	3000	3100	3150
Calcium (%)	1.0	0.95	0.92	0.90
Available phosphorus (%)	0.45	0.42	0.40	0.38
Sodium (%)	0.19	0.18	0.18	0.18

TABLE 8.13 Examples of broiler diets (kg)						
	Starter		Grower		Finisher	
Corn	563	268	582	605	652	506
Wheat	-	200	-	-	-	270
Barley	-	200	-	-	-	-
Soybean meal (48%)	336	270	305	307	238	170
Meat Meal (50%)	20	-	30	-	20	-
Fat	35	17	46	45	47	10
Ground limestone	17	16	13	15	15	15
Calcium phosphate (20% P)	15	15	10	15	15	15
Salt	3	3	3	3	3	3
Vitamin:Mineral premix[1]	10	10	10	10	10	10
Methionine	1.2	1.0	0.8	0.6	0.6	1.0
Calculated analysis						
Crude protein (%)	22.0	22.0	21.8	20.0	18.0	16.1
Digestible Protein (%)	17.7	17.7	17.7	16.2	14.2	12.9
Crude Fat (%)	5.9	5.9	7.0	7.0	7.3	3.4
Metabolizable Energy (kcal/kg)	3060	3060	3145	3146	3200	3050
Calcium (%)	1.00	1.00	0.98	0.95	0.94	0.96
Av. Phosphorus (%)	0.42	0.42	0.42	0.42	0.41	0.41
Sodium (%)	0.17	0.17	0.18	0.17	0.17	0.18
Methionine (%)	0.48	0.48	0.46	0.40	0.37	0.37
Methionine & cystine (%)	0.82	0.82	0.80	0.71	0.64	0.61
Tryptophan (%)	0.31	0.31	0.30	0.28	0.25	0.22
Lysine (%)	1.25	1.25	1.27	1.10	0.96	0.78
Threonine (%)	0.94	0.94	0.94	0.86	0.78	0.65

[1]Use additional choline chloride if vitamin premix does not contain this vitamin

TABLE 8.14 Broiler breeder diet specifications

	Starter	Grower	Breeder (peak feed/bird/day, g)			Male feed
			165	155	140	
Approximate protein level (%)	18.0	16.0	15.5	16.0	16.5	12.0
Amino acids (% of diet)						
Arginine	.92	.82	.73	.78	.82	.58
Lysine	.90	.72	.60	.64	.68	.50
Methionine	.42	.38	.30	.33	.35	.23
Methionine + cystine	.74	.63	.53	.57	.60	.40
Tryptophan	.18	.14	.11	.12	.13	.10
Histidine	.19	.17	.14	.15	.16	.12
Leucine	.92	.84	.71	.75	.80	.60
Isoleucine	.75	.67	.51	.58	.62	.40
Phenylalanine	.62	.55	.41	.46	.49	.30
Phenylalanine + tyrosine	.95	.90	.65	.70	.79	.50
Threonine	.75	.70	.52	.59	.63	.40
Valine	.80	.70	.60	.62	.65	.50
Metabolizable energy (kcal/kg)	2850	2800	2850	2900	2950	2700
Calcium (%)	0.95	0.90	3.25	3.35	3.50	0.85
Available phosphorus (%)	0.42	0.40	0.38	0.39	0.40	0.35
Sodium (%)	0.18	0.18	0.18	0.18	0.19	0.18

TABLE 8.15 Examples of broiler breeder diets (kg)

	Starter	Grower	Breeder		Separate Male Feed
Corn	322	456	578	674	431
Barley	409	305	120		280
Wheat shorts	-	-	-	-	200
Soybean meal (48%)	220	190	197	210	42
Fat	10	10	10	20	10
Limestone	14	15	71	70	16
Calcium phosphate	15	15	15	14	12
Salt	3	3	3	3	3
Vitamin:Mineral premix[1]	5	5	5	5	5
Methionine	1.4	1.0	0.8	2.5	0.2
L-Lysine HCL	-	-	-	1.3	0.5
Calculated analysis					
Crude protein (%)	18.1	16.5	16.0	16.1	12.3
Digestible protein (%)	14.2	12.4	13.0	12.8	8.2
Crude fat (%)	3.1	3.3	3.3	4.3	4.3
Crude fiber (%)	4.7	3.8	3.5	2.8	4.8
Metabolizable energy (kcal/kg)	2840	2820	2850	2900	2760
Calcium (%)	0.95	0.95	3.3	3.3	0.92
Av. Phosphorus (%)	0.42	0.41	0.42	0.42	0.36
Sodium (%)	0.16	0.16	0.16	0.16	0.16
Methionine (%)	0.44	0.38	0.35	0.42	0.23
Methionine + cys (%)	0.74	0.63	0.60	0.68	0.40
Lysine (%)	0.93	0.80	0.81	0.90	0.50
Tryptophan (%)	0.27	0.23	0.23	0.24	0.17
Threonine (%)	0.73	0.66	0.67	0.72	0.46

[1]Use additional choline if premix does not contain this vitamin

example the energy level of the layer diet in Table 8.10 is changed from 2800 → 2900 kcal/kg for a bird eating 100g, then the amino acid levels etc. will have to be increased proportionally. This adjustment is necessary because it is expected that birds will eat less feed (<100g) of the higher energy diet. If the energy specification is lowered from 2800 → 2700 kcal/kg for example, then other nutrient levels are correspondingly decreased, in anticipation of birds eating more feed.

All chicken diets will contain premixes that are composed of vitamins and trace minerals. These premixes are designed to accommodate losses due to storage time, feed processing conditions and any potential anti nutrients. Specific premixes will be produced for each age and class of bird, and as an example Table 8.16 shows the specifications for young chicks and adult laying hens.

Table 8.16 Vitamin and mineral premix specifications (units per kg diet)		
	Young birds	**Laying hens**
Vitamin A (I.U)	8,000	8,000
Vitamin D$_3$ (I.U)	3,500	3,500
Vitamin E (I.U)	30	40
Vitamin K (mg)	2.0	2.0
Thiamin (mg)	4.0	2.0
Riboflavin (mg)	6.0	4.0
Pantothenic acid (mg)	14.0	10.0
Vitamin B$_{12}$ (μg)	12	10
Biotin (μg)	200	75
Niacin (mg)	40	35
Pyridoxine (mg)	4.0	3.0
Folic acid (mg)	1.0	1.0
Choline (mg)	700	1200
Manganese (mg)	70	70
Iron (mg)	80	80
Zinc (mg)	70	70
Copper (mg)	10	8
Selenium (mg)	0.3	0.3
Iodine (mg)	0.4	0.4

The premix levels may have to be adjusted depending upon the choice of ingredients. Biotin levels for example will necessarily be increased for diets containing >10% wheat. Breeder hens will likely require additional levels of some critical vitamins such as E and riboflavin. Choline is included in Table 8.16. However because it is very hygroscopic, and needed in such large quantities relative to the other vitamins, it is often added as a separate ingredient.

Measurement of Diet and Ingredient Nutrient Quality

O ptimizing the nutrient intake of all classes of poultry requires extensive information on the coment and availability of nutrients in ingredients used in formulation. While biological assay procedures are usually the most accurate and precise options, they are usually time consuming and expensive to conduct. Nutritionists are continually striving to develop rapid *in vitro* systems that mimic biological systems and in some instances these now provide reliable information.

A major decision involving nutrient analyses is frequency of assay. All assays must be conducted for a specific end point, and it is uneconomical to conduct analyses if the data does not provide useful information for the nutritionist. The frequency of sampling will obviously vary with the significance of a particular ingredient in the feed. For example, when meat meal is used extensively and represents a significant proportion of dietary amino acids, then amino acid analyses should be done more frequently. On the other hand, where a history of consistent analyses is developed, then testing can be less frequent. Table 9.1 shows a proposed schedule for chemical and biological assay of some common feed ingredients.

TABLE 9.1 Quality control schedule for ingredients

	Moisture	CP	Fat	Ca	P	Amino Acids Total	Amino Acids Digestible	ME	Other analyses
Corn	1	2	4	7	7	6	7	7	Molds-3; mycotoxins-4
Wheat	1	2	4	7	7	6	7	7	Pentosans-6
Barley	1	2	4	7	7	6	7	7	β-glucans-4
Milo	1	2	4	7	7	6	7	7	Tannins-3
Wheat-shorts	1	2	4	7	5	6	7	7	
Rice bran	1	2	2	1	7	6	7	7	Antioxidant-6
Bakery by-product	1	1	1	1	1	4	6	6	Salt-3
Canola meal	1	2	4	7	7	6	7	7	Glucosinolates-5
Soybean meal	1	1	3	4	3	5	7	7	Urease-4
Soybeans	1	3	3	7	7	6	7	7	Urease-3
Corn gluten meal	1	2	4	7	7	5	7	7	
Cottonseed meal	1	1	4	7	7	6	7	7	Gossypol-3
Peanut meal	1	1	4	7	7	6	7	7	Aflatoxin-3
Sunflower meal	1	1	4	7	7	6	7	7	
Meat meal	1	1	1	1	1	3	6	5	Salmonella-4
Fish meal	1	1	1	1	3	3	6	6	Gizzard erosion-3
Poultry by-product	1	1	1	3	3	4	6	6	
Feather meal	1	1	3	7	7	3	6	6	
Fats and oils	1		1					5	Fatty acids-3; stability-4
Limestones	1			1					
Phosphates	1			1					Vanadium-6
Salt	1								

1 = each delivery; 2 = weekly; 3 = monthly; 4 = 6x each year; 5 = 3x each year; 6 = 2x each year; 7 = yearly

For assay results to be meaningful, ingredients must be sampled accurately. For bagged ingredients, at least 4 bags per tonne, to a maximum of 20 samples per delivery, should be taken, and then these sub-samples pooled to give one or two samples that are subsequently assayed. It is always advisable to retain a portion of this mixed sample, especially when assays are conducted by outside laboratories. For bulk ingredients, there should be about 10 sub-samples taken from each delivery and again this mixed to give a representative composite for assay.

9.1 PROXIMATE ANALYSES

The most widely used method is a system termed "proximate analysis", developed by workers at the Weende Experiment station in Germany. By this method, a feedstuff is partitioned into six fractions: water, ether extract, crude fiber, nitrogen-free extract, crude protein and ash. Some of the information from proximate analyses (usually the protein, ether extract, fiber and ash values) are shown on labels, which accompany feedstuffs and complete feeds. These values represent the guarantees of quality used by the feed manufacturing industry. The methods for conducting proximate analyses are briefly described in the following paragraphs. Details can be found in Methods of Analysis, published by the Association of Official Analytical Chemists, 16th Edition (1997).

Water is usually determined by the loss in weight that occurs in a sample upon drying to a constant weight in an oven. The official methods involve drying a representative sample in a vacuum oven at 95-100°C or for 2 hours at 135°C at atmospheric pressure. The moisture content of some ingredients, which contain other volatile compounds, particularly short chain fatty acids or fat decomposition products, cannot be determined by these methods. For these feedstuffs distillation of the moisture in toluene is an acceptable method.

Although water is considered a utrient, it effectively is a diluent. Increase in moisture, therefore, reduces the total nutritional value of a feedstuff. Because water content can vary, ingredients should be compared for their nutrient content on a dry matter basis.

Ether extract is determined by extracting the dry sample with ether; the weight of the extract is determined after distilling the ether and weighing the residue. The ether extraction may be conducted with a suitable apparatus such as a Soxhlet or a Goldfisch extractor. Although this is the usual method for determining fat in feeds, ether extraction does not remove all the fats, especially phospholipids or fats bound to protein. Often acid hydrolysis followed by extraction of the hydrolysate with chloroform or ether is necessary to obtain "total" lipid values. Acid hydrolysis also liberates fat present as soap, and is more likely to liberate fat from bacterial cell walls.

Crude fiber refers to the organic residue of a feed that is insoluble after successive boiling with 0.255N H_2SO_4 and 0.313N NaOH solutions according to specified procedures. The determination of crude fiber is an attempt to separate the more readily digestible carbohydrates from those less readily digestible. Boiling with dilute acid and alkali is an attempt to imitate the process that occurs in the digestive tract. This procedure is based on the supposition that carbohydrates, which are readily dissolved by this procedure, also will be readily digested by animals, and that those not soluble under these conditions are not readily digested. At best, this is an approximation of the indigestible material in feedstuffs. Nevertheless, it is used as a general indicator in estimating the energy value of feeds. Feeds high in fiber will be low in available energy.

Crude protein is determined by measuring the nitrogen content of the feed and multiplying this by 6.25. This factor is based upon the observation that on average a pure protein contains 16% nitrogen. Thus $100/16 = 6.25$. Although this value does not give a completely accurate picture of the protein content of feeds, particularly of certain specific ingredients, it is universally used.

The nitrogen content of a feedstuff is determined usually by the Kjeldahl method. This involves conversion of the nitrogen in feedstuffs to an ammonium salt by digestion with concentrated sulfuric acid in the presence of a suitable catalyst. The ammonia is distilled from the digestion mixture into a collecting vessel after the sample is made alkaline. The amount of ammonia is determined by titration with standard acid.

Ashing of a feed sample combusts all organic constituents, leaving behind the non-volatile mineral elements. Some elements such as selenium and arsenic form volatile oxides at this temperature. These losses can be avoided if the ash is made alkaline by addition of known quantities of calcium oxide prior to ashing.

Nitrogen-free extract (NFE) is determined by subtracting from 100 the sum of the percentages of ash, crude protein, crude fiber, ether extract and water. The NFE is considered to be a measure of the digestible carbohydrates.

Proximate analysis gives some indication of the nutritive value of a feedstuff in poultry feeding. For example, a material very high in crude fiber is likely to have a low energy value, while feedstuffs low in crude fiber and high in ether extract are likely to be of high-energy value. The crude protein content of material is a good indicator of its potential value as a protein source. Unless the amino acid composition is known, however, the actual quality of the protein cannot be determined.

Certain materials such as meat meals normally contain high quantities of ash. In meatmeal and fishmeal, calcium and phosphorus may be estimated from the ash value since it consists mainly of bone ash. Thus a determination of the ash of these materials may be very useful. The proximate analysis of feedstuffs is not a precise measurement of nutritional value. Coupled with other measurements, however, and with some background as to the expected value of the ingredient, proximate analysis values are useful and provide a starting point for consideration of other in depth nutrient analyses.

Feed control programs of government agencies usually require certain information about the proximate analysis on each feed label. This usually consists of standards for crude protein, fat, fiber and ash. Feed manufacturers also conduct proximate analysis of incoming ingredients to assess their quality. It must be kept in mind, however that the proximate analysis is really an approximate analysis, and by itself cannot be considered a reliable estimate of feeding value for any particular ingredient or diet.

9.2 SEPARATION OF PLANT CONSTITUENTS INTO CELL WALL COMPONENTS AND CELL CONTENTS

The limitations of the system of proximate analysis have led to the development by Dr. P.J. Van Soest of analytical systems for the estimation of nutrient availability in plant materials. This system separates plant components on the basis of their solubility in detergent solutions. By extraction of plant materials with a neutral detergent solution, the cell contents can be separated from the cell wall constituents. Cell contents contain proteins, starches, sugars, free amino acids and lipids, which can be readily digested and absorbed by most animals. The cell walls contain cellulose, hemicellulose and lignin, which are essentially undigested by poultry. This fraction may represent the true "indigestible fiber" content of feedstuffs for poultry and other nonruminant animals.

If the plant material is extracted with an appropriate acidic detergent solution, the principle components of the residue are lignin and cellulose. These substances are essentially indigestible by poultry. The Van Soest system for determination of the indigestible components of plants is widely used in the analysis of forages and other ingredients fed to ruminant animals. To date, relatively few investigators have examined its value for predicting energy value of feed ingredients for poultry.

9.3 STARCH AND SUGAR ANALYSIS

The determination of the readily digestible carbohydrates in feeds is an alternative to chemically determining the indigestible carbohydrate components. A starch and sugar analysis has been used by Southgate (1969) to attempt to define the digestible and indigestible components of human foods. Methods for total sugars in feedstuffs are described by the AOAC (1997). Basically these methods involve water extraction of the feedstuff and the determination of total reducing sugar in the extract. A plant amylase is used to hydrolyze the starch and the resulting sugar released by the enzyme is quantitated.

9.4 CHEMICAL METHODS FOR ESTIMATION OF METABOLIZABLE ENERGY

An important measure of the relative usefulness of a feed ingredient is its metabolizable energy value. The biological procedure required to determine the metabolizable energy value of an ingredient is lengthy and expensive. An accurate method of estimating metabolizable energy value from chemical composition would be useful, particularly when new ingredients are encountered. Unfortunately, measurement of the metabolizable energy value of a feed cannot be done by determination of simple chemical compounds.

Probably the most successful method for estimation of metabolizable energy from chemical analyses was developed by Carpenter and Clegg (1956). Since this time many variations of this prediction have been developed, yet the accuracy of prediction is little improved. This method, used to estimate the energy value of cereals and cereal byproducts, is based on proximate analysis and determination for the starch and sugar content of ingredients. The equation developed by these workers is: M.E. in kcal/kg = 53 + 38 (% crude protein + 2.25 x % ether extract + 1.1 x % starch + %sugar).

The standard deviation between estimated metabolizable energy value by this formula and the biologically determined metabolizable energy is around ± 190 kcal/kg or about 5-8% of the values obtained. This prediction equation is much better than a similar formula based on NFE instead of starches plus sugars, although the prediction of ME is much less accurate for high fiber materials. Greater accuracy with such an equation for cereals could be developed if the various carbohydrate fractions other than sugar and starch, such as pectin, hemicellulose and cellulose, were considered. In view of the time involved in the measurement of ME by bioassay (see Section 9.10), such regression equations are of use in providing an initial indication of the ME value of an ingredient. However, their limitations for less commonly used ingredients should be recognized.

If all energy yielding components provide consistent amounts of energy, simple equations with no intercept or interactions seem attractive. However, this is unlikely to be the case in practical situations, because of factors such as nutrient synergism and interaction. Fiber is a good example of this situation. Fiber *per se* is likely to provide little energy to poultry, yet incorporation of fiber components into equations, invariably increases accuracy. It is likely that fiber components adversely influence digestibility of other nutrients, and this may be an age dependent effect.

A concern about chemical prediction equations is whether or not different equations are required to predict ME values for different ages of bird or different classes of ingredient or whether a single equation is sufficient. In reviewing all encompassing equations reported for complete feed, Fisher (1983) shows residual standard deviation of predicted means to range from 75 to 470 kcal/kg. Accuracy of prediction for individual ingredients are substantially less. In developing many hundreds of equations to describe ME, Fisher (1983) concludes that the so-called best equation has a standard deviation of just less than 60 kcal/kg, or about 2% for most diets. However, this equation is based on analyses for fat, protein, NDF, starch and fatty acid saturations. The latter analyses are not routinely conducted, and hence cost-benefit and time involved are less attractive.

9.5 AMINO ACID ANALYSES

E arly progress in protein nutrition was made difficult by the lack of good methods for readily determining the amino acids present in proteins. Microbiological assays of amino acids, using organisms requiring various amino acids for their growth, were very useful in obtaining values for the amino acid composition of feedstuffs, prior to the 1950's. These assay procedures, which are still very useful when many samples are to be analyzed for only a few amino acids, gave good information on the amino acid content of feed ingredients.

However, in 1954, Moore and Stein of the Rockefeller Institute published methods for determining nearly all of the amino acids in a protein hydrolysate following separation by chromatography on sulfonated polystyrene-ion exchange resins. The amino acids are separated by changing pH and ionic strength of buffers and determined quantitatively by a characteristic color reaction with ninhydrin. A reliable gas-liquid chromatographic separation and measurement of the twenty amino acids of proteins was developed by Gehrke, *et al.* (1971). For gas-liquid chromatography, it is necessary to esterify the amino acids with a volatilizing compound. Roach and Gehrke (1969) have described the procedure for the direct esterification of protein amino acids to form N-trifluoroacetyl (TFA)-N-butyl esters. These chromatographic procedures have since been automated, and it is now possible to determine the amino acids in a protein hydrolysate using highly automated analyzers. Physiological fluids can also be analyzed for free amino acids by these procedures.

The major factor influencing the precision of amino acid analyses is the destruction that occurs during hydrolysis of the protein. Tryptophan is almost completely destroyed by acid hydrolysis and can only be determined following alkaline or enzymatic hydrolysis. The acid buffers used in amino acid analyses also cause losses of tryptophan. Special precautions also must be taken against loss of methionine and cystine during hydrolysis. Performic acid oxidation is usually carried out prior to hydrolysis; such that methionine is converted to methionine sulfone and cystine to cysteic acid. Amino acids are then liberated from the proteins by hydrolysis with 6N HCl. The hydrolysate is diluted with sodium citrate buffer adjusting pH to 2.20 and individual amino acids then separated by ion exchange chromatography. For tryptophan, the protein is hydrolyzed under vacuum with 4.2N NaOH.

9.6 FATTY ACID ANALYSIS

Fatty acids are determined by gas-liquid chromatography following hydrolysis of the fat into glycerol and fatty acid components. The measurement of the fatty acid composition of fats involves the use of techniques of gas-liquid chromatography. For this determination the fat must be hydrolyzed to glycerol and its accompanying fatty acids. These fatty acids are then converted to methyl esters to enable them to be volatilized at relatively low temperatures. These mixtures of methyl esters are separated and measured in a gas chromatograph.

In principle, gas chromatography is quite simple. The column used consists of a solid inert absorbent on which a suitable liquid phase is held. This liquid phase is chosen so that the sample to be analyzed will "partition" between the gas and liquid phase, that is, will have certain affinity or solubility for the liquid phase but also show a significant vapor pressure as the sample is carried through the column by an inert carrier gas. Mixtures to be separated must have components that have different affinities or that partition between the liquid and gas phases. All common fatty acids present in the usual feed fats can be determined by appropriate chromatographic techniques.

9.7 VITAMIN ASSAYS

Because vitamins are usually present in feeds in very small amounts, and may exist in several active forms or in bound forms, their analysis may be complicated and is a very specialized task. A brief description of the general nature of the analytical methods used for the various vitamins is given in this section. These methods may involve chemical assays or biological procedure using microbes or chicks.

9.7.1 Vitamin A

The common procedure for measuring vitamin A makes use of the blue color which the vitamin gives with antimony-trichloride in the Carr-Price Reaction. While the reaction is very sensitive, it is not very specific as a number of compounds related to vitamin A will influence the results obtained, with carotenoids being the major variable. The procedure for determining vitamin A requires that saponification of the sample takes place to remove fatty acids, and then column chromatography be employed to separate the vitamin A from carotene and other related compounds and finally the reaction of the purified vitamin with antimony-trichloride. While chemical methods for determining vitamin A are quite useful in measuring the potential value of a feedstuff as a source of this vitamin, there are biological assays that have been developed which give a more precise measurement of the availability of the vitamin. Such biological assays are specially useful in determining the biological activity of vitamin A related compounds such as carotenoids.

9.7.2 Vitamin D

While there are chemical procedures for measuring vitamin D activity and more recent ones have proven fairly reliable for assaying feedstuffs, the method of choice is still a biological assay and the chick is the bird of choice in assessing supplements for poultry due to the unequal activity of vitamins D_2 and D_3 for poultry as compared to mammals. The chick assay has been standardized by the AOAC and involves feeding a standard rachitogenic ration to young chicks for 21 days. Supplements to be tested are then fed to these chicks and bone ash values compared to chicks receiving a reference standard of known vitamin D potency.

9.7.3 Vitamin E

Chemical determinations of vitamin E are complicated by the fact that many biological materials contain numerous tocopherols which differ in their biological activity as a source of this vitamin for the chick. The determination of vitamin E in feeds usually involves extraction of the feed with a lipid solvent, saponification of the extracted lipid and isolation of the α-tocopherol by thin layer chromatography, and then isolation of the tocopherol by a colorimetric reaction. Care must be taken during the assay procedure to avoid α-tocopherol losses due to oxidation.

9.7.4 Vitamin K

While chemical methods are available for determining vitamin K, these are complicated and generally unsatisfactory due to several vitamin K active compounds found in feedstuffs as well as many non-vitamin K substances that interfere with such assays. The assay of choice is thus the biological procedure using young chicks. This assay measures prothrombin time since prothrombin is the most limiting vitamin K dependent blood clotting factor in chicks. The bioassay involves adding excess thromboplastin and calcium to the blood of chicks receiving a dietary supplement of the test substances, measuring clotting time, and comparing this to clotting time of chicks receiving a standard quantity of vitamin K added to the test diet. While this method does not give an indication of the type of vitamin K active compound present, it does give a reasonable indication of the vitamin K activity of the feed or ingredient. Menadione content of feeds can be determined by chromatography (AOAC, 1997).

9.7.5 Vitamin B$_1$ (Thiamin)

The common method for determining thiamin is the thiochrome procedure. Oxidation of thiamin in an alkaline solution produces a yellow pigment which shows intense blue fluorescence under ultraviolet light. Before thiamin can be determined, it must be released from its coenzyme form, thiamin pyrophosphate which is the most common form found in feeds. This can be accomplished by the additions of protease or a suitable phosphatase, or by absorbing interfering substances on a specialized column. The eluate obtained is then oxidized by K$_3$ Fe(CN)$_6$ in the presence of a strong base. This produces the thiochrome which is dissolved in isobutanol and determined with a fluorometer.

A number of microbiological methods are used to determine thiamin. The mold *Phycomyces blakesleeanus* and a yeast, *Saccharomyces cerevisiae*, have been used successfully. The bacterium *Lactobacillus fermenti*, is sensitive to free thiamin in small quantities and 5 to 50 μg can be assayed using this organism. The flagellate protozoan, *Ochromonas donica*, is also very sensitive, measuring quantities between 0.1 and 30 μg, and it also has the advantage of measuring only true thiamin because it is insensitive to the coenzyme or the thiamin moieties. For feed control purposes, however, the thiochrome procedure is usually preferred.

9.7.6 Vitamin B$_2$ (Riboflavin)

The chemical determination of riboflavin was one of the first reliable chemical methods for estimation of a vitamin in feeds. This method, developed by Scott *et al.* (1946), is based upon several unique properties of riboflavin. (1) Riboflavin gives off an intense greenish fluorescence when exposed to light in wavelengths ranging from 440 to 500 mμ, and the intensity of the fluorescence is proportional to the concentration of riboflavin. (2) Riboflavin is stable to heat and acid and can be released from proteins by boiling in acid solution. (3) Riboflavin is stable to treatment with oxidizing agents such as potassium permanganate, which destroys most other materials capable of fluorescence in blue light. (4) Riboflavin is readily reduced to the non-fluorescent leuco form by treatment with SnCl$_2$ or Na$_2$S$_2$O$_4$. These properties are useful in a fluorometric method for determining riboflavin. Further purification of low concentrations of riboflavin by adsorption on activated magnesium silicate columns and elution with pyridine prior to treatment with potassium permanganate improves the accuracy of the method for certain high pigment materials.

Microbiological methods for riboflavin assay have also been widely used. Growth and production of lactic acid by *Lactobacillus casei* is dependent upon the presence of riboflavin in the medium. This assay is particularly useful when large numbers of samples are to be assayed.

9.7.7 Nicotinic acid (Niacin)

A colored compound formed by the rupture of the pyridine nucleus of nicotinic acid by cyanogen bromide is the basis for the AOAC method for the analysis of niacin in feedstuffs. The material in question must be hydrolyzed by strong acids to free the nicotinic acid from bound forms present in most feedstuffs. The concentration of niacin is measured colorimetrically by comparison with a standard concentration curve. Microbiological methods are used widely for assay of nicotinic acid. As in the chemical method, the nicotinic acid must be freed from bound forms before assay. *Lactobacillus plantarum* responds to both nicotinic acid and nicotinamide, whereas *Leuconostoc mesenteroides* measures only nicotinic acid.

9.7.8 Vitamin B_6 (Pyridoxine)

Since the vitamin B_6 group consists of three separate components namely, pyridoxol, pyridoxal and pyridoxamine, chemical assays for the vitamin are complicated. Thus for determination of the vitamin B_6 content in feedstuffs, animal or microbial growth assays are preferred. The amount of protein and type of carbohydrate in the diet can also affect chick bioassays if proteins containing large amounts of tryptophan, methionine or cysteine are present in a diet since the requirement for pyridoxine is increased under these conditions. The type of carbohydrate in a diet affects the response to vitamin B_6 apparently due to its effect on intestinal synthesis of the vitamin. Microbiological assays for the vitamin are complicated because most forms of vitamin B_6 are bound to various proteins, from which they must be freed. The actual method of freeing the vitamin from each type of material often needs to be investigated thoroughly before the microbiological method can be applied with confidence.

9.7.9   Pantothenic acid

Biological assays, both animal or microbiological are the only satisfactory methods for determining pantothenic acid in feedstuffs. Chick bioassays involve growth responses for chicks fed a diet containing a pantothenic supplement and comparing this with responses when chicks are fed a known quantity of the vitamin. A microbiological assay uses specific organisms that respond only to free pantothenic acid and not to the coenzyme or to the conjugated forms of the vitamin found in natural feedstuffs. Thus, it is necessary to liberate free pantothenic acid by treatment with enzymes prior to the assay. Such enzymes are required to hydrolyze the amine bond between pantothenic acid and the mercaptoethylamine in coenzyme A.

9.7.10 Biotin

No satisfactory chemical test has been developed for the determination of biotin in feedstuffs and so microbiological tests are used. Biotin, like other vitamins is found in coenzyme forms and so it must be released from these forms prior to assay by autoclaving with sulfuric acid. The preferred organism for microbiological assay is *Lactobacillus plantarum*. Since unsaturated fatty acids such as oleic acid can replace biotin as a growth factor for this microorganism, ether extraction of the sample must be carried out prior to assay. Biological assays using chick growth also can be used.

9.7.11 Folic acid

The chemical determination of folic acid is complicated because of the variety of forms that exist in feed ingredients. Microbiological assays are often used to determine its concentration in feedstuffs. As with other vitamins, it must be freed from its conjugated forms before it can be adequately assayed. Biological assays using rats or chicks can also be used to estimate folic acid content of feedstuffs. The biological responses may be survival, prevention of perosis, blood hemoglobin levels, growth or feathering. Growth assays or measurements of blood hemoglobin responses are probably the most reproducible and simplest of the biological assays using chicks.

Folic acid in tissues and serum also can be measured using a radiometric assay that makes use of a folic acid binding protein in cow's milk. The method is based on the principle that the amount of radioactive folate taken up by the binding protein will vary with the level of nonradioactive folate present in the sample. The method is highly specific and very sensitive. It may be used for assay of folate in feeds as the assay methodology is improved. Similar types of radiometric assays have been developed for a number of the B vitamins.

9.7.12 Vitamin B_{12}

While chemical assays have been developed for vitamin B_{12} for pharmaceutical preparations they are usually not sensitive enough to be used routinely for assaying feed ingredients. The protozoan, *Ochromonas malhamens* is commonly used for the assay of true vitamin B_{12} since it does not respond to deoxyribonucleosides or pseudo forms of vitamin B_{12} but appears to respond to the compounds required by animals as compared to other microorganisms.

Extraction of B_{12} from natural materials requires the use of techniques which can differ for various materials. Steaming and autoclaving in a buffer between pH 4.5 and 7 in the presence of cyanide has been found to be effective in releasing B_{12} from bound forms and maintains the cobalamines in the more stable cyano forms. A biological growth assay using chicks from B_{12} deficient breeders has also been developed.

9.7.13 Choline

A widely used method for assaying feed ingredients for choline involves the precipitation of choline as choline reineckate by the addition of a reinecke salt. Choline is first extracted from the sample with methanol, followed by hydrolysis to liberate choline from its phospholipid forms. Choline in the hydrolysate is then precipitated as the reinecke salt either in acid or alkaline solution. After washing, the precipitate is dissolved in acetone and measured spectrophotometrically. Sensitive microbiological methods have also been developed to assay for choline.

9.8. METHODS FOR MINERAL ANALYSIS

The analysis for mineral elements are in general relatively easy to perform as they usually involve only a single chemical entity. Advances in analytical instrumentation have simplified the analysis of many mineral elements. Because trace minerals are often present in minute amounts, one of the biggest problems affecting their precise determination is the possible contamination from other sources like water and airborne particles, and also sampling procedures from large quantities of feedstuff.

Atomic absorption spectroscopy is a powerful analytical tool available for analyzing most nutritionally important minerals. The element to be analyzed is introduced into a flame where it becomes dissociated from its chemical bonds into an unexcited, un-ionized ground state as individual atoms. The element in this state is capable of absorbing radiation at discrete bands of narrow wavelength. When a beam of light at one of these wavelengths is directed through the flames, the amount of the light absorbed is proportional to the concentration of the element being analyzed. Atomic absorption spectroscopy is very precise and very sensitive as each element has its own characteristic absorption wavelength.

Conventional wet lab analysis of feeds and feed ingredients for calcium, phosphorus, sodium, potassium, chorine, zinc, magnesium and manganese have been in use for many years. Again, such methods are fully reviewed in the latest AOAC (1997) publication. Selenium, one of the more recent and important trace minerals shown to be essential to normal well being of animals, can be detected at extremely low levels (0.01 ppm) by the latest technology developed.

A more recent development in mineral analyses has been x-ray fluorescence. Used commonly in the mining industry, this technique seems to have great potential for rapid assay of minerals in feed, following minimal sample preparation (Valdes and Leeson, 1990). Minerals fluoresce at various frequencies when bombarded with x-rays that are produced by radioactive isotopes. Much like near infrared analysis, the technique relies on a calibration of spectral intensity data which is converted to analytical concentrations by use of calibration curves or mathematical relationships. Valdes *et al.* (1985) also applied near infrared analysis for minerals in poultry feeds.

9.9 NEAR INFRARED SPECTROSCOPY (NIRS)

As detailed in the previous section, NIRS has been used to assay feeds for minerals. However, the greatest potential for this technique lies in assay of organic molecular bonds, which suggests potential for measuring protein, carbohydrates, water, fats and perhaps energy.

The use of near infrared reflectance analysis (NIRA) for determining simple components in grains and oilseeds has been used routinely over the last few years. The principle of NIRA was developed by Karl F. Norris at the U.S. Department of Agriculture, some 30 years ago and was eventually established as a new branch of agricultural chemistry. In 1976, Norris and his coworkers applied the technique for the first time in the evaluation of forage quality parameters. NIRA quickly became an ideal laboratory technique because it is very fast, inexpensive, and does not require chemical reagents or produce fumes or waste products. Similarly, there is no sample preparation except grinding and the technique does not need trained people after the calibrations are developed. Several nutrients in a sample can also be analyzed simultaneously.

NIRA relies on chemometrics, or the application of mathematics to analytical chemistry. The technique is an integration of light spectroscopy, statistics, and computer science. Mathematical models are constructed that relate composition of active chemical groups to energy absorption in the near infrared region of the spectrum (700-2500 nm). In this region, we essentially measure vibrations of hydrogen attached to atoms, such as nitrogen, oxygen or carbon. Absorption of light energy follows the Beer-Lambert Law which describes the light absorption properties of a substance in relation to the concentration of a particular constituent. Because most feedstuffs are opaque, NIRA usually uses reflectance of light instead of transmittance through the sample. The reflected light from a sample is used to indirectly quantitate the amount of light energy absorbed in a sample. NIRA measures the absorption of infrared radiation by sample components, for example, peptide bonds, at specific wavelengths in the near infrared spectrum. Other components of the sample absorb energy as well, however, and have the effect of interfering. This interference effect is eliminated by mathematical treatment of the spectral data and by multiple linear regression or other statistical procedures.

Because each molecule usually exists in its lowest energy state, absorption of energy will "excite" the molecule and raise its energy state. Such energy absorption occurs at a wavelength that is characteristic for that particular molecule. For samples of mixed composition, whether it be ingredients or complete feeds, very subtle analysis must be used to differentiate all the various chemical groupings. In the weaker absorbing NIR range of wavelengths, it is "secondary" absorption wavelengths that are considered, most often referred to as "overtones". By considering a spectra of wavelengths, a characteristic pattern of absorption (reflectance) energy is given for each major component of the sample. Chemometrics then involves calculation of correlation coefficients at each wavelength and simultaneously selecting both the best fit with the nutrient under study, and also the "best fit" of all other absorption frequencies so as to remove all interference problems.

NIRA, therefore, correlates "real" data established for a diet with energy-absorbing bands within the light spectrum under study. Why is this technique different from simple correlation with chemical analysis as described previously? Hopefully, NIRA will do more than just analyze for protein, fat, fiber, etc. and correlate with some component such as ME. For example, proteins that are complexed with carbohydrates, or fiber, will have different energy absorption characteristics and presumably such proteins may be of varying availability to the bird. NIRA, therefore, has the potential to correlate with more than just total level of constituent nutrients, or in other words, considers facets of availability. For this reason, NIRA has potential for prediction of ME, although because of the complexity of this nutrient, it does pose a major challenge (Valdes and Leeson 1991, 1992, 1994).

The usefulness of NIRA depends entirely on careful and conscientious calibration of the equipment. To some extent this exercise has been simplified through introduction of scanning machines that cover a wide band of NIR. Prior to this technology, only fixed wavelength equipment was available and so *a priori* knowledge of likely absorption bands or tedious testing of numerous wavelengths was essential in order to develop useful calibrations.

9.10 DETERMINATION OF METABOLIZABLE ENERGY

Although chemical methods are useful for analysis of feed ingredients and diets for individual nutrients, or for estimating energy value of feeds, they do not measure animal response directly. Therefore, most chemical evaluation of feedstuffs must be backed up by biological tests of the usefulness of feeds and feed ingredients. The three basic measures of the energy value of diets and of feedstuffs are digestible energy, metabolizable energy and net energy. Their relation to each other and to the gross energy of the diet was illustrated previously in Figure 2.2.

For most animals, digestible energy is easy to determine. With avian species however, true digestibility is very difficult to measure because undigested residues and urinary wastes are excreted.together. It is more convenient to determine the metabolizable energy of a diet by treating the pooled excreta as a single material representing the unutilized portion of the feed energy.

9.10.1 Classical bioassays

The method in general use for measurement of metabolizable energy of feed ingredients was developed by Hill and associates at Cornell University in the 1950's. Other methods of estimating the metabolizable energy value of feedstuffs include the "True Metabolizable Energy" (TME) value developed by Guillaume and Summers (1970) and popularized by Sibbald and colleagues. Bioassays involve the feeding of complete diets to birds over a 5-7 d period, with estimation of energy intake as feed and energy output via the excreta over this time period. Retained energy is metabolizable energy. Studies in ruminant nutrition predominated at the time when the various systems of energy evaluation were originally developed and introduced, and for this reason ME was not initially proposed as a useful system, due mainly to the practical difficulties involved in the measurement with ruminants. Of such difficulties, eructation of gaseous products of rumen metabolism was most problematic. Axelsson (1939) and Halnan (1949) indicated that production of such gases by the fowl is almost non-existent and hence the main disadvantage of using ME with ruminants, does not apply to poultry. In addition, for avian species, a system based on ME has the attraction that ME is relatively simple to determine because feces and urine are voided together. In experiments carried out with chicks, Hill and Anderson (1958) concluded that ME was "a highly precise measure of food energy for the chick" and was unaffected by plane of nutrition, whilst the estimation of productive energy (PE) was associated with a high degree of variation due to the incorrect assumptions of Fraps (1946) that PE per unit weight of diet is unaffected by plane of nutrition and that maintenance requirement per unit body weight is constant.

In the practical determination of ME by bioassay, a number of important considerations must be accommodated in the procedure. Failure to fully understand such criteria can greatly influence the final ME value, and so negate usefulness of comparative data. In considering published data, nutritionists should critically evaluate such potential variations in experimental procedures.

a) Methods of relating food intake and excreta output

As previously described, ME represents the ingested energy which becomes available for metabolic processes, and in practice is determined by a balance procedure in which food intake over a period, is related to the excreta output over the same period. Such measurements may be conducted either by measurement of the quantities of feed eaten and excreta voided, or by relating excreta voided to a unit weight of feed consumed by use of an unabsorbed marker material. In theory, a total balance procedure is preferable, as the method measures ME directly. In practice however, total feed intake can be difficult to measure because of spillage, and measurement of total excreta output can also be difficult. If an unabsorbed marker substance is used, the necessity for measurement of total feed intake and total excreta output is obviated. A comparison of the concentrations of the marker substance in the dry matter of feed and excreta allows the calculation of the quantity of excreta voided per unit of feed eaten. In practice, the marker most usually used is chromic oxide (Cr_2O_3). The assumption that Cr_2O_3 is completely unabsorbed has been questioned (Vohra and Kratzer, 1967) and the methods used for the determination of (Cr_2O_3) have not always yielded accurate and consistent results. When added to a diet, Cr_2O_3 must be mixed with wheat flour (Kane *et al,* 1950) or a similar carrier, to counteract its electrostatic properties. Incorporation of Cr_2O_3 directly into a diet results in a substantial loss during the mixing process, due to electrostatic precipitation, whilst the production and incorporation of Cr_2O_3 wheat flour "bread" counteracts, but does not totally nullify such effects (Vohra, 1972). Barium sulphate has been suggested as an alternate marker, however its measurement is difficult in the presence of calcium.

In practical situations where Cr_2O_3 is used as an indicator, the reasons for any discrepancies in ME values are difficult to identify, in that problems of dietary mixing due to its electrostatic properties, absorption or retention by experimental animals or variability in procedures of its analytical determination may be involved. Of such factors, the main concern is that Cr_2O_3 may be absorbed by the animal. Studies using radioactive labeled Cr (Cr^{51}) (Duke *et al.*, 1968) suggests that Cr is not totally inert in this respect, and in the former study only some 88% of administered Cr^{51} was recovered in the excreta. Crude fiber (CF) or various fractions of the CF complex have been proposed as unabsorbed marker materials suitable for ME determinations.

b) Application of a nitrogen correction factor

An ME value determined by any procedure is termed the classical ME value while allowances made for nitrogen (N) retention will yield a corrected ME value. If during an ME determination, nitrogen is retained by the animal, the excreta will contain less urinary N and hence less energy than from an animal which is not retaining N. As the extent of N retention differs with age and species, a correction factor is essential if comparisons of ME values for the same ingredient with different animals are to be made.

Hill and Anderson (1958) assumed that if N is not retained it will appear as uric acid, and proposed that a correction value of 8.22 kcal/g nitrogen retained be used, because this is the energy obtained when uric acid is oxidized completely. This assumption has been criticized since only 60-80% of the nitrogen of chicken urine is in the form of uric acid. In support of using the energy value of uric acid, Hill and Anderson (1958) suggested that the assumption that oxidation of body protein would yield a similar pattern of nitrogenous excretory products to that normally found in chicken urine, is no more correct than the assumption that all nitrogen is excreted as uric acid. From a practical viewpoint, the uric acid value has been used most frequently and is generally quoted.

Sibbald and Slinger (1963) questioned the validity of correcting for N retention, suggesting that correction does little to improve the usefulness of classical ME values and that the extra work involved is not justified. Contrary to these findings, Leeson *et al.* (1977) indicate the need for nitrogen correction in interpretation of bioassay data.

c) Methods of dietary formulation

When the ME value of an ingredient is to be determined, two or more diets must be used. These consist of a basal diet of known composition and one or more test diets in which portions of the basal diet or an ingredient of the basal diet are replaced by the test ingredient. Differences in the determined ME values of the basal and test diets can then be related to the proportions of test ingredient substituted. Lockhart *et al.* (1967) showed that the ME value obtained for wheat was similar when obtained by this method to that obtained when wheat was fed alone. The nutrient balance and palatability of various other ingredients often precludes the method of feeding the test ingredient alone however, and therefore the latter method does not find general applicability. Feeding ingredients alone also fails to identify potential synergism between fatty acids and between amino acids, and is one of the limitations of the TME assay (see Section 9.10.2).

The two methods most frequently used in substituting the test ingredient are those proposed by Anderson *et al.* (1958) and Sibbald and Slinger (1963). In the method of Anderson *et al.* (1958) the test ingredient is substituted for glucose, whilst in the later method, the test ingredient is substituted for all the energy-yielding ingredients of the basal diet. Anderson *et al.* (1958) proposed that the value of 3.65 kcal/g be used as the standard value for glucose. The basal diet used by Anderson *et al.* (1958), containing about 50% glucose and assigned the number E9, has been used extensively in ME determinations. In the method of Sibbald and Slinger (1963), the test ingredient is substituted essentially for part of the complete basal diet. However, to avoid mineral and vitamin deficiencies, substitution does not include this part of the diet. Also, in an attempt to maintain the protein contents of substituted diets within an acceptable range, the use of two basal diets of differing protein contents was proposed. The authors stated that basal diets composed of practical feed ingredients were preferable to those formulated with purified or semi-purified materials, since the ultimate aim of an ME assay is the production of ingredient values for use in the formulation of commercial diets containing non-purified ingredients. As previously noted, Anderson *et al.* (1958) quoted an ME for glucose of 3.65 kcal/g dry matter. An error in the ME of glucose would be reflected in the ME of the test ingredient commensurate with the proportion of test ingredient substituted. An advantage of the substitution method of Sibbald and Slinger (1963) is that the ME value of the reference basal diet is necessarily determined in each ME assay. While samples of glucose are likely to be less variable than samples of practical ingredients, the ME of glucose may vary under different dietary conditions and its ME value should be determined under the experimental conditions used.

The test ingredient may be substituted at one or more levels. Regardless of the basal diet used, the accuracy of the ME value obtained is dependent to some extent upon the proportions of the test ingredient substituted into test diets. The error of determination of the test diet is therefore multiplied by a factor of

$100 \div \%$ substitution, in extrapolating to calculate the test ingredient ME value. This explains the need for as high a proportion of the test ingredient in the test diets as is possible. Usually nutrient balance and palatability determine the maximum inclusion which can be used in practice for a particular ingredient.

Potter *et al.* (1960) proposed a linear regression procedure for the calculation of ME values for ingredients substituted at several levels. The ingredient ME value is derived by extrapolation to 100% inclusion from a regression equation relating test diet ME values to proportion of test ingredient in such diets. During the bioassay therefore, basal and test diets are fed for a 3-4d acclimatization period, followed by a 2-4d collection period. If Cr_2O_3 is added to the feed, there is no need to measure feed intake or excreted output. If no marker is used, then total feed intake must be carefully monitored over the test period, and excreta carefully collected. Using a 2-4d collection period there will be minimal loss of nutrients from the excreta and so they can be simply collected on open trays beneath the bird. For more extensive collection times it may be necessary to collect excreta under acid solutions. Feed is assayed for gross energy and nitrogen and excreta dried and likewise assayed. All analytical data is usually expressed on a moisture free basis.

Table 9.2 shows calculation of AMEn of wheat shorts where measurement of feed intake and excreta output replace the use of a marker.

TABLE 9.2 Sample calculation of AMEn of wheat shorts when tested at 40% substitution of a basal diet		
Analytical values	**Diet**	**Excreta**
a) Basal diet:		
Nitrogen (g/g)	0.035	0.080
GE (kcal/g)	4.500	4.800
Feed intake 1000g		
Excreta output 300g		
b) Test diet:		
Nitrogen (g/g)	0.030	0.060
GE (kcal/g)	4.300	4.600
Feed intake 750g		
Excreta output 280g		

Calculations are as follows:

1. AMEn of basal diet

$$\frac{1,000g \times 4.50 - [300 \times 4.80 + (1,000 \times 0.035 - 300 \times 0.080) 8.22]}{1,000 \text{ g}}$$

= 2,970 kcal/kg

2. AMEn of test diet (containing 40% wheat shorts)

$$\frac{750g \times 4.30 - [280 \times 4.60 + (750 \times 0.03 - 280 \times 0.06) 8.22]}{750g}$$

= 2,520 kcal/kg

3. AMEn of wheat shorts

$$2970 - \frac{(2970 - 2520)}{0.40}$$

= 1,845 kcal/kg

Table 9.3 shows calculation of the AMEn of safflower meal from a bioassay involving a basal diet and a test diet composed of 30% safflower and 70% basal. Cr_2O_3 was used as a marker.

TABLE 9.3 Calculation of metabolizable energy of safflower meal (Safflower meal substituted at 30% of test diet)		
Analytical values	Diet	Excreta
a) Basal diet:		
Nitrogen, grams/gram	0.0425	0.1181
Chromium, milligrams/gram	2.83	16.64
Gross energy, kilocalories/gram	4.211	3.114
b) Test diet (30% safflower):		
Nitrogen, grams/gram	0.0670	0.1115
Chromium, milligrams/gram	2.83	7.58
Gross energy, kilocalories/gram	4.481	3.430

i) Basal diet

Excreta energy/gram diet
$$= 3.114 \times \frac{2.83}{16.64} = 0.530 \text{ kcal}$$

Nitrogen retained per gram of diet
$$= 0.0425 - (0.1181 \times \frac{2.83}{16.64}) = 0.0224 \text{ g}$$

Nitrogen correction
$$= 0.0224 \times 8.22 = 0.184 \text{ kcal/g}$$

ME of basal diet
$$= 4.211 - (0.530 + 0.184) = 3.497 \text{ kcals/g}$$

ii) Test diet:

Excreta energy/gram diet
$$= 3.430 \times \frac{2.83}{7.58} = 1.279 \text{ kcal}$$

Nitrogen retained per gram of diet
$$= 0.0670 - (0.1115 \times \frac{2.83}{7.58}) = 0.0254 \text{ g}$$

Nitrogen correction
$$= 0.0254 \times 8.22 = 0.209 \text{ kcal/g}$$

ME of substituted diet
$$= 4.481 - (1.279 + 0.209) = 2.993 \text{ kcal/g}$$

iii) Therefore, ME of safflower meal
$$= 3.497 - \frac{(3.497 - 2.993)}{0.30} = 1.82 \text{ kcal/g}$$

9 10.2 TME and rapid bioassays

True Metabolizable Energy (TME) is quoted by Harris (1966) in describing an estimate of ME in which correction is made for metabolic fecal and endogenous urinary energy. These energy components are not directly of dietary origin, and as suggested by Sibbald (1980), their accommodation in bioassays leads to TME.

In addition to correcting for these anomalies, the method is quite rapid in that it takes only a 48h collection period. The method also has a major advantage in requiring only very small quantities of feed, and so is very useful in screening products from pilot projects and seed breeding experiments. Although the method is referred to as a "rapid" procedure, it is still quite time consuming, relative to conventional proximate analyses. It is difficult to routinely arrive at TME values in less than a week, and almost as expensive as regular ME assays at $1,000 per sample.

A major criticism of this procedure is that ingredients are most often fed alone (since there is little potential for feed refusal) and so synergism between ingredients cannot be accommodated. Such synergism is known to occur between fatty acids (Leeson and Summers, 1976) and there is good evidence for synergism between protein concentrates (Woodham and Deans, 1977).

Farrell (1978) overcame problems of force-feeding by training birds to consume their daily food allowance in a 1 hour period. Analyses of excreta collected over the next 24h is then reported to allow for estimation of ME within 36h of receipt of a feed sample. Many other researchers have been unsuccessful in training birds to consume feed within this time period, and since this original publication, it is now generally accepted that certain ingredients will not be cleared from the gut within 24h. Obtaining routine data within 36h may therefore be optimistic.

9.10.3 Available energy by growth assay

Squibb (1971) suggested a method for the "standardization and simplification" of ME determination procedures. The method is a modification of that described by Yoshida and Morimoto (1970) based on the premise that rapidly growing immature animals restricted in terms of energy intake but given adequate protein, will show an increase in growth in direct proportion to energy added to the diet. Squibb (1971), restricted the feed intake of chicks to 40-60% of *ad libitum* intake of a diet deficient in energy but adequate in protein. During the test period, additional energy in the form of 10% corn oil or 10% of a test ingredient is added to the diet. From consideration of growth rates and on the assumption that the corn oil provides 8.76 kcal/kg ME, the ME of the test ingredient is extrapolated. Squibb (1971) suggested that this method required no complicated calculations, chemical analyses or collections, and that it is accurate to with ± 1%. Considering the restricted feeding of the energy deficient diet used by Squibb, the adequacy of the protein in terms of quantity and quality can be questioned. Also the usefulness of corn oil as a standard material in view of the problems and variability associated with the determination of ME values of such materials, (Leeson and Summers, 1976) may be questioned. The fact that the animal is deficient in energy also raises the question of its state of protein nutrition since under such conditions protein is likely to be used as an energy source. The assay has greatest application for fats and other liquid ingredients.

9.10.4 *In vitro* systems for energy

Apart from pepsin digestibility measurements, few attempts have been made at developing *in vitro* techniques for monogastrics. A fairly rapid two-stage *in vitro* technique that uses pepsin digestion followed by incubation with pig intestinal fluid was developed by Furuya *et al.* (1979). While this original method was designed to predict digestible dry matter (DDM) and digestible crude protein (DCP) with pigs, Clunies and Leeson (1984) showed that with certain modifications, the system is even more accurate with poultry diets. The system attempts to simulate digestion up to the level of the small intestine, and so this is perhaps why the system works for poultry because pig and poultry digestive systems are comparable up to this level of the intestine. While the method essentially measures digestibility, ME can be estimated from consideration of the gross energy input and output of the system (Clunies and Leeson, 1984). Because the *in vitro* method gives a good estimate of digestibility, there seems to be potential for predicting energy avail ability. The premise for this work is based upon reports by Nelson *et al.* (1975) that the digestibility of DM correlates well with ME_n for sorghum grains. Also ME_n of ingredients may be predicted from metabolizable dry matter (Han *et al.*, 1976).

An obvious limitation to the *in vitro* system, is dependence on porcine intestinal fluid. Replacement of this biological fluid with a synthetic medium will reduce costs and increase general acceptance of the system. Fisher (1983) cites preliminary work on such an *in vitro* system. Using 28 different diets, mean *in vitro* DE was 3.51 kcal/kg DM relative to an AME_n of 3.39 kcal/kg DM, with SD of ± 2.2%. However, regressing AME on *in vitro* DE, a SD of 240 kcal/kg was obtained, which is substantially greater than that obtained with regression involving conventional proximate-type analyses. Leeson and Clunies (1987) have also investigated the use of pancreatin/amylase/bile mixtures in the second stage of the *in vitro* system showing a fair degree of accuracy in prediction.

9.11 PRODUCTIVE ENERGY

Prior to the mid 1950's 'productive energy values' were the primary measure of energy content of poultry feedstuffs. Fraps (1946) at Texas A & M University, published an extensive set of productive energy values for feed ingredients.

"Productive energy" measurements are an attempt to determine the net energy value of a feed, which is the quantity of energy actually available for maintenance and production. The major difference between metabolizable and net energy is the specific dynamic action or the heat lost in utilization of the food. The basic procedure for productive energy determination involves obtaining data to fit the equation:

WM + G = FX
W: Average chick weight for experimental period (usually 14 days)
M: Maintenance requirement of chick
G: Gain in carcass energy during feeding period
F: Food intake
X: Productive energy value of diet per unit weight

'W' can be determined by weighing chicks at appropriate intervals during the experiment. 'G' is estimated by determining the difference in carcass energy between a representative group of chicks sacrificed at the start of the experiment and the experimental groups killed at the end of the experiment. 'F' is measured during the course of the experiment. The diet to be studied is fed at two planes of intake. Some groups of chicks are full-fed while others are restricted to 60 or 70% of the intake of the full-fed groups. 'M' is extrapolated from data when 'F=0.

Two separate sets of data, therefore, are obtained at the two planes of intake. By using these data in two sets of the equation, WM + G = FX, the method of solution of simultaneous equations can be used to solve for the unknown X, the productive energy of the diet per unit weight. As serious drawback of this method is the necessity of assuming that the maintenance energy requirement of the chicks on both planes of nutrition, is equal.

Because many of the measurements involved in the determination of productive energy values are difficult to obtain with precision, the productive energy value of a specific diet is much less reproducible than the metabolizable energy value. Metabolizable energy values have been used extensively in recent years since they are highly correlated with net energy value in well balanced diets.

9.12 CALCULATED NET ENERGY VALUES

DeGroote (1974,) proposed a method for calculating net energy from determined ME values. The metabolic efficiency of utilization of metabolizable energy from protein, fat and carbohydrate is known to differ. ME for carbohydrates has a net availability of around 75%, protein 60% and fat 90%. Thus, the net energy values of diets high in fat may be underestimated compared to diets high in carbohydrates unless some correction factor is applied to the ME values. DeGroote proposed a method whereby the percentage of dietary protein, fat and carbohydrate is multiplied by their appropriate efficiency factor (75, 90 and 60). Therefore, when the ME value of an ingredient is multiplied by the appropriate efficiency values a net energy value is obtained. DeGroote claimed that this method was superior to the ME system in that it allows a more accurate energy evaluation of feed ingredients and thus a better prediction of gains and feed conversions expected from different diets. Any error inherent in ME estimate obviously influences the NE estimate.

9.13 DETERMINATION OF DIGESTIBILITY

A classical method for evaluation of feed ingredients is measurement of digestibility. Basically, measurements of digestibility are an attempt to determine the amount of given nutrient absorbed in the gastro-intestinal tract from a given quantity of feed. This involves both the processes of digestion, i.e., hydrolysis to release nutrients in a form in which they can be absorbed, and absorption from the intestinal lumen. Some investigators have used the term "absorbability" rather than "digestibility" to describe the process.

Digestibility can be determined by accurately measuring feed intake and fecal output. From these measurements, together with chemical analysis for the nutrient, the digestibility is calculated. For example, the % digestibility of protein is calculated as:

$$\frac{[(\text{Feed intake x \% Diet protein}) - (\text{Fecal output x \% Feces protein})]100}{(\text{Feed intake x \% Diet protein})}$$

A similar procedure may be used to determine the digestibility of fat, crude fiber, dry matter, energy or any other nutrient. To avoid the necessity of making total collections of excreta, an indicator method, such as the chromic oxide procedure used for determining metabolizable energy, may be used. "Apparent" digestibility is that obtained from data uncorrected for endogenous losses (e.g., losses of protein in feces of birds receiving a protein-free diet). "True" digestibility is determined by correcting for these losses.

A refinement of these digestibility assays is determination of ileal digestibility. If birds are fed an inert marker, such as Cr_2O_3, then the bird can be sacrificed and digesta samples from the terminal ileum collected. These samples are 'uncomplicated' by microbial cecal activity, and are handled and assayed in the same manner as are feces or excreta.

The digestibility of fats can be readily determined in chickens using mixed excreta since essentially no fat is present in chicken urine. Thus, the digestible energy value of fats is preferred over ME values since fats cannot be substituted in test diets at levels high enough to obtain accurate ME values. In this case the digestible energy value is, equivalent to the metabolizable energy value.

In order to get a reliable estimate of true digestibility for poultry, procedures were initiated to separate feces and urine. The most satisfactory method is a colostomy where an opening is made for the large intestine outside of the body. A second procedure is where the ureters are exposed by surgery so that an appropriate collecting vessel can be attached to collect the urine. In general, if long term collections from adult birds are anticipated then the colostomy method is preferred, whereas exteriorizing the ureters is preferred for short term collections, especially for young birds.

9.14 SPECIALIZED INGREDIENT ANALYSES

There a number of rapid tests available for evaluating specific ingredients. The decision to carry out any of these tests is based on significance of the ingredient in the diet, and so the relative contribution of constituents under test. Developing historical data on ingredients is also a useful way of determining the need and frequency of various testing procedures. The following tests or methodologies are assumed to be in addition to more extensive chemical testing that will routinely be used for most nutrients as described in previous sections of this Chapter 9.

a) Soybeans and soybean meal

Levels of the enzyme urease are used as an indicator of trypsin inhibitor activity. Urease is much easier to measure than is trypsin inhibitor and both molecules show similar heat-sensitivity characteristics. A rapid qualitative screening test for urease can be carried out using conversion of urea to ammonia in the presence of an indicator.

A qualitative test for urease activity can be carried out using a simple colorimetric assay. Urea-phenol red test solution is brought to an amber color by using either 0.1N HCl or 0.1N NaOH. About 25g of soybean meal is then added to 50 ml of indicator in a petri dish. After 5 minutes the sample is viewed for presence of red particles. If the sample has no red particles showing, the mixture should stand another 30 minutes, and if again no red color is seen, it suggests overheating of the meal. If up to 25% of the surface is covered in red particles, it is an indication of acceptable urease activity, while 25-50% coverage suggest need for more detailed analysis. Over 50% incidence of red colored particles suggests an under-heated meal.

When proteins are heated, their solubility in various solutes changes. Plant proteins are normally soluble in weak alkali solution. However, if these proteins are heat treated, as normally occurs during processing of many ingredients, the solubility of protein will decline. Dale and co-workers at Georgia have developed a fairly rapid test which seems to give a reasonable estimate of protein solubility and hence protein quality in soybean meal. The assay involves adding just 1.5g of soybean meal to 75 ml of 0.2% potassium hydroxide solution, and stirring for 20 minutes. Soluble proteins will be in the liquid phase, and so all or a portion of the centrifuged liquid is assayed for crude protein, and protein content relative to the original 1.5g sample calculated accordingly. By knowing the crude protein content of the original sample of soybean meal, percentage solubility can easily be calculated. Typical results are shown by Araba and Dale (1990) showing that as heating time is increased, there is a decrease in protein solubility. Values of 75-80% solubility seem to be ideal, with higher values suggesting under heating, and lower values overheating of the protein.

More recently there has been renewed interest in Protein Dispersibility Index (PDI). This measure of availability is simply the solubility in water, and Batal et al. (2000) suggest that PDI is a more consistent and sensitive indicator of soybean processing conditions than are measures of urease or KOH solubility.

b) Protein and amino acid dye binding

Proteins will bind with a number of dyes and so this provides the basis for colorimetric assays. These dye binding techniques can be used to test protein *per se*, or used to test for protein in various extractions involved in assays of solubility or digestibility. Dye-binding can therefore replace the Kjeldahl analysis depending upon sensitivity needs. The most commonly used methods are as follows:

Cresol Red	J. Amer. Assoc. Anal. Chem. 43:44Q
Orange G	J. Nutr. 79:239
Coomassie Blue	Anal. Biochem. 72:248

Lysine also reacts with certain dyes to give a colorimetric assay. Carpenter (1960) suggested that if the e-amino group of lysine is free to react with dye, then the lysine can be considered as "available". The most commonly used dye is Fluoro-2,4 dinitrobenzene (FDNB), which gives a yellow/orange color when combined with lysine.

c) Fishmeal gizzard erosion factor

In some countries, fishmeal is an economical feed ingredient to use in poultry diets. As previously described, some samples of fishmeal will cause severe gizzard erosion in young birds. Where fishmeal is an integral part of a broiler diet, it is common to carry out a chick growth test with each shipment of fishmeal. About 50 chicks are fed a broiler starter diet, usually without any fishmeal, for 5-7 days. At this time, the diet is mixed with 40-50% of the test fishmeal, and this diet fed for another 7-10 days. Birds are then sacrificed and the gizzards examined for erosion, often using a subjective scale as follows:

1. very mild erosion, with good gizzard color
2. mild erosion, with evidence of destruction of the lining in some areas
3. erosion in localized areas, with cracks in the thinner lining
4. severe erosion, cracking, thinning and discoloration
5. sloughing of the gizzard lining with hemorrhage

Because 40-50% fishmeal is used, some gizzard erosion is expected with most samples. Scores of 4-5 are often used to reject samples, although this decision will, to some extent, depend upon the level of fishmeal to be used in the commercial diet.

d) Sorghum tannins

Tannins are detrimental to protein utilization, and so levels should be minimized in poultry diets. Sorghum is a potential source of tannin, and this is usually found in the outer seed coats. Unfortunately there is not a clear relationship between seed coat color and tannin content. High tannin sorghums are usually darker in color, but some dark colored sorghums are also low in tannin. The tannins are present in the testa, which is the layer immediately beneath the outer pericarp. One quick test is therefore to cut into the seed and observe for presence of a pigmented (tannin) testa. More recently, a bleach test has been developed which again shows presence or not of a pigmented testa. About 20 g of sorghum is mixed with 5 g potassium hydroxide and 75 ml of household bleach. The mixture is shaken until the KOH dissolves, and then a set aside for 20 minutes. Sorghum grains are then strained, rinsed with water and placed on a paper towel. The KOH will remove the outer pericarp, and expose the testa. High tannin grains will appear dark brown/black while low tannin sorghum will be bleached white/yellow.

e) Gossypol in eggs

Feeding gossypol to laying hens can result in discoloration of both the yolk (green-brown) and albumen (pink). Gossypol is usually found in cottonseed meal and as described previously for this ingredient there are ways to minimize the effects of this compound by diet modification. However, egg discoloration occurs periodically and cottonseed meal or cottonseed oil is often suspected. Placing egg yolks in a petri dish with ammonia quickly causes varying degrees of brown discoloration depending upon gossypol content.

f) Fat assays

Fat quality is best assessed by measurement of moisture, impurities and individual fatty acids. However, there are a number of less extensive tests that can be used to give some idea of fat composition and quality. Fat titre is a measure of hardness, and simply relates to melting point. The break-point between tallows and greases is about 40°C. The higher the melting point, the more saturated the fat. Titre should obviously be consistent for an individual class of fat or fat blend from any one supplier. Iodine value can also be used as a measure of hardness. Each double bond (unsaturated) will take up a molecule of iodine, and so higher values mean more unsaturation, which in turn should relate to lower titre (Table 2.6). Iodine value is greatly influenced by levels of palmitic, oleic and linoleic acid in most fats and oils. Generally, as titre increases by 10 units over the range of 50-100, then palmitic acid content decreases by about 2%. Also as a rule of thumb iodine value = 0.9 x % oleic acid + 1.8% linoleic acid.

g) Rice hulls

Rice bran, sometimes called rice pollards, is used extensively in rice growing areas of the world. The major variable affecting nutritive value, is the content of hulls, which are essentially indigestible for poultry. A major component of hulls is lignin, and this reacts with the reagent phloroglucinol to produce a color reaction. The reagent is produced by combining 1 g of phloroglucinol with 80 ml 2M HCl and 20 ml ethanol. The rice by-product is mixed 1:2 with reagent and held at about 25°C for 10 minutes. Development of red color will be directly proportional to hull content. Actual hull content and a color score card are necessary to "calibrate" the assay.

h) Mineral solubility

Neutralizing mineral salts with various acids can be used to give some idea of mineral availability, and when an assay is monitored over time, then information on rate of solubility is also obtained. Hopefully all mineral sources will be total-ly available to the bird, although at least with calcium sources there is concern about solubilization occurring too quickly. With laying hens for example, a moder-ate rate of solubility is preferable to very rapid solubilization, because the former more closely matches the prolonged duration of need for calcium supply to the shell gland.

Limestone solubility can easily be measured by monitoring pH of the mineral in dilute acid (Cheng and Coon, 1990; Zhang and Coon, 1997). After recording the original pH of a 90 ml aliquot of 0.1N HCl, 10 g of limestone is gradually added, and without stirring, pH measured after time intervals of say 10, 20, 30 and 60 minutes. Limestone will result in an increase in pH, as H^+ ions are liberated from solution. A pH change of +0.1 relates to a 20% solubility, while changes of 0.2, 0.3, 0.4, 0.5, 0.6, 0.7,0.8, 0.9 and 1.0 relate to about 37, 50, 60, 70, 75, 80, 84, 87 and 90% solubility respectively. A high solubility after 60 minutes is expect-ed from a quality limestone, whereas the rate of achieving 95-99% solubility will give an indication of the rate of calcium release in the proventriculus. Particle size and particle porosity are the factors most likely to affect rate of change of solubility. Optimum eggshell quality, and perhaps bone development in young birds, are dependent upon a consistent pattern of calcium solubility. Neutralization of ammonium citrate has also been used to assess solubility of phosphate sources and also of manganese and zinc salts. Coon and Leske (1996) proposed a straight forward bioassay for assessment of phosphorus in feed grade minerals. Chicks are intubated with dicalcium phosphate or the test ingredient and phosphorus balance determined over a 48 hr period.

9.15 PURIFIED DIETS IN NUTRITION RESEARCH

Diets in which levels of nutrients are well defined are extremely useful in nutrition research. The development of these purified diets has led to the discovery of the various nutrient requirements and an understanding of their inter-relationship. Three such diets used in studies with chicks are shown in Table 9.4. These are based on isolated soybean protein, casein or crystalline amino acids to

TABLE 9.4 Purified diets for use in studies with growing chicks			
Ingredients	A	B	C
		%	
Isolated soybean protein		25.00	
Casein	25.00		
Amino acid premix*			23.64
L-Arginine HCl	1.50		
DL-Methionine	0.40	0.60	
Glycine	1.00	0.40	
Refined corn oil	4.00	4.00	5.00
Sucrose			59.46
Glucose	57.54	60.17	
Cellulose	3.00	3.00	3.00
Vitamin premix	1.20	1.20	1.20
Mineral premix	6.36	5.63	7.70

*L-arginine HCl, 1.33; L-histidine HCl:H_2O, 0.41; L-lysine HCl, 1.40; L-tyrosine, 0.63; L-tryptophan, 0.22; L-phenylalanine, 0.68; DL-methionine, 0.55; L-cystine, 0.35; L-threonine, 0.65; L-leucine, 1.20; L-isoleucine, 0.80; L-valine, 0.82; glycine, 1.60; L-glutamic acid, 12.00; L-proline, 1.00.

supply the amino acids, and purified carbohydrates, refined vegetable oil, vitamins and minerals to supply the remainder of the nutrients. Deficiencies of virtually all nutrients known to be required by chickens can be produced by omission of the appropriate nutrient from one of these diets.

The diet based on amino acids is the most highly purified of the three. Isolated soybean protein and casein contain quantities of some nutrients that must be considered as contaminants when preparing purified diets for specific purposes. Rates of growth achieved by chicks are normally best with the diet containing isolated soybean protein, and somewhat less than maximum with the diet based on pure amino acids.

Vitamin and mineral premixes for these diets are shown in Tables 9.5 and 9.6 respectively. These are designed to provide nutrients required in sufficient quantities to prevent a deficiency. The use of bicarbonate salts in the mineral premix, used in conjunction with the amino acid diet, is done to neutralize amino acid hydrochlorides.

TABLE 9.5 Vitamin premix for use in purified diets shown in Table 9.4	
Vitamin	Amount per 100g diet
Thiamine HCl, mg	1.5
Riboflavin, mg	1.5
Nicotinic acid, mg	5.0
Folic acid, mg	0.6
Pyridoxine, mg	0.6
Biotin, mg	0.06
Vitamin B_{12}, μg	2.0
Choline Cl, mg	200
d-Calcium pantothenate, mg	2.0
Menadione sodium bisulfite, mg	0.15
Vitamin E, IU	5.0
Vitamin D_3 IU	450
Vitamin A, IU	450
Antioxidant (butylated hydroxytoluene or ethoxyquin), mg	≤10
Glucose to make	1.20 grams

TABLE 9.6 Mineral premixes for purified diets. A, B, C as shown in Table 9.4			
Mineral	Diet A*	Diet B	Diet C
	g/100g premix		
$CaHPO_4\ 2H_2O$	1.80	2.07	3.40
$CaCO_3$	1.90	1.48	1.50
KH_2PO_4	1.40	1.00	
$NaHCO_3$	0.88		1.10
$KHCO_3$			1.10
KCl		0.10	
NaCl		0.60	
$MnSO_4H_2O$	0.035	0.035	0.055
$FeSO_47H_2O$	0.05	0.05	0.05
$MgCO_3$			0.50
$MgSO_4$	0.30	0.30	
KIO_3	0.0002	0.0002	0.0002
$CuSO_45H_2O$	0.003	0.003	0.003
$ZnCO_3$	0.015	0.015	0.015
$CoCl_2$	0.00017	0.00017	0.0002
$NaMoO_42H_2O$	0.00083	0.00083	0.0008
Na_2SeO_3	0.00002	0.00002	0.00002

*This mineral mixture contains no added chloride. When L-arginine HCl is omitted from diet A (Table 9.4), additional chloride must be provided.

SELECTED REFERENCES

AOAC, 1997. Methods of Analyses. Association of Official Analytical Chemists. 16th Ed. Publ. AOAC.

Anderson, D.L., F.W. Hill and R. Renner, 1958. Studies of the metabolizable and productive energy of glucose for the growing chick. J. Nutr. 65:561-574.

Araba, M. and N. Dale, 1990. Evaluation of protein solubility as an indicator of overprocessing of soybean meal. Poultry Sci. 69:1749-1752.

Axelsson, J., 1939. The general nutritive value of poultry feed. Proc. 7th Wlds. Poult. Congr. Cleveland, Ohio. 165-167.

Batal, A.B., M.W. Douglas, A.E. Engram and C.M. Parsons 2000. Protein Dispersibility Index as an indicator of adequately processed soybean meal. Poultry Sci. 79:1592-1596.

Carpenter, K.J., 1960. The estimation of available lysine in animal protein foods. Biochem. J. 77:604.

Carpenter, K.J. and K.M. Clegg, 1956. The metabolisable energy of feeding stuffs in relation to their chemical composition. J. Sci. Fd. Agric. 7:45-51.

Cheng, T.K. and C.N. Coon, 1990. Comparison of various *in vitro* methods for the determination of limestone solubility. Poultry Sci. 69:2204-2208.

Clunies, M. and S. Leeson, 1984. *in vitro* estimation of dry matter and crude protein digestibility. Poultry Sci. 63:82-88.

Coon, C.N. and K.L. Leske, 1996. An evaluation of phosphorus bioavailability. A phosphorus retention approach. Proc. BASF Symposium. Atlanta, Georgia, Jan 23. pp 1-18.

DeGroote, G., 1974. A comparison of a new NE system with the ME system in broiler diet formulation, performance and profitability. Br. Poultry Sci. 15;75-95.

Duke, G.E., G.A. Petrides and R.K. Ringer, 1968. Cr-51 in food metabolizability and passage rate studies with the Ring-necked pheasant. Poultry Sci. 47:1356-1363.

Farrell, D.J., 1978. Rapid determination of metabolizable energy of foods using cockerels. Br. Poultry Sci. 19:303-308.

Fisher, C., 1983. Energy evaluation of poultry rations. Recent Advances in Animal Nutrition. Ed. Haresign. Publ. Butterworths, London.

Fraps, G.S., 1946. Composition and productive energy of poultry feeds and rations. Tex. Agr. Exp. Sta. Bul. 678.

Furuya, S., K. Sakamoto and S. Takahashi, 1979. A new *in vitro* method for the estimation of digestibility using the intestinal fluid of the pig. Br. J. Nutr. 41:511-520.

Gehrke, C.W., K. Kuo and R.W. Zumwalt, 1971. The complete gas-liquid chromatographic separation of the 20 protein amino acids. J. Chromatography 57:209.

Guillaume, J. and J.D. Summers, 1970. Maintenance energy requirement of the rooster and influence of plane of nutrition on ME. Can. J. Anim. Sci. 50:363-369.

Halnan, E.T., 1949. The architecture of the avian gut and tolerance to crude fiber. Br. J. Nutr. 3:245-253.

Han, Y.K., H.W. Hockstetler and M.L. Scott, 1976. Metabolizable energy values of some poultry feeds determined by various methods and their estimation using metabolizability of dry matter. Poultry Sci. 55:1335-1342.

Harris, L.E., 1966. Biological energy interrelationships and glossary of energy terms. NAS-NRC. Washington, D.C.

Hill, F.W. and D.L. Anderson, 1958. Comparison of ME and PE determination with growing chicks. J. Nutr. 64:587-604.

Kane, E.A., W.C. Jacobson and L.A. Moore, 1950. A comparison of techniques used in digestibility studies with dairy cattle. J. Nutr. 41:583-596.

Leeson, S. and J.D. Summers, 1976. Fat ME values – effect of fatty acid saturation. Feedstuffs 48:(46) 26-28.

Leeson, S., K.N. Boorman, D. Lewis and D.H. Shrimpton, 1977. Metabolizable energy studies with turkeys. A study of the nitrogen correction factor. Br. Poultry Sci. 18:373-379

Leeson, S. and M. Clunies, 1987. in vitro estimation of digestibility and ME. Proc. Maryland. Nutr. Conf., Baltimore March 19-20, pp 95.

Lockhart, W.C., R.L. Bryant and D.W. Bolin, 1967. A comparison of several methods in determining the ME content of Durum wheat and wheat cereal by chicks. Poultry Sci. 46:805-810.

Moore, S. and W.H. Stein, 1954. Procedures for the chromatographic determination of amino acids on four per cent cross-linked sulfonated polystyrene resins. J. Biol. Chem. 211:893.

Nelson, T.S., E.L. Stephenson, A. Burgos, J. Floyd and J. York, 1975. Effect of tannin content and dry method digestion on energy utilization and average amino acid availability of hybrid sorghum grains. Poultry Sci. 54:1620-1623.

Norris, K.F., R.F. Barnes, D.E. Moore and J.S. Shenk, 1976. Predicting forage quality by NIRS. J. Anim. Sci. 43:889-897.

Potter, L.M., L.D. Matterson, A.W. Arnold, W.J. Pudelkiewicz and E.P. Singsen, 1960. Studies in evaluating content of feeds for the chick. 1. The evaluation of the metabolizable energy and productive energy of alpha cellulose. Poultry Sci. 39:1166-1178.

Roach, D. and C.W. Gehrke, 1969. Direct esterification of protein amino acids – GLC of N-TFA-N-butyl esters. J. Chromatography 44:269.

Scott, M.L., F.W. Hill, L.C. Norris and G.F. Heuser, 1946. Chemical determination of riboflavin. J. Biol. Chem. 165:65-68.

Sibbald, I.R., 1980. Metabolizable energy evaluation of poultry diets. Recent Advances in Animal Nutrition. Ed. Haresign and Lewis. Publ. Butterworths, London.

Sibbald, I.R. and S.J. Slinger, 1963. A biological assay of ME in poultry feed ingredients together with findings which demonstrate some of the problems associated with the evaluation of fats. Poultry Sci. 42:313-325.

Southgate, D.A.T., 1969. Determination of carbohydrates in foods. I. Available carbohydrate. J. Sci. Food Agr. 20:236.

Squibb, R.L., 1971. Estimating the metabolizable energy of foodstuffs with an avian model. J. Nutr. 101:1211-1216.

Valdes, E.V. and S. Leeson, 1990. Use of x-ray fluorescence spectroscopy to analyze calcium and phosphorus in poultry feeds. Poultry Sci. 69:1803-1805.

Valdes, E.V. and S. Leeson, 1991. Measurement of ME in poultry feeds by an in vitro system. Poultry Sci. 71:1493-1503.

Valdes, E.V. and S. Leeson, 1992. Use of NIRA to measure ME in poultry feeding ingredients. Poultry Sci. 71:1559-1563.

Valdes, E.V. and S. Leeson, 1994. Measurement of ME, GE, and moisture in feed grade fats by NIRA. Poultry Sci. 73:163-171.

Valdes, E.V., L.G. Young, S. Leeson, I. McMillan, F. Portella and J.E. Winch, 1985. Application of NIRS to analyses of poultry feeds. Poultry Sci. 64:2136-2142.

Vohra, P. and F.H. Kratzer, 1967. Absorption of barium sulphate and chromic oxide from the chicken gastrointestinal tract. Poultry Sci. 46:1603-1604.

Vohra, P., 1972. Evaluation of metabolisable energy for poultry. Wlds. Poultry Sci. J. 28(2):204-214.

Woodham, A.A. and P.S. Deans, 1977. Nutritive value of mixed proteins. Br. J. Nutr. 37:289-308.

Yoshida, M. and H. Morimoto, 1970. Biological assay of available energy with growing chicks. II. Development of a mini-test applicable to the small amount of sample. Agr. Biol. Chem. 34:683.

Zhang, B. and C.N. Coon, 1997. Improved *in vitro* methods for determining limestone and oystershell solubility. J. Appl. Poultry Res. 6:94-99.

10

Naturally Occurring Toxins Relevant to Poultry Nutrition

A variety of antinutritional and/or toxic compounds are present in cereal grains, legume seeds and other plants used in poultry nutrition. Most of these substances are normal constituents of varying chemical composition (e.g. proteins, fatty acids, glycosides, alkaloids) which can be distributed throughout or in specific parts of the plant. Some of these compounds can be inactivated by different processes such as washing, soaking, and/or heating. When heat is used, care must be taken to assure that the treatment is neither too weak to leave the substances still biologically active, nor too strong so that it alters the nutritional quality of the ingredient. In a few instances, extreme thermal processing can also lead to the formation of toxic compounds. In addition to the toxic components present in some ingredients, another potential source for toxic substances in grains and legumes is the contamination with toxic weed seeds during harvest, transportation and storage. Examples of common weed seeds which contaminate feed crops are crotalaria, jimson weed, and castor seeds.

10.1 PROTEINS, DIPEPTIDES AND AMINO ACIDS

10.1.1 Proteins

The two major groups of proteins with toxicological or antinutritional effects are the protease (e.g. trypsin) inhibitors and the lectins. Protease inhibitors alter the normal regulatory process of the exocrine pancreatic secretion, while lectins cause death of the intestinal epithelial cells by inactivating their ribosomes, thus arresting protein synthesis. Protease inhibitors and lectins are usually denatured by heat, although the specific proteins present in such legume seeds as Jack beans (*Canavalia ensiformis*) are particularly resistant to heat inactivation. Several studies have been conducted to determine the possibility of using Jack beans in poultry diets (reviewed by Belmar *et al.*, 1999). However, the use of Jack beans is restricted by the presence of several antinutritional factors, particularly the lectin known as concanavalin-A. Improvement in the nutritional value of Jack beans can be obtained from different treatments, but processed beans still contain a residual toxic component which results in depression of growth rate and feed intake.

a. Protease inhibitors

Chemical substances capable of inhibiting trypsin and chymotrypsin (protease inhibitors) are present in many plants but their levels are usually low. Such legume seeds as soybeans (*Glycine max*), however, tend to contain higher levels of protease inhibitors. Other legume seeds with protease inhibitors include lima beans (*Phaseolus lunatus*), kidney, navy, pinto and common garden beans (*Phaseolus vulgaris*), cow peas (*Vigna sinensis*), fava beans (*Vicia fava*), and green peas (*Pisum sativum*). In general, protease inhibitor content in cereals is much lower than in legume seeds. Among cereal grains the content of protease inhibitors is greater in rye and lowest in wheat, while barley and oats contain intermediate levels (Sosulski *et al.*, 1998).

The protease inhibitors present in soybeans have been extensively studied and are usually used as models for all other plant protease inhibitors. The biochemistry and physiological significance of the trypsin inhibitors present in soybeans was reviewed by Liener (1994). The protease inhibitors found in soybeans have been grouped into two main groups. The first group includes proteins with an average molecular weight of about 20,000 with two disulfide bridges, and with specificity mainly against trypsin (Kunitz inhibitor). The second group of proteins include those having an average molecular weight of 8,000 with a relatively high number of disulfide bridges and with specificity towards both trypsin and chymotrypsin (Bowman-Birk inhibitor). Table 10.1 summarizes the most important features of these inhibitors.

TABLE 10.1 Main characteristics of the protease inhibitors present in soybeans					
Inhibitor type	Molecular weight	Amino acid residues	Disulfied bridges	Active sites	Main substrate
Kunitz	20,000	181	2	1	Trypsin
Bowman-Birk	8,000	71	7	2	Trypsin, chymotrypsin

The Kunitz inhibitor has one active site that combines with trypsin in a stoichiometric irreversible manner. The Bowman-Birk inhibitor has two different active sites: a trypsin-binding site and a chymotrypsin-binding site. Inhibition of trypsin activity affects protein digestion since trypsin is the common activator of all the pancreatic enzymes that are secreted as zymogens, including trypsinogen, chymotrypsinogen, proelastase and carboxypeptidase. However, the major pathophysiological effect caused by trypsin inhibitors is not the impairment of protein digestion but an excessive secretion of the exocrine pancreas. Cholecystokinin (CCK) is a peptide that mediates pancreatic enzyme secretion and is secreted by the proximal small intestine under the control of a negative feedback loop. An increase in the level of trypsin activity in the intestinal lumen results in decreased secretion of CCK. A peptide known as "monitor peptide" is secreted in the pancreatic juice as a stimulus for CCK secretion by the intestinal mucosa. When protein digestion is complete, the monitor peptide is destroyed by trypsin and CCK secretion ceases. However, in the presence of a trypsin inhibitor in the diet the pancreas is continuously stimulated by CCK because the monitor peptide is not destroyed. Excessive stimulation of the pancreas causes hypertrophy and hyperplasia. Feeding raw soybeans causes an increase in the relative weight of the pancreas in most animal species, including chickens. In a recent study, broilers fed a diet containing 41% raw soybeans had an average pancreas weight of 5.6 g/kg body weight, while birds fed a similar diet containing 41% wet-extruded soybeans had an average pancreas weight of 1.8 g/kg body weight (Perilla et al., 1997). Figure 10.1 shows the pancrease from chickens fed raw soybeans and soybeans processed at different temperatures of wet extrusion.

The excreta of chickens fed diets containing raw soybeans have a higher water content and are much more sticky than the excreta of chickens fed heat processed soybeans. It should be noted, however, that protease inhibitors alone do not account for all of the growth inhibition caused by raw soybeans. Another group of compounds that are considered to play a significant role in the antinutritional effect of raw soybeans are the lectins.

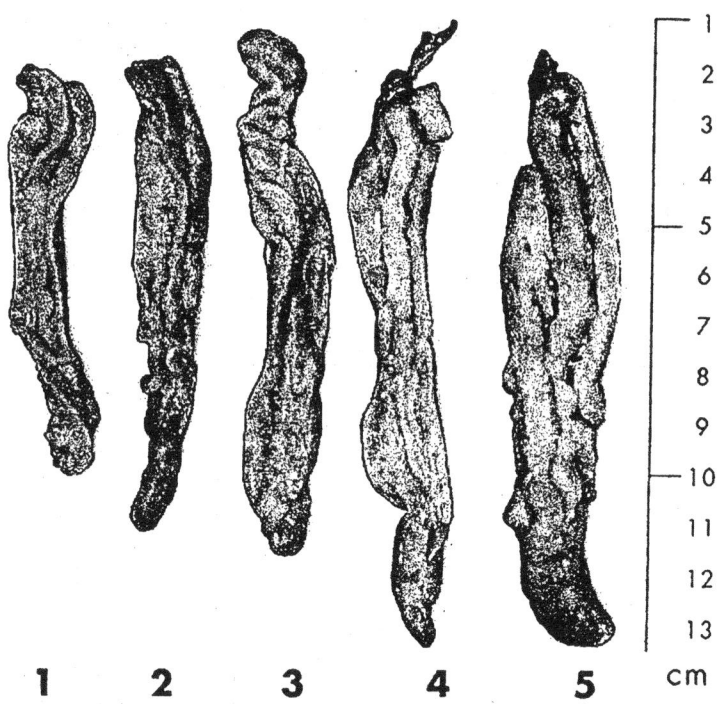

Figure10.1 Pancreata from chickens fed full-fat soybeans processed at different temperatures of wet extrusion, as follows: 1,126°C;2,122°C; 3,120°C;4, 118°C; and 5, raw soybeans. (Courtesy of G.J. Diaz).

Protease inhibitors are thermolabile and their activity is easily counteracted by heating. The extent to which trypsin inhibitor activity is destroyed depends upon the heating temperature and time, and the particle size and moisture content of the soybean meal. These variables are carefully controlled during the commercial processing of soybeans in order to ensure a product having maximum nutritional value. Although the urease test is a simple assay useful to estimate the protease inhibitor content in soybeans, it is only an indirect assay which does not measure the actual protease inhibitor activity. The most common assay employed to measure the trypsin inhibitor activity in soybean and soybean products is based on the inhibition of bovine trypsin activity on the synthetic substrate N--a- DL-arginine-p-nitroanilide or casein (Kakade *et al.*, 1974). A more specific enzyme linked immunoassay (ELISA) for the Kunitz trypsin inhibitor was developed using monoclonal antibodies.

b. Lectins

Many plant species, including several important crop and food plants, contain carbohydrate-binding proteins, better known as lectins, agglutinins or hemagglutinins. Lectins have the ability to agglutinate red blood cells from various animal species, due to the interaction of multiple binding sites on the lectin molecule with specific sugars (glycoproteins) present on the cell membrane surface. This type of interaction occurs not only with red blood cells but also with other cells.

The toxicity of the different lectins varies greatly. For example, the lectins in maize and barley are relatively nontoxic but feeding high levels of raw kidney beans (*Phaseolus vulgaris*) to rats will cause their death due to the toxic effects of the lectins. The most toxic and widely studied plant lectins are those from the seeds of the castor bean plant (*Ricinus communis*) and the jequirity bean plant (*Abrus precatorius*), known as ricin and abrin, respectively. The mechanism of action of these lectins, including the mechanisms of entry, translocation of the toxic subunit into the cytoplasm, and the mechanism by which ribosomes are inactivated by the toxic subunit were reviewed by Wiley (1991). Ricin, abrin and related lectins are composed of two different subunits (A and B) linked together by a single disulfide bridge. The B-chain (B, binding) is the actual lectin (agglutinin) that binds to cell surface receptors containing terminal galactose residues. Binding of the B-chain to the cell surface is an obligatory step in order to exert the toxic action on intact cells. However, the toxic action is caused by the A-chain (A, active), which is actually an enzyme with catalytic activity (RNA N-glycosidase). The A-chain damages ribosomes in eukaryotic cells by destroying the major rRNA, thus inhibiting protein synthesis. A single molecule of A-chain inside the cytosol is capable of killing a cell. Some lectins, known as type 1 ribosome-inactivating proteins (RIPs) are only composed of an A-chain (Barbieri *et al.*, 1993). Type 1 RIPs are generally much less toxic than the two-chain lectins (type 2 RIPs) and are found in several crop plants including barley and corn.

Castor beans are highly toxic due to the presence of ricin in all parts of the plant, particularly the seeds. Consumption of castor seeds cause violent purgation, straining with bloody diarrhea, weakness, salivation, trembling and incoordination. The castor bean plant originates from Asia and Africa but it is now also growing in Europe and America. In the United States the castor plant is distributed in the South Central States and castor beans have been found contaminating soybeans (List *et al.*, 1979). Castor bean seeds are oval and have a dark brown shiny cuticle with multiple light patches (Figure 10.2). The toxic effects of dietary castor beans in growing chickens were investigated by Diaz and co-workers (unpublished data) who fed one day old broiler chicks a commercial diet containing 0, 2, and 4% ground castor beans for 3 weeks. Dietary castor seeds caused a dramatic effect on growth: the average body weight at 21 days was 677, 240, and 148 g for chicks receiving 0, 2 and 4% castor seeds, respectively. Clinical signs in birds fed castor seeds included depression, abnormal feathering, dehydration, feed refusal, pasted vents, hemorrhagic diarrhea, and mortality. Gross pathological examination of dead birds revealed severe congestion of major organs, increased vascularization and hyperemia of the gut and hemorrhagic or catarrhal enteritis. Histological examination showed congestion and oval cell proliferation in the liver, while the mucosal layer of the duodenum showed hemorrhaging, necrosis of the microvilli, and sloughed cells.

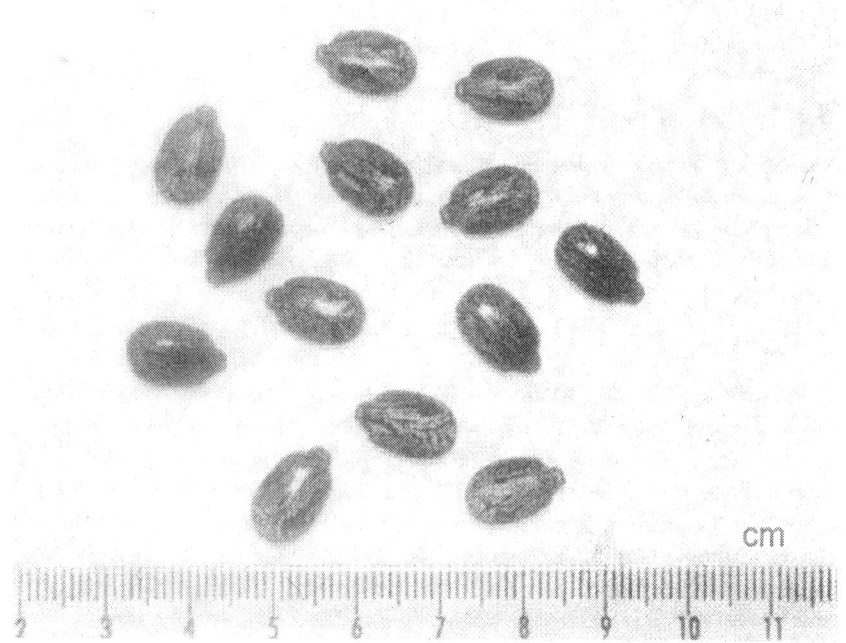

Figure 10.2 Castor bean (Ricinus communis) seeds. (Courtesy of G.J. Diaz).

In addition to ricin and abrin, another lectin that has received special attention is the soybean lectin or soybean agglutinin (SBA). SBA exists in several different isoforms (isolectins) that can be distinguished immunochemically but exhibit similar properties. In studies conducted with rats, it was observed that the SBA accounted for about 25% of the growth inhibition produced by raw soybeans. Some 60% of dietary lectin is not inactivated in the gastrointestinal tract and becomes bound to the intestinal mucosal epithelium causing disruption of the brush border, atrophy of the microvilli and decreased viability of the epithelial cells. The interaction of the lectin with the intestinal epithelium causes an increase in the relative weight of the small intestine due to hyperplasia of the crypt cells. Other pathological effects attributed to SBA include decreased blood insulin levels, inhibition of disaccharidases and proteases in the intestine, degenerative changes in liver and kidney and interference with the absorption of nonheme iron and lipid from the diet (Liener, 1994).

Lectins are heat sensitive and their biological activity is destroyed by moist heat but not by dry heat. In order to obtain all their nutritional potential, kidney and other beans should be soaked prior to cooking to ensure moisture penetration of the whole seed. In soybeans, the inactivation of SBA by moist heat treatment parallels the destruction of protease inhibitors and the inhibition of hemagglutinating activity can be used to monitor the improvement in the nutritional value of the treated soybeans.

10.1.2 Toxic dipeptides

Two toxic dipeptides are particularly relevant to poultry nutrition: gizzerosine and linatine. Gizzerosine is not of plant origin but it occurs in certain fish meals and causes severe gizzard erosions and ulcerations in broiler chickens. Linatine is present in linseed meal and upon bioactivation (hydrolysis) produces a vitamin B_6 antagonist.

a. Gizzerosine

Gizzerosine [2-amino-9-(4-imidazolyl)-7-azononanoic acid] has been identified as the causative agent of the toxicosis known as black vomit in broiler chickens because the contents of the esophagus and crop of the chickens turn black due to presence of acid-digested blood from the gizzard. Gizzerosine is formed by the reaction of the ε-amino group of lysine with the imidazolylethyl group of histidine (or histamine) during the heat processing of fish meal. It is important to note that gizzerosine is formed only during the dry heating of certain fish, especially those having red meat and free histidine in the soluble fraction of the protein. Heat processing of white fish with low levels of free histidine does not lead to gizzerosine formation. The chemical structure of gizzerosine is shown in Figure 10.3.

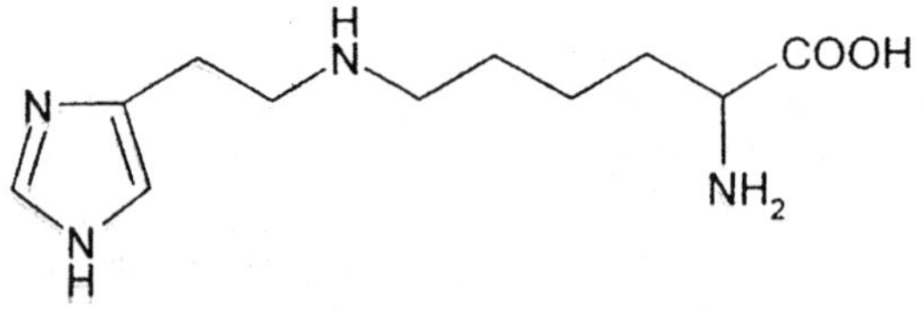

Figure 10.3 Gizzerosine

Gizzerosine is a highly toxic compound for broiler chickens. Sugahara *et al.* (1988) suggested that the maximum tolerable concentration of L-gizzerosine in practical diets should be less than 0.4 ppm. Dietary levels of gizzerosine above 0.5 ppm induce erosions, ulcerations and even perforation of the gizzard and/or duodenum. Erosions and ulcerations of the gizzard lead to extensive bleeding, while perforation of the gizzard and/or duodenum causes death within hours. Early signs of toxicosis include anorexia, ruffled feathers, and decreased growth. The mechanism of action of gizzerosine was elucidated by Masumura *et al.* (1985). Gizzerosine is a potent stimulator of histamine H_2- receptors at oxynticopeptic cells of the proventriculus. The stimulation of H_2-receptors causes an excessive gastric acid secretion (HCl) and a severe decrease in pH at the proventriculus and gizzard. The extremely low pH causes damage to the koilin layer and submucosa of the gizzard that leads to erosion, ulceration and perforation.

Several dietary treatments for gizzerosine toxicosis have been tested including the supplementation of the H_2-histamine receptor antagonist cimetidine and the antacid compounds sodium bicarbonate and magnesium trisilicate. The results have been inconclusive and poor or no protection has been obtained. Omeprazole is a potent inhibitor of gastric acid secretion which inhibits the H^+-K^+-ATPase pump in oxynticopeptic cells in chickens (Guinotte *et al.*, 1993). The ability of this compound to decrease and/or control the gastric acid secretion induced by gizzerosine has not been tested and should be investigated.

Gizzerosine levels in fish meals and complete feeds can be determined by high-performance liquid chromatography (Ohta *et al.*, 1988) and radioimmunoassay (Torres *et al.*, 1999). Alternatively, a reliable and simple bioassay with broiler chicks can be used (Diaz and Sugahara, 1995) to estimate gizzerosine levels and determine whether a fish meal can be incorporated into a chicken diet or not. Gizzerosine may interact with other toxic compounds found in the diet such as mycotoxins. Diaz and Sugahara (1995) observed that high dietary levels of aflatoxin B_1 (3 ppm) can potentiate the lethal effects of gizzerosine.

b. Linatine

Linatine, a dipeptide formed by the condensation of 1-amino-D-proline and glutamic acid is an antagonist of pyridoxal phosphate (vitamin B_6). Linatine (Figure 10.4) is present in flaxseed meal and in all parts of the immature flax plant (*Linum usitatissimum*) and upon hydrolysis yields 1- amino-D-proline and glutamic acid. Flax meal may also contain cyanogenic glycosides such as linustatin, neolinustatin, and linamarin (see section 10.6.1).

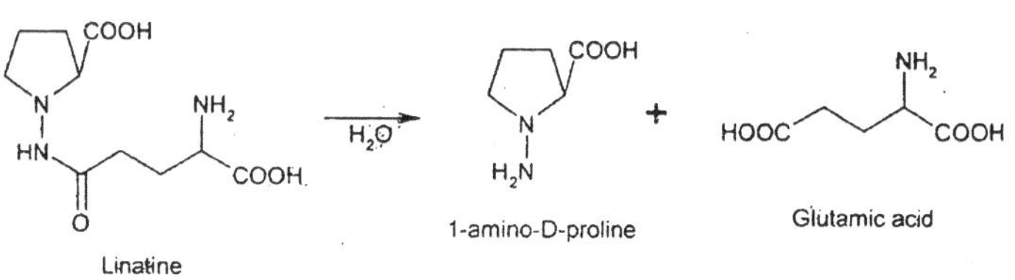

Figure 10.4 Linatine and its constitutive amino acids, 1-amino-D-proline and glutamic acid.

The toxic component of linatine is the amino acid 1-amino-D-proline, an asymmetrically substituted secondary hydrazine that condenses readily with pyridoxal and pyridoxal phosphate forming stable hydrazones. Pyridoxal phosphate is involved in transamination, decarboxylation, and other reactions of amino acid metabolism. Chicks fed high doses of linatine or 1-amino-D-proline develop signs indistiguishible from those of classical vitamin B_6 deficiency (or hydrazine poisoning) including anorexia, poor growth, perosis, and convulsions. These adverse effects can be overcome by the administration of any form of vitamin B_6. Interestingly, this toxic effect has not been observed in mature poultry.

10.1.3 Toxic amino acids

Non-protein amino acids with toxic or antinutritional effects are found in many legumes, some of which are used as protein sources. These amino acids occur in unconjugated form and usually interfere with the metabolism of structurally related essential amino acids.

a. Canavanine and indospicine

Canavanine and indospicine are non-protein amino acids structurally similar to the essential amino acid arginine (Figure 10.5). Canavanine is found in the tropical legume jack bean (*Canavalia ensiformis*) and also in legumes from the genus *Robinia* and *Sesbania*. The L-canavanine content in jackbean seeds ranges from 1.2 to 3.7% (Belmar and Morris, 1994; Michelangeli and Vargas, 1994), while sesbania seeds contain about 0.6% L-canavanine. Indospicine is present in the plant creeping indigo (*Indigofera spicata*), which also contains canavanine.

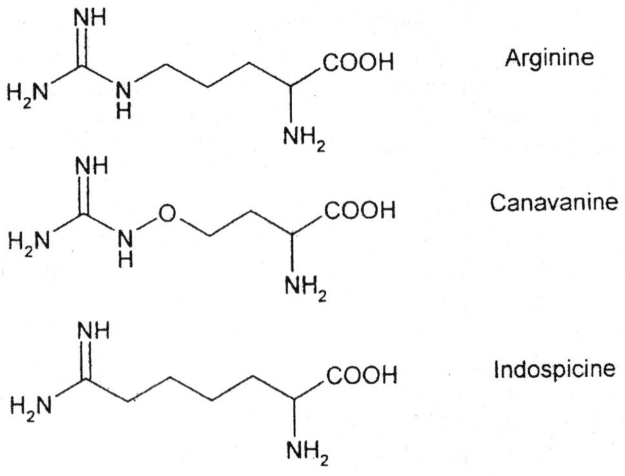

Figure 10.5 Arginine, canavanine, and indospicine.

When nutritional studies are conducted using the whole jackbean seed it is not possible to discriminate the adverse effect of L-canavanine from the effects of other toxic compounds present in the legume, particularly the lectin concanavalin A (see section 10.1.1). Therefore, it has been necessary to investigate the effect of canavanine in poultry by adding the purified amino acid to complete diets which do not contain jack beans. The effects of dietary supplementation of purified L-canavanine (either as the sulfate or the free base form) on performance parameters in broiler chickens are summarized in Table 10.2.

TABLE 10.2 Effects of dietary supplementation of the toxic amino acid L-canavanine on broiler chicken performance			
Dietary L-canavanine	Duration of treatment	Effect on performance	Reference
0.03%	2 weeks	No effect on growth, survival or feed intake	Shqueir *et al.*, 1989
0.35%	7 weeks	No effect on growth, feed intake, and protein utilization	Belmar and Morris, 1994
1.0%	11 days	25% decrease in feed intake and growth	Michelangeli and Vargas, 1994

Dietary levels of 0.35% L-canavanine or less have no adverse effects on broiler performance but levels of 1.0% decrease growth and feed intake. The mechanism of action of canavanine was reviewed by D'Mello (1995). Chickens are particularly susceptible to canavanine because they have a non-functional urea cycle and therefore have no means of synthesizing arginine. Increased excretion of urea, indicative of increased arginase activity, has been reported in chickens consuming canavanine. The elevated arginase activity serves to metabolize canavanine but a concomitant loss of arginine may occur in a manner similar to that seen in the lysine-arginine antagonism. This loss of arginine causes adverse effects on the bird since arginine is an essential amino acid for poultry. Canavanine may also act by competing with arginine and lysine for transport across cell membranes. High levels of ornithine have also been detected in birds consuming canavanine. This effect is attributed to the synthesis of a canavanine derivative (canaline), which binds to and inactivates ornithine decarboxylase. Chicks fed jack bean diets exhibit hepatic ornithine decarboxylase activity of only 19% of that detected in control birds. Canavanine content in raw and processed jackbean seeds can be detected using a simple colorimetric method or by high-performance liquid chromatography (Viroben and Michelangeli-Vargas, 1997).

Indospicine, another arginine analog, is a competitive inhibitor of arginase. This mechanism of action affects mostly mammalian species because in uricotelic species such as birds, arginase plays a minor role in the overall nitrogen elimination. The seeds of *Indigofera spicata*, however, are toxic to chicks due to the presence of

3-nitropropanoic acid, a highly specific and irreversible inhibitor of succinate dehydrogenase, a key enzyme of the Krebs cycle.

Recent studies have shown that both canavanine and indospicine are inhibitors of the constitutive and inducible nitric oxide synthetases (Pass *et al.*, 1996). Nitric oxide synthetases generate nitric oxide from arginine and nitric oxide has important biochemical functions including relaxation of blood vessels, neutralization of superoxide, inhibition of platelet aggregation, modulation of neurotransmission and immune responses and killing of tumor cells and parasites. It has been suggested that the toxic action of canavanine and indospicine might be related to the inhibition of nitric oxide synthetases (Pass *et al.*, 1996).

b) Mimosine

Leucaena leucocephala is a tropical legume native to Central America and Mexico but now widely distributed in the high-rainfall regions of South America, Africa, Asia and northern Australia. *Leucaena* can be included in the diet of non-ruminants at a 5-10% inclusion level without signs of toxicosis. The nutritional composition of *Leucaena* and the factors limiting its use in poultry were reviewed by D'Mello and Acamovic (1989). Dried *Leucaena* leaf meal is equivalent to cottonseed meal as a source of protein; however, dietary *Leucaena* depresses growth in broilers and egg production in layers. The relatively poor nutritive value of *Leucaena* is considered to be due mainly to the presence of mimosine, -[*N*-(3-hydroxy-4-oxo-pyridyl)]-a-aminopropionic acid (Figure 10.6). *Leucaena* contains about 3-5% mimosine on a dry matter basis but it also contains other antinutritional compounds including protease inhibitors, tannins and galactomannans.

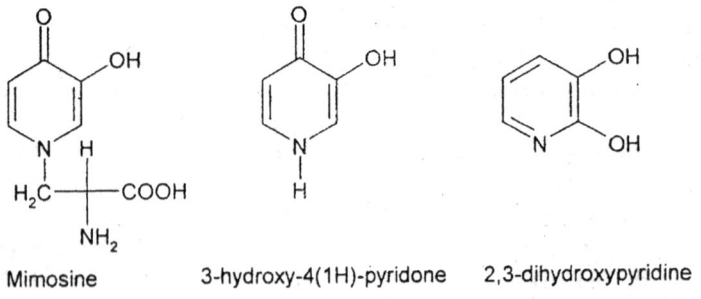

Mimosine   3-hydroxy-4(1H)-pyridone   2,3-dihydroxypyridine

Figure 10.6 Mimosine and its degradation products, 3-hydroxy-4(IH)-pyridone (3,4-DHP) and 2,3-dihydroxypyridine (2,3-DHP).

Studies conducted to determine the toxic effects of mimosine in chickens have shown that young chicks are more sensitive than adult birds. Growth rate and feed intake are severely affected in chickens receiving a diet containing 0.33% pure mimosine (D'Mello and Acamovic, 1989). However, an adult bird is capable of metabolizing a single oral dose of mimosine without exhibiting adverse effects. Recently, the effects of pure mimosine on performance and bone integrity in broiler chicks were investigated by Kamada *et al.* (1998). Chicks fed a diet containing 1% mimosine for 12 days gained only 50% of the weight gained by controls and developed osteopathy characterized by decreased bone strength and mineral density.

c. Lathyric amino acids: β-Aminopropionitrile (BAPN), β-N-oxalylamino-L-alanine (BOAA) and β-cyano-L-alanine (BCA)

Osteolathyrism and neurolathyrism are degenerative diseases affecting the connective tissue and nervous system. Osteolathyrism, the main form of lathyrism affecting livestock, causes skeletal deformities and aortic rupture. Figure 10.7 shows the structures of the lathyric amino acids.

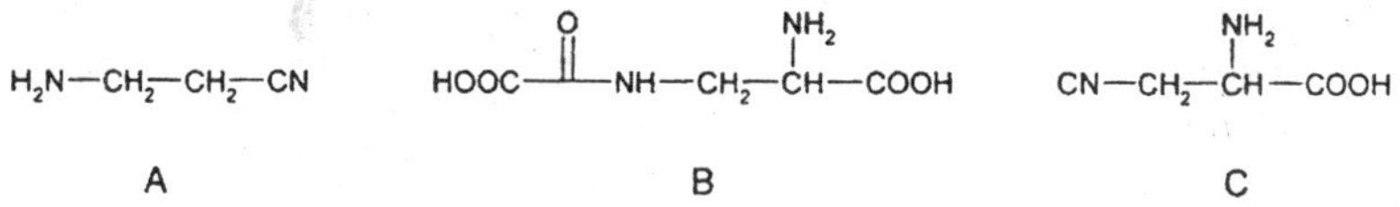

$$H_2N-CH_2-CH_2-CN$$

$$HOOC \overset{O}{\overset{\|}{-}} -NH-CH_2-\overset{NH_2}{\overset{|}{CH}}-COOH$$

$$CN-CH_2-\overset{NH_2}{\overset{|}{CH}}-COOH$$

A   B   C

Figure 10.7 Lathyric amino acids: (A) β-aminopropionitrile, (B) β-N-oxalylamino-L-alanine, and (C), β-cyano-L-alanine.

The amino acid β-aminopropionitrile (BAPN) is a naturally occurring osteolathyrogen present in the seeds of *Lathyrus odoratus* (sweet pea), *L. sylvestris* (flat pea), *L. pusillus* (singletary pea), *L. hirsutus* (caley pea) and *L. roseus*. Consumption of these type of *Lathyrus* seeds (or purified BAPN) causes extensive abnormalities in bones and the vascular system due to the impairment of the cross linkage of collagen and elastin fibers. In chickens, BAPN produces a common pattern manifested by increased collagen solubility, bone deformation, and modification of arterial elastin with subsequent reduction in the tensile strength of the aorta. Signs of osteolathyrism in broiler chicks receiving diets containing *Lathyrus odoratus* seeds include ruffled feathers, enlarged hock joints, curled toes, ataxia, leg paralysis and death (Raharjo *et al.*, 1988). In laying hens BAPN affects the normal development of the egg membranes and shell. Ultrastructural alterations include widespread separation of fibers (which are highly branched in normal eggs), uneven pore size and distribution, large interstitial spaces and late fusion of the palisade layer (Chowdhury and Davis, 1995). These changes result in a loss of tensile strength of the membranes and in a highly porous and weak shell. In the chicken embryo skin, BAPN affects the normal skin development and alters the size and shape of the feather rudiments (Marsh and Gallin, 1994).

Vicia sativa (common vetch), *Vicia villosa* (hairy vetch), and *Vicia angustifolia* (narrow leaf vetch) contain the neurolathyrogen β-cyano-L-alanine (BCA). BCA can be present in the form of a dipeptide of glutamic acid (α-glutamyl-β-cyano-L-alanine). BCA appears to be much more toxic than the neurolathyrogen BOAA for poultry. The incorporation of 20-40% *V. sativa* seed into practical type diets for chicks causes high mortality (70-100%) and decreased growth (Harper and Arscott, 1962). Affected birds show a high degree of excitability, nervous signs, convulsions and opisthotonos prior to death. *V. villosa* seed is less toxic than *V. sativa* seed. Laying hens are also susceptible to the adverse effects of *V. sativa*. Farran *et al.* (1995) found that the incorporation of 22.5% raw *V. sativa* seed into a layer ration decreases egg production, body weight and feed intake. However, when the seeds are autoclaved they could be safely incorporated up to 25% in rations for layers. It should be noted that the toxicology of BCA in poultry species has not been adequately documented.

d. Selenoamino acids

Several plants contain toxic structural analogues of the sulfur-containing amino acids in which the sulfur atom is replaced by selenium (Se-Met and Se-Cys). In *Astragalus* species (Milk vetch), the predominant selenoamino acids are *Se*-methylselenocysteine and selenocystathione. *Astragalus spp.* are toxic plants known as selenium accumulators (also known as primary selenium indicators) and can accumulate large amounts of selenium ranging from 1,000 to 10,000 ppm (air-dried basis). The toxicosis caused by the ingestion of plants containing large amounts of selenoamino acids is due to the selenium moiety and is actually a selenium toxicosis.

10.2 FATTY ACIDS

A number of fatty acids are known to cause adverse effects on poultry health and/or performance.

10.2.1 Cyclopropene fatty acids

Cyclopropene fatty acids (CPFA) are naturally occurring plant fatty acids that contain a propene ring in their carbon chains (Figure 10.8). Two CPFA are present in the seeds and other parts of plants of the *Malvales* order: Malvalic acid (2-octyl-1-cyclopropene-1-heptanoate) and sterculic acid (2-octyl- 1-cyclopropene-1-octanoate). Plants of the *Malvales* order include species that are economically important for humans and livestock such as cotton and kapok.

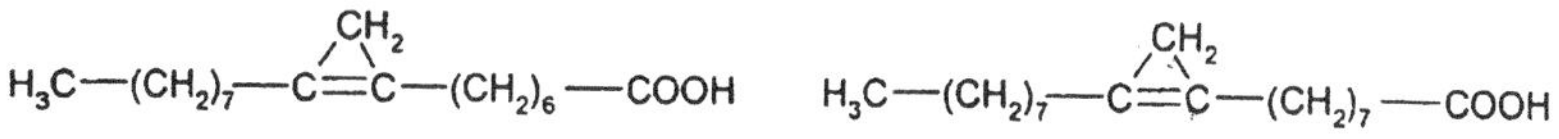

$$H_3C-(CH_2)_7-C\overset{CH_2}{\underset{}{=}}C-(CH_2)_6-COOH \qquad H_3C-(CH_2)_7-C\overset{CH_2}{\underset{}{=}}C-(CH_2)_7-COOH$$

Malvalic acid   Sterculic acid

Figure 10.8 Cyclopropene fatty acids malvalic and sterculic.

CPFA occur in crude cottonseed oil at levels of 1-2% and are also present in cotton-seed meal. Malvalic acid is present at a higher concentration than is sterculic acid. CPFA are important in egg production due to their potential adverse effects on egg quality. In laying hens, CPFA intensify the effect of gossypol in causing olive green egg yolks (see section 10.5.3) and also cause a pink discoloration of the egg albumen. Further, when large amounts of CPFA are fed to laying hens, the egg yolks develop a rubbery, pasty, and viscous appearance after a short period of cold storage. This alteration is caused by an increased concentration of satu-rated fatty acids in the egg yolk. Egg yolks and tissue lipids from hens fed CPFA have been found to contain low iodine values and high levels of stearic (C18:0) and palmitic (C16:0) acid, associated with low levels of palmitoleic (C16:1, ω-7) and oleic acid (C18:1, ω-9) (Keshavarz, 1993). The increased content of saturat-ed fatty acids is due to a direct inhibitory effect of CPFA on Δ^6 and Δ^5-desaturation reactions in liver microsomes, which prevents the desaturation of stearic and palmitic acids to their corresponding monounsaturated fatty acids. The inhibitory effect is thought to be caused by the irreversible reaction of the propene ring of CPFA with thiol groups present in the liver desaturase system. Alternatively, inhibition may be the result of competition between CPFA and the normal substrate and/or prod-uct of desaturation during the microsomal synthesis of phospholipids (Cao *et al.*, 1993).

Dietary CPFA not only influence the fatty acid composition of the egg yolk but also alter the permeability of the vitelline membrane. As a result of this altered permeability, iron from the egg yolk diffuses to the albumen and binds to ovotrans-ferrin (conalbumin), which acts as an iron chelator. The reaction between ovotransferrin and iron is responsible for the pink discoloration of the albumen mentioned above. Some ovotransferrin may also diffuse to the egg yolk where it combines with iron causing a brownish-salmon colored yolk. The pink albumen discoloration is more prevalent in eggs that have been stored for several weeks.

10.2.2 Erucic acid

Erucic acid (docosenoic acid, C22:1, ω-9) is a major fatty acid present in rape-seed and mustard seed oils. The erucic acid content of rapeseed oil in older varieties of *Brassica campestris* and *B. napus* ranges from 25 to 45%; however, cultivars selected in Canada are practically free from erucic acid. Canola is the registered name for rapeseed containing less than 2% total fatty acids in the oil as erucic acid and less than 30 μmoles of alkenyl glucosinolates per gram of oil free dry matter of the seed (see section 10.6.2). The factors affecting the nutritional value of canola meal include not only erucic acid and glucosinolates but also sinapine, tannins and phytates. These antinutritional factors are described in other sections of the present chapter (sections 10.5.4, 10.5.2, and 10.4.1, respectively).

Erucic acid is mainly a cardiotoxic compound capable of causing fatty degeneration and fibrosis of myocardial cells. In chickens, adverse effects of dietary erucic acid are reflected in feed consumption, growth, and apparent digestibility of total lipids and individual fatty acids (Sim *et al.,* 1985); additionally, chicks fed diets containing erucic acid deposit less fat and utilize energy less efficiently (Renner *et al.,* 1979). In laying hens, 10 to 20% of a high erucic acid rapeseed oil in the diet depresses feed intake, egg production, egg weight, yolk weight and hatchability, when compared with the performance of hens fed tallow or corn oil. In addition, when layers are fed a diet containing 10% rapeseed oil, no particular flavor or odor is detected, but the eggs are consistently given a lower score by a taste panel (Leslie *et al.,* 1973).

10.3 CARBOHYDRATES

Non-starch polysaccharides (β-glucans and arabinoxylans) and α-galactoside oligosaccharides (raffinose and stachyose) are not digested by the enzymes secreted into the digestive tract of chickens. These compounds do not cause overt signs of toxicity but instead have anti-nutritive properties that may affect the performance of broilers and layers.

10.3.1 Non-starch polysaccharides (β-glucans, arabinoxylans)

Non-starch polysaccharides (NSP), such as β-glucans and arabinoxylans (pentosans), are complex structural carbohydrates present in the endosperm cell walls of cereal grain seeds. Although it was initially thought that NSP contributed to the nutrition of the chicken through cecal fermentation, it is currently considered that NSP's have anti-nutritive effects even at concentrations as low as 5% in broiler diets. The adverse nutritional effects of NSP are primarily due to their effect on the viscosity of the digesta. The absorption of fatty acids and monoglycerides is particularly affected and a fat malabsorption syndrome is produced. Clinical manifestations of dietary NSP in poultry include decreased growth, increased feed conversion, sticky droppings, watery excreta and pasty vents; birds may appear dull and less responsive to the environment (Annison and Choct, 1991). Other NSP polysaccharides capable of causing adverse effects in poultry include pectin, and the guar, xantham and locust bean gums. The adverse effects of NSP in poultry diets can be minimized by adding exogenous β-glucanases and pentosanases of fungal origin to the diet; these enzymes cause partial breakdown of β-glucan and pentosan polymers, reducing their viscosity (Campbell and Bedford, 1992). These enzymes have been extensively described in Chapter 6.

10.3.2 Oligosaccharides (raffinose, stachyose)

The α-galactosides of sucrose, raffinose and stachyose, are low molecular weight oligosaccharides containing α-1,6-galactosidic bonds. These compounds are present in soybeans and other beans and are not digested due to lack of α-1,6-galactosidase. Unlike soluble fiber constituents, oligosaccharides do not significantly alter the viscosity of the digesta. However, undigested oligosaccharides pass through the small intestine to the lower gut, where they serve as substrates for bacterial fermentation and cause explosive bacterial growth.

10.4 CHELATES (MINERAL-BINDING COMPOUNDS)

Nonpolysaccharide components of the plant cell walls such as silicates, phytates, and oxalates are capable of binding certain metal ions, thereby making them biologically unavailable. Chelates do not generally cause overt signs of toxicity but due to their metal binding capacity they may induce mineral deficiencies. The only chelates capable of inducing an acute toxic response are the soluble oxalates, which bind to serum calcium ions forming crystals; calcium oxalate crystals may block the renal tubules and induce acute renal failure. Complex carbohydrates, especially those containing uronic and phenolic acid groups or sulfated residues (e.g. pectins and alginates) may bind magnesium, calcium, zinc, and iron.

10.4.1 Phytic acid

Phytic acid is considered to be the chief storage form of phosphate and inositol in mature seeds. The proper chemical designation for phytic acid is myoinositol 1,2,3,4,5,6-hexakis (dihydrogen phosphate). The occurrence, bioavailability and implications of phytic acid in poultry nutrition were reviewed by Ravindran *et al.* (1995), and described in Figure 5.12. Phytic acid is a strong chelating agent that can bind divalent metal ions to form complex phytate, rendering minerals unavailable for intestinal absorption. Poor bioavailability of zinc, calcium, magnesium, and iron has been reported in diets containing high phytate levels.

10.4.2 Oxalates

Oxalic acid is found in many plants forming salts with alkaline or alkaline-earth metals (Figure 10.9). Oxalic acid salts formed with potassium and sodium are soluble and are absorbed through the gastro-intestinal tract. In contrast, oxalic acid salts of calcium and magnesium are insoluble crystals, which are not absorbed. In plants having a very acid cell content (pH 2), the oxalate is present as soluble potassium acid oxalate. Plants having a slightly acid cell medium (pH 6) contain soluble sodium oxalate and insoluble calcium and magnesium oxalates.

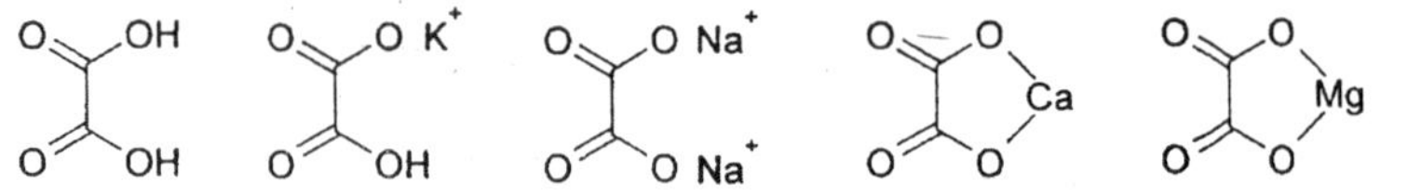

Figure 10.9 Oxalic acid and oxalates

The solubility of the oxalic acid salt present in the plant determines the mechanism of toxic action of the oxalate. Soluble oxalates are absorbed into the systemic circulation where they combine with plasma calcium ions forming insoluble calcium oxalate. Chelation of calcium leads to hypocalcemia, tetany and eventually death when high doses of oxalate are consumed. When intake is low, poor bone growth or egg shell formation are observed. Also, calcium oxalate may crystallize within the blood vessels and cause vascular necrosis and hemorrhages. The precipitation of calcium oxalate crystals within the renal tubules leads to anuria, uremia and acute renal failure. Soluble oxalate is classified as a slightly toxic compound for chickens since the LD_{50} of soluble oxalate in one week old chicks is 984 mg/kg body weight (Williams and Olsen, 1992).

Plants in the Araceae family are notorious for containing insoluble oxalates in their leaves and other parts of the plant (Table 10.3). In contrast with soluble salts, insoluble oxalates are not absorbed into the systemic circulation. However, insoluble crystals of calcium or magnesium oxalate penetrate the tongue and pharynx and cause severe local irritation and inflammation when the plant is eaten. Some plants (e.g. *Dieffenbachia spp.*) also contain proteolytic enzymes which trigger the release of kinins and histamine causing an inflammatory response.

Plants which accumulate oxalates are used as energy or protein sources in poultry rations, particularly in developing countries (Samarasinghe and Rajaguru, 1992). A list of plants capable of accumulating oxalates is shown in Table 10.3. In order to avoid their potential toxic effects, these plants must be used with caution if they are intended to be used in poultry diets. It is important to note that besides toxic plants, another source of soluble oxalate are grains and grasses infected with fungi capable of producing large quantities of oxalic acid (e.g. *Aspergillus niger*).

10.5 PHENOLIC COMPOUNDS

Phenolic compounds are widely distributed in plant tissues. Some phenolic compounds are simple essential metabolites while others are complex structures of unknown function. Phenolic compounds relevant to poultry nutrition include free phenolic acids, polymeric phenols (tannins), and microconstituent phenolics such as gossypol and sinapine.

| TABLE 10.3 Plants which accumulate toxic levels of oxalates | | | |
| Plants which accumulate soluble oxalates | | Plants which accumulate insoluble oxalates (family Araceae) | |
Latin name	Common name	Latin name	Common name
Amaranthus retroflexus	red-root pigweed	*Alocasia spp.*	alocasia
Centhrus ciliaris	buffel grass	*Caladium arboreum*	caladium
Chenopodium album	lamb's quarters	*Colocasia esculenta*	taro, cocoyam
Digitaria decumbens	pangola grass	*Dieffenbachia picta*	dieffenbachia
Halogeton glomeratus	halogeton	*Dieffenbachia sequine*	dumb cane
Oxalis cernua	soursob	*Monstera deliciosa*	monstera
Panicum maximum	elephant grass	*Philodendron cordatum*	philodendron
Rheum rhaponticum	rhubarb		
Rumex spp.	sorrels and docks		
Sarcobatus vermiculatus	greasewood		

10.5.1 Phenolic acids

Phenolic acids are simple phenols containing one or more carboxyl groups located either on the aromatic ring or in the side chain. Phenolic acids include the benzoic and cinnamic acid-based phenolics (Figure 10.10). Benzoic acid-based phenolics are widely distributed in nature. The simpler types include *p*-hydroxybenzoic, protocatechuic, vanillic, gallic and syringic acids. Cinnamic acid- based phenolics are found in most oil seeds and tend to occur as esters with quinic acid or sugars. Chlorogenic acid, a well-known phenolic present in sunflower, is an ester of caffeic and quinic acids and is found in several isomeric and derivatized forms.

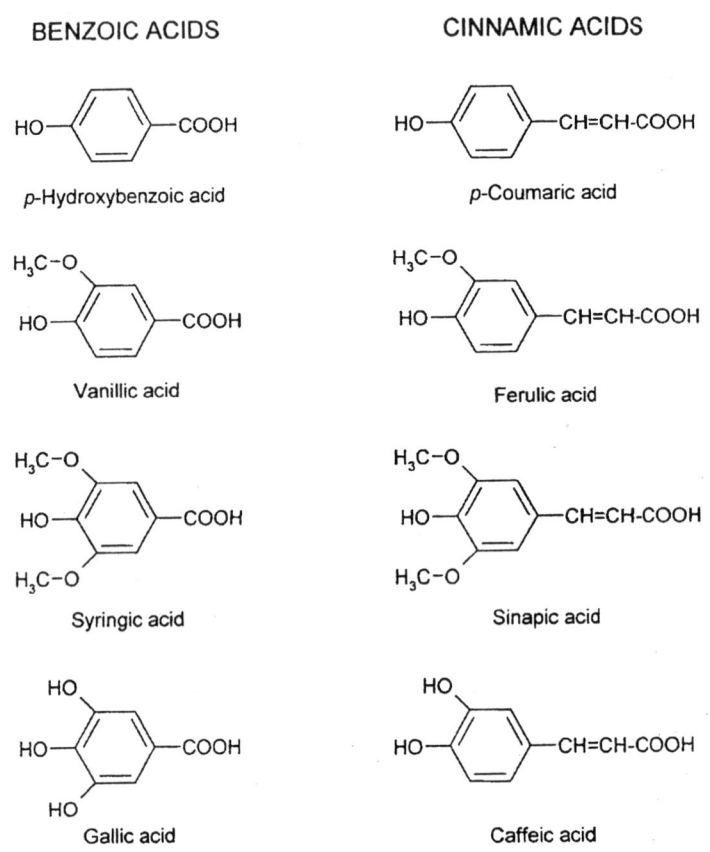

Figure 10.10 Common phenolic acids.

Free phenolic acids are of particular relevance in poultry nutrition because they can generate *o*- quinones capable of binding lysine and methionine residues in proteins. Cinnamic acids and their esters present in oilseeds are particularly relevant because they are easily oxidized by phenol oxidase (phenolase, polyphenol oxidase) to form *o*-quinones (e.g. chlorogenoquinone). Once formed, o- quinones may react non-enzymatically to polymerize or may reduce or bind covalently to such functional groups as amino, thiol or methylene. The ε-amino group of lysine and the thioester group of methionine are commonly attacked by *o*-quinones, rendering these essential amino acids unavailable for the bird (Figure 10.11).

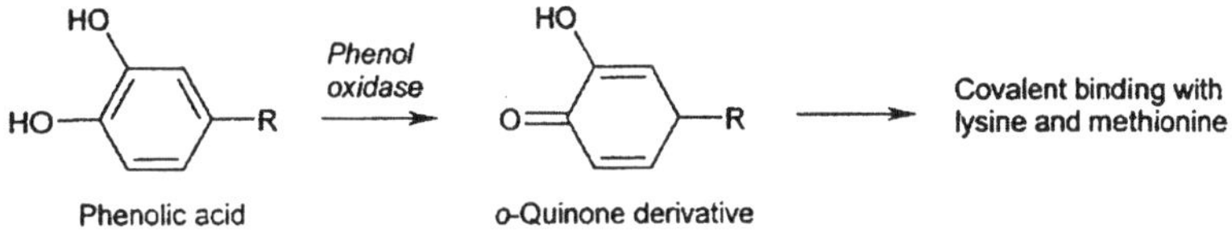

Figure 10.11 Phenol oxidase-catalyzed oxidation of phenolic acids to o-quinone derivatives followed by covalent binding of amino and thioester groups in amino acid residues.

Formation of o-quinone derivatives is particularly important in sunflower meal, which may contain up to 3.0-3.5% phenolic acids. Chlorogenic and caffeic acids account for about 70% of the phenolics found in sunflower meal.

10.5.2 Tannins

Tannins are defined as naturally occurring water soluble polyphenolic compounds with a molecular weight between 500 and 3000, capable of precipitating proteins from aqueous solutions. Tannins are not well defined substances but rather a group of compounds sharing some common properties and capable of forming stable crosslinks with other molecules. Although the chemistry of tannins is complex, they are usually divided into two groups, namely, hydrolyzable and condensed tannins. Hydrolyzable tannins contain a central carbohydrate core (glucose or quinic acid) esterified to phenolic carboxylic acids, such as gallic acid. Figure 10.12 shows an example of a hydrolyzable tannin. Hydrolyzable tannins occur in several tropical legumes used as forage such as *Acacia spp.* Tannic acid is a well-known gallotannin that contains 8-10 moles of gallic acid per mole of glucose and has been extensively used in *in vivo* trials. Condensed tannins are polymers of flavan-3-ols linked by carbon-carbon bonds. In most grain legumes tannins are present as condensed tannins, where they are mainly present in the testa of the colored seeds.

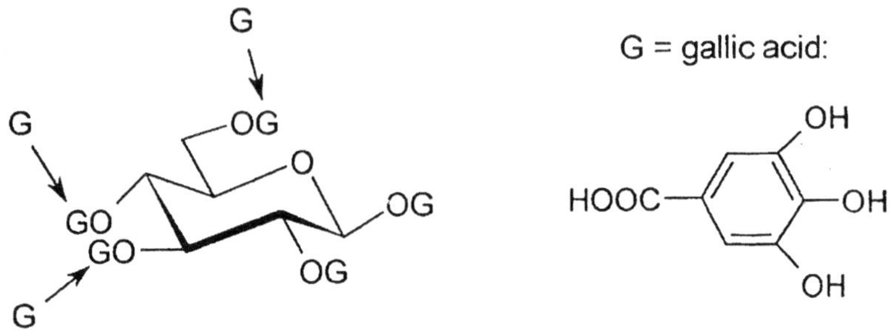

Figure 10.12 Hydrolyzable tannin with a glucose core.

Some of the ingredients used in poultry nutrition contain considerable amounts of condensed tannins including grain sorghum, millet, rapeseed, fava beans, and some oil seeds. Cottonseed meal contains considerable amounts of condensed tannins (1.6% dry matter), while barley, triticale and soybean meal contain almost non-detectable levels of tannins (0.1% dry matter). Among poultry feed ingredients, the highest content of tannins is present in sorghum grain (*Sorghum bicolor*). Tannin content in high tannin sorghum cultivars has been reported to range between 2.7 and 10.2% catechin equivalents (Jansman, 1993).

Sorghum cultivars with high levels of condensed tannins are widely grown because they are resistant to bird predation, preharvest germination, mold production and weathering. The polyphenols from sorghum are of the condensed type only and consist of 2-40 monomeric units. The tannin content in sorghum is often considered to correlate with the darkness of the seed coat. However, a study conducted with 24 varieties of sorghum ranging in tannin content from 0.05 to 3.67% (catechin equivalents) showed that seed color is not an adequate indicator of tannin content (Boren and Waniska, 1992).

Feeding high tannin sorghum cultivars to chickens has been associated with reduced growth rate and feed efficiency in broilers and reduced egg production in layers. An increased incidence of leg abnormalities (valgus-varus) was reported in chickens fed a high tannin sorghum as compared to those receiving a low tannin sorghum diet (Elkin *et al.,* 1978).

Means to control the adverse effects of dietary tannins include dietary supplementation of DL-methionine and supplementation of tannin-binding agents. Gelatin, polyvinylpyrrolidone (PVP), and polyethyleneglycol have a high affinity for tannin, which are capable of binding and detoxifying the tannin.

10.5.3 Gossypol

The use of cotton seed meal (CSM) in monogastric animals is limited by its high fiber content and the presence of toxic compounds such as tannins and gossypol, a yellow polyphenolic pigment. Gossypol occurs in the pigment glands of the cotton-seed and the pigment glands found in the foliage parts of the plant. The concentration of gossypol in the seed varies considerably among cotton species and among cultivars within species, and may range between 0.3% and 3.4% (Percy *et al.*, 1996). Typically, CSM contains about 0.5% free gossypol. Any cottonseed protein product intended for human consumption must contain less than 0.045% free gossypol. Gossypol may be found in a free, toxic form, or in a bound form, which is non-toxic. Free gossypol is highly reactive due to the presence of both phenolic and aldehydic groups (Figure 10.13). The phenolic groups react readily to form esters and ethers. The aldehyde groups react with amines to form Schiff bases and with organic acids to form heat labile compounds. During high temperature oil extraction or meal processing, the aldehyde groups of gossypol may react with the ε-amino group of lysine and other amino acid residues in the cottonseed globulins. Bound gossypol is not absorbed and is non-toxic, but the biological availability of lysine in the CSM is reduced. The method of processing of the cottonseed determines the protein value and free gossypol content of the CSM. During screwpress extraction (expeller) most of the free gossypol binds to amino acids, reducing the value of the protein. Extraction by prepress solvent and direct solvent produces CSM of higher protein quality but considerably increases the free gossypol content. Free gossypol content in solvent extracted CSM ranges from 0.1 to 0.5%, while for expeller processed meal the typical free gossypol content is about 0.05%. Whole seed has almost all the gossypol in the free form.

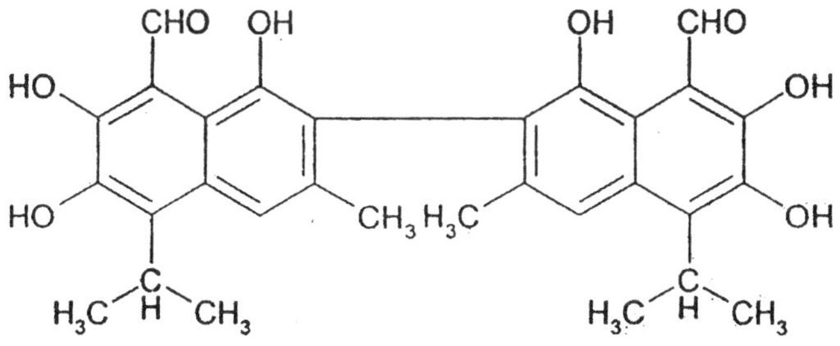

Figure 10.13 Gossypol.

Broilers can safely tolerate up to 100 ppm of dietary free gossypol without exhibiting adverse effects on performance. Layer rations should contain less than 50 ppm gossypol in order to prevent the occurrence of a green discoloration of the egg yolks, particularly after storage. In addition to causing green discoloration of the yolks, high dietary levels of gossypol decrease the hatchability of fertile eggs. Iron salts (e.g. ferric sulfate) can be added to CSM diets to detoxify gossypol by binding the reactive groups with iron. A 1:1 ratio of free gossypol to iron is recommended, but even with iron supplementation the level of free gossypol should not exceed 400 ppm for broilers and 150 ppm for layers. High dietary protein also has protective effects, especially in pelleted diets, presumably by binding of free gossypol with amino acid residues. Gossypol may react with the ε-amino group of lysine and arginine and with the thiol group of cysteine.

10.5.4 Sinapine

Sinapine (Figure 10.14), the choline ester of the sinapic acid (see section 10.5.1), is a bitter component of *Brassica* and *Crambe spp*. Canola meal contains between 2.5 and 3.0% sinapine, while crambe meals contain about 0.5% sinapine. Fishy taint in eggs has been reported after feeding rapeseed to certain strains of laying hens, particularly those that lay brown shelled eggs. The fishy taint is caused by the presence of trimethylamine typically at levels of 1-5 $\mu g/g$ egg.

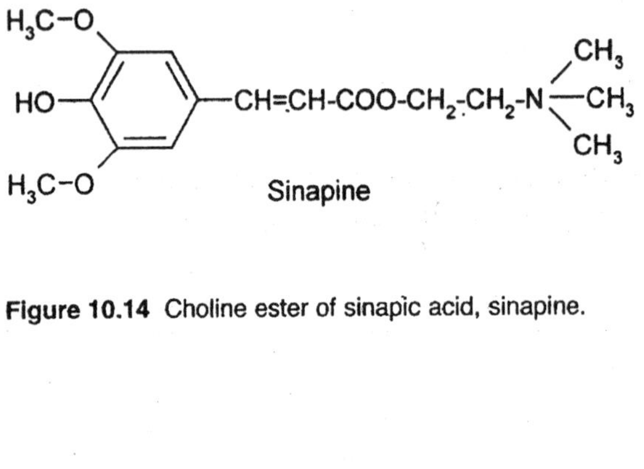

Figure 10.14 Choline ester of sinapic acid, sinapine.

The fishy taint problem is further complicated by the fact that certain glucosinolates (see section 10.6.2) present in canola meal inhibit the hepatic enzyme trimethylamine oxidase. This effect was shown when 200 ppm 5-vinyloxazolidone-2-thione and 2-hydroxybut-3-enyl glucosinolate were added to rapeseed meal-free rations (Fenwick et al., 1989). The fishy taint in eggs can be eliminated by feeding the hens diets containing less than 0.1% sinapine. When the canola meal contains 3% sinapine, its maximum level of inclusion in the diet should be 3%.

10.5.5 Photodynamic phenols: hypericin and fagopyrin

Hypericin and fagopyrin (Figure 10.15) are well known plant toxins capable of causing primary photosensitization. Hypericin is present in the leaves, stems, and flowers of *Hypericum spp.*, with *Hypericum perforatum* (St. John's wort) being the most toxic weed species of the genus. Fagopyrin is found both in the seed and foliage of buckwheat.

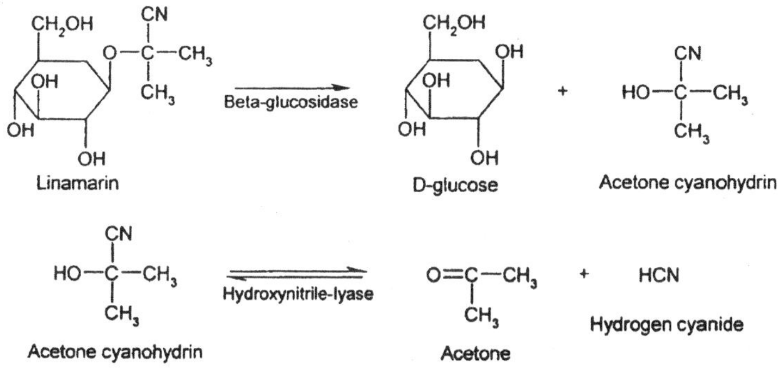

Figure 10.15   Primary photosensitizing compounds, hypericin and fagopyrin.

Photosensitization is a condition in which lightly pigmented skin is hyperreactive to sunlight due to the presence of a photodynamic compound in the skin. Photodynamic compounds adsorb ultraviolet energy from the sun and transfer it to receptor molecules that readily initiate chemical reactions in skin macromolecules. Lesions produced by photodynamic agents include inflammation, erythema, edema, serum exudation, scab formation and skin necrosis. Tissue injury probably results from the production of reactive oxygen and/or through alterations in cell membrane integrity. Several cases of photosensitization caused by hypericin and fagopyrin have been documented in livestock, but no natural outbreaks of this condition have been reported in poultry. However, other photoactive compounds chemically unrelated to hypericin and fagopyrin have been implicated in primary photosensitization in poultry. Furocoumarins (psoralens) are photoactive substances present in plants in the families *Umbelliferae* and *Rutaceae*. One plant capable of accumulating psoralens is bishop's weed (*Ammi majus*, Umbelliferae) and severe photosensitization with erythema and blistering on the beak and feet, and eye lesions have occurred in poultry fed grain containing bishop's weed seeds.

10.6 GLYCOSIDES

Glycosides are substances composed of a sugar moiety and a non-sugar moiety known as the aglycone. Some glycosides, (e.g. the cardiac glycosides) are toxic as such, while others (e.g. cyanogenic glycosides) need to be hydrolyzed in order to become toxic. Upon hydrolysis, these latter type of glycosides release the aglycone, which might be toxic *per se* or might rearrange into a toxic or antinutritional substance. Glycosides are widely distributed in the plant kingdom and many crop plants important in poultry nutrition are known to contain potentially toxic glycosides.

10.6.1 Cyanogenic glycosides (cyanoglycosides, cyanogens)

Cyanogenic glycosides, cyanoglycosides or cyanogens are compounds which on treatment with acid or following hydrolysis by specific enzymes release hydrogen cyanide (HCN). Cyanoglycosides occur in more than 2000 species of plants, cassava being the major food crop containing high amounts of cyanogens. Cassava is traditionally processed by chopping the root under running water to wash away the cyanogens. Alternatively, the cassava root may be chopped, crushed, and dried under the sun until the HCN evaporates. Plants relevant to poultry nutrition which accumulate significant amounts of cyanoglycosides are listed in Table 10.4.

TABLE 10.4 Plants relevant to poultry nutrition which accumulate cyanogenic glysosides	
Ingredient	Cyanoglycoside(s)
Flax (linseed)	Linustatin, neolinustatin, linamarin
Cassava	Linamarin, lotaustralin
Lima bean	Linamarin, lotaustralin
Forage sorghum	Dhurrin
Vetches	Vicianin

The cyanoglycosides are not toxic *per se* but the enzymes responsible for their hydrolysis and later synthesis of HCN (β-glucosidase and hydroxynitrile-lyase, respectively) are present in all cyanogenic plants. Cyanogens occur in the epithelial cells while the enzymes are present only in mesophyll cells. Even though enzyme and substrate are physically separated in the plant, damage to the plant from wilting, trampling, frost, or drought causes the glycoside to come into contact with the enzymes and HCN is released. Linamarin is a common cyanoglycoside found in trefoils (*Lotus spp.*), white clover (*Trifolium repens*), and important crops including cassava, lima bean, and, to a lesser extent, flax. The reactions leading to the release of HCN from linamarin are shown in Figure 10.16.

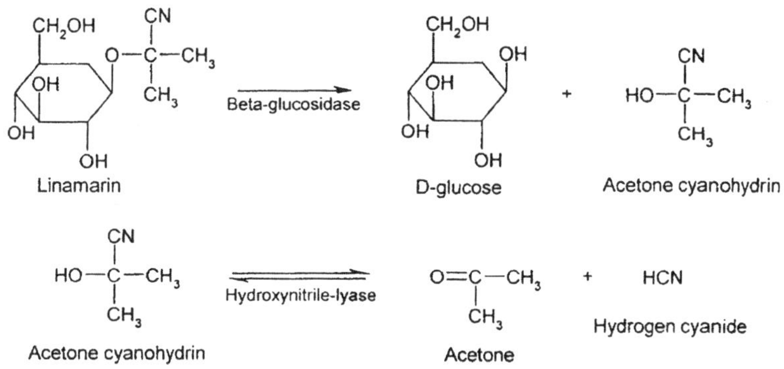

Figure 10.16 Formation of hydrogen cyanide (HCN) from the cyanoglycoside linamarin. Following hydrolysis of linamarin by β-glucosidase, HCN is synthesized by the enzyme hydroxynitrile-lyase.

Once released, HCN is rapidly absorbed from the gastro-intestinal tract, but is a weak acid and dissociates in the blood. The cyanide ion (CN^-) is a very strong ligand to heme iron and reacts with the ferric (oxidized) form of cytochrome oxidase in the mitochondria, forming a stable complex and blocking the respiratory chain. As a result, hemoglobin cannot release its oxygen to the electron transport system and death occurs due to cellular hypoxia (cytotoxic anoxia). The blood has a characteristic bright cherry red color. Mortality occurs only when the cyanogenic plants are offered in the fresh, unprocessed form. Performance of poultry on cassava diets is not affected as long as the HCN content in the final ration is less than 100 ppm.

Small amounts of cyanide can be tolerated by animals. Non-lethal doses of cyanide are detoxified to thiocyanate (SCN^-) by the ubiquitous enzyme rhodanese. In chickens, rhodanese activity is detected in all tissues (Aminlari and Shahbazi, 1994). It has been suggested that in chickens, the high activity of rhodanese in the proventriculus plays a key role in the detoxication of cyanide before it is absorbed systemically. Rhodanese transfers sulfur from various donors (mainly thiosulfate) to cyanide to form thiocyanate. Even though thiocyanate is much less toxic than cyanide, thiocyanate is goitrogenic (see section 10.6.2.) and chronic exposure to low levels of cyanide may lead to the development of goiter. Additionally, the detoxication of HCN by the formation of thiocyanate uses a significant proportion of the daily intake of sulfur; increased sulfur utilization for detoxication of cyanide may cause a sulfur deficiency which manifests itself by reduced feed intake and body weight gain.

10.6.2 Thioglycosides (glucosinolates)

Thioglycosides, more commonly known as glucosinolates, are a large group of toxic compounds present in many plants, particularly in members of the family *Cruciferae*. Examples include mustard, horseradish, cabbage, brussels sprouts, broccoli, cauliflower, kale, turnips, and rapeseed. Non-selected cultivars of rapeseed contain 110-150 moles of aliphatic glucosinolates per gram of oil-free dry matter. In general, the maximum level of glucosinolates in a diet for poultry should be less than 2.5 moles per gram. The chemistry, occurrence, methods of analysis, and toxic and antinutritional effects of glucosinolates in several species were reviewed by Fenwick *et al.* (1989) and Duncan (1991).

As with cyanoglycosides (see section 10.6.1), intact glucosinolates are not toxic *per se*, however, glucosinolates are always accompanied in plant tissue by the enzyme myrosinase, which catalyzes the cleavage of the thioglucoside bond of glucosinolates. Hydrolysis by myrosinase (or non-enzymatically by heat or low pH) yields a variety of toxic compounds produced by rearrangement of the aglycone moiety. Most glucosinolates can be classified into three groups according

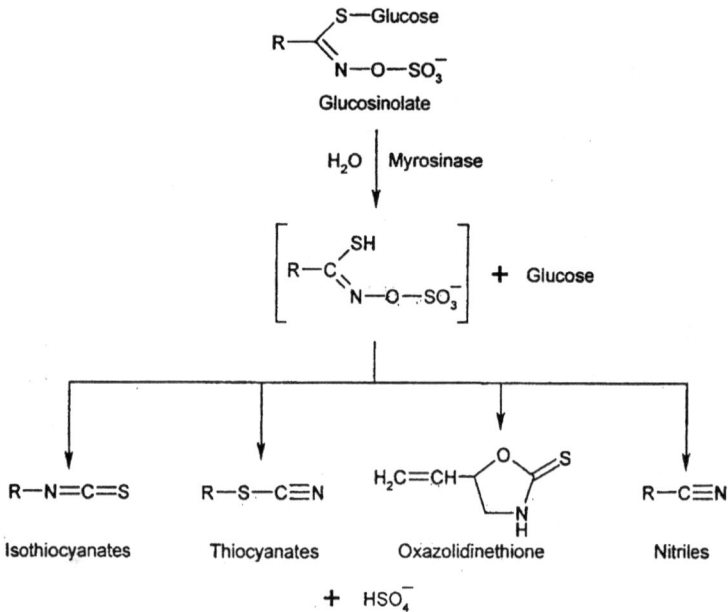

Figure 10.17 Formation of biologically active compounds following enzymatic hydrolysis of glucosinolates.

to the final products of their hydrolysis. The largest group comprise the glucosinolates, generally having an alkyl or alkenyl side chain, which upon hydrolysis yield mainly isothiocyanates. The second group, being much smaller than the first one, includes glucosinolates having a β-hydroxyl radical that forms unstable hydroxyisothiocyanates which spontaneously cyclize to goitrogenic oxazolidinethiones. The third group comprise glucosinolates having an indole nucleus (indole glucosinolates or glucobrassicins), which yield thiocyanates. Additionally, and depending on the pH of the reaction, these three groups of glucosinolates can also lead to the formation of nitriles. Figure 10.17 shows the main compounds produced following hydrolysis of glucosinolates.

The toxic or antinutritional effect of glucosinolates depends on the type of compound produced after the enzymatic hydrolysis of the parent compound. In general, glucosinolates that produce cyanates (isothiocyanates and thiocyanates) and oxazolidinethiones (Figure 10.17) cause impaired thyroid function as measured by reduced plasma levels of thyroid hormones and increased thyroid weight. In contrast, glucosinolates that yield nitriles upon hydrolysis are mainly nephrotoxic and hepatotoxic. Oxazolidinethiones, also known as goitrins, are potent goitrogenic compounds. Goitrins inhibit the incorporation of iodine into the precursors of the thyroid hormone thyroxine (T_4) and also interfere with T_4 secretion. The altered secretion of T_4 is accompanied by reduced growth rate and hyperplasia and hypertrophy of the thyroid gland (goiter). The adverse effect of goitrins is not overcome by adding more dietary iodine. Thiocyanates and isothiocyanates also inhibit iodine uptake by the thyroid gland but their effect is less severe than that caused by goitrins. The effect of cyanates is most pronounced with diets low in iodine and can be overcome by the addition of iodine to the diet. Nearly half of the glucosinolates present in the canola cultivars are precursors of thiocyanate. Nitriles are more toxic than goitrins and cyanates. In general, it can be considered that the toxicity of the glucosinolate-derived compounds is nitriles > oxazolidinethiones > cyanates.

In layers, feeding high glucosinolate rapeseed meal has been associated with increased mortality, decreased egg production, and decreased egg size. The maximum recommended level of inclusion of a high glucosinolate rapeseed meal in layer rations is 5%. However, this level can be raised up to 10% when a low glucosinolate rapeseed meal is fed. In broilers, a dose-response relationship between glucosinolates and decreased body weight is observed, and dietary glucosinolate levels between 3.1 and 4.5 mg/g cause a 10% decrease in body weight gain (Fenwick et al., 1989). No effective treatment or inactivating procedure has been developed to control glucosinolates.

10.6.3 Saponins

Saponins are a large group of structurally-related substances with properties resembling those of soaps and detergents. Chemically, saponins are triterpene or steroidal glycosides and thus, two main groups of saponins are recognized: those having a triterpenoid aglycone and those with a steroidal aglycone. Most of the saponins found in grains and forage feeds are of the triterpenoid type. Saponins occur in hundreds of plants including alfalfa, guar, sunflowers, lupins, chick peas, soybeans, navy beans and peanuts. Particularly high levels of saponins are found in alfalfa (specially in immature sprouts), chick peas and soybeans. Even though saponins comprise a variety of different compounds, all saponins have several common characteristics including bitter taste, mucosal irritating properties, foaming properties, *in vitro* hemolytic properties, and ability to form complexes with bile acids and cholesterol.

Dietary saponins cause feed refusal in poultry. Decreased feed intake is caused not only by the bitter taste of saponins, but also because of the irritation caused by saponins on the oral mucosa and gastro-intestinal tract. Saponins have also been implicated in reduced growth, and interference with the absorption of cholesterol, fatty acids, and lipid-soluble vitamins. Jenkins and Atwal (1994) showed that chicks fed 0.9% dietary triterpenoid saponins had reduced feed intake, weight gain, and digestibility of fat, and a marked increased in the excretion of cholesterol and reduced absorption of vitamin A and vitamin E. In contrast to triterpenoid saponins, feeding a steroidal saponin had no effect on any of the parameters measured (Jenkins and Atwal, 1994).

10.6.4 Hemolytic glycosides (vicine, convicine)

Vicine and convicine are pyrimidine β-glucosides present in faba beans (*Vicia faba*), common vetch (*Vicia sativa*) and other *Vicia* species. Vicine and convicine are hydrolyzed by anaerobic microflora of the lower gastro-intestinal tract to the highly reactive aglycones, divicine and isouramil, respectively (Figure 10.18). Divicine and isouramil have been implicated in a type of hemolytic anemia called "favism" in humans genetically deficient in glucose-6-phosphate dehydrogenase (G6PD) activity. The increased sensitivity of G6PD-deficient individuals to suffer from favism is due to the oxidative stress caused by divicine and isouramil (or their metabolites) on the red blood cell (RBC). Decreased RBC G6PD activity results in impaired NADPH generation, depletion of reduced glutathione, reduced ability to scavenge free radicals, and increased sensitivity to oxidative stress.

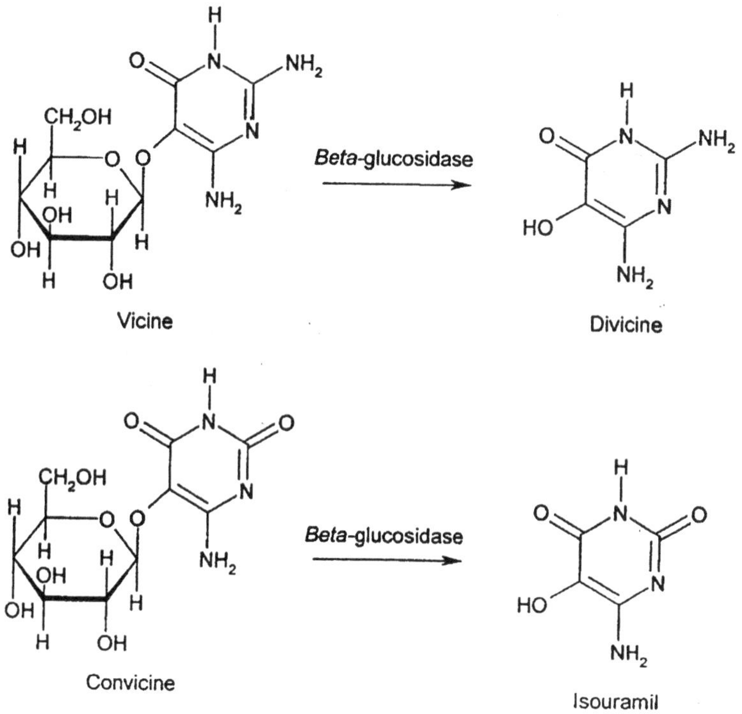

Figure 10.18 Vicine, convicine, and their aglycones.

Marquardt *et al.* (1974) reported that unprocessed faba beans decrease chicken growth and feed efficiency. Muduuli *et al.* (1981) found that dietary vicine isolated from faba beans affects the reproductive performance of laying hens. In this later study, vicine caused a reduction in fertility and hatchability and depressed egg and yolk mass production by reducing egg weight and, to a lesser extent, the rate of lay. Vicine also decreased yolk membrane strength and increased the number of blood spots in the yolk. Interestingly, this study demonstrated that vicine is also capable of causing RBC hemolysis and oxidative stress in the chicken. Increased oxidative stress was evidenced by increased levels of plasma lipid peroxides, decreased ratio of vitamin E:lipid, and increased erythrocyte hemolysis (Muduuli *et al.*, 1981).

10.7 ALKALOIDS

Alkaloids are secondary plant metabolites widely distributed in nature. Alkaloids are colorless, generally basic (pK_a 7-9), insoluble in water (but soluble in organic solvents), and can form salts with acids. All alkaloids contain nitrogen, generally forming part of a heterocyclic structure. There are thousands of known alkaloids but most are not considered toxic. The most relevant toxic alkaloids in poultry nutrition are the pyrrolizidine, piperidine, and tropane alkaloids.

10.7.1 Pyrrolizidine alkaloids (monocrotaline, senecionine)

Pyrrolizidine alkaloids (PA) are a large group of naturally occurring hepatotoxins containing a pyrrolizidine nucleus (Figure 10.19). The highest level of PA are found in *Crotalaria spectabilis* and *C. retusa* seeds, with 3.85 and 2.69%, respectively. PA in plants can be of three general types: monoesters (e.g. heliotrine), diesters (e.g. lasiocarpine), and cyclic diesters (e.g. monocrotaline, jacobine, senecionine). The most toxic ones are cyclic diesters, while monoesters are the least toxic. In order to be potentially toxic, a PA must have a 1,2 insaturation in the pyrrolizidine nucleus and there must be a branch in the ester group. PA are not toxic *per se*: They are bioactivated to highly reactive pyrrol metabolites by cytochrome P450 enzymes (Figure 10.19). Enzymatic bioactivation occurs mainly in the liver but it can also occur in other organs or systems containing cytochrome P450 enzymes such as the lung, kidney, heart, and gastro-intestinal tract. The toxic metabolites formed enzymatically are known as pyrroles or dihydropyrrolizidine derivatives (DHP). Pyrroles are very reactive molecules and powerful alkylating agents that react with macromolecular components inside the cell. Pyrroles from diester PA may act as bifunctional alkylating agents capable of crosslinking DNA, thereby inhibiting cell replication. This mechanism of action could explain the antimitotic effect of PA. Pyrroles may be detoxified by binding nucleophiles such as glutathione or through hydrolysis of the ester groups by esterases.

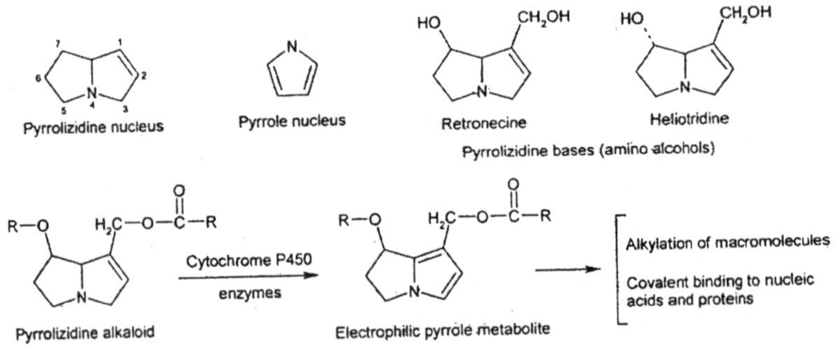

Figure 10.19 Bioactivation of pyrrolizidine alkaloids to electrophilic metabolites

The toxicosis caused by the ingestion of PA in animals has been well characterized. In chickens, PA toxicosis is caused primarily by consumption of *Senecio* and *Crotalaria spp*, whose seeds are rich in senecionine and monocrotaline, respectively. *Crotalaria spectabilis* (showy rattlebox) is very toxic for poultry. *C. spectabilis* plants are readily recognized for their yellow flowers, which have a typical humming-bird-like shape (Figure 10.20). This plant was introduced into the United States in 1921 and the first report of *Crotalaria* toxicosis was made in 1934 when 34 hens kept in a pen with mature *C. spectabilis* plants were found dead. The crops and gizzards of the dead birds contained *C. spectabilis* seeds. Further experiments showed that the seeds were toxic for chickens. In 1959, several layer and broiler flocks in South Carolina and Georgia were affected by feed contaminated with *C. spectabilis* seeds. The following year, Allen and co-workers characterized the toxicosis produced by *C. spectabilis* in chickens. Practical diets containing *Crotalaria* seeds at concentrations greater than 0.3% caused a 100% mortality within 18 days. Dead birds had hemorrhages in the liver, lungs and pericardium. Ascites was observed in all birds, accompanied by a marked reduction in the relative size of the liver (Allen *et al.*, 1960). Numerous clinicopathological studies have since been conducted to characterize the effects of PA in poultry species. The clinical signs, effects on performance and gross and histopathological findings of PA intoxication are usually common to all species of poultry; ducks, however, appear to be more sensitive than chickens. Two clinical forms of the disease are observed: acute and chronic. Early clinical signs of PA toxicosis include depression, anorexia, inactivity and depressed growth. At gross pathology, an acute intoxication is characterized by enlarged, friable and mottled red, yellow or brown livers. The gall bladder is always distended with clear, green bile. Chronic toxicosis causes atrophy and severe irregularity in the shape and size of the liver lobes, which are also firm, and sometimes covered by fibrin. Splenomegaly is a common finding with the spleen usually enlarged 2-3 times its normal size. The kidneys are pale and enlarged. Due to the severe hepatic fibrosis, chickens develop ascites during chronic toxicosis. *Crotalaria spp.* seeds have been found as contaminants in soybean and sorghum.

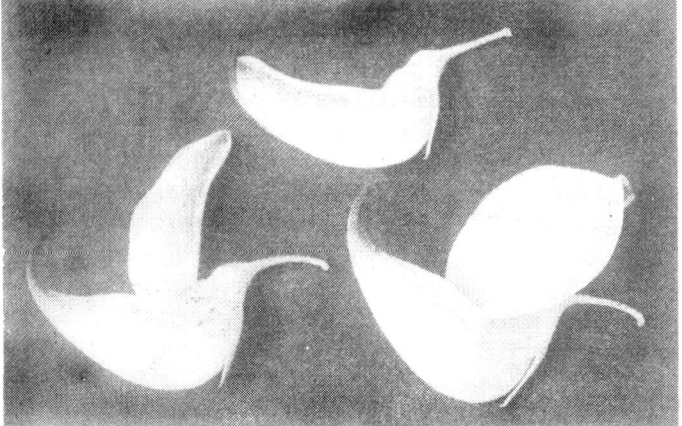

Figure 10.20   Showy rattlebox (Crotalaria spectabilis) flowers.
(Courtesy of G.J. Diaz.)

10.7.2 Piperidine alkaloids (coniine, γ-coniceine)

Most naturally occurring alkaloids found in plants and microorganisms contain the piperidine ring in their structure (Figure 10.21). The most important piperidine alkaloids are those present in the seeds and other parts of the poison hemlock (*Conium maculatum*). This plant is a large biennial herb originally from Europe but currently naturalized in North and South America and Asia. In North America, poison hemlock is also known as poison food parsley, hemlock, spotted hemlock, and California or Nebraska fern. Poison hemlock contains at least 8 piperidine alkaloids (Panter and Keeler, 1989). The two major ones are coniine, which predominates in the seeds, and γ-coniceine, which is more abundant in vegetative parts of the plant (Figure 10.21). Coniine is of historical interest because it was the first alkaloid to be discovered (1827) and the first one to be chemically synthesized (1886).

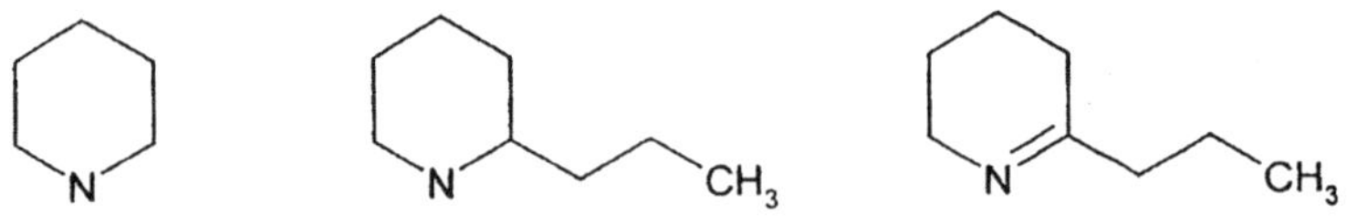

Piperidine   Coniine   Coniceine
nucleus

Figure 10.21   Piperidine nucleus and structure of the two major piperidine alkaloids from Conium maculatum: coniine and γ-coniceine.

Reports of poison hemlock intoxication in poultry are rare. Frank and Reed (1986) reported a case of poison hemlock toxicosis in a flock of range turkeys. Clinical signs included tremors, paralysis and increased mortality. Gross examination revealed hepatic congestion and enteritis and numerous *Conium maculatum* seeds were found in the crop, proventriculus and gizzard. Histopathologic alterations were limited to catarrhal enteritis. In later studies, Frank and Reed (1990) investigated the toxicity of coniine in chickens. Coniine toxicosis was manifested by characteristic nicotinic signs including excitement, depression, hypermetria (hyperextension of the right leg), seizures, opisthotonos, and flaccid paralysis. No gross or microscopic lesions were observed. The sensitivity to coniine in the three species studied, appeared to be: quails > chickens > turkeys. Frank and Reed (1990) also investigated the residuality of coniine in edible tissues of birds dying from coniine intoxication. Ingestion of poison hemlock seeds by birds is of concern for human health as it has been reported that European quails consume the seeds with impunity and are capable of causing intoxication in humans consuming these quail. Coniine was detected in the liver and muscle of birds 7 days after ingestion and the authors suggested caution when deciding the fate of birds that have had access to *Conium maculatum* seeds.

10.7.3 Datura alkaloids (atropine, scopolamine)

The *Datura* genus belongs to the Solanaceae family and includes more than 1600 species of plants. Some of these plants produce alkaloids with a tropane ring in their structure (Figure 10.22) which exhibit both toxicological and pharmacological properties. Other Solanaceae plants containing tropane alkaloids are the deadly nightshade (*Atropa belladonna*), henbane (*Hyoscyamus niger*), and mandrake (*Mandragora officinarum*). Seeds of *Datura spp.* have been found as contaminants in feedstuffs including soybeans, linseed, corn, wheat, and sorghum. In fact, *Datura* is considered to be the most toxic and most prevalent weed seed contaminant of soybeans (List *et al.*, 1979). *Datura spp.* are originally from tropical and warm temperate climates.

The major tropane alkaloids present in *Datura spp.* are hyoscine (scopolamine) and *dl*-hyoscyamine (atropine) (Figure 10.22), although the content of each alkaloid varies according to the plant species. In *D. stramonium*, for example, atropine predominates, while in *D. ferox*, scopolamine is the major alkaloid. List *et al.* (1979) analysed jimsonweed seeds isolated from soybeans and found them to contain atropine, scopolamine, and total alkaloids at 0.29, 0.05, and 0.34%, respectively. According to these results, the scopolamine:atropine ratio in jimsonweed seeds is about 15:85. In contrast, in *D. ferox* seeds the scopolamine:atropine ratio has been reported to be 98:2 (Kovatsis *et al.*, 1993). Tropane alkaloids are present in every part of the plant, with greater amounts found in younger plants. In tropical areas *Datura spp.* is a perennial plant; however, in temperate zones it is an annual and can be readily controlled by cutting it before it goes to seed.

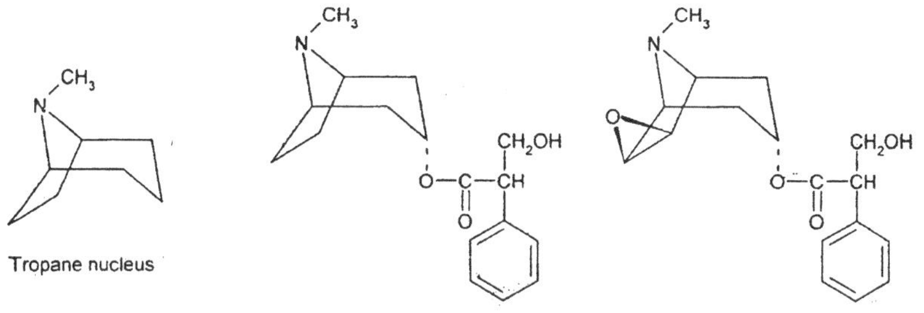

Tropane nucleus

dl-Hyoscyamine (atropine)

Hyoscine (scopolamine)

Figure 10.22 Tropane nucleus and major tropane alkaloids found in Datura spp.

In broilers, dietary *Datura* seeds adversely affect growth, without causing overt signs of toxicosis. Day and Dilworth (1984) added jimsonweed seeds to broiler diets and found decreased growth at dietary levels of 3% or higher. At 3 weeks of age, the mean body weight of chicks receiving 3% dietary jimsonweed seed was only 67% of the controls, while the body weight of chicks receiving 6% seed was 62% of the controls. No clinical signs were reported and the authors concluded that about 1% jimsonweed seed meal was the maximum dietary level that could be safely incorporated into the diet of young broilers. In later studies, Kovatsis et al. (1993, 1994) fed the main alkaloids of D. ferox to broilers and layers. A mixture of scopolamine:hyoscyamine (98:2) was incorporated at four dietary levels (1.5, 15, 75 or 150 ppm) to broilers or layers for 90 days. In broilers, alkaloid feeding caused a significant dose dependent decrease in growth. No significant differences in cardiac rate and breathing frequency were noted between alkaloid-fed chickens and controls, and no gross or histological lesions were found in birds receiving the alkaloids. In layers, alkaloid levels of 150 ppm reduced egg production but lower levels had no effect. Egg weight, shell thickness, and body weight of hens was unaffected at all levels tested. Heart rate was increased in hens fed 150 ppm alkaloids after 5 weeks, but no effect on the respiratory rate was observed. It was concluded that a total alkaloid concentration of up to 75 ppm is safe for laying hens.

10.8   MYCOTOXINS

Mycotoxins are secondary metabolites produced by certain species of fungi growing under specific environmental conditions. Primary metabolites are those produced by all fungi for both the synthesis of biomass and to generate the energy necessary for primary metabolism. In contrast, secondary metabolism is usually restricted to a small number of species (may be even strain specific) and it occurs mainly after a phase of balanced growth, usually associated with morphogenetic changes like sporulation. Secondary metabolites include pigments and compounds active against microorganisms (antibiotics), plants (phytotoxins) or animals/humans (mycotoxins). The biological role of secondary metabolism in fungi is still unknown. The environmental factors that determine fungal growth and mycotoxin production in feeds and feedstuffs are related both to the substrate itself (intrinsic factors) and to the storage conditions of the substrate (extrinsic factors). Table 10.5 summarizes the major factors determining mold growth and mycotoxin production in cereal grains. Some of these factors can be manipulated to reduce mold growth and therefore, mycotoxin production. For example, when grain moisture level is about 12% or lower, fungal growth is severely decreased (Krabbe et al., 1995).

TABLE 10.5 Factors affecting mold growth and mycotoxin production in cereal grains	
Intrinsic factors	**Extrinsic factors**
Ingredient composition (lipids, carbohydrates, trace metals, etc.).	Relative humidity: RH greater than 70% favors fungal growth.
pH:Fungal growth decreases with decreasing pH. This is the basis for the use of organic acids (e.g. propionic acid) as feed additives to control fungal growth in stored grain.	Environmental temperature: The optimal temperature for fungal growth and mycotoxin production varies with the species and often the optimal temperature for fungal growth differs from the optimal temperature for mycotoxin production. In general, *Aspergillus* and *Penicillium* fungi grow better at higher temperatures than do Fusarium fungi.
Grain moisture: The optimal grain moisture is >13% for saprophytic fungi (e.g. *Aspergillus* and *Penicillium spp.*) and >20% for phytopathogenic fungi (e.g. Fusarium spp.).	Oxygen/CO_2: Fungi are aerobic organisms. Studies conducted with mycotoxigenic Fusaria have shown that when the storage atmosphere of the grain contains only 5% oxygen and 40% CO_2, fungal growth is severely affected and no mycotoxins are produced.
Water activity (a_w): This parameter is related to the water that is actually available for the fungi to grow. Some ingredients (e.g. peanuts) may have low moisture (ca. 9%) but very high water activity and can easily support Aspergillus growth and aflatoxin production.	Surface area of grain. Smaller particles, such as fines, have relatively increased surface area, which predisposes mold growth.

When mycotoxigenic fungi contaminate the grain, two types of fungi can be recognized: those that preferentially infect stored grain (saprophytic) and those which attack the plant in the field (phytopathogenic). The most important species of saprophytic fungi are *Aspergillus* and *Penicillium*, while *Fusarium spp.* are the most relevant mycotoxigenic phytopathogens. It should be emphasized that not all strains of a particular species of fungus are capable of producing mycotoxins. For instance, it is considered that only about 10% of the *Aspergillus flavus* strains are capable of producing aflatoxins. Therefore, contamination of a given substrate with fungi does not necessarily imply mycotoxin contamination.

Many mycotoxins, with different chemical structures and biological activities, have been identified. Mycotoxins may be carcinogenic (e.g. aflatoxin B_1, ochratoxin A, fumonisin B_1), estrogenic (zearalenone and zearalenols), neurotoxic (fumonisin B_1), nephrotoxic (ochratoxins, citrinin, oosporeine), dermonecrotic (trichothecenes) or immunosuppressive (T-2 toxin, ochratoxin A, and aflatoxin B_1). Mycotoxins can be found in feed ingredients such as corn, sorghum, barley, wheat, rice, cottonseed, and groundnut. Most mycotoxins are relatively stable compounds which are not destroyed by processing of feed and may even be concentrated in screenings. The chemistry, natural occurrence, and general toxicology of the major mycotoxins affecting poultry were reviewed by Leeson et al. (1995).

Even though extensive research has been conducted in the field of mycotoxins and mycotoxicosis in poultry in the past four decades, there is still much confusion and misleading information. Aflatoxins have been traditionally considered as potent hepatotoxins in chickens; however, rigorous toxicological studies have shown that chickens are relatively resistant to these compounds. Sensitive animal species such as trout are affected by aflatoxin dietary levels as low as 20 ppb; however, levels above 1200 ppb are required to induce any measurable toxic effect in chickens, and 2500 ppb is the minimum level capable of affecting growth. Diaz *et al.* (1995) showed that young chicks can tolerate up to 3000 ppb aflatoxin for 7 days without noticeable effects. The relative resistance of broiler chickens and laying hens to aflatoxins was also demonstrated by the studies of Kan *et al.* (1989). A diet containing 100 ppb aflatoxin B_1 from naturally contaminated corn was fed to broiler chickens for 6 weeks and to laying hens for 3 weeks. No difference in performance was observed compared with controls and no residues were found in breast muscle, eggs or chicken livers at a detection limit of 5 ppt (Kan *et al.*, 1989). In a recent survey conducted in Colombia it was found that 32% of the poultry feed and feedstuff samples analyzed contained detectable levels of aflatoxin B_1; however, the average content in positive samples was less than 20 ppb (Céspedes and Diaz, 1997). These results are in agreement with those from surveys conducted in other countries including the United States and Canada. In spite of these results, it is still common to see diagnosis of aflatoxiosis. Diagnosis of mycotoxicosis is usually based on non-specific lesions or signs such as low body weight, poor feathering, decreased rate of lay, presence of subcutaneous petechial or ecchymotic hemorrhages, etc. In addition, the determination of the toxic substance in the feed at levels that are potentially toxic, constitutes an integral part of the toxicologic diagnosis. In many instances, controlled studies have shown that nutrition, management, infectious or toxic problems different from mycotoxins have been the real etiologic agents in suspect cases of mycotoxicosis.

Ochratoxin A is another mycotoxin traditionally considered to be of importance in chickens. However, it occurs very sporadically (<10%) and at low levels (<10 ppb). Trichothecene mycotoxins, on the other hand, are *Fusarium* produced toxins that occur naturally at levels potentially toxic for chickens. The most important mycotoxins of this group are T-2 toxin, HT-2 toxin and diacetoxyscirpenol (DAS). Diaz et al. (1994) showed that T-2 toxin and DAS, at dietary levels likely to be found in naturally contaminated feeds (2 ppm), can significantly reduce egg production and feed intake in commercial layers and to increase the incidence of soft-shelled eggs. Typical type A tricothecene-induced oral lesions are also observed at these dietary levels (Figure 10.23).

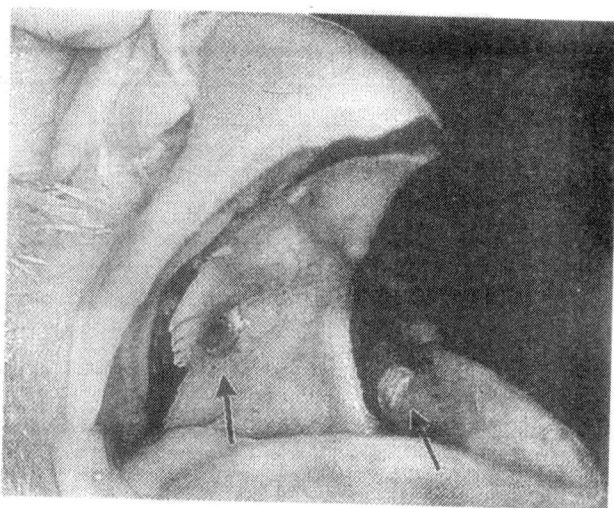

Figure 10.23 Lesions in the oral cavity induced by dietary T-2 toxin at 2ppm in commercial laying hens. (Courtesy of G.J. Diaz).

A critical analysis of the mycotoxin research conducted in chickens in the past decade suggests that aflatoxins and ochratoxin A, at the levels likely to be found in practical diets, are not a concern for the chicken producer. Consideration must be given, however, to type A trichothecene mycotoxins such as T-2 toxin and DAS, which are found in nature at potentially toxic levels. Table 10.6 summarizes the minimum dietary levels of these three groups of mycotoxins capable of inducing adverse effects on poultry.

It is important to note that fungi can adversely affect poultry performance by altering the nutritional composition of the substrate during their primary metabolism, without necessarily producing secondary metabolites. Unfortunately this field of research has received little attention compared to that on mycotoxins. Fungal growth decreases the density and energy content of the grain, and alters its vitamin and amino acid content. One vitamin that is commonly affected by fungi is thiamin. *Fusarium proliferatum, F. moniliforme*, and *Aspergillus flavus* have been demonstrated to severely decrease the thiamin content of poultry feeds and feedstuffs (Fritz *et al.,* 1973; Kao and Robinson, 1972; Nagaraj and Wu, 1994) and to induce signs of thiamin deficiency in chickens consuming them. Thiamin deficiency is induced by the degradation of the vitamin by fungal thiaminases. The amino acid profile of substrates infected with fungi is also altered. In studies conducted by Kao and Robinson (1972), cystine, lysine, histidine, arginine, aspartic acid, and glutamic acid all decreased in *Aspergillus flavus*-contaminated wheat. Cystine content decreased the most, with only about 26% remaining. Methionine was the only amino

TABLE 10.6 Clinical guide to major mycotoxins in poultry

Mycotoxin	Type of bird	Dietary level	Main effects
Aflatoxin	Broiler chicks	3 ppm	No detrimental effect on performance after 2 weeks of exposure.
	Laying hens	2.5 ppm	Minimal dietary concentration capable of affecting performance when given for 3 weeks or more.
Ochratoxin A	Broiler chickens	1.5-2 ppm	Minimal dietary level capable of reducing weight gain.
		2-4 ppm	Increased relative weight of kidney, liver and proventriculus; decreased relative weight of thymus and bursa.
Trichothecenes: T-2 toxin and DAS	Broiler chickens	400 ppb	Oral lesions; no adverse effect on performance
		1-4 ppm	Oral lesions; decreased feed intake and weight gain; abnormal feathering.
	Laying hens	1-2 ppm	Oral lesions; decreased feed intake and egg production; low incidence (<2%) of soft-shelled eggs.
	Broiler breeders	5 ppm	Oral lesions; decreased feed intake and body weight; no detrimental effect on fertility or hatchability.

acid that increased in moldy grain, probably at the expense of cystine. The energy content in contaminated grain is also affected by mold growth. During their normal metabolism, fungi use triglycerides as an energy source, releasing CO_2 during this process. Krabbe *et al.* (1995) showed that fungal activity in corn is negatively correlated with the energy content of the grain. After 60 days of storage, corn with low, intermediate and high fungal activity (as measured by CO_2 release) had residual ether extract values of 4.8, 4.0, and 2.2%, respectively. The adverse effects on health and performance caused by the nutritional deficiencies induced by molds growing on poultry feeds are usually non specific, and are similar to those reported for several poultry mycotoxicosis (Leeson *et al.*, 1995). Therefore, the effect of fungal growth on the nutritional quality of feeds and feedstuffs needs to be considered as a possible differential diagnosis in suspect field cases of mycotoxicosis.

10.9   OTHER COMPOUNDS

10.9.1 Nitrates

The nitrate content of cereal grains and legume seeds varies with species, strain, and growing conditions and commonly ranges from 0.5 to 18 ppm. Nitrate can be reduced to the more toxic nitrite ion by the microorganisms in the lower gastro-intestinal tract of monogastrics. Also, nitrate in plants can be reduced to nitrite by bacterial metabolism. Nitrite is readily absorbed from the gastro-intestinal tract and diffuses into the red blood cells where it oxidizes the ferrous iron (Fe^{2+}) of the oxyhemoglobin molecule to the ferric state (Fe^{3+}) forming methemoglobin. Methemoglobin is not capable of carrying oxygen and therefore the oxygen supply to body tissues is reduced. Because methemoglobinemia results in tissue hypoxia, Diaz *et al.* (1995) investigated whether administration of dietary nitrite played any role on the incidence of two conditions that have been related with chronic hypoxemia: broiler pulmonary hypertension and spontaneous turkey cardiomyopathy (STC). Levels of dietary nitrite were 0, 200, 400, 800, 1200, and 1600 ppm, and were fed to broiler chickens and turkey poults for 35 and 14 days, respectively. Both poults and chicks developed a transient significant increase in methemoglobinemia after 7 days of exposure to dietary nitrite; however, the levels returned to normal afterwards in spite of the presence of nitrite in the diet. No effect on pulmonary hypertension (as measured by the right ventricle weight to total ventricle weight ratio) was observed in chickens receiving dietary nitrite, but the turkey poults fed 1200 ppm nitrite had a numerically higher incidence of STC than did controls (20 vs 5%). Interestingly, both chicks and poults developed anemia; poults appeared to be more sensitive to the adverse effects of nitrite on blood hemoglobin content since the minimum dietary level causing anemia was 800 ppm in poults and 1200 ppm in chicks. Decreased performance was observed with the highest dietary concentration. The results of this study indicate that the dietary nitrite levels required to induce an adverse effect in poultry (methemoglobinemia, anemia, and decreased body weight) are probably too high compared to the nitrate levels expected to be present in cereal grains and legume seeds. It should be noted, however, that nitrate and nitrite may also be present at significant levels in water sources.

10.9.2 Biogenic amines

Animal by-product meals used in poultry nutrition are susceptible to bacterial contamination, both before and after processing. Bacterial growth and metabolism can enzymatically modify some of the nutrients present in the meals. Biogenic amines (also known as ptomaines), are decarboxylated compounds produced during the bacterial catabolism of certain amino acids. Biogenic amines or substances derived from them may also be found as naturally occurring compounds with pharmacological activity. Examples of these amines include histamine, which is derived from histidine, and the catecholamine hormones (DOPA, dopamine, norepinephrine, and epinephrine), which are derived from phenylethylamine. Common biogenic amines formed in animal by-products by decarboxylation include cadaverine (from lysine), tryptamine (from tryptophan), agmatine (from arginine), tyramine (from tyrosine), phenylethylamine (from phenylalanine), histamine (from histidine), and putrescine (from ornithine). Putrescine is the precursor of two more biogenic amines namely spermine and spermidine. These three biogenic amines (putrescine, sper mine and spermidine) are collectively known as polyamines (Figure 10.24). Polyamines are considered to be important promoters of DNA, RNA, and protein synthesis, cell division, and tissue growth.

$$H_3\overset{+}{N}-(CH_2)_4-\overset{+}{N}H_3$$

Putrescine

$$H_3\overset{+}{N}-(CH_2)_3-\underset{H}{N}-(CH_2)_4-\overset{+}{N}H_3$$

Spermidine

$$H_3\overset{+}{N}-(CH_2)_3-\underset{H}{N}-(CH_2)_4-\underset{H}{N}-(CH_2)_3-\overset{+}{N}H_3$$

Spermine

Figure 10.24 Polyamine Structures.

It has been common to assume that biogenic amines are toxic for chickens; however, recent studies indicate no serious concern for poultry producers. Bermudez and Firman (1998) investigated the effect of dietary phenylethylamine (4.8 ppm), putrescine (49 ppm), cadaverine (107 ppm), and histamine (131 ppm) or a combination of these four amines on broiler chicken health and performance. The dietary levels of biogenic amines used in this study corresponded to the maximum levels that could potentially be found in practical diets (based on the highest levels of biogenic amines reported in the United States and assuming that no more than 10% animal by-product meal would be used to formulate a ration). No adverse effects on performance and no gross lesions were observed for any of the treatments. The authors concluded that these four biogenic amines, fed at the highest levels likely to occur in the United States, are unlikely to produce adverse effects on health or performance.

The results of Bermudez and Firman (1998) confirmed previous reports demonstrating that low levels of histamine and putrescine are not detrimental to chicken performance. In fact, depending on the dietary concentration, putrescine may even have beneficial effects. In studies conducted with broiler chickens, Harry et al. (1975) reported that histamine is capable of causing gizzard erosions and ulcerations similar to those induced by gizzerosine (see section 10.1.2). However, the levels required to induce such lesions were extremely high (1,000 – 10,000 ppm), and levels as high as 500 ppm did not cause adverse effects. It should be noted that gizzerosine is not a biogenic amine, as it is not produced by decarboxylation of any amino acid. Gizzerosine is formed by the non-peptidic union of histidine (or histamine) and lysine under extreme heating temperatures used during the processing of certain fish meals. The biogenic polyamine putrescine is of particular interest because it has been shown to have growth-promoting activity (Smith, 1990). Addition of putrescine to a complete crystalline amino acid diet elicited a growth response in growing chicks, suggesting that putrescine may be an essential nutrient for chicks. When 2,000 and 4,000 ppm putrescine were added, a significant improvement in body weight was observed. Levels of 8,000 and 10,000 ppm, however, caused a significant decrease in body weight compared with controls. The toxicity of the polyamines increases with molecular weight and charge. Spermidine shows very little growth-promoting effect, while spermine is highly toxic for chickens (Smith *et al.,* 1996).

10.9.3 Toxic myopathy (Senna spp.)

The genus *Senna* (family Leguminosae), formerly known as *Cassia*, comprise a wide array of annual and perennial herbs, shrubs, wood vines, and trees found in the tropics and subtropics, particularly in tropical America. Various species of *Senna spp.* are known to produce myopathy in livestock as a result of being grazed, or by contamination of feed by seeds. Toxic species of *Senna* include *S. occidentalis* (coffee senna, coffeeweed, coffee-pod, "cafelillo"), *S. obtusifolia* (sickle-pod), *S. reticulata* ("bajagua"), *S. tora* ("bicho"), and *S. roemeriana*. *S. occidentalis* is a widely distributed weed common in corn, sorghum, and soybean fields and *Senna* seeds have been found as contaminants in these three feedstuffs. Contamination in sorghum is particularly difficult to detect because sorghum grains and *Senna* seeds are of similar color, size and density (Figure 10.25).

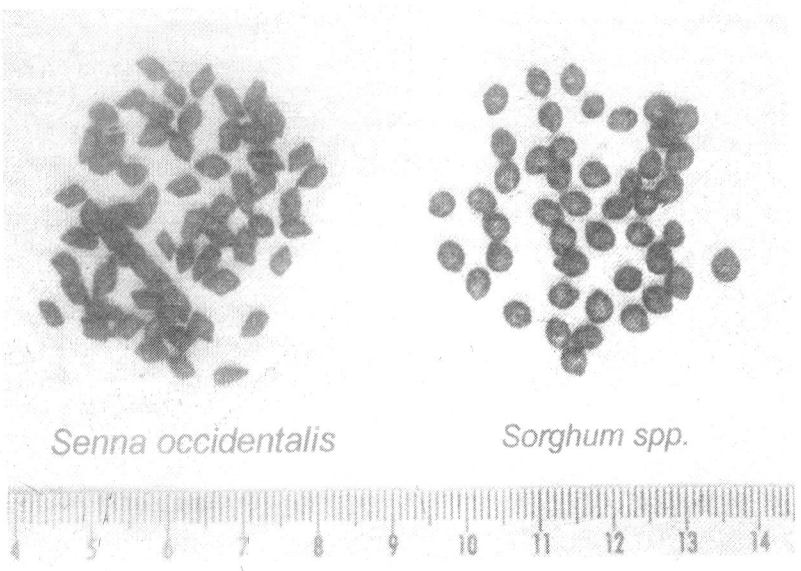

Figure 10.25 Senna occidentalis seeds found as contaminants in corn grain. Senna seeds are similar to sorghum seeds in color, size, and density. (Courtesy of G.J. Diaz).

Simpson *et al.* (1971) fed chicks diets containing 0, 0.5, 1, 2, or 4% *S. occidentalis* seeds for 3 weeks. A dose-dependent decrease in body weight was observed with increasing dietary levels of *Senna* seeds. The body weight of birds receiving 2% and 4% seeds was about 53% and 63% below that of controls, respectively. Feed intake was also inversely related to the dietary concentration of *Senna* seeds. Mortality was 0, 2.5, 2.5, 5 and 65%, for chicks fed 0, 0.5, 1, 2 and 4% seeds, respectively. Most birds fed 2% or 4% seeds were ataxic or partially paralyzed before death. Gross lesions were found only in birds fed 2 or 4% seeds and were restricted to the semitendinosus muscle, which was pale and edematous. Microscopic examination revealed focal swelling, fragmentation and necrosis of myofibers, accompanied by swelling and proliferation of sarcolemmic nuclei. The lesions were similar to those seen in vitamin E-selenium deficiency in chicks. Muscle damage due to consumption of *Senna* seeds has also been reported in layers. Page *et al.* (1977) fed White Leghorns diets containing 0, 2, 5, or 10% *S. obtusifolia* seeds. All levels of seed decreased feed intake, egg production, and egg size; egg yolks from hens receiving seeds were platinum colored. At post-mortem examination the semitendinosus and pectoralis superficialis muscles were pale and edematous. In another experiment with hens, *S. obtusifolia* seeds were fed to White Leghorn layers at 0, 2, 3, 4, 5, 6, or 7% (Flunker *et al.*, 1989). Egg production and feed intake were significantly reduced with 2% of seed. Within the first 24 h, feed intake was decreased to 37% below that of controls by the highest seed level. Egg specific gravity decreased significantly at dietary levels of 5% or higher. It was concluded that complete diets contaminated with 2% or more *S. obtusifolia* seeds can adversely affect performance in laying hens. Haraguchi *et al.* (1998) characterized the muscle degeneration caused by *S. occidentalis* seeds in growing chicks. Seven-day-old chicks were fed a diet containing 4% *S. occidentalis* seeds for 15 days. Intense muscle atrophy and acid phosphatase activity in muscle cells was consistent with a severe degenerative process. High accumulation of lipids was also observed, along with dilation of the sarcoplasmic reticulum and enlarged mitochondria with abnormal cristae. The identity of the myotoxin of *Senna* plants is still unknown.

SELECTED REFERENCES

Allen, J.R., Childs, G.R., and Cravens, W.W. 1960. *Crotalaria spectabilis* toxicity in chickens. Proceedings for the Society of Experimental Biology and Medicine, 104:434-436.

Aminlari, M., and Shahbazi, M. 1994. Rhodanese (thiosulfate:cyanide sulfurtransferase) distribution in the digestive tract of chicken. Poultry Science, 73:1465-1469.

Annison, G., and Choct, M. 1991. Anti-nutritive activities of cereal non-starch polysaccharides in broiler diets and strategies minimizing their effects. World's Poultry Science Journal, 47:232-242.

Arnold, R.L., Olson, O.E., and Carlson, C.W. 1972). Dietary selenium and arsenic additions and their effects on tissue and egg selenium. Poultry Science, 52:847-854.

Barbieri, L., Battelli, M.G., and Stirpe, F. 1993. Ribosome-inactivating proteins from plants. Biochimica et Biophysica Acta, 1154:237-282.

Belmar, R., and Morris, T.R. 1994. Effects of the inclusion of treated jack beans *Canavalia ensiformis*) and the amino acid canavanine in chick diets. Journal of Agricultural Science, 123:393- 405.

Belmar, R., Nava-Montero, R., Sandoval-Castro, C., and McNab, J.M. 1999. Jack bean (*Canavalia ensiformis* L.) in poultry diets: antinutritional factors and detoxification studies – A review. World's Poultry Science Journal, 55:37-59.

Bermudez, A.J., and Firman, J.D. 1998. Effects of biogenic amines in broiler chickens. Avian Diseases, 42:199-203.

Boren, B., and Waniska, R.D. 1992. Sorghum seed color as an indicator of tannin content. Journal of Applied Poultry Research, 1:117-121.

Campbell, G.L., and Bedford, M.R. 1992. Enzyme applications for monogastric feeds: A review. Canadian Journal of Animal Science, 72:449-466.

Cao, J., Blond, J.P., and Bézard, J. 1993. Inhibition of fatty acid Δ^6 and Δ^5 desaturation by cyclopropene fatty acids in rat liver microsomes. Biochimica et Biophysica Acta, 1210:27-34.

Céspedes, A.E., and Diaz, G.J. 1997. Analysis of aflatoxins in poultry and pig feeds and feedstuffs used in Colombia. Journal of the AOAC International, 80:1215-1219.

Chowdhury, S.D., and Davis, R.H. 1995. Influence of dietary osteolathyrogens on the ultrastructure of shell and membranes of eggs from laying hens. British Poultry Science, 36:575-583.

Day, E.J., and Dilworth, B.C. 1984. Toxicity of jimson weed seed and cocoa shell meal to broilers. Poultry Science, 63:466-468.

Diaz, G.J., Julian, R.J., and Squires, E.J. 1995. Effect of graded levels of dietary nitrite on pulmonary hypertension in broiler chickens and dilatory cardiomyopathy in turkey poults. Avian Pathology, 24:109-120.

Diaz, G.J., Squires, E.J., Julian, R.J., and Boermans, H.J. 1994. Individual and combined effects of T-2 toxin and DAS in laying hens. British Poultry Science, 35:393-405.

Diaz, G.J., and Sugahara, M. 1995. Individual and combined effects of aflatoxin and gizzerosine in broiler chicke s. British Poultry Science, 36:729-736.

D'Mello, J.P.F. 1995. Anti-nutritional substances in legume seeds. In: D'Mello, J.P.F., and Devendra, C. (Eds). Tropical legumes in animal nutrition. CAB International, Wallingford, pp. 135-172.

D'Mello, J.P.F., and Acamovic, T. 1989. *Leucaena leucocephala* in poultry nutrition – A review. Animal Feed Science and Technology, 26:1-28.

Duncan, A.J. 1991. Glucosinolates. In: D'Mello, J.P.F., Duffus, C.M., and Duffus, J.H. (Eds). Toxic substances in crop plants. The Royal Society of Chemistry, Cambridge, pp. 126-147.

Elkin, R.G., Featherson, W.R., and Rogler, J.C. 1978. Investigations of leg abnormalities in chicks consuming high tannin sorghum grain diets. Poultry Science, 57:757-765.

Farran, M.T., Uwayjan, M.G., Miski, A.M.A., Sleiman, F.T., Adada, F.S., and Ashkarian, V.M. 1995. Effect of feeding raw and treated common vetch seed (*Vicia sativa*) on the performance and egg quality parameters of laying hens. Poultry Science, 74:1630-1635,

Fenwick, G.R., Heaney, R.K., and Mawson, R. 1989. Glucosinolates. In: Cheeke, P.R. (Ed.) Toxicants of Plant Origin, Vol. II. Glycosides. CRC Press, Boca Raton, pp. 1-41.

Flunker, L.K., Damron, B.L., and Sundlof, S.F. 1989. Response of white leghorn hens to various dietary levels of Cassia obtusifolia and nutrient fortification as means of alleviating depressed performance. Poultry Science, 68:909-913.

Frank, A.A., and Reed, W.M. 1986. Conium maculatum (poison hemlock) toxicosis in a flock of range turkeys. Avian Diseases, 31:386-388.

Frank, A.A., and Reed, W.M. 1990. Comparative toxicity of coniine, an alkaloid of Conium maculatum (poison hemlock), in chickens, quails, and turkeys. Avian Diseases, 34:433-437.

Fritz, J.C., Mislivec, P.B., Pla, G.W., Harrison, B.N., Weeks, C.E., and Dantzman, J.G. 1973. Toxigenicity of moldy feed for young chicks. Poultry Science, 52:1523-1530.

Guinotte, F., Gautron, J., Soumarmon, A., Robert, J.C., Peranzi, G., and Nys, Y. 1993. Gastric acid secretion in the chicken: effect of histamine H2 antagonists and H^+/K^+-ATPase inhibitors on gastro-intestinal pH and of sexual maturity calcium carbonate level and particle size on proventricular H^+/K^+ ATPase activity. Comparative Biochemistry and Physiology, 160A:319- 327.

Haraguchi, M., Górniak, S.L., Calore, E.E., Cavaliere, M.J., Raspantini, P.C., Calore, N.M.P., and Dagli, M.L.Z. 1998. Muscle degeneration in chicks caused by *Senna occidentalis* seeds. Avian Pathology, 27:346-351.

Harper, J.A., and Arscott, G.H. 1962. Toxicity of common and hairy vetch seed for poults and chicks. Poultry Science, 41:1968-1974.

Harry, E.G., Tucker, J.F., and Laursen-Jones, A.P. 1975. The role of histamine and fish meal in the incidence of gizzard erosion and proventricular abnormalities in the fowl. British Poultry Science, 16:69-78.

Jansman, A.J.M. 1993. Tannins in feedstuffs for simple-stomached animals. Nutrition Research Reviews, 6:209-236.

Jenkins, K.J., and Atwal, A.S. 1994. Effects of dietary saponins on fecal bile acids and neutral sterols, and availability of vitamins A and E in the chick. Journal of Nutritional Biochemistry, 5:134-137.

Kakade, M.L., Rackis, J.J., McGhee, J.E., and Puski, G. 1974. Determination of trypsin inhibitor activity of soy products: collaborative analysis of an improved procedure. C real Chemistry, 51:376-382.

Kamada, Y., Oshiro, N., Miyagi, M., Okum H., Hongo, F., and Chinen, I. 1998. Osteopathy in broiler chicks fed toxic mimosine in Leucaena leucocephala. Bioscience, Biotechriology and Biochemistry, 62:34-38.

Kan, C.A., Rump, R. and Kosutzky, J. 1989. Low level exposure of broilers and laying hens to aflatoxin B1 from naturally contaminated corn. Archives fur Geflugelkunde, 53:204-206.

Kao, C., and Robinson, R.J. 1972. Aspergillus flavus deterioration of grain: its effect on amino acids and vitamins in whole wheat. Journal of Food Science, 37:261-263.

Keshavarz, K. 1993. Effect of corn contaminated with velvetweed seeds on eggs. Journal of Applied Poultry Research, 2:232-238.

Kovatsis, A., Flaskos, J., Nikolaidis, E., Kotsaki-Kovatsi, V.P., Papaioannou, N., and Tsafairs, F. 1993. Toxicity study of the main alkaloids of *Datura ferox* in broilers. Food and Chemical Toxicology, 31:841-845.

Kovatsis, A., Kotsaki-Kovatsi, V.P., Nikolaidis, E., Flaskos, J., Tzika, S., and Tzotzas, G. 1994. The influence of Datura ferox alkaloids on egg-laying hens. Veterinary and Human Toxicology, 36:89-92.

Krabbe, E.L., Reginatto, M.F., and Penz, A.M. 1995. Effects of different moisture and propionic acid levels during storage on corn nutritional value, fungal activity, and broiler chicken performance. Abstracts, 16th Annual Meeting of the Southern Poultry Science Society, p. 39.

Leeson, S., Diaz, G.J., and Summers, J.D. 1995. Poultry Metabolic Disorders and Mycotoxins. University Books, Guelph, pp. 190-332.

Leslie, A.J., Pepper, W.F., Brown, R.G., and Summers, J.D. 1973. Influence of rape-seed products on egg quality and laying hen performance. Canadian Journal of Animal Science, 53:747-752.

Liener, I.E. 1994. Implications of antinutritional components in soybean foods. Critical Reviews in Food Science and Nutrition, 34:31-67.

List, G.R., Spencer, G.F., and Hunt, W.H. 1979. Toxic weed seed contaminants in soybean processing. Journal of the American Oil Chemist's Society, 56:706-710.

Marquardt, R.R., Campbell, L.D., Stothers, S.C., and McKirdy, J.A. 1974. Growth responses of chicks and rats fed diets containing four cultivars of raw and autoclaved faba beans. Canadian Journal of Animal Science, 54:177-182.

Marsh, R.G., and Gallin, W.J. 1994. Toxic effects of -aminopropionitrile treatment on developing chicken skin. Journal of Experimental Zoology, 268:381-389.

Masumura, T., Sugahara, M., Noguchi, T., Mori, K., and Naito, H. 1985. The effect of gizzerosine, a recently discovered compound in overheated fish meal, on the gastric secretion of the chicken. Poultry Science, 64:356-361.

Michelangeli, C., and Vargas, R.E. 1994. L-canavanine influences feed intake, plasma basic amino acid concentrations and kidney arginase activity in chicks. Journal of Nutrition, 124:1081-1987.

Muduuli, D.S., Marquardt, R.R., and Guenter, W. 1981. Effect of dietary vicine on the reproductive performance of laying hens. Canadian Journal of Animal Science, 61:757-764.

Nagaraj, R.Y., and Wu, W.D. (1994). Toxicity of *Fusarium proliferatum* M-7176 and nutritional intervention in chicks. Poultry Science, 73:617-626.

Ohta, Y., Ohashi, H., Enomoto, S., and Machida, Y. 1988. Simple measurement of gizzerosine in fish meals by high-performance liquid chromatography. Agricultural and Biological Chemistry, 52:2817-2821.

Page, R.K., Vezey, S., Charles, O.W., and Hollifield, T. 1977. Effects on feed consumption and egg production of coffee bean seed (*Cassia obtusifolia*) fed to White Leghorn hens. Avian Diseases, 21:90-96.

Panter, K.E., and Keeler, R.F. 1989. Piperidine alkaloids of poison hemlock (*Conium maculatum*). In: Cheeke, P.R. (Ed.) Toxicants of Plant Origin, Vol. I. Alkaloids. CRC Press, Boca Ratón, pp. 109-132.

Pass, M.A., Arab, H., Pollitt, S., and Hegarty, M.P. 1996. Effects of the naturally occurring arginine analogs indospicine and canavanine on nitric oxide mediated functions in aortic endothelium and peritoneal macrophages. Natural Toxins, 4:135-140.

Percy, R.G., Calhoun, M.C., and Kim, H.L. 1996. Seed gossypol variation within *Gossypium barbadense* L. cotton. Crop Science, 36:193-197.

Perilla, N.S., Cruz, M.P., de Belalcázar, F., and Diaz, G.J. 1997. Effect of temperature of wet extrusion on the nutritional value of full-fat soyabeans for broiler chickens. British Poultry Science, 38:412-416.

Ravindran, V., Bryden, W.L., and Kornegay, E.T. 1995. Phytates: occurrence, bioavailability and implications in poultry nutrition. Poultry and Avian Biology Reviews, 6:125-143.

Raharjo, Y.C., Cheeke, P.R., and Arscott, G.H. 1988. Effects of butylated hydroxyanisole and cysteine on toxicity of *Lathyrus odoratus* to broiler and Japanese quail chicks. Poultry Science, 67:153-155.

Renner, R., Innis, S.M., and Clandinin, M.T. 1979. Effects of high and low erucic acid rapeseed oils on energy metabolism and mitochondrial function in the chick. Journal of Nutrition, 109:378-387.

Samarasinghe, K., and Rajaguru, A.S.B. 1992. Raw and processed wild colocasia corm meal (*Colocasia esculenta* (L.) Schott, var. esculenta) as an energy source for broilers. Animal Feed Science and Technology, 36: 143-151.

Shqueir, A.A., Brown, D.L., and Klasing, K.C. 1989. Canavanine content and toxicity of sesbania leaf meal for growing chicks. Animal Feed Science and Technology, 25:137-147.

Sim, J.S., Toy, B., Crick, D.C., and Bragg, D.B. 1985. Effect of dietary erucic acid on the utilization of oils or fats by growing chicks. Poultry Science, 64:2150-2154.

Simpson, C.F., Damron, B.L., and Harms, R.H. 1971. Toxic myopathy in chicks fed Cassia occidentalis seeds. Avian Diseases, 15:284-290.

Smith, T.K. 1990. Effect of dietary putrescine on whole body growth and polyamine metabolism. Proceedings for the Society of Experimental Biology and Medicine, 190:332-336.

Smith, T.K., Mogridge, J.L., and Sousadias, M.G. 1996. Growth-promoting potential and toxicity of spermidine, a polyamine and biogenic amine found in foods and feedstuffs. Journal of Agricultural and Food Chemistry, 44:518-521.

Sosulski, F.W., Minja, L.A., and Christensen, D.A. 1998. Trypsin inhibitors and nutritive value of cereals. Plant Food for Human Nutrition, 38:23-34.

Sugahara, M., Hattori, T., and Nakajima, T. 1988. Effect of synthetic gizzerosine on growth, mortality, and gizzard erosion in broiler chickens. Poultry Science, 67:1580-1584.

Torres, M., Manosalva, H., Carrasco, L., De Ioannes, A.E., and Becker, M.I. 1999. Procedure for radiolabeling gizzerosine and basis for a radioimmunoassay. Journal of Agricultural and Food Chemistry, 47:4231-4236.

Viroben, G., and Michelangeli-Vargas, C. 1997. Determination of canavanine in raw and processed jackbean seeds. Sciences des aliments, 17:299-307.

Wiley, R.G. 1991. Ricin and related plant toxins: Mechanism of action and neurobiological applications. In: Keeler, R.F., and Tu, A.T. (Eds). Handbook of Natural Toxins. Volume 6. Toxicology of Plant and Fungal Compounds. Marcel Dekker, New York, pp. 243-268.

Williams, M.C., and Olsen, J.D. 1992. Toxicity to chicks of combinations of miserotoxin, nitrate, selenium, and soluble oxalate. In: James, L.F., Keller, R.F., Bailey, Jr., E.M., Cheeke, P.R., and Hegarty, M.P. (Eds). Poisonous plants. Proceedings of the Third International Symposium. Iowa State University Press, Ames, pp. 143-147.